Functional Neurosurgery: A Clinical Approach

Functional Neurosurgery: A Clinical Approach

Edited by Arthur Colfer

hayle medical

New York

Hayle Medical,
750 Third Avenue, 9th Floor,
New York, NY 10017, USA

Visit us on the World Wide Web at:
www.haylemedical.com

ISBN: 978-1-64647-518-6

Cataloging-in-Publication Data

Functional neurosurgery : a clinical approach / edited by Arthur Colfer.
p. cm.
Includes bibliographical references and index.
ISBN 978-1-64647-518-6
1. Nervous system--Surgery. 2. Nervous system--Diseases. I. Colfer, Arthur.
RD593 .F86 2023
617.480 025 73--dc23

Table of Contents

Preface

Any surgery that is performed on the nervous system, comprising the brain or spinal cord, is known as neurosurgery. Functional neurosurgery is a specific type of neurosurgery that aims to restore some neurological condition or function, or to treat a chronic neurological disorder that interferes with a person's day-to-day abilities or function. It entails precise surgical targeting of anatomical structures to modulate neurologic function. Functional neurosurgery covers a broad range of procedures that alter the functioning of the nervous system from the brain to peripheral nerves in the leg or arm. This can be achieved through a variety of methods including removing a seizure-causing part of the brain, utilizing an electrical stimulator on the spinal cord or brain to improve the symptoms of chronic pain or Parkinson's disease, or infusing medication directly into the spinal fluid. The success of any functional neurosurgical procedure depends on various factors such as constant monitoring, patient cooperation, as well as observation for early diagnosis and management of complications. This book explores all the important aspects of functional neurosurgery in the modern day. Different approaches, evaluations, and advanced studies on this topic have been included herein. The book will serve as a reference to a broad spectrum of readers.

This book has been the outcome of endless efforts put in by authors and researchers on various issues and topics within the field. The book is a comprehensive collection of significant researches that are addressed in a variety of chapters. It will surely enhance the knowledge of the field among readers across the globe.

It gives us an immense pleasure to thank our researchers and authors for their efforts to submit their piece of writing before the deadlines. Finally in the end, I would like to thank my family and colleagues who have been a great source of inspiration and support.

Editor

1

From Structure to Circuits: The Contribution of MEG Connectivity Studies to Functional Neurosurgery

Elizabeth W. Pang[1,2,3]* *and O. C. Snead III*[1,2,3]

[1] *Division of Neurology, Hospital for Sick Children, Toronto, ON, Canada,* [2] *Neurosciences and Mental Health, SickKids Research Institute, Toronto, ON, Canada,* [3] *Department of Paediatrics, Faculty of Medicine, University of Toronto, Toronto, ON, Canada*

Correspondence:
Elizabeth W. Pang
elizabeth.pang@sickkids.ca

New advances in structural neuroimaging have revealed the intricate and extensive connections within the brain, data which have informed a number of ambitious projects such as the mapping of the human connectome. Elucidation of the structural connections of the brain, at both the macro and micro levels, promises new perspectives on brain structure and function that could translate into improved outcomes in functional neurosurgery. The understanding of neuronal structural connectivity afforded by these data now offers a vista on the brain, in both healthy and diseased states, that could not be seen with traditional neuroimaging. Concurrent with these developments in structural imaging, a complementary modality called magnetoencephalography (MEG) has been garnering great attention because it too holds promise for being able to shed light on the intricacies of functional brain connectivity. MEG is based upon the elemental principle of physics that an electrical current generates a magnetic field. Hence, MEG uses highly sensitive biomagnetometers to measure extracranial magnetic fields produced by intracellular neuronal currents. Put simply then, MEG is a measure of neurophysiological activity, which captures the magnetic fields generated by synchronized intraneuronal electrical activity. As such, MEG recordings offer exquisite resolution in the time and oscillatory domain and, as well, when co-registered with magnetic resonance imaging (MRI), offer excellent resolution in the spatial domain. Recent advances in MEG computational and graph theoretical methods have led to studies of connectivity in the time-frequency domain. As such, MEG can elucidate a neurophysiological-based functional circuitry that may enhance what is seen with MRI connectivity studies. In particular, MEG may offer additional insight not possible by MRI when used to study complex eloquent function, where the precise timing and coordination of brain areas is critical. This article will review the traditional use of MEG for functional neurosurgery, describe recent advances in MEG connectivity analyses, and consider the additional benefits that could be gained with the inclusion of MEG connectivity studies. Since MEG has been most widely applied to the study of epilepsy, we will frame this article within the context of epilepsy surgery and functional neurosurgery for epilepsy.

Keywords: magnetoencephalography (MEG), connectivity, epilepsy surgery, intractable epilepsy, functional mapping

INTRODUCTION

With the advent of high resolution non-invasive neuroimaging, there has been improved ability to map the structure of the brain, as well as its connections. The idea that brain connections can be diagrammed as a "connectome" (Salvador et al., 2005; Sporns et al., 2005; Achard et al., 2006) has generated great hope that this "connectome" will provide the framework whereby we can understand the neural basis of human function and disease. The result was a significant paradigm shift in the field of neuroscience from a primarily modular, segregated view of brain function to a new view of integration amongst brain regions. According to this latter connectionist perspective, brain function depends on a network of widely distributed, interconnected circuits that communicate between distant brain regions to integrate incoming information and produce a coordinated output.

Understanding brain connectomics included investigations into both structural and functional connectivity, as these concepts are both interdependent and complementary. There is increasing evidence that brain areas communicate both along established physical pathways as well as functional pathways that may not be directly tied to brain structure, and thus the study of one is integral to the study of the other. In terms of structural connectivity, magnetic resonance imaging (MRI) has elucidated the anatomical arrangement of brain regions while diffusion tensor imaging (DTI) protocols in tandem with tractography algorithms, has supplied information on structural connections by tracking the course of myelinated fibers that travel between distant brain regions (Clayden, 2013).

The first methods for measuring brain functional connectivity were achieved using resting state functional MRI (fMRI) scans which identified pairs of brain regions showing time-correlated fluctuations in blood oxygen levels (Biswal et al., 1995). There are now a large number of studies which attest to the value of resting state fMRI for examining functional connections between brain regions (for reviews, see van den Heuvel and Hulshoff Pol, 2010; Van Essen, 2013). These investigations of functional connectivity are key as it is thought that it is the functional connections in the brain that are the drivers of cognitive behaviors.

Magnetoencephalography (MEG) is another imaging modality able to track functional connectivity (for a review on MEG, see Hari and Salmelin, 2012). MEG single-channel systems were developed in the 1970s with the first commercial whole-head MEG systems becoming available in the 1990s. It was only in the early 2000s that MEG use gained traction and attention with more standardized scanning and analysis protocols (Stufflebeam, 2011; Hari and Salmelin, 2012). The technique of MEG is based upon the elemental principle of physics that an electrical current generates a magnetic field. Hence, MEG uses highly sensitive biomagnetometers to measure extracranial magnetic fields produced by intracellular neuronal currents. Source localization of epileptic spikes and evoked responses as determined by MEG are co-registered with MRI and termed magnetic source imaging (MSI). MEG is primarily sensitive to signals arising from regions where the apical dendrites are tangentially oriented to the skull and scalp surface. Unlike electroencephalography (EEG), MEG signals are unaffected by tissue defects of the brain and skull bone, and unlike fMRI, abnormal hemodynamics in vascular malformations do not distort the MEG signal. So, MEG is a neurophysiological modality which measures the summed neuronal activity of small cortical patches covering several millimetres with a time scale in the milliseconds. Localization of this activity allows mapping of brain regions involved in specific functions. However, the high sampling rate of MEG recordings also allows for measurement of a wide bandwidth of oscillatory responses, and the computation of the correlated (by phase and/or amplitude) oscillatory activity between distinct cortical patches also gives a metric of functional connectivity. Thus, like fMRI, MEG can offer both localization and connectivity information.

Table 1 provides a comparison between the neuroimaging modalities discussed thus far. As can be seen, each neuroimaging modality presents with its own set of advantages and disadvantages, and in all likelihood, it will be the convergence of these methods that will generate the next big leaps of knowledge in the field. As fMRI is a more mature technology, much has been written about it; however, MEG, as a younger technology, is not as well known but holds promise. We think it important that clinician neuroscientists, and not just basic neuroimaginers, understand the potential that MEG has to address some of the gaps in our understanding of neural circuitry and functional connectivity. Further, while using a segregationist model, MEG has become an established clinical tool for localizing epilepsy foci and basic functions. With the paradigm shift to a network perspective of the brain, we think there is room for developing studies of MEG functional connectivity to assess whether MEG can accurately identify functional networks, and whether the applications of MEG

TABLE 1 | Comparison of non-invasive neuroimaging methods for acquiring connectome data.

Modality and substrate	Advantage	Disadvantage
MRI: anatomy	• High resolution images of brain structure	• Only provides anatomical information
DTI: water diffusion	• High resolution images of fiber tracts	• Only provides information on structural connectivity
fMRI: blood oxygen consumption	• High spatial resolution • Able to localize function • Measures resting state and task-based functional connectivity	• Relatively slower timing resolution • Only measures lower frequency oscillations
MEG: synchronous firing of neuronal populations	• Millisecond temporal resolution • Broadband measurement of spectral data • Relatively good spatial localization when used with a good source reconstruction algorithm • Measures resting state and task-based functional connectivity	• Uncertain as to sensitivity for $n = 1$ measurements and clinical decisions

functional connectivity studies can be expanded into other domains, including neurosurgery.

In summary, the high resolution of MEG in the spatial, temporal and spectral/oscillatory domains allows tracking of synchronous neuronal firing (i.e., measuring evoked responses) and computations of oscillatory connectivity (i.e., measuring induced or intrinsic networks across a wide bandwidth of frequencies) as it relates to functions and behaviors. Further, advances in neurochemistry link the substrates of neurotransmission with the neuronal oscillatory activity such that a comprehensive picture of brain function, from chemistry to neuronal activity to blood flow and metabolism, is emerging. These represent the additional important contributions that MEG can offer to our understanding of cognition-related brain dynamics.

The information gained from MEG connectivity studies is synergistic with, and complementary to, the information gained from MR connectivity studies (Brookes et al., 2011), and together, these can offer new perspectives on brain function and structure. The paradigm shift in neuroscience, which conceives of the brain as holistic and integrated (as opposed to functionally segregated as will be described below), raises questions both as to the impact of neurosurgery on the function of the whole brain circuit and the ability of the rest of the circuitry to re-shape itself to compensate and maintain function in the face of brain injury and disease. These questions are important to the neurosurgical community because the answers invite a broader perspective on brain organization of function which can translate into new thinking about functional neurosurgery and possibly improved outcomes. MEG is a tool which is directly relevant to exploring and addressing these questions.

In this article, we begin by describing the traditional use of MEG for functional neurosurgery, particularly within the context of pre-surgical mapping for epilepsy surgery. We continue with a discussion of recent advances in MEG connectivity analyses and its application to the identification of both functional and dysfunctional networks. We end with our assessment of these MEG methods and present our thoughts on future applications of these methods to functional neurosurgery.

MEG FOR PRE-SURGICAL FUNCTIONAL MAPPING: THE LOCALIZATION MODEL

Traditional neurosurgery has relied on the visual identification of neuroanatomical landmarks. In fact, neurosurgery as a specialty has grown from increasing empirical support for the idea that specific brain functions were linked to discrete areas of the cortex (Penfield and Jasper, 1954). With contributions from histological, lesional and functional studies, the primary sensory cortices were located: to the striate cortex for visual functions, Heschl's gyrus for auditory functions, and the post- and pre-central gyri for sensorimotor functions (for a review, see Mesulam, 1998). Using post-mortem and lesion studies, early clinicians elucidated specific left hemisphere brain centers allocated to speech production and comprehension; the first higher-order cognitive function to be localized (for a historical overview, see de Almeida et al., 2014). These findings supported a localization model of function.

As stated above, MEG sensors capture magnetic signals generated by the synchronous firing of a group of neurons. These data are visualized, like an EEG, as a plot of time on the x-axis against the size of the magnetic field strength on the y-axis. Source reconstruction algorithms have been developed that can compute the location of the brain source(s) that could have generated the observed signal. By asking the participant to complete a task, it is expected that segments of the recording corresponding to task processing would show regional increases in magnetic activity relative to a "baseline" or a time period with no task activity. Identification of the sites showing increased magnetic field strength (that is, neuronal activity) above baseline is thought to "localize" the generators involved in producing the function of interest. This computational process is referred to as "solving the inverse problem", and this solution can be applied at every active time point so that a spatiotemporal activation profile is created (for a review, see Simos et al., 2000). While there are several valid approaches to solving the inverse problem, each has its own set of limitations and as long as users are aware of the unique limitations of their selected algorithm and interpret their results with these limitations in mind, any source reconstruction algorithm could be used (Stufflebeam, 2011).

The use of MEG to localize basic sensory functions is well established (for a review, see Stufflebeam et al., 2009) and a set of clinical guidelines (Burgess et al., 2011) are available that outline the minimum standards required for routine clinical recordings of somatosensory, basic hand motor, auditory and visual function. The first studies to map the somatosensory cortex using somatosensory evoked fields (SEF) in the MEG were conducted in control adults and recorded median and ulnar nerve stimulations, as well as stimulation of the individual digits. The results showed an orderly somatotopic representation on the posterior bank of the central fissure, and it was concluded that MEG recordings had sufficient sensitivity to resolve finger and hand topography in the somatosensory region of the brain (Baumgartner et al., 1991). These methods were applied to identify the central sulcus pre-surgically, and confirmed with direct cortical mapping (Gallen et al., 1993), as well as visual inspection of MR images (Sobel et al., 1993). In one of the first reports using pre-surgical SEF recordings in adult patients with drug-resistant frontal lobe partial seizures, the authors demonstrated high accuracy for localization of the post-central gyrus and central sulcus (Smith et al., 1994), a finding later confirmed in children (Minassian et al., 1999). In fact, in cases of cortical dysplasia, where cerebral function may not be in expected anatomical areas, MEG has demonstrated utility for identifying somatosensory cortices even when they are located outside the Rolandic areas (Burneo et al., 2004). The propensity of sensorimotor cortices to functionally reorganize makes it imperative to identify the central sulcus and map sensory and motor cortical regions (Nakasato and Yoshimoto, 2000).

In tandem with studies designed to map the somatosensory cortex, groups interested in motor function have used voluntary finger and hand movements in the MEG to identify the location of the pre-central gyrus (Weinberg et al., 1990; Kristeva et al., 1991; Nagamine et al., 1994; Pang et al., 2008). The accuracy of these methods is greatly improved with the application of electromyography electrodes on the limb of interest, as this allows precise identification of movement onset (Gaetz et al., 2009; Pang et al., 2009). However, while voluntary finger and hand movements can be easily completed by cooperative adults, repetitive voluntary movements are challenging in young children, and in clinical conditions where there may be involuntary movements, movement disorders, or reduced motor control (e.g., stroke, epilepsy). Thus, there is interest in finding alternative ways to activate the motor cortex, for example using motor imagery (Burianová et al., 2013; Kraeutner et al., 2014) or passive movements (e.g., Onishi et al., 2013). These methods are still under development but hold promise for their potential utility in patients unable to comply with the requirements for completing repetitive voluntary movements.

Like the SEF, both the auditory evoked fields (AEF) and visual evoked fields (VEF) are straight forward and easy to map. Using tone stimulation, the primary auditory cortex on the superior temporal gyrus is identifiable (Papanicolaou et al., 1990) and has been found to have a tonotopic organization (Pantev et al., 1995). Further, there is evidence that epilepsy in the primary auditory cortex impairs auditory processing ability in adults (Kubota et al., 2007) and children (Korostenskaja et al., 2010); however, it is only in extreme cases, such as deafness where there is dramatic functional reorganization of auditory areas (for a review, see Gordon et al., 2011). Using binocular (Harding et al., 1994) and monocular (Seki et al., 1996) pattern-reversal stimulation, the topographic organization of the primary visual cortex within the calcarine fissure can be identified. In cases where there is loss of visual function, as in patients with a partial or homonymous hemianopsia, the unaffected function continues to show reliable localization and excellent correlation with the cortical anatomy (Nakasato et al., 1996), and again, there is not substantial reorganization of visual cortices except in cases of a complete loss of function as in blindness (for a review, see Kupers and Ptito, 2014).

In summary, for identification of primary sensory areas around major anatomical landmarks such as the central sulcus, superior temporal gyrus or calcarine fissure, visual identification during functional neurosurgery may be sufficient. However, in cases where there is concern about cortical re-organization, MEG is invaluable because it is an easy, non-invasive method to quickly confirm the adequacy of the localization model although other non-invasive functional mapping methods (for example, fMRI) would also suffice for basic sensory mapping.

WHEN LOCALIZATION MODELS ARE INSUFFICIENT: MAPPING LANGUAGE IN THE BRAIN

The localization model of language has been the backbone of language research for decades. A framework for basic language function was built upon lesion studies whereby injuries to specific brain areas produced stereotyped deficits in the affected patients. Those data suggested that in a healthy adult, language is subsumed in the left hemisphere within two perisylvian regions. The anterior region, also known as Broca's area, is located in the pars opercularis and pars triangularis of the inferior frontal gyrus while the posterior region, known as Wernicke's area, is located in the posterior portion of the superior temporal gyrus and adjacent parietal cortex. At its most basic level, the former region is thought to be involved in the production of speech while the latter is involved in the comprehension of language (Geschwind, 1970).

The advent of fMRI allowed intact persons to have their language tested non-invasively, and the first reports were that the Broca-Wernicke model mostly held true (Binder et al., 1995). While language was dominant in the left hemisphere, the borders of the classic Broca and Wernicke Areas were broader than originally thought, and there was greater intermixing of function and less sharp distinctions between expressive and receptive language (Binder et al., 1997; Binder, 1997).

Early MEG studies centered around receptive language function and it was demonstrated that by presenting words in the auditory modality, posterior language areas could be activated, and a laterality index calculated to determine the language dominant hemisphere (Breier et al., 2000). This calculation of language dominance showed high concordance with the intracarotid amobarbital procedure in children (Breier et al., 2001) and adults with epilepsy (Papanicolaou et al., 2004), as well as with fMRI (Billingsley-Marshall et al., 2007). More recently, protocols were developed to enable localization of frontal cortical areas involved in language production (Herdman et al., 2007) and validated against fMRI (Pang et al., 2011). Most recently, methods have been developed for assessing receptive language dominance under sedation (Rezaie et al., 2014) or sleep (Van Poppel et al., 2012). Because these new advances are in the research domain and still require extensive validation, the current clinical MEG guidelines recommend using language studies to index language laterality, but do not give definitive recommendations for methods to localize language (Burgess et al., 2011).

As more language neuroimaging studies are conducted, it has become increasingly apparent that there is a higher prevalence of atypical language lateralization and localization in patients with a neurological condition. For example, patients with mesial temporal lobe epilepsies (Pataraia et al., 2004), complex partial seizures (Breier et al., 2005), medically refractory epilepsy (Kadis et al., 2007) or stroke (Breier et al., 2004) were often found to show atypical language representation. Further, an initial case study (Kamada et al., 2006), followed by a set of case series (Gage et al., 2011; Eliashiv et al., 2014), reported a dissociation of language dominance. In all of these MEG studies, patients with left temporal lobe epilepsy showed receptive language dominance shifted to the right hemisphere while expressive language dominance was lateralized to the left. As well, studies of language lateralization using MEG (Kadis et al., 2011) and fMRI (Holland et al., 2007) in the typically developing brain showed bilateral and diffuse language representation in the young brain that became more left lateralized with age and expertise. Clearly, the left hemisphere frontal-temporal perisylvian model of language localization is inadequate in patients with disease and in developing children, and neurosurgery based solely on visual identification of language-related neuroanatomical landmarks would place the patient at increased risk for incurring language deficits post-operatively.

FROM SEGREGATION TO INTEGRATION: MAPPING BRAIN FUNCTIONAL NETWORKS

The major shortcoming of the localization model is the premise that function is subsumed in an anatomically distinct region of the cerebral cortex, without consideration of the connections between and within regions. For example, we know that Broca's area is connected to Wernicke's area via the arcuate fasciculus, we know there are also connection to primary sensory and secondary association areas, and we know that these areas communicate and feedback to each other; however, localization models using a segregation approach cannot account for this complexity. Recent advances in computational neuroscience and improvements in computational processing power, have made it possible to augment studies of structural connectivity, which are anchored in physical anatomical pathways, to include measures of functional and effective connectivity, which describe network communication and integration (for a review, see Friston, 2011).

Therefore, in order to gain a fuller understanding of brain function and dynamics, there has been a shift towards connectionist paradigms which provide metrics to describe the level of communication and integration between distinct brain areas. Further, this shift has been driven by new understanding that the resting brain is not truly "at rest" (for a review, see Raichle, 2015). The traditional experimental approaches using brain evoked responses treated the non-task-related activity as "noise", which required time-locked averaging to enhance the signal and decrease the noise. However, it is now known that there are active functional networks when the brain is "at rest", and these involve not just the default mode network, but intrinsic networks for sensory, motor, language and attentional functions (e.g., Lowe et al., 1998; Cordes et al., 2001; Seeley et al., 2007). The elucidation of the relation between small cell assemblies containing as few as 600–800 cortical neurons and their relation to activation patterns in fMRI as seen by the blood-oxygen level (BOLD) contrast (Logothetis et al., 2001; Logothetis and Pfeuffer, 2004), led to later findings that, in fact, network communication was driven by neuronal oscillatory signals (Ikegaya et al., 2004). Thus, we have seen a convergence whereby we increasingly understand the relation between the hemodynamic signal, intrinsic neuronal oscillations and basic neurophysiological function (Lu et al., 2007; He et al., 2008; Khader et al., 2008).

DEFINITIONS AND COMPUTATIONS: FUNCTIONAL AND EFFECTIVE CONNECTIVITY

There is excellent body of foundational work describing the initial investigations into fMRI and MEG functional connectivity. **Table 2** provides a list of the seminal works in this field. As well, to aid the interested reader, we include also a list of recommended articles that give either a comprehensive overview or present thoughtful critiques on this topic. The following paragraphs are intended to give a brief summary of basic concepts and introduce frequently used terminology.

Functional connectivity is defined as the "temporal correlations between remote neurophysiological events", and effective connectivity is defined as "the influence [that] one neural system exerts over another" (Friston, 1994, p. 57). Thus, functional connectivity is a statistical measure that deals with the observation of correlated activity between remote brain areas under the assumption that areas behaving in a highly correlated manner must be working together. Functional connectivity does not provide insight into how these correlations are mediated and whether they are both essential to the process, or just correlated outputs driven by another process. Effective connectivity, on the other hand, deals with directions of influence and causality (Friston, 1994). **Figure 1** illustrates a generic MEG connectivity pipeline from acquisition through connectivity computation to data visualization, characterization and statistic comparisons. The figure legend provides specifics on each of the steps.

Because of the high temporal resolution of MEG, this technique can capture neuronal activity in the time domain as well as neuronal oscillatory activity in the time-frequency domain (for a review, see Pizzella et al., 2014). Thus, MEG connectivity can be computed based on correlated amplitude changes, which to some extent mimics fMRI functional connectivity (Brookes et al., 2011), and/or correlated oscillatory changes in the phase of the signals, which is a measure of synchronization and desynchronization (Schnitzler and Gross, 2005) between populations of neurons. This ability to quantify correlated amplitude and spectral changes between regions offers a perspective of the mechanisms and dynamics of brain connectivity that were not accessible without this level of temporal resolution. As well, the application of MEG functional connectivity patterns to graph theoretical analysis, organizes and visualizes the output into networks where important properties, such as node strength and path length can be identified (Stam, 2004). **Figure 2** illustrates a graph or network and provides definitions for a number of common terms used in describing neural networks using graph theory terminology.

When initial studies suggested that brain functional connectivity did not overlay exactly onto brain structural connectivity via large fiber tracts, the question of which mechanisms underlie brain communication was brought to

TABLE 2 | Recommended list of (a) seminal papers and (b) reviews and commentaries on functional connectivity, in chronological order.

(a) Seminal papers: modality, authors, title

Modality	Authors	Title
MRI	Friston (1994)	Functional and effective connectivity in neuroimaging: a synthesis
	Bullmore et al. (1996)	Functional magnetic resonance image analysis of a large-scale neurocognitive network
	Biswal et al. (1997)	Simultaneous assessment of flow and BOLD signals in resting state functional connectivity maps
	Büchel and Friston (2001)	Interactions among neuronal systems assessed with functional neuroimaging
	Koch et al. (2002)	An investigation of functional and anatomical connectivity using magnetic resonance imaging
	Greicius et al. (2003)	Functional connectivity in the resting brain: a network analysis of the default mode hypothesis
	Salvador et al. (2005)	Neurophysiological architecture of functional magnetic resonance images of human brain
MEG	Gross et al. (2001)	Dynamic imaging of coherent sources: studying neural interactions in the human brain
	Stam (2004)	Functional connectivity patterns of human magnetoencephalographic recordings: a "small-world" network?
	Schnitzler and Gross (2005)	Functional connectivity analysis in magnetoencephalography

(b) Reviews and commentaries: authors, title

Authors	Title
Horwitz (2003)	The elusive concept of brain connectivity.
Sporns et al. (2005)	The human connectome: a structural description of the human brain.
Friston (2005)	Models of brain function in neuroimaging.
Bassett and Bullmore (2006)	Small-world brain networks
Hagmann et al. (2010)	MR Conectomics: principles and challenges
Yeo et al. (2011)	The organization of the human cerebral cortex estimated by functional connectivity.
He et al. (2011)	Electrophysiological imaging of brain activity and connectivity—challenges and opportunities.
Toga et al. (2012)	Mapping the human connectome.
van Diessen et al. (2015)	Opportunities and methodological challenges in EEG and MEG resting state functional brain network research.

Full citations are contained in reference list.

the forefront. The surprising answer came from the field of cellular electrophysiology and neuronal oscillations. It is known that neural populations can be coupled via chemical or electrical synapses, and once coupled, cell populations will engage in synchronized rhythmic activity. This oscillatory activity provides windows of alternating reduced and enhanced excitability that serve as a dynamic gating mechanism for the exchange of information. The dynamic gating of communication can occur between distributed nodes but have an overall organization based on a relatively stable structural connectome, and in fact, are organized in a hierarchical system that is responsible for the local-global integration of information whereby lower frequencies are involved in long-range global communication and higher frequencies in local interactions (von Stein and Sarnthein, 2000). At rest, neuronal populations have a preferred oscillatory frequency but when engaged in a task, the oscillatory dynamics of that structure will change and other oscillation frequencies will become dominant. These oscillations within distributed cell assemblies can co-occur, interact with and modulate each other thereby transmitting information over long distances (for a review, please see Buzsáki et al., 2013). Further, the disruption of these processes, at either the neurophysiological or neuroanatomical level, can lead to cognitive dysfunction and/or brain disease.

MEG STUDIES OF FUNCTIONAL CONNECTIVITY IN PATIENTS WITH EPILEPSY

The most widespread clinical application of MEG has been in patients with localization-related epilepsy in whom surgical treatment of the epilepsy is being considered (see Bagić et al., 2011 for clinical guidelines for epilepsy recordings). Epilepsy surgery is the standard of care for appropriately selected adults and children with medically refractory epilepsy (Wiebe and Jetté, 2012). Surgical treatment for epilepsy is highly effective, has durable benefits, and can result in far better outcomes with respect to seizure freedom, improved quality of life, and reduction of the psychosocial comorbidities that accompany drug resistant epilepsy than continued medical treatment (Wiebe and Jetté, 2012; Jette et al., 2014).

A successful outcome from epilepsy surgery is generally defined as a seizure-free state with no imposition of neurological

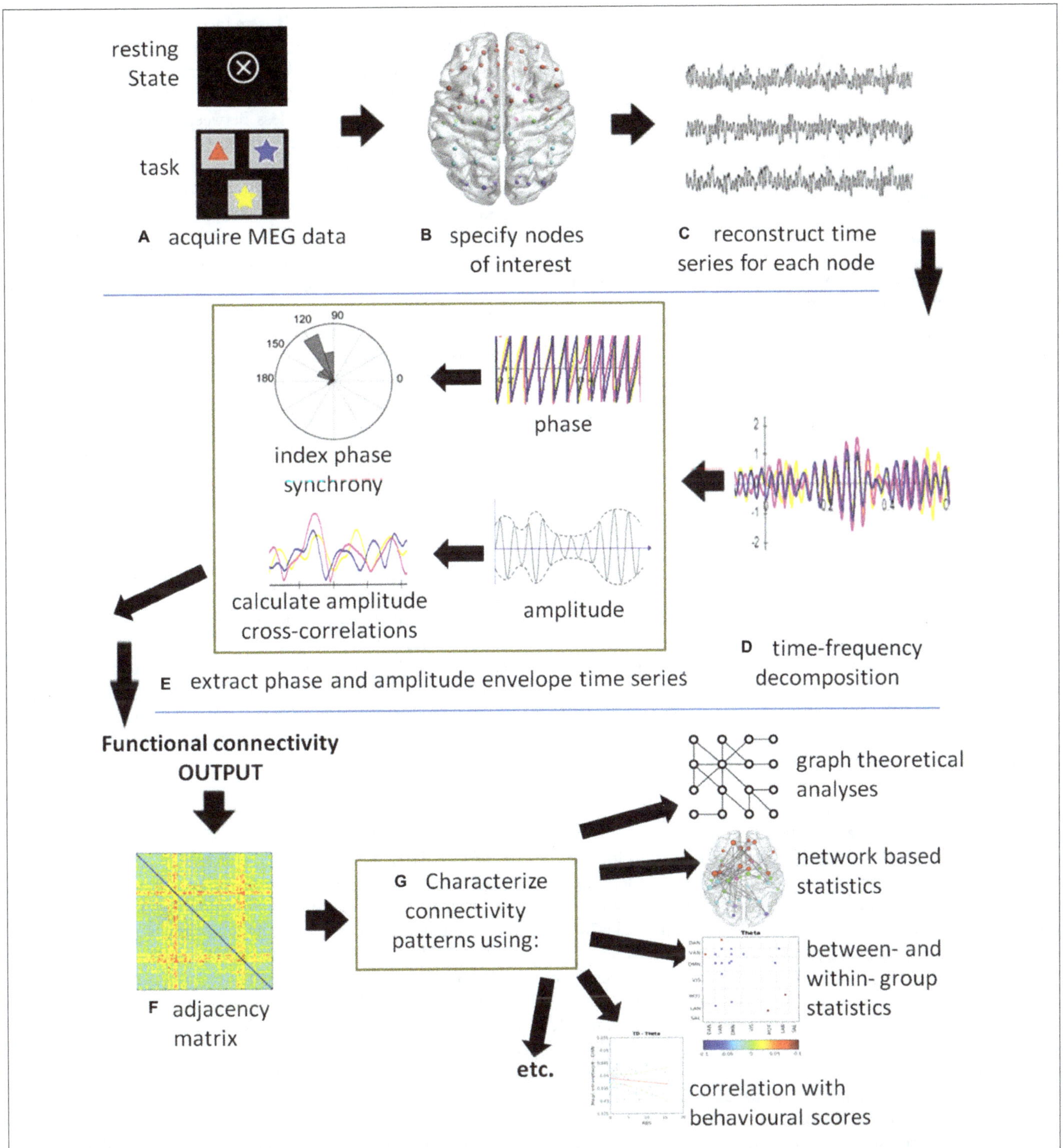

FIGURE 1 | A schematic of a generic magnetoencephalography (MEG) connectivity pipeline. (A) MEG data can be acquired with or without a task. **(B)** Nodes of interest can be derived from specific coordinates obtained by source analysis, from the literature, or using either a grid- or atlas-based approach. **(C)** A time series is reconstructed for each node of interest. **(D)** Time-series decomposition is most commonly completed using a Hilbert or wavelet transform, although other methods can be used. At this stage, the data could be submitted to causality analysis to compute effective connectivity. **(E)** The phase and/or amplitude envelope information is extracted and correlations computed between all node pairs at each time point. Commonly used are the phase lag index (PLI), weighted PLI (wPLI), sometimes the phase locking value (PLV), and amplitude correlations. **(F)** The resultant output is an adjacency matrix showing connectivity between all node pairs. In this example, a color plot is used where red indicates highly connected nodes, although other types of plots may be used. **(G)** The connectivity results can be submitted to statistics depending on the question of interest. For example, graph theoretical metrics and network based statistics can be used to characterize the connectivity patterns in the networks. Group level statistics can be conducted using partial-least squares (PLS) or permutation testing. Individual scores on behavioral and neuropsychological assessments can be correlated with connectivity measures and submitted to a regression analysis.

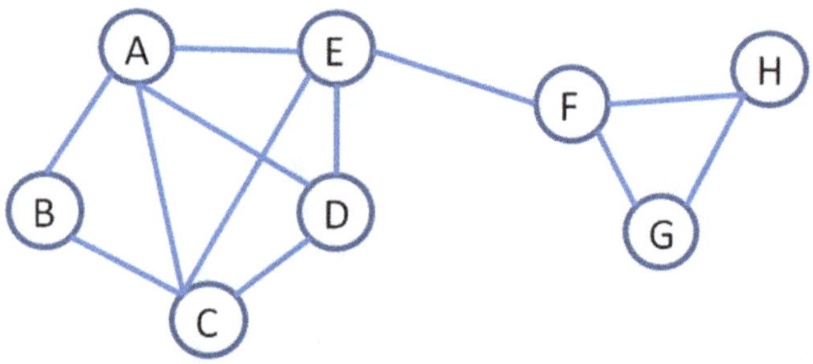

FIGURE 2 | An example of a network to illustrate terminology used in graph theory (Stam, 2004). *Nodes* are the objects in the graph and are represented by a letter. Nodes are connected by *edges*, represented by the lines. *Path length* is the number of edges between two pairs of nodes, for example, the path length between B to H is 4. *Degree* is a measure of centrality and refers to the number of edges joining into a node, for example, A has a degree of 4 while H has a degree of 2. *Hub* is a measure of importance and nodes that are hubs have a high number of edges, for example, A and C are both hubs. *Neighborhood* refers to a set of adjacent nodes; thus, there are two neighborhoods in this example (A–E) and (F–H). The edge between E and F is referred to as a *bridge*, as it joins two neighborhoods. Node *strength* is another important concept and is a measures of the connectedness of a node's neighbors to each other.

deficit (Snead, 2001). The key to this goal is to identify precisely the epileptogenic zone, which is defined as the area necessary and sufficient for the generation of habitual seizures, and the smallest amount of tissue that can be removed to achieve a seizure-free outcome (Obeid et al., 2009; Engel, 2013). In order to achieve seizure-freedom without an imposition of a neurologic deficit, one needs to lateralize and then localize the epileptogenic zone as well as localize eloquent function in the involved hemisphere. The use of MEG in the pre-surgical diagnostic evaluation of epilepsy candidacy in adults and children with medically refractory localization-related epilepsy contributes significantly to all three of these goals. Specifically, potential roles for MEG in epilepsy surgery include localization of the epileptogenic zone in conjunction with other non-invasive neurophysiological and imaging modalities (Lim et al., 2013; Jayakar et al., 2014), contribution to the decision making relevant to the indication for invasive monitoring and guidance of intracranial electrode placement as well as localization of eloquent function (Paetau and Mohamed, 2013). There are ample data from multiple centers that attest to the high sensitivity of MEG for epileptic activity and the importance of this modality in surgical decision-making (for example: Sutherling et al., 2008; Knowlton et al., 2009; Otsubo et al., 2010; Widjaja et al., 2013).

Despite the increasing and improved use of MEG, often in conjunction with other localization methods such as PET, SPECT and subdural grids, seizure control following epilepsy surgery even in carefully selected patients is not always optimal. In fact, it is estimated that epilepsy surgery only achieves complete and sustained seizure control in approximately 50% of patients with a focal neocortical epilepsy (Najm et al., 2013) and 75% with a mesial temporal lobe epilepsy (Spencer and Huh, 2008; Englot et al., 2013). These failures in surgical treatment are thought to stem from both an incomplete delineation, and thus resection, of the epileptogenic zone, as well as an incomplete understanding of the brain network in epilepsy (Englot et al., 2015). However, all that said, MEG does have a predictive value in epilepsy surgery. The complete resection of MEG clusters (defined as 6 or more spike sources with 1 cm or less between adjacent sources) has been shown to be correlated with post-surgical seizure freedom (Iida et al., 2005; Knowlton et al., 2009; Otsubo et al., 2010; Jung et al., 2013; Albert et al., 2014). Conversely, diffuse MEG spike sources indicate less likelihood for a localized seizure onset zone; therefore, this finding should weigh against invasive monitoring in the decision making process (Jung et al., 2013). Finally, it should be noted that MEG has been shown to be helpful in delineating an area of epileptogencity for subsequent resection in patients with an MRI-negative epilepsy (Rheims et al., 2013).

Some of the first MEG functional connectivity studies have reported abnormal increased connectivity in the theta-alpha range in patients with absence seizures (Chavez et al., 2010), increased connectivity in the beta range in patients with complex partial seizures (Madhavan et al., 2013), increased connectivity in the beta-gamma bands in focal cortical dysplasia (Jeong et al., 2014), increased connectivity in idiopathic generalized epilepsy (Elshahabi et al., 2015), and increases in functional connectivity between the default mode and medial temporal areas indicated the laterality of temporal lobe epilepsy (Hsiao et al., 2015). As well, in patients with epilepsy secondary to a brain tumor, increased connectivity was correlated with an increased numbers of seizures, and seizure vulnerability was related to a disorganized brain network topology (Douw et al., 2010). Clearly, epileptic cortex is associated with aberrant network connectivity within and between brain regions although the exact nature of this relation is not yet known.

It has been suggested that increased connectivity across small distances, that is, aberrant local connectivity amongst a small group of neurons, might be indicative of an irregularity in neuronal excitability (Laufs, 2012) and may thus be an important factor in epileptiform spike generation. For this reason, mapping the connectivity pattern around seizure onset zones might provide information about how seizures propagate and the extent of the epileptic network. At this time, these ideas have only been explored with electrocorticography (ECoG) and high-density EEG data. For example, one study measured effective connectivity from ECoG to discriminate connectivity associated with epileptic vs. eloquent cortex (Asano et al., 2013), while another used changes in patterns of functional connectivity to predict upcoming seizures and localize the seizure onset zone (van Mierlo et al., 2014). A study using high-density EEG found that neuropsychological deficits were related to different patterns of connectivity dysfunctions in right vs. left temporal lobe epilepsies (Coito et al., 2015). These ideas have not yet been applied to MEG although these electrophysiological studies suggest that these methods would be effective in MEG and would allow this information to be gathered non-invasively. However, MEG connectivity analysis of atypical expressive language laterality has been shown to be associated with the alteration of large-scale network integration in children with medically-refractory localization-related epilepsy (Ibrahim et al., 2015). Similarly MEG analysis has shown an association between network perturbations and neurocognitive outcome in children with medically refractory epilepsy (Ibrahim et al., 2014a,b).

MEG functional connectivity studies have not yet been applied to pre-surgical functional mapping protocols, although studies in controls are being reported and will lay the foundation for clinical studies. In a group of control adults performing a verb generation task, left hemisphere language networks were identified that included canonical and extra-canonical language areas which interacted through short-range synchronization in the gamma band with long range modulation in the theta band (Doesburg et al., 2012). Effective connectivity measurements in a group of typically developing school-aged children confirmed posterior-to-anterior flow of information, from visual fusiform areas to language areas in the supramarginal and angular gyri to inferior frontal areas (Simos et al., 2013) with measures of effective connectivity correlating with age (Kadis et al., 2016). Further, left hemisphere connectivity in the theta band correlated with performance on receptive language tasks in pre-school children (Kikuchi et al., 2011) while task-dependent theta-band synchronization for expressive language increased with age through adolescence and correlated with neuropsychological assessments of language ability (Doesburg et al., 2016). Finally, a study has demonstrated concordance between MEG and fMRI measures of functional connectivity on a naming task, with MEG providing additional information from different frequency bands (Liljeström et al., 2015b) that support specific functional roles for the different frequency bands with beta frequencies playing a more facilitatory role and gamma oscillatory synchronization playing a more inhibitory role in speech production (Liljeström et al., 2015a).

With these first studies of MEG language-related functional connectivity in control adults and typically developing children, the stage is set for translation of these methods into the clinical realm to examine the impact of disease on network changes. The patterns of network changes will inform us as to how the injured brain has re-organized itself or compensated so as to preserve function.

FUNCTION BEYOND STRUCTURE: THE VALUE OF ADDING MEG STUDIES TO FUNCTIONAL NEUROSURGERY

Hart et al. (2016) have provided a comprehensive overview of the relevance of graph theoretical analysis and functional connectivity computations to neurosurgical practice. The authors emphasize the current paradigm shift where brain function is considered a product of information exchange between members of a neural network, and functional mapping includes a description of the network properties.

It follows that abnormalities in brain connectivity may be responsible for a number of brain dysfunctions. In situations where there are known structural abnormalities, for example, a brain tumor, there is a non-specific but observable loss of functional connectivity (Bartolomei et al., 2006; Guggisberg et al., 2008) which could be related to a decrease in neurocognitive function (Bosma et al., 2008). A recent study used resting state MEG connectivity analyses to assess the impact of tumors in eloquent areas (Martino et al., 2011) concluded that these methods held promise as a potential avenue for non-invasive pre-surgical planning. In fact, there are now a number of studies examining MEG functional connectivity changes in a variety of neurological and psychiatric conditions (e.g., Stam, 2010; Dunkley, 2015; Pang et al., 2016). The data accumulating from these studies increasingly illustrate the value of exploring functional network abnormalities that are not observable at the level of structural connectivity. That is, there are an increasing numbers of examples where the brain's gross anatomy and structure are normal on MRI but investigations at the brain's microstructural level demonstrate alterations that impair neuronal output and connectivity with a resultant impairment of function.

While most clinical studies show connectivity differences at the group level, recent new approaches allow the correlation of network metrics with individual neuropsychological and/or behavioral scores. For example, in a study from our lab, soldiers with post-traumatic stress disorder were found to have significantly higher connectivity in the right parietal cortex, and the extent of this hyper-connectivity was directly correlated with their clinical symptoms of depression and anxiety (Dunkley et al., 2015). This is one recent example which demonstrates the possibility of extracting network metrics at an "$n = 1$" level to allow correlation and interpretation for a single patient.

While far from being ready to take this approach into the operating room, it is a curious mind and the persistent movement forward in small steps that culminates in a large leap of knowledge. The journal *Neurosurgery* published a special article entitled "Mapping the Human Connectome" (Toga et al., 2012) which summarizes, "For the foreseeable future, a comprehensive description of the complete connectome of even a single human brain might be viewed as unattainable. But the science of connectomics is devoted to filling in the gaps". We think, at this stage, neurosurgeons can play a significant role in "filling in the gaps" to test the multitude of functional connectivity hypotheses and findings that are filling the literature. The classic lesion studies by Broca, or stimulation studies by Penfield, were instrumental in developing the localization models of function. Like these pioneers, modern day neurosurgeons can parlay their observations of brain disease to answer questions regarding the characteristics, integrity and plasticity of functional neural networks and brain dynamics. At that time, we hope that MEG will be included in the repertoire of neuroimaging studies. MEG, with its high resolution in the temporal and oscillatory domains, is ideally suited to explore the oscillatory dynamics that underlie brain functional communication and complements the information obtained by other neuroimaging modalities.

With regards to functional neurosurgery, the increasing evidence that data acquired from MEG can model neural networks with high fidelity raises the possibility of simulating the impact of a resection and predicting functional outcome. For example, using MEG data collected from a patient with epilepsy, connectivity algorithms would identify the hubs and connections within the epilepsy and functional (i.e., language or motor) networks for that individual. With this information, a model of these networks could be created and subjected to simulated resections. A simulated resection may involve removal of a putative epileptogenic zone that impinges on functional cortex. The model could then predict whether the core epileptogenic zone was identified and whether sufficient disconnections were made to preclude seizure propagation. At the same time, the model could predict whether key hubs, or compensatory hubs, with sufficient connections were retained within the functional network to preserve core behaviors. Various simulated resection margins could be tested until the right balance of disease removal and functional sparing was achieved. While MEG studies of functional connectivity are not ready for this level of translation, the ability of MEG to record true neurophysiological activity with high fidelity brings the possibility of neural network modeling and simulations into the realm of possibility. This potential advancement raises exciting possibilities for future applications and approaches in functional neurosurgery.

SUMMARY

With access to new neuroimaging tools and methods for understanding brain function, the field of neurosurgery has an opportunity to grow in its ability to offer more precise surgical margins that approach disease more aggressively while better preserving functional networks. The measurement of structural and functional connectivity will open a window on brain function, communication and organization that will offer both theoretical and practical insights. The addition of MEG studies, with its high resolution in the time, space and oscillatory domain, will allow a look into brain communication that augments and fine tunes what can be learned from brain structure.

Within the field of neuroscience, a multi-layered paradigm shift has been occurring. First, our traditional segregationist view of function, while adequate for identifying "hubs" of activity, is woefully inadequate for describing the complexity of function. Rather, the introduction of metrics which describe the properties of both the hubs and connections seem to provide a more accurate picture of how function is subsumed in the brain. Second, our traditional view of a "resting" brain is now thought to be incorrect. In his recent review of this topic, Raichle (2015) uses the term "restless" brain, reflecting the shift from considering non-task-related activity as "noise", to a new understanding that the brain is always working and there are functional brain networks active during non-task periods. Finally, it is now understood that these intrinsic functional brain networks are organized and can be identified by high inter-regional correlations in phase or amplitude. Network communication occurs by modulation and integration of these inter- and intra-regional oscillations. The MEG is well poised for exploring questions of intrinsic brain networks and neuronal oscillations.

The application of computational neuroscience, and the identification of functional connections will improve our understanding of how distinct brain regions interact, and whether a region is essential or collateral to a function, Understanding the role that a particular region and its network connections play in a function will be very helpful in neurosurgical decision making, especially in a diseased brain, where developmental and neuroplastic processes may have shifted aspects of a function to another region. While the field of computational neuroscience is still very young, it already holds great promise for what it may offer to the field of neurosurgery for pre-surgical planning and the improvement of neurosurgical care.

AUTHOR CONTRIBUTIONS

EWP and OCS contributed equally to the writing of this article.

ACKNOWLEDGMENTS

The authors would like to thank Dr. Benjamin T. Dunkley and Mr. Simeon M. Wong for contributing images and assisting with the creation of **Figure 1**.

REFERENCES

Achard, S., Salvador, R., Whitcher, B., Suckling, J., and Bullmore, E. (2006). A resilient low-frequency small world human brain functional network with highly connected association cortical hubs. *J. Neurosci.* 26, 63–72. doi: 10.1523/JNEUROSCI.3874-05.2006

Albert, G. W., Ibrahim, G. M., Otsubo, H., Ochi, A., Go, C. Y., Snead, O. C. III, et al. (2014). Magnetoencephalography-guided resection fo epileptogenic foci in children. *J. Neurosurg. Pediatr.* 14, 532–537. doi: 10.3171/2014.8.peds13640

Asano, E., Brown, E. C., and Juhász, C. (2013). How to establish causality in epilepsy surgery. *Brain Dev.* 35, 706–720. doi: 10.1016/j.braindev.2013.04.004

Bagić, A. I., Knowlton, R. C., Rose, D. F., and Ebersole, J. S. (2011). American clinical magnetoencephalography society clinical practice guideline 1: recording and analysis of spontaneous cerebral activity. *J. Clin. Neurophysiol.* 28, 348–354. doi: 10.1097/WNP.0b013e3182272fed

Bartolomei, F., Bosma, I., Klein, M., Baayen, J. C., Reijneveld, J. C., Postma, T. J., et al. (2006). How do brain tumors alter functional connectivity? A magnetoencephalography study. *Ann. Neurol.* 59, 128–138. doi: 10.1002/ana.20710

Bassett, D. S., and Bullmore, E. (2006). Small-world brain networks. *Neuroscientist* 12, 512–523. doi: 10.1177/1073858406293182

Baumgartner, C., Doppelbauer, A., Deecke, L., Barth, D. S., Zeitlhofer, J., Lindinger, G., et al. (1991). Neuromagnetic investigation of somatotopy of human hand somatosensory cortex. *Exp. Brain Res.* 87, 641–648. doi: 10.1007/bf00227089

Billingsley-Marshall, R. L., Clear, T., Mencl, W. E., Simos, P. G., Swank, P. R., Men, D., et al. (2007). A comparison of functional MRI and magnetoencephalography for receptive language mapping. *J. Neurosci. Methods* 161, 306–313. doi: 10.1016/j.jneumeth.2006.10.020

Binder, J. R. (1997). Neuroanatomy of language processing studied with functional MRI. *Clin. Neurosci.* 4, 87–94.

Binder, J. R., Frost, J. A., Hammeke, T. A., Cox, R. W., Rao, S. M., and Prieto, T. (1997). Human brain language areas identified by functional magnetic resonance imaging. *J. Neurosci.* 17, 353–362.

Binder, J. R., Rao, S. M., Hammeke, T. A., Frost, J. A., Bandettini, P. A., Jesmanowicz, A., et al. (1995). Lateralized human brain language systems demonstrated by task subtraction functional magnetic resonance imaging. *Arch. Neurol.* 52, 593–601. doi: 10.1001/archneur.1995.00540300067015

Biswal, B. B., Van Kylen, J., and Hyde, J. S. (1997). Simultaneous assessment of flow and BOLD signals in resting state functional connectivity maps. *NMR Biomed.* 10, 165–167. doi: 10.1002/(sici)1099-1492(199706/08)10:4/5<165::aid-nbm454>3.0.co;2-7

Biswal, B., Yetkin, F. Z., Haughton, V. M., and Hyde, J. S. (1995). Functional connectivity in the motor cortex of resting human brain using echo-planar MRI. *Magn. Reson. Med.* 34, 537–541. doi: 10.1002/mrm.1910340409

Bosma, I., Douw, L., Bartolomei, F., Heimans, J. J., van Dijk, B. W., Postma, T. J., et al. (2008). Synchronized brain activity and neurocognitive function in patients with low-grade glioma: a magnetoencephalography study. *Neuro Oncol.* 10, 734–744. doi: 10.1215/15228517-2008-034

Breier, J. I., Castillo, E. M., Boake, C., Billingsley, R., Maher, L., Francisco, G., et al. (2004). Spatiotemporal patterns of language-specific brain activity in patients with chronic aphasia after stroke using magnetoencephalography. *Neuroimage* 23, 1308–1316. doi: 10.1016/j.neuroimage.2004.07.069

Breier, J. I., Castillo, E. M., Simos, P. G., Billingsley-Marshall, R. L., Pataraia, E., Sarkari, S., et al. (2005). Atypical language representation in patients with chronic seizure disorder and achievement deficits with magnetoencephalography. *Epilepsia* 46, 540–548. doi: 10.1111/j.0013-9580.2005.48904.x

Breier, J. I., Simos, P. G., Wheless, J. W., Constantinou, J. E., Baumgartner, J. E., Venkataraman, V., et al. (2001). Language dominance in children as determined by magnetic source imaging and the intracarotid amobarbital procedure: a comparison. *J. Child Neurol.* 16, 124–130. doi: 10.2310/7010.2001.7010

Breier, J. I., Simos, P. G., Zouridakis, G., and Papanicolaou, A. C. (2000). Lateralization of activity associated with language function using magnetoencephalography: a reliability study. *J. Clin. Neurophysiol.* 17, 503–510. doi: 10.1097/00004691-200009000-00010

Brookes, M. J., Hale, J. R., Zumer, J. M., Stevenson, C. M., Francis, S. T., Barnes, G. R., et al. (2011). Measuring functional connectivity using MEG: methodology and comparison with fcMRI. *Neuroimage* 56, 1082–1104. doi: 10.1016/j.neuroimage.2011.02.054

Büchel, C., and Friston, K. (2001). Interactions among neuronal systems assessed with functional neuroimaging. *Rev. Neurol. (Paris)* 157, 807–815.

Bullmore, E. T., Rabe-Hesketh, S., Morris, R. G., Williams, S. C., Gregory, L., Gray, J. A., et al. (1996). Functional magnetic resonance image analysis of a large-scale neurocognitive network. *Neuroimage* 4, 16–33. doi: 10.1006/nimg.1996.0026

Burgess, R. C., Funke, M. E., Bowyer, S. M., Lewine, J. D., Kirsch, H. E., and Bagic, A. I. (2011). American clinical magnetoencephalography society clinical practice guideline 2: presurgical functional brain mapping using magnetic evoked fields. *J. Clin. Neurophysiol.* 28, 355–361. doi: 10.1097/WNP.0b013e3182272ffe

Burianová, H., Marstaller, L., Sowman, P., Tesan, G., Rich, A. N., Williams, M., et al. (2013). Multimodal functional imaging of motor imagery using a novel paradigm. *Neuroimage* 71, 50–58. doi: 10.1016/j.neuroimage.2013.01.001

Burneo, J. G., Kuzniecky, R. I., Bebin, M., and Knowlton, R. C. (2004). Cortical reorganization in malformations of cortical development: a magnetoencephalographic study. *Neurology* 63, 1818–1824. doi: 10.1212/01.wnl.0000144179.87918.2f

Buzsáki, G., Logothetis, N., and Singer, W. (2013). Scaling brain size, keeping timing: evolutionary preservation of brain rhythms. *Neuron* 80, 751–764. doi: 10.1016/j.neuron.2013.10.002

Chavez, M., Valencia, M., Navarro, V. V., Latora, V., and Martinerie, J. (2010). Functional modularity of background activities in normal and epileptic brain networks. *Phys. Rev. Lett.* 104:118701. doi: 10.1103/physrevlett.104.118701

Clayden, J. D. (2013). Imaging connectivity: MRI and the structural networks of the brain. *Funct. Neurol.* 28, 197–203. doi: 10.11138/FNeur/2013.28.3.197

Coito, A., Plomp, G., Genetti, M., Abela, E., Wiest, R., Seeck, M., et al. (2015). Dynamic directed interictal connectivity in left and right temporal lobe epilepsy. *Epilepsia* 56, 207–217. doi: 10.1111/epi.12904

Cordes, D., Haughton, V. M., Arfanakis, K., Carew, J. D., Turski, P. A., Moritz, C. H., et al. (2001). Frequences contributing to functional connectivity in the cerebral cortex in 'resting-state' data. *Am. J. Neuroradiol.* 22, 1326–1333.

de Almeida, A. N., Alho, E. J., and Teixeira, M. J. (2014). Models of functional cerebral localization at the dawning of modern neurosurgery. *World Neurosurg.* 81, 436–440. doi: 10.1016/j.wneu.2013.01.033

Doesburg, S. M., Tingling, K., MacDonald, M. J., and Pang, E. W. (2016). Development of network synchronization predicts language abilities. *J. Cogn. Neurosci.* 28, 55–68. doi: 10.1162/jocn_a_00879

Doesburg, S. M., Vinette, S. A., Cheung, M. J., and Pang, E. W. (2012). θ-modulated γ-band synchronization among activated regions during a verb generation task. *Front. Psychol.* 3:195. doi: 10.3389/fpsyg.2012.00195

Douw, L., van Dellen, E., de Groot, M., Heimans, J. J., Klein, M., Stam, C. J., et al. (2010). Epilepsy is related to θ band brain connectivity and network topology in brain tumor patients. *BMC Neurosci.* 11:103. doi: 10.1186/1471-2202-11-103

Dunkley, B. T. (2015). Differential intrinsic coupling modes in psychological and physical trauma. *Front. Psychiatry* 6:140. doi: 10.3389/fpsyt.2015.00140

Dunkley, B. T., Sedge, P. A., Doesburg, S. M., Grodecki, R. J., Jetly, R., Shek, P. N., et al. (2015). θ, mental flexibility and post-traumatic stress disorder: connecting in the parietal cortex. *PLoS One* 10:e0123541. doi: 10.1371/journal.pone.0123541

Eliashiv, D. S., Kurelowech, L., Quint, P., Chung, J. M., Otis, S. M., and Gage, N. M. (2014). Atypical cortical language organization in epilepsy patients: evidence for divergent hemispheric dominance for receptive and expressive language function. *J. Clin. Neurophysiol.* 31, 208–217. doi: 10.1097/WNP.0000000000000058

Elshahabi, A., Klamer, S., Sahib, A. K., Lerche, H., Braun, C., and Focke, N. K. (2015). Magnetoencephalography reveals a widespread increase in network connectivity in idiopathic/genetic generalized epilepsy. *PLoS One* 10:e0138119. doi: 10.1371/journal.pone.0138119

Engel, J. Jr. (2013). Why is there still doubt to cut it out? *Epilepsy Curr.* 13, 198–204. doi: 10.5698/1535-7597-13.5.198

Englot, D. J., Hinkley, L. B., Kort, N. S., Imber, B. S., Mizuiri, D., Honma, S. M., et al. (2015). Global and regional functional connectivity maps of neural oscillations in focal epilepsy. *Brain* 138, 2249–2262. doi: 10.1093/brain/awv130

Englot, D. J., Lee, A. T., Tsai, C., Halabi, C., Barbaro, N. M., Auguste, K. I., et al. (2013). Seizure types and frequency in patients who 'fail' temporal lobectomy for intractable epilepsy. *Neurosurgery* 73, 838–844. doi: 10.1227/NEU.0000000000000120

Friston, K. J. (1994). Functional and effective connectivity in neuroimaging: a synthesis. *Hum. Brain Mapp.* 2, 56–78. doi: 10.1002/hbm.460020107

Friston, K. J. (2005). Models of brain function in neuroimaging. *Annu. Rev. Psychol.* 56, 57–87. doi: 10.1146/annurev.psych.56.091103.070311

Friston, K. J. (2011). Functional and effective connectivity: a review. *Brain Connect.* 1, 13–36. doi: 10.1089/brain.2011.0008

Gaetz, W., Cheyne, D., Rutka, J., Drake, J., Benifla, M., Strantzas, S., et al. (2009). Pre-surgical localization of primary motor cortex in paediatric patients with brain lesions by the use of spatially filtered MEG. *Neurosurgery* 64, ons177–ons185; discussion ons186. doi: 10.1227/01.NEU.0000316433.10913.32

Gage, N. M., Eliashiv, D. S., Isenberg, A. L., Fillmore, P. T., Kurelowech, L., Quint, P. J., et al. (2011). Rethinking clinical language mapping approaches: discordant receptive and expressive hemispheric language dominance in epilepsy surgery candidates. *J. Clin. Neurophysiol.* 28, 278–288. doi: 10.1097/WNP.0b013e31821c321d

Gallen, C. C., Sobel, D. F., Waltz, T., Aung, M., Copeland, B., Schwartz, B. J., et al. (1993). Noninvasive presurgical neuromagnetic mapping of somatosensory cortex. *Neurosurgery* 33, 260–268; discussion 268. doi: 10.1097/00006123-199308000-00012

Geschwind, N. (1970). The organization of language and the brain. *Science* 170, 940–944. doi: 10.1126/science.170.3961.940

Gordon, K. A., Wong, D. D., Valero, J., Jewell, S. F., Yoo, P., and Papsin, B. C. (2011). Use it or lose it? Lessons learned from the developing brains of children who are deaf and use cochlear implants to hear. *Brain Topogr.* 24, 204–219. doi: 10.1007/s10548-011-0181-2

Greicius, M. D., Krasnow, B., Reiss, A. L., and Menon, V. (2003). Functional connectivity in the resting brain: a network analysis of the default mode hypothesis. *Proc. Natl. Acad. Sci. U S A* 100, 253–258. doi: 10.1073/pnas.0135058100

Gross, J., Kujala, J., Hamalainen, M., Timmermann, L., Schnitzler, A., and Salmelin, R. (2001). Dynamic imaging of coherent sources: studying neural interactions in the human brain. *Proc. Natl. Acad. Sci. U S A* 98, 694–699. doi: 10.1073/pnas.98.2.694

Guggisberg, A. G., Honma, S. M., Findlay, A. M., Dalal, S. S., Kirsch, H. E., Berger, M. S., et al. (2008). Mapping functional connectivity in patients with brain lesions. *Ann. Neurol.* 63, 193–203. doi: 10.1002/ana.21224

Hagmann, P., Cammoun, L., Gigandet, X., Gerhard, S., Grant, E. P., Wedeen, V., et al. (2010). MR conectomics: principles and challenges. *J. Neurosci. Methods* 194, 34–45. doi: 10.1016/j.jneumeth.2010.01.014

Harding, G. F., Degg, C., Anderson, S. J., Holliday, I., Fylan, F., Barnes, G., et al. (1994). Topographic mapping of the pattern onset evoked magnetic response to stimulation of different portions of the visual field. *Int. J. Psychophysiol.* 16, 175–183. doi: 10.1016/0167-8760(89)90044-5

Hari, R., and Salmelin, R. (2012). Magnetoencephalography: from SQUIDs to neuroscience: neuroimage 20th anniversary special edition. *Neuroimage* 61, 386–396. doi: 10.1016/j.neuroimage.2011.11.074

Hart, M. G., Ypma, R. J. F., Romero-Garcia, R., Price, S. J., and Suckling, J. (2016). Graph theory analysis of complex brain networks: new concepts in brain mapping applied to neurosurgery. *J. Neurosurg.* 124, 1665–1678. doi: 10. 3171/2015.4.jns142683

He, B. J., Snyder, A. Z., Zemple, J. M., Smyth, M. D., and Raichle, M. E. (2008). Electrophysiological correlates of the brain's intrinsic large-scale functional architecture. *Proc. Natl. Acad. Sci. U S A* 105, 16039–16044. doi: 10.1073/pnas. 0807010105

He, B., Yang, L., Wilke, C., and Yuan, H. (2011). Electrophysiological imaging of brain activity and connectivity-challenges and opportunities. *IEEE Trans. Biomed. Eng.* 58, 1918–1931. doi: 10.1109/tbme.2011.2139210

Herdman, A. T., Pang, E. W., Ressel, V., Gaetz, W., and Cheyne, D. (2007). Task-related modulation of early cortical responses during language production: an event-related synthetic aperture magnetometry study. *Cereb. Cortex* 17, 2536–2543. doi: 10.1093/cercor/bhl159

Holland, S. K., Vannest, J., Mecoli, M., Jacola, L. M., Tillema, J.-M., Karunanayaka, P. R., et al. (2007). Functional MR of language lateralization during development in children. *Int. J. Audiol.* 46, 533–551. doi: 10. 1080/14992020701448994

Horwitz, B. (2003). The elusive concept of brain connectivity. *Neuroimage* 19, 466–470. doi: 10.1016/s1053-8119(03)00112-5

Hsiao, F.-J., Yu, H.-Y., Chen, W.-T., Kwan, S.-Y., Chen, C., Yen, D.-J., et al. (2015). Increased intrinsic connectivity of the default mode network in temporal lobe epilepsy: evidence from resting-state MEG recordings. *PLoS One* 10:e0128787. doi: 10.1371/journal.pone.0128787

Ibrahim, G. M., Cassel, D., Morgan, B. R., Smith, M. L., Otsubo, H., Ochi, A., et al. (2014a). Resilience of brain networks to interictal epileptiform discharges is associated with cognitive outcome. *Brain* 137, 2690–2702. doi: 10. 1093/brain/awu214

Ibrahim, G. M., Morgan, B. R., Doesburg, S. M., Taylor, M. J., Pang, E. W., Donner, E., et al. (2015). Atypical language laterality is associated with large-scale disruption of network integration in children with intractable focal epilepsy. *Cortex* 65, 83–88. doi: 10.1016/j.cortex.2014.12.016

Ibrahim, G. M., Morgan, B. R., Lee, W., Smith, M. L., Donner, E. J., Wang, F., et al. (2014b). Impaired development of intrinsic connectivity networks in children with medically-intractable localization-related epilepsy. *Hum. Brain Mapp.* 35, 5686–5700. doi: 10.1002/hbm.22580

Iida, K., Otsubo, H., Matsumoto, Y., Ochi, A., Oishi, M., Holowka, S., et al. (2005). Characterizing magnetic spike sources by using magnetoencephalo-graphy-guided neuronavigation in epilepsy surgery in pediatric patients. *J. Neurosurg.* 102, 187–196. doi: 10.3171/ped.2005.102.2.0187

Ikegaya, Y., Aaron, G., Cossart, R., Araonov, D., Lampl, I., Ferster, D., et al. (2004). Synfire chains and cortical songs: temporal modules of cortical activity. *Science* 304, 559–564. doi: 10.1126/science.1093173

Jayakar, P., Gaillard, W. D., Tripathi, T., Libenson, M. H., Mathern, G. W., and Cross, H. (2014). Diagnostic test utilization in evaluation for respective epilepsy surgery in children. *Epilepsia* 55, 507–518. doi: 10.1111/epi.12544

Jeong, W., Jin, S.-H., Kim, M., Kim, J. S., and Chung, C. K. (2014). Abnormal functional brain network in epilepsy patients with focal cortical dysplasia. *Epilepsy Res.* 108, 1618–1626. doi: 10.1016/j.eplepsyres.2014. 09.006

Jette, N., Reid, A. Y., and Wiebe, S. (2014). Surgical management of epilepsy. *CMAJ* 186, 997–1004. doi: 10.1503/cmaj.121291

Jung, J., Bouet, R., Delpeuch, C., Ryvlin, P., Isnard, J., Guenot, M., et al. (2013). The value of magnetoencephalography for seizure-onset zone localization in magnetic resonance imaging-negative partial epilepsy. *Brain* 136, 3176–3186. doi: 10.1093/brain/awt213

Kadis, D. S., Dimitrijevic, A., Toro-Serev, C. A., Smith, M. L., and Holland, S. K. (2016). Charaterizing information flux within the distributed pediatric expressive language network: a core region mapped through fMRI-constrained MEG effective connectivity analyses. *Brain Connect.* 6, 76–83. doi: 10. 1089/brain.2015.0374

Kadis, D. S., Iida, K., Kerr, E. N., Logan, W. J., McAndrews, M. P., Ochi, A., et al. (2007). Intrahemispheric reorganization of language in children with medically intractable epilepsy of the left hemisphere. *J. Int. Neuropsychol. Soc.* 13, 505–516. doi: 10.1017/s1355617707070397

Kadis, D. S., Pang, E. W., Mills, T., Taylor, M. J., McAndrews, M. P., and Smith, M. L. (2011). Characterizing the normal developmental trajectory of expressive language lateralization using magnetoencephalography. *J. Int. Neuropsychol. Soc.* 17, 896–904. doi: 10.1017/s1355617711000932

Kamada, K., Takeuchi, F., Kuriki, S., Todo, T., Morita, A., and Sawamura, Y. (2006). Dissociated expressive and receptive language functions on magnetoencephalography, functional magnetic resonance imaging and amobarbital studies. Case report and review of the literature. *J. Neurosurg.* 104, 598–607. doi: 10.3171/jns.2006.104.4.598

Khader, P., Schicke, T., Röder, B., and Rösler, F. (2008). On the relationship between slow cortical potentials and BOLD signal changes in humans. *Int. J. Psychophysiol.* 67, 252–261. doi: 10.1016/j.ijpsycho.2007.05.018

Kikuchi, M., Shitamichi, K., Yoshimura, Y., Ueno, S., Remijn, G. B., Hirasawa, T., et al. (2011). Lateralized θ wave connectivity and language performance in 2- to 5-year-old children. *J. Neurosci.* 31, 4984–4988. doi: 10.1523/JNEUROSCI. 2785-11.2011

Knowlton, R. C., Razdan, S. N., Limdi, N., Elgavish, R. A., Killen, J., Blount, J., et al. (2009). Effect of epilepsy magnetic source imaging on intracranial electrode placement. *Ann. Neurol.* 65, 716–723. doi: 10.1002/ana.21660

Koch, M. A., Norris, D. G., and Hund-Georgiadis, M. (2002). An investigation of functional and anatomical connectivity using magnetic resonance imaging. *Neuroimage* 16, 241–250. doi: 10.1006/nimg.2001.1052

Korostenskaja, M., Pardos, M., Fujiwara, H., Kujala, T., Horn, P., Rose, D., et al. (2010). Neuromagnetic evidence of impaired cortical auditory processing in pediatric intractable epilepsy. *Epilepsy Res.* 92, 63–73. doi: 10.1016/j.eplepsyres. 2010.08.008

Kraeutner, S., Gionfriddo, A., Bardouille, T., and Boe, S. (2014). Motor imagery-based brain activity parallels that of motor execution: evidence from magnetic source imaging of cortical oscillations. *Brain Res.* 1588, 81–91. doi: 10.1016/j. brainres.2014.09.001

Kristeva, R., Cheyne, D., and Deecke, L. (1991). Neuromagnetic fields accompanying unilateral and bilateral voluntary movements: topography and analysis of cortical sources. *Electroencephalogr. Clin. Neurophysiol.* 81, 284–298. doi: 10.1016/0168-5597(91)90015-p

Kubota, Y., Otsuki, T., Kaneko, Y., Niimura, K., Nakama, H., and Okazaki, M. (2007). Delayed N100m latency in focal epilepsy associated with spike dipoles at the primary auditory cortex. *J. Clin. Neurophysiol.* 24, 263–270. doi: 10. 1097/wnp.0b013e3180556685

Kupers, R., and Ptito, M. (2014). Compensatory plasticity and cross-modal reorganization following early visual deprivation. *Neurosci. Biobehav. Rev.* 41, 36–52. doi: 10.1016/j.neubiorev.2013.08.001

Laufs, H. (2012). Functional imaging of seizures and epilepsy: evolution from zones to networks. *Curr. Opin. Neurol.* 25, 194–200. doi: 10.1097/WCO. 0b013e3283515db9

Liljeström, M., Kujala, J., Stevenson, C., and Salmelin, R. (2015a). Dynamic reconfiguration of the language network preceding onset of speech in picture naming. *Hum. Brain Mapp.* 3693, 1202–1216. doi: 10.1002/hbm.22697

Liljeström, M., Stevenson, C., Kujala, J., and Salmelin, R. (2015b). Task- and stimuls-related cortical networks in language production: exploring similarity of MEG- and fMRI-derived functional connectivity. *Neuroimage* 120, 75–87. doi: 10.1016/j.neuroimage.2015.07.017

Lim, M. E., Bowen, J. M., Snead, O. C., III, Elliott, I., Donner, E., Weiss, S., et al. (2013). Access to surgery for paediatric patients with medically refractory epilepsy: a systems approach. *Epilepsy Res.* 107, 286–296. doi: 10.1016/j.eplepsyres.2013.08.010

Logothetis, N. K., Pauls, J., Augath, M., Trinath, T., and Oettermann, A. (2001). Neurophysiological investigation of the basis of the fMRI signal. *Nature* 412, 150–157. doi: 10.1038/35084005

Logothetis, N. K., and Pfeuffer, J. (2004). On the nature of the BOLD fMRI contrast mechanism. *Magn. Reson. Imaging* 22, 1517–1531. doi: 10.1016/j.mri.2004.10.018

Lowe, M. J., Mock, B. J., and Sorenson, J. A. (1998). Functional connectivity in single and multislice echoplanar imaging using resting-state fluctuations. *Neuroimage* 7, 119–132. doi: 10.1006/nimg.1997.0315

Lu, H., Zuo, Y., Gu, H., Waltz, J. A., Zhan, W., Scholl, C. A., et al. (2007). Synchronized δ oscillations correlate with the resting-state function MRI signal. *Proc. Natl. Acad. Sci. U S A* 104, 18265–18269. doi: 10.1073/pnas.0705791104

Madhavan, D., Heinrichs-Graham, E., and Wilson, T. W. (2013). Whole-brain functional connectivity increases with extended duration of focal epileptiform activity. *Neurosci. Lett.* 542, 26–29. doi: 10.1016/j.neulet.2013.02.052

Martino, J., Honma, S. M., Findlay, A. M., Guggisberg, A. G., Owen, J. P., Kirsch, H. E., et al. (2011). Resting functional connectivity in patients with brain tumors in eloquent areas. *Ann. Neurol.* 69, 521–532. doi: 10.1002/ana.22167

Mesulam, M. M. (1998). From sensation to cognition. *Brain* 121, 1013–1052. doi: 10.1093/brain/121.6.1013

Minassian, B., Otsubo, H., Weiss, S., Elliott, I., Rutka, J. T., and Snead, O. C. (1999). Magnetoencephalographic localization in pediatric epilepsy surgery: comparison with invasive intracranial electroencephalography. *Ann. Neurol.* 46, 627–633. doi: 10.1002/1531-8249(199910)46:4<627::aid-ana11 >3.0.co;2-c

Nagamine, T., Toro, C., Balish, M., Deuschl, G., Wang, B., Sato, S., et al. (1994). Cortical magnetic and electrid fields associated with voluntary finger movements. *Brain Topogr.* 6, 175–183. doi: 10.1007/bf01187707

Najm, I., Jehi, L., Palmini, A., Gonzalez-Martinez, J., Paglioli, E., and Bingaman, W. (2013). Temporal patterns and mechanisms of epilepsy surgery failure. *Epilepsia* 54, 772–782. doi: 10.1111/epi.12152

Nakasato, N., Seki, K., Fujita, S., Hatanaka, K., Kawamura, T., Ohtomo, S., et al. (1996). Clinical application of visual evoked fields using an MRI-linked whole head MEG system. *Front. Med. Biol. Eng.* 7, 275–283.

Nakasato, N., and Yoshimoto, T. (2000). Somatosensory, auditory and visual evoked magnetic fields in patients with brain disease. *J. Clin. Neurophysiol.* 17, 201–211. doi: 10.1097/00004691-200003000-00009

Obeid, M., Wyllie, E., Rahi, A. C., and Mikati, M. A. (2009). Approach to pediatric epilepsy surgery: state of the art, Part I: general principles and presurgical workup. *Eur. J. Paediatr. Neurol.* 13, 102–114. doi: 10.1016/j.ejpn.2008.05.007

Onishi, H., Sugawara, K., Yamashiro, K., Sato, D., Suzuki, M., Kirimoto, H., et al. (2013). Neuromagnetic activation following active and passive finger movements. *Brain Behav.* 3, 178–192. doi: 10.1002/brb3.126

Otsubo, H., Ochi, A., and Snead, O. C. (2010). "Magnetoencephalography," in *Pediatric Epilepsy Surgery: Preoperative Assesment and Surgical Treatment*, eds O. Cataltepe and G. I. Jallo (New York, NY: Thieme Medical Publishers), 53–58.

Paetau, R., and Mohamed, I. S. (2013). "Magnetoencephaloagraphy (MEG) and other neurophysiological investigations," in *Handbook of Clinical Neurology*, (3rd Series, Pediatric Neurology Part I) eds O. Dulac, M. Lassonde and H. B. Sarnat (Elsevier BV: Netherlands), 461–465.

Pang, E. W., Drake, J., Otsubo, H., Martineau, A., Strantzas, S., Cheyne, D., et al. (2008). Intraoperative confirmation of hand motor area identified preoperatively by magnetoencephalography: case report. *Pediatr. Neurosurg.* 44, 313–317. doi: 10.1159/000134923

Pang, E. W., Dunkley, B. T., Doesburg, S. M., da Costa, L., and Taylor, M. J. (2016). Reduced brain connectivity and mental flexibility in mild traumatic brain injury. *Ann. Clin. Transl. Neurol.* 3, 124–131. doi: 10.1002/acn3.280

Pang, E. W., Gaetz, W., Drake, J. M., Strantzas, S., MacDonald, M. J., Otsubo, H., et al. (2009). Patient with post-central gyrectomy demonstrates reliable localization of hand motor area using magnetoencephalography (MEG): case report. *Pediat. Neurosurg.* 45, 311–316. doi: 10.1159/000235749

Pang, E. W., Wang, F., Malone, M., Kadis, D. S., and Donner, E. J. (2011). Localization of Broca's area using verb generation tasks in the MEG: validation against fMRI. *Neurosci. Lett.* 490, 215–219. doi: 10.1016/j.neulet.2010.12.055

Pantev, C., Bertrand, O., Eulitz, C., Verkindt, C., Hampson, S., Schuierer, G., et al. (1995). Specific tonotopic organizations of different areas of the human auditory cortex revealed by simultaneous magnetic and electric recordings. *Electroencephalogr. Clin. Neurophysiol.* 94, 26–40. doi: 10.1016/0013-4694(94)00209-4

Papanicolaou, A. C., Baumann, S., Rogers, R. L., Saydjari, C., Amparo, E. G., and Eisenberg, H. M. (1990). Localization of auditory response sources using magnetoencephalography and magnetic resonance imaging. *Arch. Neurol.* 47, 33–37. doi: 10.1001/archneur.1990.00530010041016

Papanicolaou, A. C., Simos, P. G., Castillo, E. M., Breier, J. I., Sarkari, S., Pataraia, E., et al. (2004). Magnetoencephalography: a noninvasive alternative to the Wada procedure. *J. Neurosurg.* 100, 867–876. doi: 10.3171/jns.2004.100.5.0867

Pataraia, E., Simos, P. G., Castillo, E. M., Billingsley-Marshall, R. L., McGregor, A. L., Breier, J. I., et al. (2004). Reorganization of language-specific cortex in patients with lesions or mesial temporal epilepsy. *Neurology* 63, 1825–1832. doi: 10.1212/01.WNL.0000144180.85779.9a

Penfield, W., and Jasper, H. (1954). Epilepsy and the functional anatomy of the human brain. *JAMA* 155:86. doi: 10.1001/jama.1954.03690190092039

Pizzella, V., Marzetti, L., Della Penna, S., de Pasquale, F., Zappasodi, F., and Romani, G. L. (2014). Magnetoencephalography in the study of brain dynamcies. *Funct. Neurol.* 29, 241–253.

Raichle, M. E. (2015). The restless brain: how intrinsic activity organizes brain function. *Philos. Trans. R. Soc. Lond. B Biol. Sci.* 370:20140172. doi: 10.1098/rstb.2014.0172

Rezaie, R., Narayana, S., Schiller, K., Birg, L., Wheless, J. W., Boop, F. A., et al. (2014). Assessment of hemispheric dominance for receptive language in pediatric patients under sedation using magnetoencephalography. *Front. Hum. Neurosci.* 8:657. doi: 10.3389/fnhum.2014.00657

Rheims, S., Jung, J., and Ryvlin, P. (2013). Combination of PET and magnetoencephalography in the presurgical assessment of MRI-negative epilepsy. *Front. Neurol.* 4:188. doi: 10.3389/fneur.2013.00188

Salvador, R., Suckling, J., Coleman, M. R., Pickard, J. D., Menon, D., and Bullmore, E. (2005). Neurophysiological architecture of functional magnetic resonance images of human brain. *Cereb. Cortex* 15, 1332–1342. doi: 10.1093/cercor/bhi016

Schnitzler, A., and Gross, J. (2005). Functional connectivity analysis in magnetoencephalography. *Int. Rev. Neurobiol.* 68, 173–195. doi: 10.1016/s0074-7742(05)68007-5

Seeley, W. W., Menon, V., Schatzberg, A. F., Keller, J., Glover, G. H., Kenna, H., et al. (2007). Dissociable intrinsic connectivity networks for salience processing and executive control. *J. Neurosci.* 27, 2349–2356. doi: 10.1523/JNEUROSCI.5587-06.2007

Seki, K., Nakasato, N., Fujita, S., Hatanaka, K., Kawamura, T., Kanno, A., et al. (1996). Neuromagnetic evidence that the P100 component of the pattern reversal visual evoked response originates in the bottom of the calcarine fissure. *Electroencephalogr. Clin. Neurophysiol.* 100, 436–442. doi: 10.1016/0168-5597(96)95098-4

Simos, P. G., Papanicolaou, A. C., Breier, J. I., Fletcher, J. M., Wheless, J. W., Maggio, W. W., et al. (2000). Insights into brain function and neural plasticity using magnetic source imaging. *J. Clin. Neurophysiol.* 17, 143–162. doi: 10.1097/00004691-200003000-00004

Simos, P. G., Rezaie, R., Fletcher, J. M., and Papanicolaou, A. C. (2013). Time-constrained functional connectivity analysis of cortical networks underlying phonological decoding in typically developing school-aged children: a magnetoencephalography study. *Brain Lang.* 125, 156–164. doi: 10.1016/j.bandl.2012.07.003

Smith, J. R., Gallen, C. C., and Schwartz, B. J. (1994). Multichannel magnetoencephalographic mapping of sensorimotor cortex for epilepsy surgery. *Stereotact. Funct. Neurosurg.* 62, 245–251. doi: 10.1159/000098627

Snead, O. C. III (2001). Surgical treatment of medically refractory epilepsy in childhood. *Brain Dev.* 23, 199–207. doi: 10.1016/s0387-7604(01)00204-2

Sobel, D. F., Gallen, C. C., Schwartz, B. J., Waltz, T. A., Copeland, B., Yamada, S., et al. (1993). Locating the central sulcus: comparison of MR anatomic and magnetoencephalographic functional methods. *Am. J. Neuroradiol.* 14, 915–925.

Spencer, S., and Huh, L. (2008). Outcomes of epilepsy surgery in adults and children. *Lancet Neurol.* 7, 525–537. doi: 10.1016/S1474-4422(08)70109-1

Sporns, O., Tononi, G., and Kötter, R. (2005). The human connectome: a structural description of the human brain. *PLoS Comput. Biol.* 1:e42. doi: 10.1371/journal.pcbi.0010042

Stam, C. J. (2004). Functional connectivity patterns of human magnetoencephalographic recordings: a 'small-world' network? *Neurosci. Lett.* 355, 25–28. doi: 10.1016/j.neulet.2003.10.063

Stam, C. J. (2010). Use of magnetoencephalography (MEG) to study functional brain networks in neurodegenerative disorders. *J. Neurol. Sci.* 289, 128–134. doi: 10.1016/j.jns.2009.08.028

Stufflebeam, S. M. (2011). Clinical magnetoencephalography for neurosurgery. *Neurosurg. Clin. N. Am.* 22, 153–167. doi: 10.1016/j.nec.2010.11.006

Stufflebeam, S. M., Tanaka, N., and Ahlfors, S. P. (2009). Clinical applications of magnetoencephalography. *Hum. Brain Mapp.* 30, 1813–1823. doi: 10.1002/hbm.20792

Sutherling, W. W., Mamelak, A. N., Thyerlei, D., Maleeva, T., Minazad, Y., Philpott, L., et al. (2008). Influence of magnetic source imaging for planning intracranial EEG in epilepsy. *Neurology* 71, 990–996. doi: 10.1212/01.wnl.0000326591.29858.1a

Toga, A. W., Clark, K. A., Thompson, P. M., Shattuck, D. W., and Van Horn, J. D. (2012). Mapping the human connectome. *Neurosurgery* 71, 1–5. doi: 10.1227/NEU.0b013e318258e9ff

van den Heuvel, M. P., and Hulshoff Pol, H. E. (2010). Exploring the brain network: a review on resting-state fMRI functional connectivity. *Eur. Neuropsychopharmacol.* 20, 519–534. doi: 10.1016/j.euroneuro.2010.03.008

van Diessen, E., Numan, T., van Dellen, E., van der Kooi, A. W., Boersma, M., Hofman, D., et al. (2015). Opportunities and methodological challenges in EEG and MEG resting state functional brain network research. *Clin. Neurophysiol.* 126, 1468–1481. doi: 10.1016/j.clinph.2014.11.018

Van Essen, D. C. (2013). Cartography and connectomes. *Neuron* 80, 775–790. doi: 10.1016/j.neuron.2013.10.027

van Mierlo, P., Papadopoulou, M., Carrette, E., Boon, P., Vandenberghe, S., Vonck, K., et al. (2014). Functional brain connectivity from EEG in epilepsy: seizure prediction and epielptogenic focus localization. *Prog. Neurobiol.* 121, 19–35. doi: 10.1016/j.pneurobio.2014.06.004

Van Poppel, M., Wheless, J. W., Clarke, D. F., McGregor, A., McManis, M. H., Perkins, F. F. Jr., et al. (2012). Passive language mapping with magnetoencephlography in pediatric patients with epilepsy. *J. Neurosurg. Pediatr.* 10, 96–102. doi: 10.3171/2012.4.PEDS11301

von Stein, A., and Sarnthein, J. (2000). Different frequencies for different scales of cortical integration: from local γ to long range α/θ synchronization. *Int. J. Psychophysiol.* 38, 301–313. doi: 10.1016/s0167-8760(00)00172-0

Weinberg, H., Cheyne, D., and Crisp, D. (1990). Electroencephalographic and magnetoencephalographic studies of motor function. *Adv. Neurol.* 54, 193–205.

Widjaja, E., Shammas, A., Valli, R., Otsubo, H., Ochi, A., Snead, O. C., et al. (2013). FDG-PET and magnetoencephalography in presurgical workup of children with localization-related nonlesional epilepsy. *Epilepsia* 54, 691–699. doi: 10.1111/epi.12114

Wiebe, S., and Jetté, N. (2012). Pharmacoresistance and the role of surgery in difficult to treat epilepsy. *Nat. Rev. Neurol.* 8, 669–677. doi: 10.1038/nrneurol.2012.181

Yeo, B. T., Krienen, F. M., Sepulcre, J., Sabuncu, M. R., Sashkari, D., Hollinshead, M., et al. (2011). The organization of the human cerebral cortex estimated by functional connectivity. *J. Neurophysiol.* 106, 1125–1165. doi: 10.1152/jn.00338.2011

2

Segmentation of the Cingulum Bundle in the Human Brain: A New Perspective Based on DSI Tractography and Fiber Dissection Study

*Yupeng Wu[1], Dandan Sun[2], Yong Wang[1], Yibao Wang[1] and Shaowu Ou[1]**

[1] Department of Neurosurgery, The First Affiliated Hospital of China Medical University, Shenyang, China, [2] Department of Cardiovascular Ultrasound, The First Affiliated Hospital of China Medical University, Shenyang, China

***Correspondence:**
Shaowu Ou
cmuoushaowu@163.com

The cingulum bundle (CB) is a critical white matter fiber tract in the brain, which forms connections between the frontal lobe, parietal lobe and temporal lobe. In non-human primates, the CB is actually divided into distinct subcomponents on the basis of corticocortical connections. However, at present, no study has verified similar distinct subdivisions in the human brain. In this study, we reconstructed these distinct subdivisions in the human brain, and determined their exact cortical connections using high definition fiber tracking (HDFT) technique on 10 healthy adults and a 488-subject template from the Human Connectome Project (HCP-488). Fiber dissections were performed to verify tractography results. Five CB segments were identified. CB-I ran from the subrostral areas to the precuneus and splenium, encircling the corpus callosum (CC). CB-II arched around the splenium and extended anteriorly above the CC to the medial aspect of the superior frontal gyrus (SFG). CB-III connected the superior parietal lobule (SPL) and precuneus with the medial aspect of the SFG. CB-IV was a relatively minor subcomponent from the SPL and precuneus to the frontal region. CB-V, the para-hippocampal cingulum, stemmed from the medial temporal lobe and fanned out to the occipital lobes. Our findings not only provide a more accurate and detailed description on the associated architecture of the subcomponents within the CB, but also offer new insights into the functional role of the CB in the human brain.

Keywords: cingulum bundle, white matter, diffusion spectrum imaging, fiber dissection, Klingler's technique

INTRODUCTION

In humans, the cingulate cortex forms an arch, extending from the rostral subcallosal area anteriorly and following the curved superior surface of the corpus callosum (CC) bilaterally on the sagittal plane (Haznedar et al., 2004). The cingulum bundle (CB) is a 5–7 mm in diameter fiber bundle that locates above the CC and under the cingulate cortex (Schmahmann and Pandya, 2006).

Abbreviations: CB, cingulum bundle; DSI, diffusion spectrum imaging; DTI, diffusion tensor imaging; GQI, Generalized q-sampling imaging; HDFT, high definition fiber tracking; QA, quantitative anisotropy; ROA, Region of avoidance; ROI, region of interest.

It originates within the white matter of the temporal pole, runs posterior and superior into the parietal lobe, then turns, forming a "ring-like belt" around the CC, into the frontal lobe, terminates anterior and inferior to the genu of the CC in the orbital-frontal cortex (Agrawal et al., 2011). Numerous studies have demonstrated that the CB is involved in core processes such as executive function, decision-making, and emotion processing (Heilbronner and Haber, 2014; Adnan et al., 2016).

In 1995, based on cytoarchitectural and receptor architecture work, Vogt et al. (1995) suggested that the cingulate cortex might be subdivided into the anterior, mid, posterior and retrosplenial cortices (ACC, MCC, PCC and RSC, respectively). The ACC is characterized by neurons expressing high levels of dopamine D1 receptors, projecting to brainstem motor systems, and which is believed to be predominantly involved in emotion and autonomic regulation (Benes, 1998; Haznedar et al., 2004). The MCC has neurons projecting to the spinal cord, which play an important role in emotional processing and visceral control (Vogt, 2016). The PCC contains large numbers of neurofilament protein-containing neurons, connecting with the parietal lobe, that monitor eye movements and respond to sensory stimuli (Vogt et al., 1992). The RSC is mainly formed by neurons receiving input from the amygdala and is known to be involved in cognitive function (Vogt and Laureys, 2005). Thus, the traditional segmentation of the CB into anterior, middle, and posterior portions (Concha et al., 2005; Jang et al., 2013), has been widely suggested by studies of functional imaging, electrical stimulation, as well as some patient studies. The anterior portion is predominantly known to be involved in executive function, decision-making, and emotion (Catheline et al., 2010; Tuladhar et al., 2015). The middle portion participates in the execution of motor- and attention-related tasks (Lin et al., 2014). The posterior region is related to cognitive function (Choo et al., 2010; Sexton et al., 2011).

In the last decade, with the rapid development of the diffusion tensor imaging (DTI) technique, we have the opportunity to study the CB *in vivo*. Based on DTI tractography, some studies have revealed that the CB is a complex network structure, containing not only long fibers that potentially extend to the frontal and temporal lobes, but also short association fibers connecting adjacent cortices (Catani and Thiebaut de Schotten, 2008; Lawes et al., 2008). According to the segmentation in the anterior-middle-posterior direction, the CB resembles an uninterrupted and continuous band, regardless the presence of numerous short association fibers. Moreover, the traditional segmentations, noted above, do not adequately explain how the functional subcomponents of the CB system connect to the different cortical and subcortical regions, which performs as a "multi-task bundle" (Jones et al., 2013; Heilbronner and Haber, 2014; Sethi et al., 2015).

Although DTI tractography has provided us with a new version of the CB, there are several technical limitations, for instance, inability to map fiber endings of the CB before contacting the cortical mantle, failure to solve fiber crossings and to follow bundles within the CB, and excessive false fiber continuity generating pseudotracts (Fernandez-Miranda, 2013; Fernández-Miranda et al., 2015). Fortunately, all these DTI problems above can be addressed by some emerging fiber mapping techniques such as high-angular-resolution diffusion imaging (HARDI) and diffusion spectrum imaging (DSI). HARDI has better angular resolution and smaller voxels (Jansons and Alexander, 2003), while DSI is essentially a model-free imaging approach that has the ability to map complex fiber architecture at the scale of single MRI voxels (Wedeen et al., 2005). Recently, a novel combination of processing, reconstruction, and tractography methods called high definition fiber tracking (HDFT) has been developed (Fernandez-Miranda et al., 2012). It employs DSI reconstructed by generalized q-sampling imaging (GQI) as a high angular resolution based approach (DSI for acquisition, GQI for estimation of fiber orientation) that leverages high directional sampling of diffusion imaging space to get better resolution of underlying white matter geometry for tractography (Yeh et al., 2010). Studies have been shown that the HDFT provides accurate replication of complex known neuroanatomical features where DTI failed (Wang et al., 2013; Fernández-Miranda et al., 2015; Wu et al., 2016).

Traditionally, experimental observations in non-human primates that employ axonal tracing are considered as the "gold standard" for guiding human white matter connective patterns (Schmahmann and Pandya, 2006; Thiebaut de Schotten et al., 2012). Mufson and Pandya (1984) found three distinct fiber components of the CB in the rhesus monkey using an autoradiographic tracer technique. Subsequently, experiments in monkeys revealed both the afferent and efferent fibers that occupied specific parts in the CB system, connecting various cortical and subcortical regions (Vogt and Pandya, 1987; Kobayashi and Amaral, 2007). Evidence has accumulated suggesting that the human CB may exhibit a similar segmentation regarding corticocortical connections. Jones et al. (2013) tested the validity of dividing the CB into three subdivisions corresponding to the "para-hippocampal", "retrosplenial", and "subgenual" portions based on DTI tractography, which provided a rough framework for the possibility of subdividing the CB, although further confirmation was necessary. In the living humans, the autoradiography tract tracing is inapplicable. Although it is not possible to use autoradiographical tracing in living humans, fiber dissection in post-mortem brains has been widely employed to cross-validate *in vivo* fiber tracking results. To date, however, there have been no studies employing such strategies.

In this study, we mapped the CB in the human using HDFT. Tractography of the CB were performed using both a subject-specific approach (10 subjects) and a template approach (Human Connectome Project, HCP-488). Complemented anatomical fiber dissections were also carried out to confirm the *in vivo* fiber tracking findings. Our study provided a more accurate and detailed description on the associated architecture of the subcomponents within the CB, contributing a comprehensive morphological basis for further functional studies.

MATERIALS AND METHODS

Participants

Ten neurologically healthy volunteers (3 males, 7 females; all right handed; age range: 20–40 years; mean age, 33.5 years) participated in the experiment between September 2013 and October 2014 at the First Affiliated Hospital of China Medical University. All participants were prescreened prior to scanning to rule out any contraindications to MRI. This study was approved by the Ethics Committee of the First Affiliated Hospital of China Medical University (permit number AF-SOP-07-1, 0-01), and carried out in accordance with the Declaration of Helsinki. Written informed consent was obtained from each participant.

Except for subject-specific analysis, we also conducted fiber tracking on a template of 488 subjects from the HCP-488, which represented the largest and highest quality data available to date. The HCP consortium led by Washington University, University of Minnesota, and Oxford University, is undertaking a systematic effort to map macroscopic human brain circuits and their relationship to behavior in a large population of healthy adults. A total of 500 subjects' data was released for the first three quarters (Q1–Q3, June 2014) and 488 subjects had diffusion scans (289 females, 199 males, average age 29.15, SD ± 3.47; Van Essen et al., 2013). The reconstructed data of the 488 subjects were averaged to create a representative template (HCP 488-subjects template is freely downloadable at: http://dsi-studio.labsolver.org/download-images).

Image Acquisition and Reconstruction

We used a 3-T Tim Trio System (Siemens) with a 32-channel head coil to acquire DSI data. This involved a 43-min, 257-direction scan using a twice-refocused spin-echo echo-planar imaging sequence and multiple q values (repetition time (TR) = 9.916 ms, echo time (TE) = 157 ms, voxel size = 2.4 × 2.4 × 2.4 mm, field of view (FoV) = 231 × 231 mm, b_{max} = 7000 s/mm^2; Wedeen et al., 2005, 2008). We also included the high-resolution anatomical imaging to be the anatomical comparisons, employing a 9-min T_1-weighted axial magnetization prepared rapid gradient echo (MPRAGE) sequence (TR = 2110 ms, TE = 2.63 ms, flip angle = 8°, 176 slices, FoV = 256 × 256 mm^2, voxel size = 0.5 × 0.5 × 1.0 mm^3; Wu et al., 2016). DSI data were reconstructed with a GQI approach (Yeh et al., 2010). The orientation distribution functions (ODFs) were reconstructed to 362 discrete sampling directions and a mean diffusion distance of 1.2 mm. ODF is a probabilistic density function on the two-dimensional (2D) surface of a sphere, that can be calculated from diffusion MRI signals. The local maximums in an ODF are often regarded as the axonal fiber orientations in deterministic fiber tracking, a method that calculates the axonal trajectories between cortical areas. DSI is a diffusion MRI q-space imaging method. It acquires diffusion signals with multiple b-values to calculate average propagator and the diffusion ODF. The diffusion encoding sampling scheme of DSI is arranged as grid points in the q-space and distinguishes itself from the common-used shell arrangement which is limited to single diffusion gradient strength. The multiple diffusion gradient strength design gives DSI better coverage on both fast and slow diffusion (Yeh et al., 2013).

The Human Connectome Project 488-Subject Template (HCP-488)

The 488 subjects underwent diffusion scans in a Siemens 3T Skyra scanner using a 2D spin-echo single-shot multiband EPI sequence with a multi-band factor of three and monopolar gradient pulse. The spatial resolution was 1.25 mm isotropic, TR = 5500 ms, TE = 89 ms. A multishell diffusion scheme was used. The b-values were 1000, 2000 and 3000 s/mm^2. The total number of diffusion sampling directions was 270. The total scanning time was around 55 min (Sotiropoulos et al., 2013; Van Essen et al., 2013). The diffusion data were conducted using a GQI approach.

White Matter Fiber Tracking

For the fiber-tracking datasets, all fiber tracking was performed using DSI Studio[1]. A whole brain seeding approach using multiple or a single region of interest (ROI) and region of avoidance (ROA) masks was performed. In voxels with multiple fiber orientations, fiber tracking was initiated separately for each orientation, and fiber progression continued with a step size of 1.2 mm, minimum fiber length of 20 mm, and turning angle threshold of 60° (Wang et al., 2013). If multiple fiber orientations existed in the current progression location, the fiber orientation that was nearest to the incoming direction and forms a turning angle smaller than 60° was selected to determine the next moving direction. To smooth each track, the next moving directional estimate of each voxel was weighted by 20% of the previous incoming direction and 80% of the nearest fiber orientation (Fernández-Miranda et al., 2015). This progression was repeated until the quantitative anisotropy (QA) of the fiber orientation dropped below a preset threshold (0.03–0.06 depending on the subject) or there was no fiber selected within the 60° angular range in the progression (Yeh et al., 2013). Once tracked, all streamlines were saved in the TrackVis file format. Segmentation of the CB was performed using DSI studio software. For comparison, FreeSurfer was used to segment cortical gyral ROIs using each participant's T1-weighted MPRAGE image (Desikan et al., 2006).

For the dorsal CB reconstruction, the ROI masks included the anterior, mid-anterior, mid-posterior, post-dorsal and post-ventral cingulate cortex (defined by the Automated Anatomical Labeling (Desikan et al., 2006); **Figure 1A**). If one label was selected to serve as seed region for the fiber-tracking algorithm, its neighboring mask was chosen for the subsequent ROI. Thus, this step repeated four times. Then, for the ventral CB, we used the methods described by Jones et al. (2013) in brief, two ROIs were placed behind and below the splenium. One ROA was placed above the body of the CC (**Figure 1B**).

[1] http://dsi-studio.labsolver.org

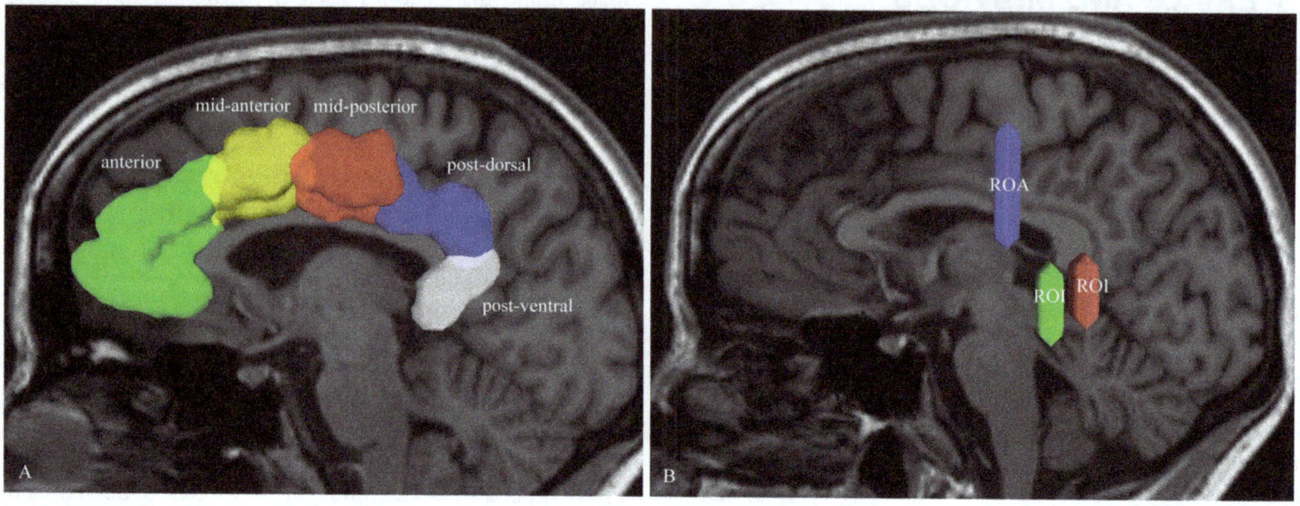

FIGURE 1 | *In vivo* fiber tractography of the cingulum bundle (CB). (A) The region of interests (ROIs) of the CB consist of five segments: anterior (green), mid-anterior (yellow color), mid-posterior (red color), post-dorsal (blue color) and post-ventral (white color) cingulate cortex. **(B)** Two ROIs and one region of avoidance (ROA) are used for reconstructing the para-hippocampal CB. The ROIs are placed behind and below the splenium. One ROA is placed above the body of the corpus callosum (CC). CB, cingulum bundle; ROI, region-of-interest; ROA, region of avoidance.

Fiber Dissection Technique

Eight hemispheres from four fresh specimens (age 38–77 years, 2 females, 2 males) were obtained from the Department of Anatomy of the First Affiliated Hospital of China Medical University. All the legal representatives signed the informed consent. The operations were approved by the Ethics Committee of the First Affiliated Hospital of China Medical University (permit number AF-SOP-07-1, 0-01). Postmortem fiber dissection was performed according to the technique originally described by Professor Josef Klingler (Ludwig and Klingler, 1965; Agrawal et al., 2011). The specimens were fixed in 10% formalin solution for four additional weeks, then frozen at −15°C for 15 days after removal of vessels, arachnoid and pia-matter. The water crystallization induced by the freezing process disrupts the structure of the gray matter (with high water content), enabling us to peel off the cortex from the brain surface. The freezing process also spreads along the white matter fibers, facilitating the dissection of

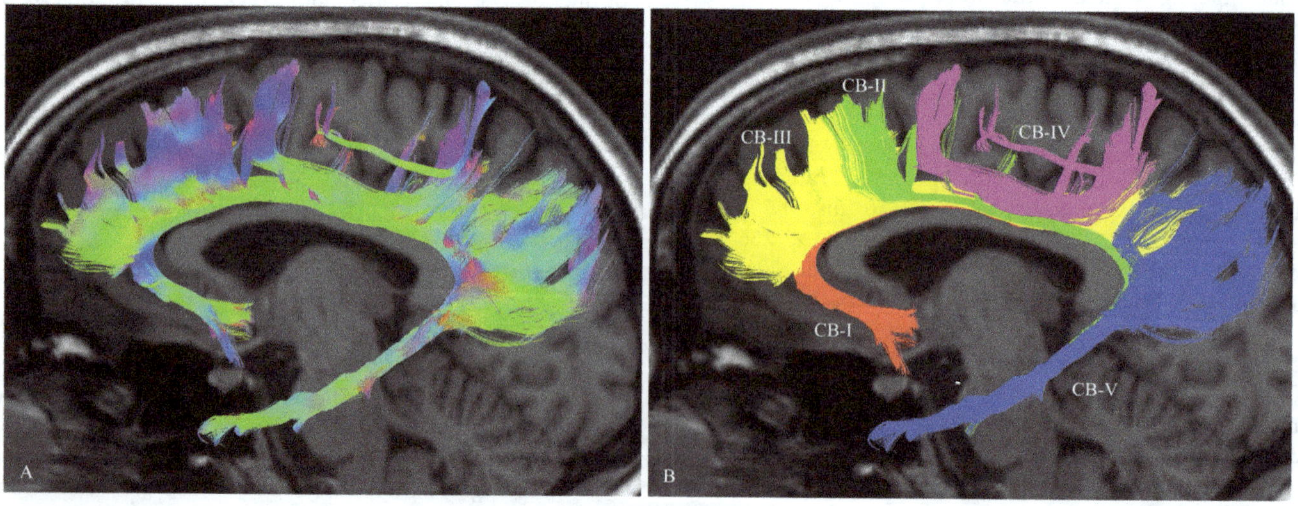

FIGURE 2 | *In vivo* fiber tractography of the CB and five potential subcomponents in the CB (subject-8, left). (A) Sagittal view of the left CB. The CB exhibits a sickle-shaped association bundle that nearly encircled the CC and extends to the temporal lobe. **(B)** Defining the subgenual areas, medial aspect of the superior frontal gyrus (SFG), precuneus, splenium and para-hippocampal gyrus as the cortex landmarks to do back-tracing for the subdivision (defined by the Automated Anatomical Labeling (Desikan et al., 2006)). Five subcomponents are identified (CB-I, red color; CB-II, green color; CB-III, yellow color; CB-IV, purple color; CB-V, blue color).

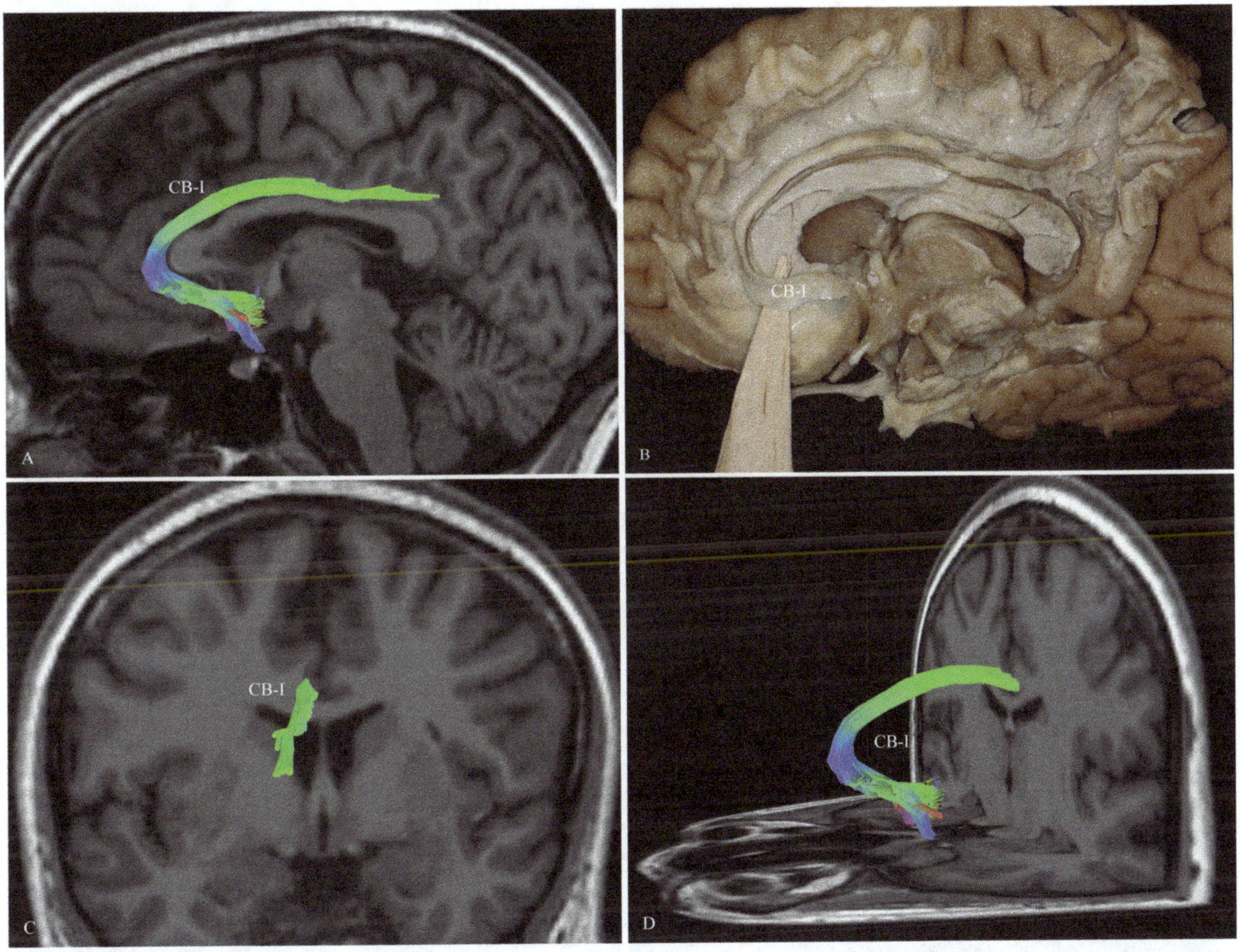

FIGURE 3 | *In vivo* fiber tractography and fiber dissection of the CB-I. (A,B) The CB-I runs from the subrostral areas in the orbital-frontal cortex anteriorly, then arches through almost 180° around the genu of the CC. **(C,D)** After that, the fibers continue above the body of the CC to the precuneus and splenium of the CC.

the fiber tracts (Martino et al., 2011). Subsequently, the specimens were washed under running water for several hours.

We performed the dissection of each specimen before the anatomy of the lateral, medial and the basal cerebral surface was carefully studied. Then, the white matter dissection was completed in a stepwise manner for the medial-to-lateral dissection process. Our dissection tools were handmade, thin, and wooden dissectors, various sized anatomic forceps. Digital images were acquired during the course of dissection. The first step of dissection was removing the cortex within the depth of the sulci, with preservation of the cortex of the hemispheres surface of the gyri. Then the short associational U shaped fibers (also known as intergyral or arcuate fibers), which interconnected neighboring gyri at the subgyral sector, were exposed. After cutting off the U fibers, the deep CB white matter was exposed. The Atlas of the fiber pathways of the brain (Schmahmann and Pandya, 2006) was used to identify and define the specific cortical connections.

We undertook the fiber dissection studies at the Surgical Neuroanatomy Lab of the China Medical University with the aid of microsurgical instrumentation and surgical microscope (6–40 magnification, Carl Zeiss, OPMI CS-NC).

RESULTS

Trajectory of the CB in the Human Brain

Subject-Specific Tractography Findings

In the fiber tractography study, the CB exhibited a sickle-shaped association bundle that nearly encircled the CC and extended to the temporal lobe. Five potential subcomponents were identified (**Figure 2**).

The CB-I ran from the orbital-frontal cortex, arched around the genu of the CC, then connected with the precuneus and splenium (**Figure 3**). Both the CB-II and the

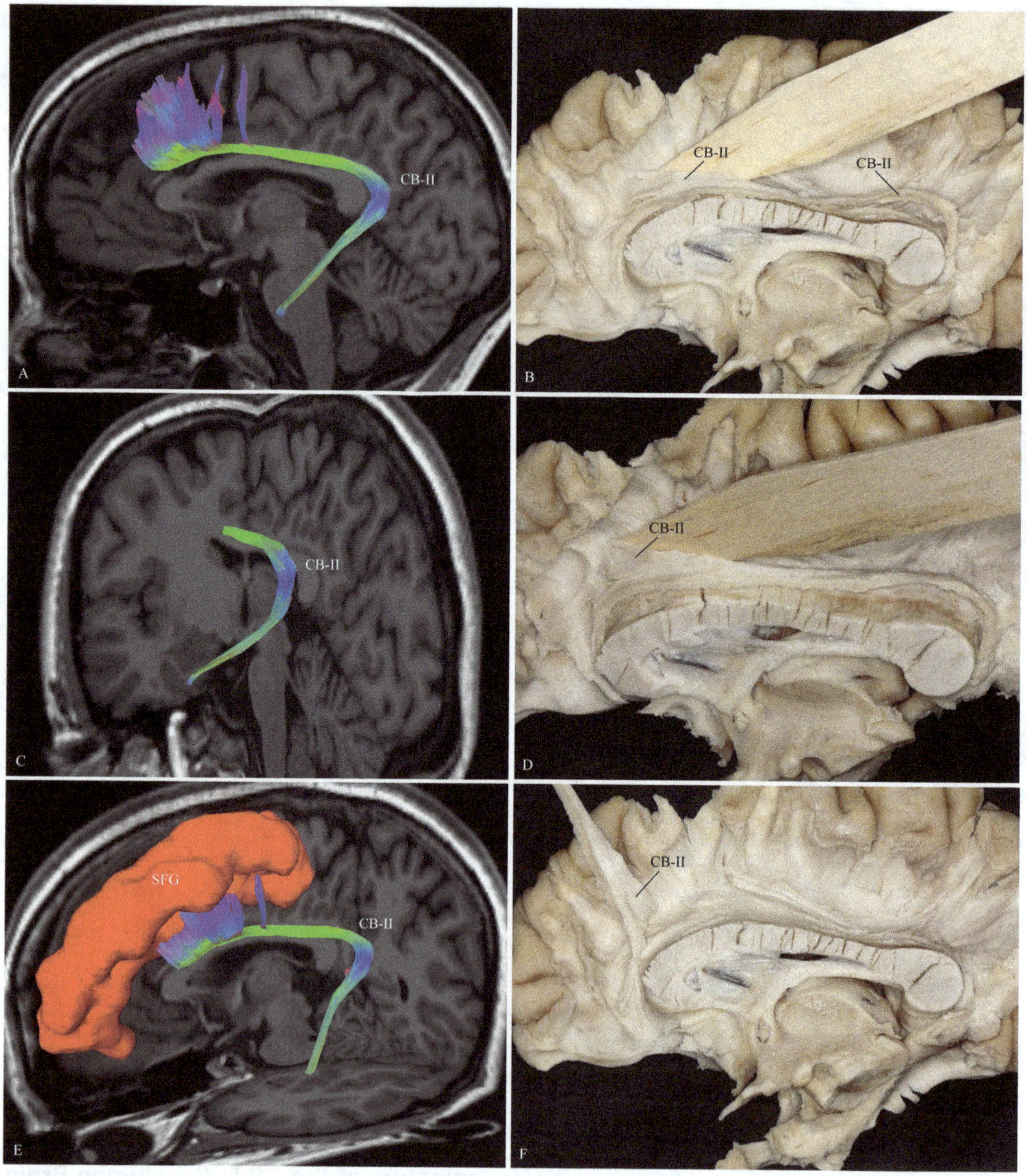

FIGURE 4 | *In vivo* fiber tractography and fiber dissection of the CB-II. (A–C) The CB-II originates from the para-hippocampal gyrus, arches around the splenium, then extends longitudinally above the CC. **(D–F)** The fibers continue anteriorly, lastly connect with the medial aspect of the SFG. SFG, superior frontal gyrus.

CB-V stemmed from the para-hippocampal gyrus. The CB-II associated with the medial aspect of the superior frontal gyrus (SFG; **Figure 4**), while the CB-V fanned out to the parietal and occipital lobes (**Figure 7**). The CB-III was the largest of the fiber bundles in the CB system and was identified in all hemispheres. These fibers originated from the

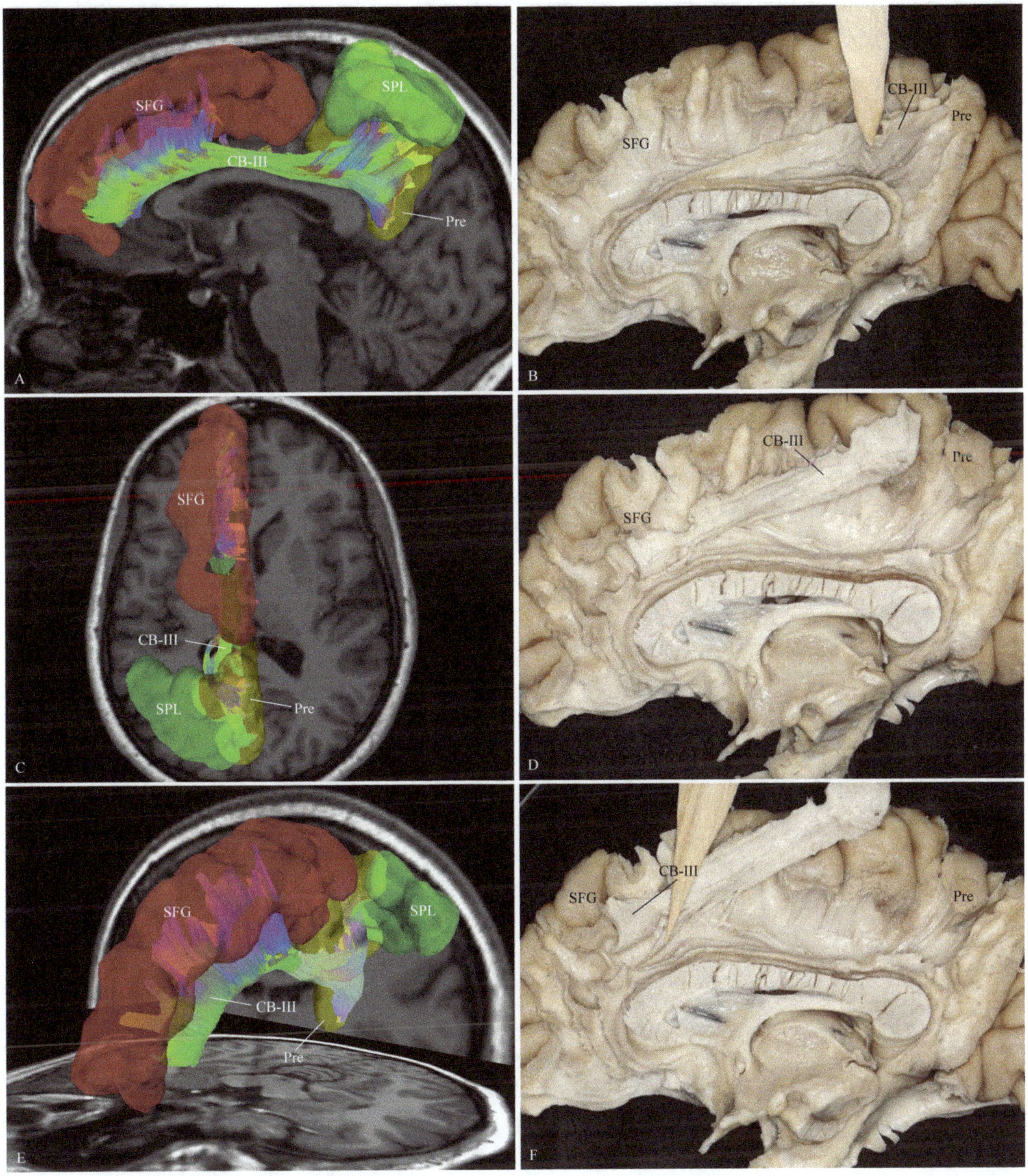

FIGURE 5 | *In vivo* fiber tractography and fiber dissection of the CB-III. (A–D) The CB-III originates from the superior parietal lobule (SPL) and precuneus, then extends along the trunk of the CC. **(E,F)** Finally, the fibers associate with the anterior and middle parts of the medial aspect of the SFG. SFG, superior frontal gyrus; SPL, superior parietal lobule; Pre, precuneus.

precuneus and terminated at the medial aspect of the SFG (**Figure 5**). The CB-IV ran in two different patterns, the para-cingulate (para-CB) and the supra-cingulate (sup-CB; **Figure 6**). Further detailed analysis showed that left and right CB had a similar location, shape and trajectory in all 20 hemispheres (**Figure 8**).

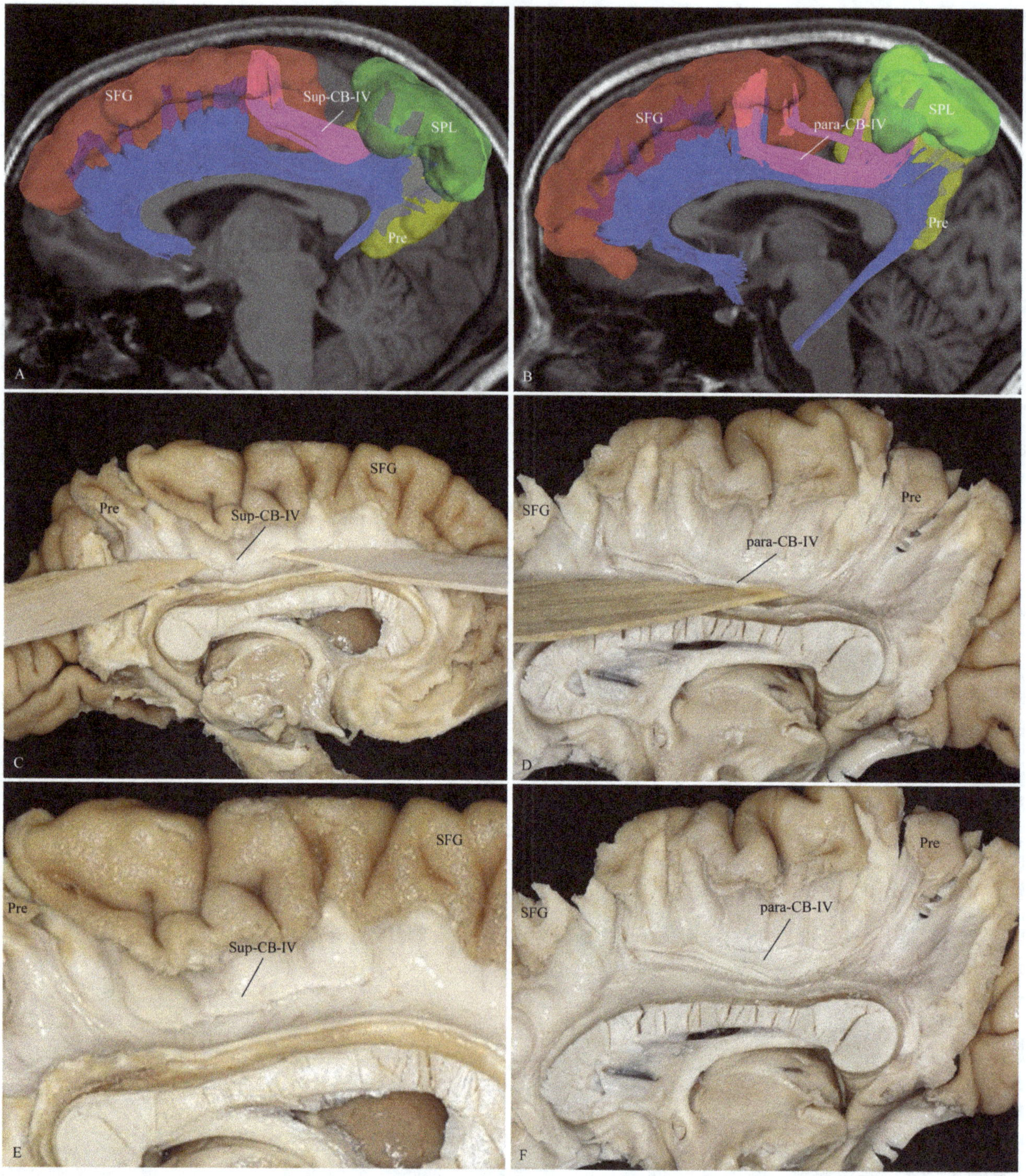

FIGURE 6 | ***In vivo*** **fiber tractography and fiber microdissection of the CB-IV.** The CB-IV is a short and minor tract that connects the SPL and precuneus with the supplementary and premotor areas. **(A,C,E)** The CB-IV (purple color) can be defined as supra-cingulate location with the other segments (blue color). **(B,D,F)** The CB-IV (purple color) can be defined as a para-cingulate location with the other segments (blue color). SFG, superior frontal gyrus; SPL, superior parietal lobule; Pre, precuneus.

Template Tractography Findings

Analysis of the HCP-488 template showed similar results to the sample subject findings above (**Figure 9**).

Fiber Dissection Findings

We first exposed the fibers originating from the precuneus that accounted for the largest part in the CB. These fibers

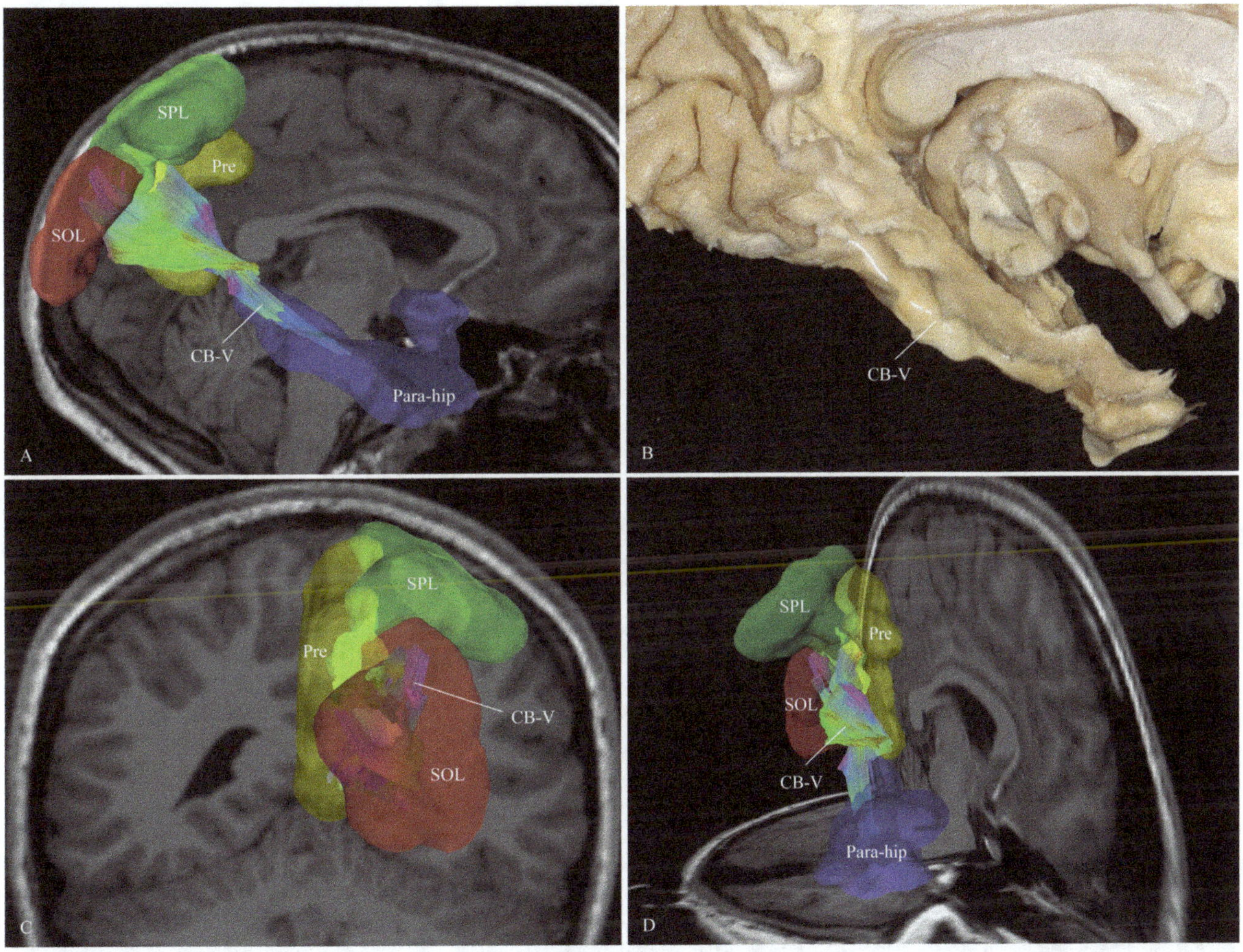

FIGURE 7 | *In vivo* fiber tractography and fiber microdissection of the CB-V. (A,B) The CB-V extends along the para-hippocampal gyrus, **(C,D)** then fans out to the parietal and occipital lobes. The scattered fibers in the parietal and occipital lobes are failed to be identified in fiber dissection. Para-hip, para-hippocampal gyrus; SPL, superior parietal lobule; Pre, precuneus; SOL, superior occipital lobule.

originated from the precuneus, ran just above the CC and terminated at the medial aspect of the SFG (**Figure 5**). Then these fibers were removed, and the dissection was continued anteriorly. We identified two groups of fibers in the front area. One was connected to the medial aspect of the SFG, while the other arched inferiorly almost 180° around the front of the genu of the CC and ended in the subcallosal gyrus and the paraterminal gyrus (**Figures 3, 4**). Both bodies of these two groups of fibers encircled the CC and extended posteriorly to the splenium. Thereafter, we identified the fibers that connected the precuneus with the supplementary and premotor areas. The two different patterns (para-CB and sup-CB) were both found in the two cerebral hemispheres (**Figure 6**).

The last step was to expose the para-hippocampal subdivision. After peeling off the gray matter of the para-hippocampal gyrus, we identified the fibers forward to the anterior para-hippocampal region. We made all efforts to expose the portion that fanned out to the occipital lobes. However, we could not identify these scattered fibers in this multiple fiber-crossing area, which may have been due to the quality of the specimens or the limitations of the fiber dissection technique (**Figure 7**).

It was hard to reveal all the subdivisions and identify the whole connections of the subcomponents in one hemisphere. For this, we showed two different hemispheres (one right and one left) for the step-by-step fiber dissection (**Figure 10**).

Spatial Relationship of the Subcomponents of the CB

A complete schematic map of the five segments was shown in **Figure 11A**. On representative T_1 sections, the CB-I was the lowest and was the closest to the midline in the subcomponents (**Figure 11B**). The CB-II extended along the bottom of the CB-III, more medial than the CB-V (**Figure 11B**).

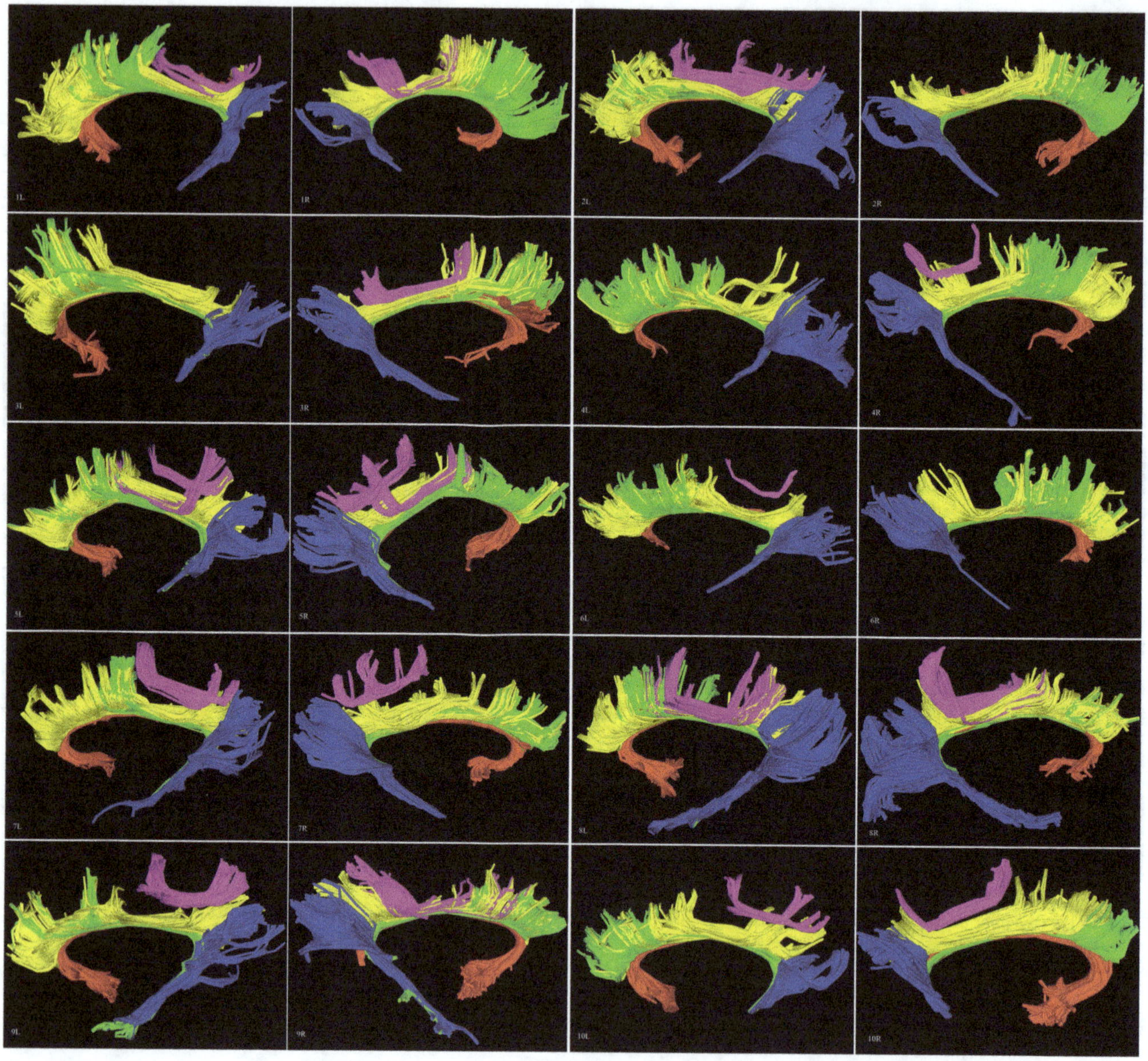

FIGURE 8 | Diffusion spectrum imaging (DSI) tractography of the CB in 20 hemispheres of 10 subjects on sagittal view. Order: subject 1, 2, 3, 4, 5, 6, 7, 8, 9, 10. Left and right CB had a similar location, shape and trajectory in all 20 hemispheres. The CB-IV can be delineated in 16 out of 20 hemispheres. On further analysis of all subjects, the CB-IV is parallel and adjacent to the others in 7 out of 16 hemispheres. In the remaining nine hemispheres, the CB-IV is located above the others in a sup-CB pattern. Red color, CB-I; green color, CB-II; yellow color, CB-III; purple color, CB-IV; blue color, CB-V; L, left; R, right.

The CB-IV was situated superficially lateral to the CB-III (**Figure 11C**). The CB-V was situated slightly more lateral (**Figure 11B**).

DISCUSSION

In the present study, we investigated the trajectory, associated architecture and anatomical connectivity of the CB in 10 subjects and a template of 488 subjects using HDFT. Compared to previous DTI reports, our study not only presented architectures of the CB with significantly higher resolution, but also demonstrated a more complete connectivity pattern of the CB. In addition, we also investigated whether there were discernible structural subdivisions in the CB based on white matter corticocortical connections. We found that there were five potentially different subcomponents within the CB, which were completely attained in both the small independent sample ($n = 10$) as well as the larger template sample ($n = 488$). The findings of fiber dissection were consistent with that of *in vivo* tractography.

The CB was originally described by Vicq d'Azyr in 1786 as one of the more complex white matter tracts in the human

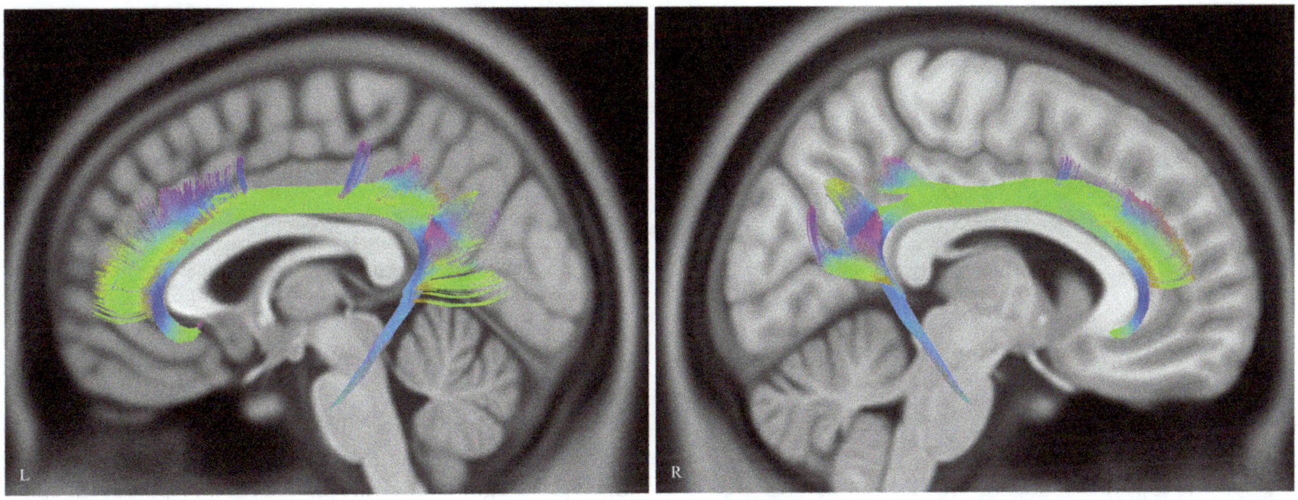

FIGURE 9 | *In vivo* fiber tractography of the CB on Human Connectome Project (HCP-488) template. CB, cingulum bundle; L, left; R, right.

brain. As the CB runs through a large extent of the brain, it had been reported that any changes in specific subregions of the CB probably resulted in different functional disorders (Jang et al., 2013). Previously, it had been widely accepted that the CB was segmented into anterior-posterior-inferior portions. However, in some autoradiographic tracing studies of the rhesus monkeys, three distinct fiber components of the CB were found. They were segmented as the connections of different cortical and subcortical regions (Mufson and Pandya, 1984). In other animal studies, both the afferent or efferent fibers were reported to occupy specific parts of the CB, connecting various cortical and subcortical regions (Vogt and Pandya, 1987; Kobayashi and Amaral, 2007). Therefore, we hypothesized that the CB system in humans might show similar corticocortical segmentation patterns. Recently, a DTI study in 20 healthy humans suggested that the CB could be subdivided into three different components (Jones et al., 2013). However, these findings needed independent confirmation at both the neuroimaging and neuroanatomical whole-brain level.

In this study, we reconstructed the CB based on the cortical ROIs defined by the Automated Anatomical Labeling (Desikan et al., 2006). The anatomic subregions are automatically generated in light of individuality which are viewed as ideal for generating tracts. After reconstructing the whole bundle, we traced back the fibers according to the cortex landmarks. Furthermore, HDFT, a high-angular-resolution-based approach employing DSI reconstructed by GQI, has been proven to be able to allow tracing from one cortical region to other cortical or subcortical regions through complex crossings areas, providing detailed evidence of the cortical site of origin or termination of the fibers without the need for approximation (Fernandez-Miranda, 2013; Fernández-Miranda et al., 2015; Wu et al., 2016). In addition, our diffusion imaging technique involves a 43 min, 176 slices and 257-direction scan, as compared with the 26 min, 60 slices and 60-direction scan used by Jones et al. (2013). All of the above are the main advantages that keep our results accurate and convincing.

On the other hand, rather than tractography results, fiber dissections can provide a more intuitive observation to represent valuable information on the anatomy of the fiber tracts. To our knowledge, it is for the first time that the complex composition of the CB is assessed in detail by fiber dissection. The two methods (tractography and fiber dissection) cross-validated here, increase the confidence that our result is not an artifact and provides a stronger support for the described connectivity of the tracing fiber than when either of the method was used alone.

Our tractographic and anatomic results suggest that the CB is not a single pathway, but rather a composition of five distinct subcomponents of white matter at different levels. We assume that each subcomponent not only contributes to the formation of a CB fiber system, but also retains its own characteristics. According to its interconnected cortical regions, we provided a detailed analysis of each subcomponent in the CB. We also described the potential role of these distinct subdivisions based on cross-species studies of monkey fiber connections, fiber trajectories from our observations and lesion-deficit correlative analysis in the human brain.

CB-I

The subgenual cingulate region (Brodmann area 25) and the orbital frontal (area 11) were suggested to play a critical role in modulating negative mood states (Seminowicz et al., 2004). In fact, previous monkey tract tracing studies showed that the connections from the orbital cortex formed at a distinct network within cingulate limbic structures (Carmichael and Price, 1995, 1996). Combining the polarized light imaging (PLI) and the macroscopical fiber dissection in the human brain, Axer et al. (2011) reported that, after running above the CC, the pregenual part of the CB curved around the genu, and then spread into the orbitofrontal white matter. All of

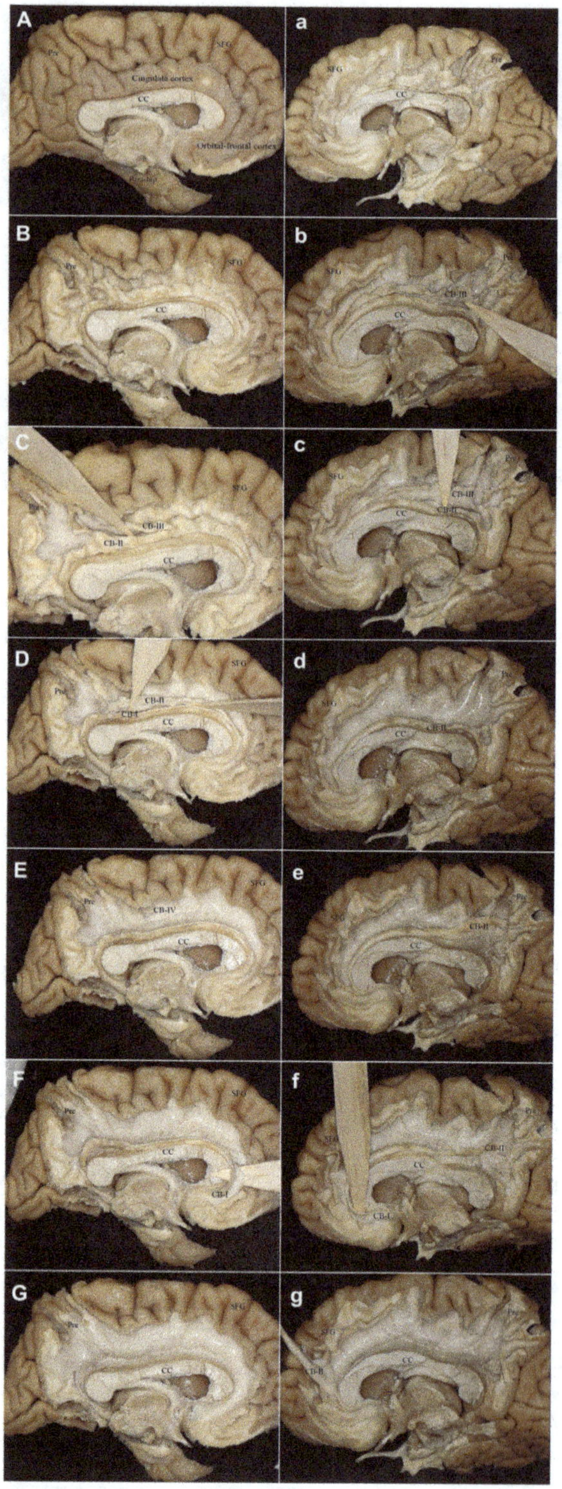

FIGURE 10 | Step-by-step fiber dissection of the CB (one left hemisphere and one right hemisphere). (A) Medial surface of the left hemisphere after removing of vessels, arachnoid and pia-matter. **(B)** Removing the cortex within the depth of the sulci only, with preservation of the cortex of the hemispheres surface of the gyri. **(C)** Identifying the CB-III fibers that originate from the precuneus and extend above the CC. **(D)** Separating *(Continued)*

FIGURE 10 | Continued
the fibers of the CB-I and CB-II above the CC. **(E)** After peeling off the CB-I, CB-II and CB-III, the supra-cingulate CB-IV can be visualized. **(F)** Identifying the CB-I fibers that originate from the subrostral areas. **(G)** Peeling off all the subcomponents. **(a)** Removing the cortex within the depth of the sulci only, with preservation of the cortex of the hemispheres surface of the gyri. **(b,c)** Separating the fibers of the CB-III and CB-II above the CC. **(d)** After peeling off the CB-III. **(e)** The body fibers of the CB-I and CB-II encircles above the CC (It is hard to separate them). **(f)** Identifying the CB-I fibers that originate from the subrostral areas. **(g)** The CB-II connects with the medial aspect of the SFG. Para-hip, para-hippocampal gyrus; Pre, precuneus; SFG, superior frontal gyrus; CC, corpus callosum.

the above are consistent with our descriptions of the CB-I (**Figure 3**).

The functional role of the CB-I remains to be ascertained. Several studies revealed that activation of the perigenual cortex and PCC might participate in affective responses to noxious stimuli (Ballantine et al., 1967; Casey et al., 1994; Vogt et al., 1996). Using electrical stimulation of the subgenual cingulate white matter on six patients, Mayberg et al. (2005) suggested that disrupting focal pathological activity in limbic-cortical circuits could effectively reverse symptoms in otherwise treatment-resistant depression. The functional imaging study found that the fiber microstructural integrity connecting the genu and splenium showed the highest significant relationship with global cognitive function and verbal memory performance (Tuladhar et al., 2015).

CB-II

Previous anatomical studies of monkeys have confirmed a long fiber component connecting with medial temporal and cingulate limbic structures, named as the "medial" network (Kondo et al., 2003). This system originates from the retrosplenial, para-hippocampal, and perirhinal cortices, extends above the CC, then ends in the medial frontal cortex (Saleem et al., 2008). The monkey "medial" network is similar to our CB-II observations in the human brain (**Figure 4**).

Path integration uses constant updation of the navigator's representation of position and orientation during movement without using landmarks, and often involves tracking a start or home location (Byrne et al., 2007). Using a novel loop closure task in 31 participants, Chrastil et al. (2015) found that the hippocampus, RSC, para-hippocampal cortex and medial prefrontal cortex (mPFC) were recruited during successful path integration. Interestingly, in our results, the course of fiber tractography of the CB-II associates with all these brain regions, suggests a potential role of the CB-II in supporting path integration.

CB-III

Our observations suggest that the CB-III is situated within the white matter of the superior parietal lobule (SPL) (area 7), the precuneus (medial area 7), the medial part of SFG (areas 8, 9 and 32) and the supplementary motor area (area 6; **Figure 5**). There is a close spatial relationship between

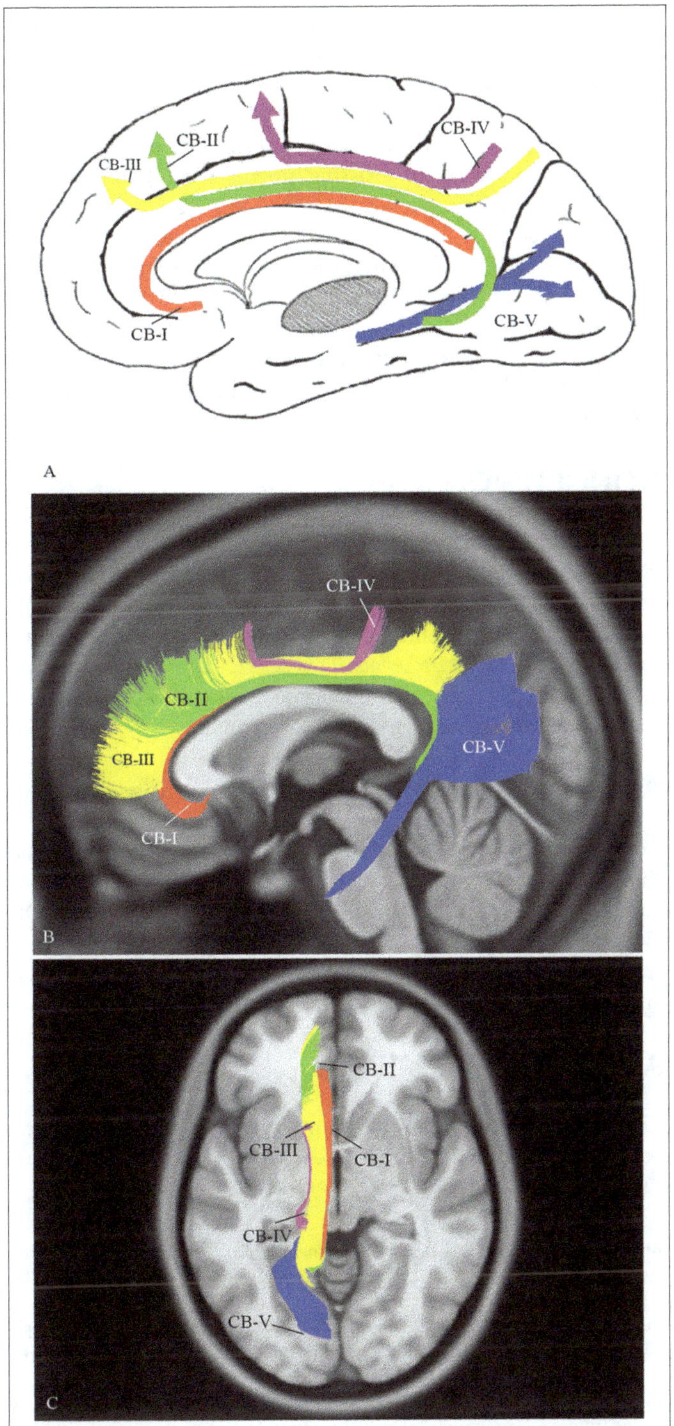

FIGURE 11 | Spatial Relationship of the subcomponents on HCP-488 template. (A) A complete schematic map of the five segments. **(B)** Depicting five segments of CB on the HCP-488 template T_1 sagittal view. The CB-I snugly curves around the genu of the CC and spreads into the orbital-frontal cortex as the lowest subdivision. For the projective scope in the medial aspect of the SFG, the CB-III is obviously larger than that of the CB-II. The body section of the CB-II extends along the bottom of the CB-III, while the caudal section is slightly more medial than the CB-V, despite their overlaps. **(C)** Axial view. The CB-I is closest to the midline in all the segments. The CB-IV is the smallest fiber tract in the CB system. It is situated superficially lateral to the CB-III.

the CB-III and the CB-II, however, the CB-III is clearly discernible from the CB as a distinctive subcomponent in our tractography analysis (**Figure 11**). The observations shown in post-mortem also correspond to the DSI results. But, it is not feasible for us to extrapolate a similar connection with the monkey experimental material. The evolution of neurocranial morphology in *Homo sapiens* is characterized by bulging of the parietal region, a feature unique to our species. Comparisons between human brains and macaque brains have shown that there are species-specific differences in the parietal cortex, such as the structural and functional connections of the intraparietal sulcal cortex (Orban et al., 2006; Scheperjans et al., 2008). Moreover, similar comparative neuroanatomical and paleontological evidence has suggested that precuneus expansion is also a neurological specialization of *Homo sapiens* (Bruner et al., 2016).

The CB-III is the largest-volume tract in the CB system. Given its multiple interconnected cortical regions and evolutional variation in brain shape among humans, we speculate that the CB-III may be the most significant part of the multi-functional CB tract, which is associated with the recent human cognitive specializations. This proposition can be supported by some functional studies. For example, white matter connectivity between the pre-SMA and the CB was associated with response conflict in healthy human subjects (Yamamoto et al., 2015). Huang et al. (2013, 2014) also found that the microstructural integrity of the white matter connecting the anterior cingulate area to the precuneus and medial superior frontal areas reflected the level of neurophysiologic dependence in tobacco withdrawal syndrome. Furthermore, several studies have proved that performance in attention-demanding cognitive tasks was related to the neural structure connecting the PCC, medial and lateral parietal cortex, and the mPFC (Raichle et al., 2001; McKiernan et al., 2003; Fox et al., 2005).

CB-IV

The CB-IV is the shortest subdivision in the CB system that connects the superior parietal lobe (area 7) and precuneus (medial area 7) with the supplementary and premotor areas (areas 8, 9 and 32). We identified both para-cingulate (para-CB) and supra-cingulate (supra-CB) patterns in fiber dissection and DSI tractography (**Figure 6**). Interestingly, the CB-IV connection is similar to the previously described superior longitudinal fasciculus I (SLF-I). Kamali et al. (2014a) assessed the trajectory and connections of the SLF-I in five subjects based on DTI technique. They described that the SLF-I located closely with the CB, which could be distinguished from the adjacent CB clearly. Another study by Jang and Hong (2012) yielded similar results, though they only reconstructed the SLF-I using the cortical ROIs without evaluating the role of CB. As previous studies have revealed that some fibers of the CB originated from the SPL and precuneus to the frontal region, our results showed that it was difficult to separate the SLF-I from the CB, especially in the para-CB location. Thus, we speculated that few fibers of the CB had been somewhat assigned to the SLF-I artificially in previous

DTI studies (Thiebaut de Schotten et al., 2011; Kamali et al., 2014a,b).

Recently, as its anatomical location was much closer to the cingulum fiber system (adjacent or just above) than to the superior longitudinal fascicle, Wang et al. (2016) suggested that this fiber bundle should be considered as part of the CB system rather than the SLF system. However, they failed to verify this assumption in fiber dissection. Our results provide important visible evidence to support this hypothesis for the first time.

CB-V

In the past decades, neuroscientists have gained insight into the anatomy of the para-hippocampal cingulum (CB-V) in humans based on tractographic and fiber anatomical studies (Fernández-Miranda et al., 2008; Jones et al., 2013). Similar connections have been found in non-human primates (Pandya et al., 1981; Kobayashi and Amaral, 2007). In agreement with previous studies of the para-hippocampal cingulum, we found a tract running from the medial temporal lobe to the parietal and occipital lobes (**Figure 7**; Sethi et al., 2015). Compared to previous reports, our results showed several important anatomical characteristics of the CB-V. First, the CB-V is situated slightly more lateral than the other subdivisions. Second, although the CB-V runs side-by-side with the CB-III, it extends further forward within the medial temporal lobe than the CB-III (**Figure 11**).

The para-hippocampal cingulum white matter connections are a target of DTI studies for early diagnosis in AD (Wisse et al., 2015). It is possible that the brain regions associated with the CB-V are the earliest to exhibit neuronal degeneration. Killiany et al. (2002) reported that the entorhinal cortex displayed early degeneration in AD patients, while the extent of hippocampal atrophy influenced episodic memory performance in AD (Ezzati et al., 2015). A relationship between para-hippocampal cingulum integrity and the decline in various domains of cognitive function, such as spatial navigation and attention-shifting tasks, was also observed in AD patients (Lin et al., 2014). For this, we assume that the CB-V constitutes a "control" pathway supporting memory, executive function and other cognitive functions (Buckner, 2004; Seeley et al., 2007).

There are several limitations in our study. First although fiber dissection can provide key macroscopic information on fiber tract anatomy, it has limited value for the study of white matter connectivity in areas of crossing fibers. Second, the subject-specific approach is performed in only 10 subjects, whereas the HCP-488 template represents an averaged map. More subjects are required to provide a more detailed understanding of CB pathway variability in the human brain, including the effects of gender and age. Nevertheless, our findings open up a new perspective for subdividing the CB, higher resolution tractography or other methods maybe uncover further dissociations in future.

CONCLUSION

Using fiber dissection and HDFT tractography, our study identified the whole CB and its five subcomponents in the human brain for the first time. Our findings provide clear evidence that the CB is not a single entity, but rather a composition of distinct subdivisions at different levels. This segmentation of the CB will offer new insights into the associated structural-functional and anatomical-clinical changes in the CB system.

AUTHOR CONTRIBUTIONS

Conceived and designed the experiments: YuW and YiW. Performed the experiments: YuW, YiW and YoW. Analyzed the data and image processing: YuW and DS. Collected the biopsy samples: YiW and YoW. Contributed reagents/materials/analyses tools: SO and YiW. Wrote the article and revised the manuscript: YuW, SO and YiW.

ACKNOWLEDGMENTS

This study was supported by grants from the National Natural Science Foundation of China (No.31540077 to Dr. YiW).

REFERENCES

Adnan, A., Barnett, A., Moayedi, M., McCormick, C., Cohn, M., and McAndrews, M. P. (2016). Distinct hippocampal functional networks revealed by tractography-based parcellation. *Brain Struct. Funct.* 221, 2999–3012. doi: 10.1007/s00429-015-1084-x

Agrawal, A., Kapfhammer, J. P., Kress, A., Wichers, H., Deep, A., Feindel, W., et al. (2011). Josef Klingler's models of white matter tracts: influences on neuroanatomy, neurosurgery and neuroimaging. *Neurosurgery* 69, 238–252; discussion 252–234. doi: 10.1227/NEU.0b013e318214ab79

Axer, H., Beck, S., Axer, M., Schuchardt, F., Heepe, J., Flucken, A., et al. (2011). Microstructural analysis of human white matter architecture using polarized light imaging: views from neuroanatomy. *Front. Neuroinform.* 5:28. doi: 10.3389/fninf.2011.00028

Ballantine, H. T. Jr. Cassidy, W. L., Flanagan, N. B., and Marino, R. Jr., (1967). Stereotaxic anterior cingulotomy for neuropsychiatric illness and intractable pain. *J. Neurosurg.* 26, 488–495. doi: 10.3171/jns.1967.26.5.0488

Benes, F. M. (1998). Model generation and testing to probe neural circuitry in the cingulate cortex of postmortem schizophrenic brain. *Schizophr. Bull.* 24, 219–230. doi: 10.1093/oxfordjournals.schbul.a033322

Bruner, E., Preuss, T. M., Chen, X., and Rilling, J. K. (2016). Evidence for expansion of the precuneus in human evolution. *Brain Struct. Funct.* doi: 10.1007/s00429-015-1172-y [Epub ahead of print].

Buckner, R. L. (2004). Memory and executive function in aging and AD: multiple factors that cause decline and reserve factors that compensate. *Neuron* 44, 195–208. doi: 10.1016/j.neuron.2004.09.006

Byrne, P., Becker, S., and Burgess, N. (2007). Remembering the past and imagining the future: a neural model of spatial memory and imagery. *Psychol. Rev.* 114, 340–375. doi: 10.1037/0033-295x.114.2.340

Carmichael, S. T., and Price, J. L. (1995). Limbic connections of the orbital and medial prefrontal cortex in macaque monkeys. *J. Comp. Neurol.* 363, 615–641. doi: 10.1002/cne.903630408

Carmichael, S. T., and Price, J. L. (1996). Connectional networks within the orbital and medial prefrontal cortex of macaque monkeys. *J. Comp. Neurol.* 371, 179–207. doi: 10.1002/(SICI)1096-9861(19960722)371:2<179::AID-CNE1>3.0.CO;2-#

Casey, K. L., Minoshima, S., Berger, K. L., Koeppe, R. A., Morrow, T. J., and Frey, K. A. (1994). Positron emission tomographic analysis of cerebral structures activated specifically by repetitive noxious heat stimuli. *J. Neurophysiol.* 71, 802–807.

Catani, M., and Thiebaut de Schotten, M. (2008). A diffusion tensor imaging tractography atlas for virtual *in vivo* dissections. *Cortex* 44, 1105–1132. doi: 10.1016/j.cortex.2008.05.004

Catheline, G., Periot, O., Amirault, M., Braun, M., Dartigues, J. F., Auriacombe, S., et al. (2010). Distinctive alterations of the cingulum bundle during aging and Alzheimer's disease. *Neurobiol. Aging* 31, 1582–1592. doi: 10.1016/j.neurobiolaging.2008.08.012

Choo, I. H., Lee, D. Y., Oh, J. S., Lee, J. S., Lee, D. S., Song, I. C., et al. (2010). Posterior cingulate cortex atrophy and regional cingulum disruption in mild cognitive impairment and Alzheimer's disease. *Neurobiol. Aging* 31, 772–779. doi: 10.1016/j.neurobiolaging.2008.06.015

Chrastil, E. R., Sherrill, K. R., Hasselmo, M. E., and Stern, C. E. (2015). There and back again: hippocampus and retrosplenial cortex track homing distance during human path integration. *J. Neurosci.* 35, 15442–15452. doi: 10.1523/JNEUROSCI.1209-15.2015

Concha, L., Gross, D. W., and Beaulieu, C. (2005). Diffusion tensor tractography of the limbic system. *AJNR Am. J. Neuroradiol.* 26, 2267–2274.

Desikan, R. S., Segonne, F., Fischl, B., Quinn, B. T., Dickerson, B. C., Blacker, D., et al. (2006). An automated labeling system for subdividing the human cerebral cortex on MRI scans into gyral based regions of interest. *Neuroimage* 31, 968–980. doi: 10.1016/j.neuroimage.2006.01.021

Ezzati, A., Katz, M. J., Lipton, M. L., Zimmerman, M. E., and Lipton, R. B. (2015). Hippocampal volume and cingulum bundle fractional anisotropy are independently associated with verbal memory in older adults. *Brain Imaging Behav.* doi: 10.1007/s11682-015-9452-y [Epub ahead of print].

Fernandez-Miranda, J. C. (2013). Editorial: beyond diffusion tensor imaging. *J. Neurosurg.* 118, 1363–1365; discussion 1365–1366. doi: 10.3171/2012.10.JNS121800

Fernandez-Miranda, J. C., Pathak, S., Engh, J., Jarbo, K., Verstynen, T., Yeh, F. C., et al. (2012). High-definition fiber tractography of the human brain: neuroanatomical validation and neurosurgical applications. *Neurosurgery* 71, 430–453. doi: 10.1227/NEU.0b013e3182592faa

Fernández-Miranda, J. C., Rhoton, A. L. Jr., Alvarez-Linera, J., Kakizawa, Y., Choi, C., and de Oliveira, E. P. (2008). Three-dimensional microsurgical and tractographic anatomy of the white matter of the human brain. *Neurosurgery* 62, 989–1026; discussion 1026–1028. doi: 10.1227/01.neu.0000333767.05328.49

Fernández-Miranda, J. C., Wang, Y., Pathak, S., Stefaneau, L., Verstynen, T., and Yeh, F. C. (2015). Asymmetry, connectivity and segmentation of the arcuate fascicle in the human brain. *Brain Struct. Funct.* 220, 1665–1680. doi: 10.1007/s00429-014-0751-7

Fox, M. D., Snyder, A. Z., Vincent, J. L., Corbetta, M., Van Essen, D. C., and Raichle, M. E. (2005). The human brain is intrinsically organized into dynamic, anticorrelated functional networks. *Proc. Natl. Acad. Sci. U S A* 102, 9673–9678. doi: 10.1073/pnas.0504136102

Haznedar, M. M., Buchsbaum, M. S., Hazlett, E. A., Shihabuddin, L., New, A., and Siever, L. J. (2004). Cingulate gyrus volume and metabolism in the schizophrenia spectrum. *Schizophr. Res.* 71, 249–262. doi: 10.1016/j.schres.2004.02.025

Heilbronner, S. R., and Haber, S. N. (2014). Frontal cortical and subcortical projections provide a basis for segmenting the cingulum bundle: implications for neuroimaging and psychiatric disorders. *J. Neurosci.* 34, 10041–10054. doi: 10.1523/JNEUROSCI.5459-13.2014

Huang, W., DiFranza, J. R., Kennedy, D. N., Zhang, N., Ziedonis, D., Ursprung, S., et al. (2013). Progressive levels of physical dependence to tobacco coincide with changes in the anterior cingulum bundle microstructure. *PLoS One* 8:e67837. doi: 10.1371/journal.pone.0067837

Huang, W., King, J. A., Ursprung, W. W., Zheng, S., Zhang, N., Kennedy, D. N., et al. (2014). The development and expression of physical nicotine dependence corresponds to structural and functional alterations in the anterior cingulate-precuneus pathway. *Brain Behav.* 4, 408–417. doi: 10.1002/brb3.227

Jang, S. H., and Hong, J. H. (2012). The anatomical characteristics of superior longitudinal fasciculus I in human brain: diffusion tensor tractography study. *Neurosci. Lett.* 506, 146–148. doi: 10.1016/j.neulet.2011.10.069

Jang, S. H., Kim, S. H., Kim, O. R., Byun, W. M., Kim, M. S., Seo, J. P., et al. (2013). Cingulum injury in patients with diffuse axonal injury: a diffusion tensor imaging study. *Neurosci. Lett.* 543, 47–51. doi: 10.1016/j.neulet.2013.02.058

Jansons, K. M., and Alexander, D. C. (2003). Persistent angular structure: new insights from diffusion MRI data. Dummy version. *Inf. Process. Med. Imaging* 18, 672–683. doi: 10.1007/978-3-540-45087-0_56

Jones, D. K., Christiansen, K. F., Chapman, R. J., and Aggleton, J. P. (2013). Distinct subdivisions of the cingulum bundle revealed by diffusion MRI fibre tracking: implications for neuropsychological investigations. *Neuropsychologia* 51, 67–78. doi: 10.1016/j.neuropsychologia.2012.11.018

Kamali, A., Flanders, A. E., Brody, J., Hunter, J. V., and Hasan, K. M. (2014a). Tracing superior longitudinal fasciculus connectivity in the human brain using high resolution diffusion tensor tractography. *Brain Struct. Funct.* 219, 269–281. doi: 10.1007/s00429-012-0498-y

Kamali, A., Sair, H. I., Radmanesh, A., and Hasan, K. M. (2014b). Decoding the superior parietal lobule connections of the superior longitudinal fasciculus/arcuate fasciculus in the human brain. *Neuroscience* 277, 577–583. doi: 10.1016/j.neuroscience.2014.07.035

Killiany, R. J., Hyman, B. T., Gomez-Isla, T., Moss, M. B., Kikinis, R., Jolesz, F., et al. (2002). MRI measures of entorhinal cortex vs. hippocampus in preclinical AD. *Neurology* 58, 1188–1196. doi: 10.1212/wnl.58.8.1188

Kobayashi, Y., and Amaral, D. G. (2007). Macaque monkey retrosplenial cortex: III. Cortical efferents. *J. Comp. Neurol.* 502, 810–833. doi: 10.1002/cne.21346

Kondo, H., Saleem, K. S., and Price, J. L. (2003). Differential connections of the temporal pole with the orbital and medial prefrontal networks in macaque monkeys. *J. Comp. Neurol.* 465, 499–523. doi: 10.1002/cne.10842

Lawes, I. N., Barrick, T. R., Murugam, V., Spierings, N., Evans, D. R., Song, M., et al. (2008). Atlas-based segmentation of white matter tracts of the human brain using diffusion tensor tractography and comparison with classical dissection. *Neuroimage* 39, 62–79. doi: 10.1016/j.neuroimage.2007.06.041

Lin, Y. C., Shih, Y. C., Tseng, W. Y., Chu, Y. H., Wu, M. T., Chen, T. F., et al. (2014). Cingulum correlates of cognitive functions in patients with mild cognitive impairment and early Alzheimer's disease: a diffusion spectrum imaging study. *Brain Topogr.* 27, 393–402. doi: 10.1007/s10548-013-0346-2

Ludwig, E., and Klingler, J. (1965). *Atlas Cerebri Humani. The Inner Structure of the Brain Demonstrated on the Basis of Macroscopical Preparations.* Boston, MA: Little Brown.

Martino, J., De Witt Hamer, P. C., Vergani, F., Brogna, C., de Lucas, E. M., Vazquez-Barquero, A., et al. (2011). Cortex-sparing fiber dissection: an improved method for the study of white matter anatomy in the human brain. *J. Anat.* 219, 531–541. doi: 10.1111/j.1469-7580.2011.01414.x

Mayberg, H. S., Lozano, A. M., Voon, V., McNeely, H. E., Seminowicz, D., Hamani, C., et al. (2005). Deep brain stimulation for treatment-resistant depression. *Neuron* 45, 651–660. doi: 10.1016/j.neuron.2005.02.014

McKiernan, K. A., Kaufman, J. N., Kucera-Thompson, J., and Binder, J. R. (2003). A parametric manipulation of factors affecting task-induced deactivation in functional neuroimaging. *J. Cogn. Neurosci.* 15, 394–408. doi: 10.1162/089892903321593117

Mufson, E. J., and Pandya, D. N. (1984). Some observations on the course and composition of the cingulum bundle in the rhesus monkey. *J. Comp. Neurol.* 225, 31–43. doi: 10.1002/cne.902250105

Orban, G. A., Claeys, K., Nelissen, K., Smans, R., Sunaert, S., Todd, J. T., et al. (2006). Mapping the parietal cortex of human and non-human primates. *Neuropsychologia* 44, 2647–2667. doi: 10.1016/j.neuropsychologia.2005.11.001

Pandya, D. N., Van Hoesen, G. W., and Mesulam, M. M. (1981). Efferent connections of the cingulate gyrus in the rhesus monkey. *Exp. Brain Res.* 42, 319–330. doi: 10.1007/bf00237497

Raichle, M. E., MacLeod, A. M., Snyder, A. Z., Powers, W. J., Gusnard, D. A., and Shulman, G. L. (2001). A default mode of brain function. *Proc. Natl. Acad. Sci. U S A* 98, 676–682. doi: 10.1073/pnas.98.2.676

Saleem, K. S., Kondo, H., and Price, J. L. (2008). Complementary circuits connecting the orbital and medial prefrontal networks with the temporal, insular and opercular cortex in the macaque monkey. *J. Comp. Neurol.* 506, 659–693. doi: 10.1002/cne.21577

Scheperjans, F., Hermann, K., Eickhoff, S. B., Amunts, K., Schleicher, A., and Zilles, K. (2008). Observer-independent cytoarchitectonic mapping of the human superior parietal cortex. *Cereb. Cortex* 18, 846–867. doi: 10.1093/cercor/bhm116

Schmahmann, J. D., and Pandya, D. N. (2006). *Fiber Pathways of the Brain*. New York, NY: Oxford UP.

Seeley, W. W., Menon, V., Schatzberg, A. F., Keller, J., Glover, G. H., Kenna, H., et al. (2007). Dissociable intrinsic connectivity networks for salience processing and executive control. *J. Neurosci.* 27, 2349–2356. doi: 10.1523/JNEUROSCI.5587-06.2007

Seminowicz, D. A., Mayberg, H. S., McIntosh, A. R., Goldapple, K., Kennedy, S., Segal, Z., et al. (2004). Limbic-frontal circuitry in major depression: a path modeling metanalysis. *Neuroimage* 22, 409–418. doi: 10.1016/j.neuroimage.2004.01.015

Sethi, A., Gregory, S., Dell'Acqua, F., Periche Thomas, E., Simmons, A., Murphy, D. G., et al. (2015). Emotional detachment in psychopathy: involvement of dorsal default-mode connections. *Cortex* 62, 11–19. doi: 10.1016/j.cortex.2014.07.018

Sexton, C. E., Kalu, U. G., Filippini, N., Mackay, C. E., and Ebmeier, K. P. (2011). A meta-analysis of diffusion tensor imaging in mild cognitive impairment and Alzheimer's disease. *Neurobiol. Aging* 32, 2322.e5–2322.e18. doi: 10.1016/j.neurobiolaging.2010.05.019

Sotiropoulos, S. N., Jbabdi, S., Xu, J., Andersson, J. L., Moeller, S., Auerbach, E. J., et al. (2013). Advances in diffusion MRI acquisition and processing in the Human Connectome Project. *Neuroimage* 80, 125–143. doi: 10.1016/j.neuroimage.2013.05.057

Thiebaut de Schotten, M., Dell'Acqua, F., Forkel, S. J., Simmons, A., Vergani, F., Murphy, D. G., et al. (2011). A lateralized brain network for visuospatial attention. *Nat. Neurosci.* 14, 1245–1246. doi: 10.1038/nn.2905

Thiebaut de Schotten, M., Dell'Acqua, F., Valabregue, R., and Catani, M. (2012). Monkey to human comparative anatomy of the frontal lobe association tracts. *Cortex* 48, 82–96. doi: 10.1016/j.cortex.2011.10.001

Tuladhar, A. M., van Norden, A. G., de Laat, K. F., Zwiers, M. P., van Dijk, E. J., Norris, D. G., et al. (2015). White matter integrity in small vessel disease is related to cognition. *Neuroimage Clin.* 7, 518–524. doi: 10.1016/j.nicl.2015.02.003

Van Essen, D. C., Smith, S. M., Barch, D. M., Behrens, T. E., Yacoub, E., Ugurbil, K., et al. (2013). The WU-minn human connectome project: an overview. *Neuroimage* 80, 62–79. doi: 10.1016/j.neuroimage.2013.05.041

Vogt, B. A. (2016). Midcingulate cortex: structure, connections, homologies, functions and diseases. *J. Chem. Neuroanat.* 74, 28–46. doi: 10.1016/j.jchemneu.2016.01.010

Vogt, B. A., Derbyshire, S., and Jones, A. K. (1996). Pain processing in four regions of human cingulate cortex localized with co-registered PET and MR imaging. *Eur. J. Neurosci.* 8, 1461–1473. doi: 10.1111/j.1460-9568.1996.tb01608.x

Vogt, B. A., Finch, D. M., and Olson, C. R. (1992). Functional heterogeneity in cingulate cortex: the anterior executive and posterior evaluative regions. *Cereb. Cortex* 2, 435–443. doi: 10.1093/cercor/2.6.435-a

Vogt, B. A., and Laureys, S. (2005). Posterior cingulate, precuneal and retrosplenial cortices: cytology and components of the neural network correlates of consciousness. *Prog. Brain Res.* 150, 205–217. doi: 10.1016/s0079-6123(05)50015-3

Vogt, B. A., Nimchinsky, E. A., Vogt, L. J., and Hof, P. R. (1995). Human cingulate cortex: surface features, flat maps and cytoarchitecture. *J. Comp. Neurol.* 359, 490–506. doi: 10.1002/cne.903590310

Vogt, B. A., and Pandya, D. N. (1987). Cingulate cortex of the rhesus monkey: II. Cortical afferents. *J. Comp. Neurol.* 262, 271–289. doi: 10.1002/cne.902620208

Wang, Y., Fernández-Miranda, J. C., Verstynen, T., Pathak, S., Schneider, W., and Yeh, F. C. (2013). Rethinking the role of the middle longitudinal fascicle in language and auditory pathways. *Cereb. Cortex* 23, 2347–2356. doi: 10.1093/cercor/bhs225

Wang, X., Pathak, S., Stefaneanu, L., Yeh, F. C., Li, S., and Fernandez-Miranda, J. C. (2016). Subcomponents and connectivity of the superior longitudinal fasciculus in the human brain. *Brain Struct. Funct.* 221, 2075–2092. doi: 10.1007/s00429-015-1028-5

Wedeen, V. J., Hagmann, P., Tseng, W. Y., Reese, T. G., and Weisskoff, R. M. (2005). Mapping complex tissue architecture with diffusion spectrum magnetic resonance imaging. *Magn. Reson. Med.* 54, 1377–1386. doi: 10.1002/mrm.20642

Wedeen, V. J., Wang, R. P., Schmahmann, J. D., Benner, T., Tseng, W. Y., Dai, G., et al. (2008). Diffusion spectrum magnetic resonance imaging (DSI) tractography of crossing fibers. *Neuroimage* 41, 1267–1277. doi: 10.1016/j.neuroimage.2008.03.036

Wisse, L. E., Reijmer, Y. D., ter Telgte, A., Kuijf, H. J., Leemans, A., Luijten, P. R., et al. (2015). Hippocampal disconnection in early Alzheimer's disease: a 7 tesla MRI study. *J. Alzheimers Dis.* 45, 1247–1256. doi: 10.3233/JAD-142994

Wu, Y., Sun, D., Wang, Y., Wang, Y., and Wang, Y. (2016). Tracing short connections of the temporo-parieto-occipital region in the human brain using diffusion spectrum imaging and fiber dissection. *Brain Res.* 1646, 152–159. doi: 10.1016/j.brainres.2016.05.046

Yamamoto, M., Kushima, I., Kimura, H., Hayashi, A., Kawano, N., Aleksic, B., et al. (2015). White matter microstructure between the pre-SMA and the cingulum bundle is related to response conflict in healthy subjects. *Brain Behav.* 5:e00375. doi: 10.1002/brb3.375

Yeh, F. C., Verstynen, T. D., Wang, Y., Fernandez-Miranda, J. C., and Tseng, W. Y. (2013). Deterministic diffusion fiber tracking improved by quantitative anisotropy. *PLoS One* 8:e80713. doi: 10.1371/journal.pone.0080713

Yeh, F. C., Wedeen, V. J., and Tseng, W. Y. (2010). Generalized q-sampling imaging. *IEEE Trans. Med. Imaging* 29, 1626–1635. doi: 10.1109/TMI.2010.2045126

3

Visualization of the Medial Forebrain Bundle using Diffusion Tensor Imaging

Ardian Hana [1], Anisa Hana [2], Georges Dooms [3], Hans Boecher-Schwarz [1] and Frank Hertel [1]*

[1] National Service of Neurosurgery, Centre Hospitalier de Luxembourg, Luxembourg City, Luxembourg, [2] Internal Medicine, Erasmus University of Rotterdam, Rotterdam, Netherlands, [3] Service of Neuroradiology, Centre Hospitalier de Luxembourg, Luxembourg City, Luxembourg

***Correspondence:**
Ardian Hana
ahana2410@gmail.com

Diffusion tensor imaging is a technique that enables physicians the portrayal of white matter tracts *in vivo*. We used this technique in order to depict the medial forebrain bundle (MFB) in 15 consecutive patients between 2012 and 2015. Men and women of all ages were included. There were six women and nine men. The mean age was 58.6 years (39–77). Nine patients were candidates for an eventual deep brain stimulation. Eight of them suffered from Parkinson's disease and one had multiple sclerosis. The remaining six patients suffered from different lesions which were situated in the frontal lobe. These were 2 metastasis, 2 meningiomas, 1 cerebral bleeding, and 1 glioblastoma. We used a 3DT1-sequence for the navigation. Furthermore T2- and DTI- sequences were performed. The FOV was $200 \times 200\,mm^2$, slice thickness 2 mm, and an acquisition matrix of 96×96 yielding nearly isotropic voxels of $2 \times 2 \times 2$ mm. 3-Tesla-MRI was carried out strictly axial using 32 gradient directions and one b0-image. We used Echo-Planar-Imaging (EPI) and ASSET parallel imaging with an acceleration factor of 2. *b*-value was 800 s/mm^2. The maximal angle was 50°. Additional scanning time was <9 min. We were able to visualize the MFB in 12 of our patients bilaterally and in the remaining three patients we depicted the MFB on one side. It was the contralateral side of the lesion. These were 2 meningiomas and one metastasis. Portrayal of the MFB is possible for everyday routine for neurosurgical interventions. As part of the reward circuitry it might be of substantial importance for neurosurgeons during deep brain stimulation in patients with psychiatric disorders. Surgery in this part of the brain should always take the preservation of this white matter tract into account.

Keywords: white matter tracts, medial forebrain bundle, diffusion tensor imaging, deep brain stimulation, cerebral lesions, neurosurgery

INTRODUCTION

Diffusion tensor imaging (DTI) is a technique that allows physicians the portrayal of white matter tracts (WMT) *in vivo* in healthy and non-healthy patients in a non-invasive way (Mesulam, 2005; Stadlbauer et al., 2006; Ciccarelli et al., 2008). It uses the differences in water molecule diffusion patterns along axon bundles throughout the brain (Basser et al., 1994; Ciccarelli et al., 2008). Using this technique we get important informations about the magnitude of diffusion anisotropy and the orientation of the maximum diffusion (Ciccarelli et al., 2008). Application areas include stroke, epilepsy, neurosurgical interventions, spinal cord disorders, or neurodegenerative disorders like

Parkinson's disease (PD) (Ciccarelli et al., 2008). Some of the WMTs which are portrayed by means of DTI include the corticospinal tract (CST), visual pathway (VP), or the medial forebrain bundle (MFB). The MFB seems to be a structure of loosely attached fibers that connects important brain areas together, among others the ventral tegmental area (VTA) of the midbrain, the lateral hypothalamus and the septal area (Coenen et al., 2009a). This WMT is composed of ascending and descending tributaries which differ in their length (Coenen et al., 2009a). Studies suggest that this WMT is situated medially of the subthalamic nucleus (STN) (Coenen et al., 2009a). This would explain why electrodes which are put in the brain for deep brain stimulation (DBS) in patients with PD provoke side effects when they lie medially of the STN (Coenen et al., 2009a). However, the concrete localization of the MFB in humans seems to be disputed between experts. Some physicians depict it as a connection between upper brain stem and the hypothalamus whereas others see it as a WMT which starts anteriorly of the STN (Coenen et al., 2009a). Physicians consider the MFB to be an important part of the mesolimbic dopamine reward system. It is considered to be the neural substrate for the reward circuitry (Gálvez et al., 2015). There have been studies in rodents concerning this WMT too. They describe it as a steak-like structure which is mainly located in the lateral wall of the hypothalamus (Coenen et al., 2009a). There it represents a compact heterogeneous pathway (Coenen et al., 2011). It starts from the VTA and ends in different forebrain structures containing myelinated and unmyelinated fibers (Furlanetti et al., 2015). In contrast to this finding, the MFB seems to be more curved in the humans. In humans it is a bipartite structure with a common trunk at the beginning which splits into two pieces in the VTA of the midbrain (Coenen et al., 2012). Before that, it connects cerebellar nuclei with the VTA (Coenen et al., 2009a, 2011, 2012). In humans we have the inferomedial (im) part which seems to correspond with the MFB of the rodents and passes from the lateral wall of the third ventricle to go to the lateral part of the hypothalamus (Coenen et al., 2012). A superolateral (sl) part leaves the VTA to ascend to the anterior limb of the internal capsule (ALIC) (Coenen et al., 2012). This part of the MFB connects to the accumbens nucleus (NAC) and the ventral striatum (Coenen et al., 2012). All species seem to have one thing in common: MFB connects the VTA with the lateral hypothalamus. The tract is composed of shorter and longer ascending and descending tributaries (Coenen et al., 2009a). They enter and leave this WMT as small fascicles (Coenen et al., 2009a). Physicians suggest that parts of the MFB might reach as far as the olfactory tubercle of the frontal lobe (Coenen et al., 2009a). Many of these stations like cingulated cortex (Brodmann area Cg25; Mayberg, 1997), ALIC (Greenberg et al., 2008), NAC (Berton and Nestler, 2006) which are connected by the MFB represent targets for DBS in patients with psychiatric disorders. DBS was first approved by the FDA in 1997 for patients with essential tremor (Karas et al., 2013). This technique was later approved for use in patients with PD, dystonia, or patients with major depression (MD) (Karas et al., 2013; Furlanetti et al., 2015). DBS delivers electrical pulses which are variable in amplitude, pulse width, and frequency, through permanently implanted electrodes (Perlmutter and Mink, 2006; Mädler and Coenen, 2012). The mechanism of DBS might consist in activation of a structure, inhibition of a structure, a combination of both, or disruption of a pathological oscillation (Karas et al., 2013). One of the major advantages of this treatment consists in the reversibility (Awan et al., 2009). The use of DBS presents an option in the treatment of MD which is reversible and at the same time adjustable (Morishita et al., 2014). MD is a common disease which has a prevalence in lifetime of 15–20% and might lead to disability of a person worldwide (Kupfer et al., 2012; Taghva et al., 2013). One of the main symptoms in patients with MD is their inability to experience pleasure (Rea et al., 2014). As the MFB seems to be a prominent structure of the reward system, different cerebral lesions like tumors (glioblastoma, meningioma, or metastasis) or bleeding might affect our behavior in a negative way by means of destroying, infiltrating, or pushing away the fibers of this tract. Glioblastoma is the most aggressive and lethal primary brain tumor (Norden et al., 2009). Its therapy consists in maximal tumor resection which is followed by radiation and chemotherapy (Cohen et al., 2009). About 25% of the patients with systemic cancer suffer from brain metastasis. The treatment consists either in surgical removal or radiation and chemotherapy, always depending on the primary cancer (Curry et al., 2005). Both lesions might affect the fibers of the MFB negatively and might be responsible for personality changes in our patients if they affect the MFB. Using special MRI modalities like DTI might help physicians distinguish between glioblatoma and metastasis (Chen et al., 2012) and furthermore be used during surgery when these lesions border the MFB in order to avoid a destruction of the tract by surgeons.

Our aim was to portray the MFB in patients with different pathologies in order to see how this WMT was affected by different lesions and whether there were clinical symptoms which could be attributed to lesions in this WMT. Furthermore, we wanted to portray the MFB in patients who would undergo a DBS in order to draw a comparison between the MFB in different patients with different diseases. An important issue was the portrayal of the MFB in relation to known and established deep brain stimulation targets like the STN. Neurosurgeons might be confronted with unwanted side effects during deep brain stimulation due to the proximity of our target and the MFB. Another important issue was to see whether there was a correlation between MFB lesions and the clinic of our patients.

MATERIALS AND METHODS

Patient Data

DTI was performed according to the guidelines and the ethical standards of the Centre Hospitalier de Luxembourg. The research protocol was approved by the Institutional Review Boards of the Centre Hospitalier de Luxembourg and was conducted according to the principles expressed in the Declaration of Helsinki. All participants provided written informed consent. We performed DTI of the brain between 2012 and 2015 on 15 consecutive patients. There were nine men and six women (**Table 1** summarizes the details). Patients can be divided into two groups. On the one hand we visualized the MFB on nine patients

TABLE 1 | Demographics of all patients.

	All	DBS	Other lesions	Men	Women	MFB depiction bilaterally	MFB depiction unilaterally	Mean age	Lesion
Patient	15	9	6	9	6	12	3	59 y	2 Metastasis 2 Meningiomas 1 Bleeding 1 Glioblastoma

TABLE 2 | Exact age of the patients.

Pat. 1	Pat. 2	Pat. 3	Pat. 4	Pat. 5	Pat. 6	Pat. 7	Pat. 8	Pat. 9	Pat. 10	Pat. 11	Pat. 12	Pat. 13	Pat. 14	Pat. 15
53 y	79 y	44 y	65 y	64 y	64 y	69 y	61 y	69 y	71 y	44 y	43 y	54 y	39 y	67 y

who would eventually undergo a DBS. Eight of these patients suffered from PD while one patient suffered from Multiple sclerosis. The other group consists of six patients. These were patients suffering from different cerebral lesions which were situated in the frontal lobe or in the vicinity of the frontal lobe. These were 2 metastasis, 2 meningiomas, 1 glioblastoma, and 1 cerebral bleeding which was mainly situated in the external capsula, but however, affected at a certain extent the frontal lobe as well. The mean age was 59 years. The youngest patient was 39 years old while the oldest patient was 79 years old. The individual age is specified in **Table 2**.

Data Acquisition

We used a 3DT1-sequence for the navigation. Furthermore T2- and DTI- sequences were performed. The FOV was $200 \times 200\,\text{mm}^2$, slice thickness 2 mm, and an acquisition matrix of 96×96 yielding nearly isotropic voxels of $2 \times 2 \times 2$ mm. 3-Tesla-MRI was carried out strictly axial using 32 gradient directions and one b0-image. We used Echo-Planar-Imaging (EPI) and ASSET parallel imaging with an acceleration factor of 2. b-value was $800\,\text{s/mm}^2$. The maximal angle was 50°. FA start value of 0.10 and ADC stop value of $0.20\,\text{mm}^2/\text{s}$ were the parameters used for tractography. Additional scanning time was less than 9 min.

DTI-preparation

After having performed a 3DT1-, T2, and DTI-sequences we transferred the data to digital imaging and communications in medicine (DICOM). The next step consists in the transfer of the data to a surgical navigation program. This step has been previously widely described in one of our previous articles (Hana et al., 2014). If we are dealing with a patient who needs a DBS, we perform the fibertracking by using two ROIs. The size of the ROI was 1 cm One ROI is put in the frontal lobe, in the medial orbitofrontal cortex, while the localization of the other ROI is in the midbrain in the ventral tegmental area. In a patient with a cerebral lesion like glioblastoma or cerebral hemorrhage, there might be necessary to segment the lesion and an eventual edema which is surrounding this lesion too (Hana et al., 2014). When the site was invaded by an edema or by a lesion then we include parts of it in the ROI. Afterwards the images are imported to operating room from the navigation system and finally they can be integrated in the operation.

DTI-limitations

It can only resolve single fiber directions but it can't depict crossing or kissing fibers (Zhang et al., 2013). Partial volume effect, like contamination with cerebrospinal fluid, is another important limitation (Zhang et al., 2013). Small tracts with different directions might not be identified. A similar effect is to be expected with an edema caused by a cerebral lesion like tumor (Wang et al., 2011). An edema infiltrates the brain tissue and hinders the portrayal of WMT in these areas. The actual size of fiber bundles might not be correctly presented even though certain parts of these tracts are identified (Kinoshita et al., 2005). Thus, WMT like the MFB might be underestimated in the presence of edema. Further limitations consist in the brain shift which remains an area that is still unsolved(Abdullah et al., 2013). Another important issue is the fact that DTI doesn't determine with accuracy the starting point or the end point of a WMT, producing multiple artifacts, and false tracts (Le Bihan et al., 2006). The possibility of false positive or false negative tracts should be kept in mind always.

RESULTS

We were able to portray the MFB in all our patients. In 12 of our patients the MFB could be visualized bilaterally and in the remaining three patients we depicted the MFB on one side. The MFB was missing on the ipsilateral side of the lesion. These were 2 meningiomas and 1 metastasis. In one case the lesion was surrounded by edema. We put our ROI as mentioned above in the VTA and in the medial orbitofrontal cortex. If one of these parts of the brain was influenced by a lesion e.g., edema we segmented the edema and included a part of it in our ROI. We assume that the fibers which could be portrayed were indeed correct and for sure but we never forgot that other fibers might be there too which couldn't be depicted due to the lesion. One case showed the MFB running laterally of the glioblastoma which was situated in between of the two MFB (**Figure 1**). Here we have the MFB depicted in blue and green. What is striking here, is the fact that a good part of the fibers are identified despite the big tumoral

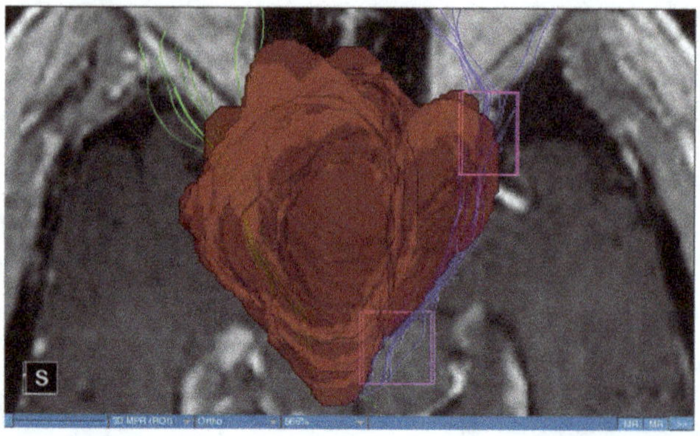

FIGURE 1 | MRI axial view, T1, red: Glioblastoma, blue: right MFB, green: left MFB.

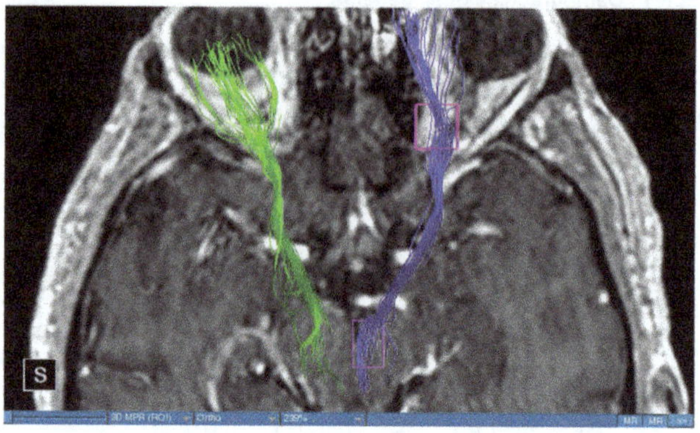

FIGURE 4 | MRI axial view, T1, DBS, blue: right MFB, green: left MFB.

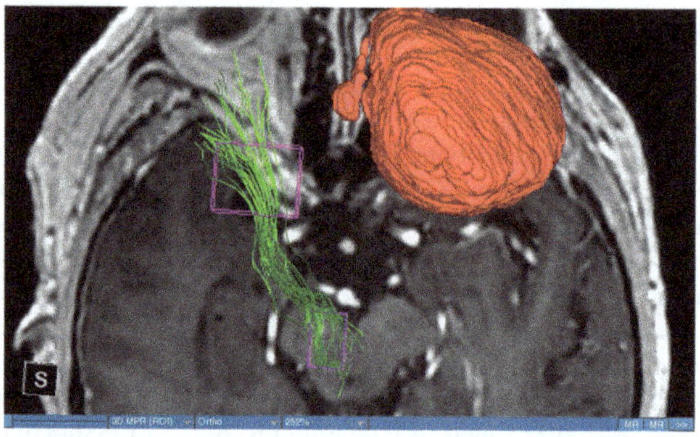

FIGURE 2 | MRI axial view, T1, red: Meningioma, green: left MFB, right MFB is missing.

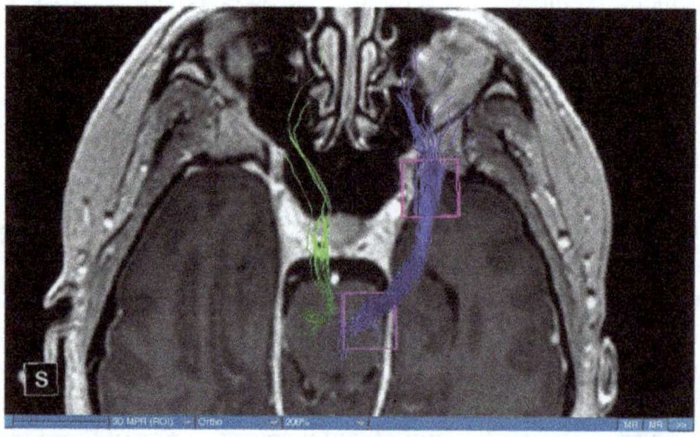

FIGURE 3 | MRI axial view, T1, DBS, blue: right MFB, green: left MFB.

lesion, however they seem to have a small volume in comparison with **Figure 3** or **Figure 7**. This might be due to the tumor which has invaded or destructed them or due to the limitation of DTI to depict WMT next to cerebral lesions completely. With other words we are sure about the correctness of the depicted fibers, however, there might be other fibers which are destroyed or disrupted by this tumor which couldn't be depicted with the DTI. This fact should always be kept in mind when visualizing WMT by means of DTI. This patient was put under antidepressive treatment in the follow up. In this respect it might be possible that the fibers of both MFB were compromised. When a certain number of fibers isn't working then symptoms might appear. The fibers pass through the superior cerebellar penduncle. They ascend through the pons and pass through two important areas. One of them is the area posterior of the red nucleus and the other one is the periaqueductal gray. The tract reaches furthermore the lateral hypothalamus. Furthermore, its fibers run through the lateral wall of the third ventricle and are situated next to the anterior horn of the lateral ventricle The fibers of this WMT are localized under the thalamus before they border the anterior limb of the internal capsule. The STN seems to be situated laterally and posteriorly of the MFB. Partially the MFB is directed latero-caudally at the level of the substantia nigra. The MFB ran from the VTA to the NAC, the medial and lateral orbitofrontal contex, and the dorsolateral prefrontal cortex. Ultimately it seems that the fibers reach out to the olfactory bulb. The MFB was situated cranially to the optic chiasm and the optical tract in his part concerning the frontal lobe. In **Figure 2** we depicted the MFB on the healthy side only. On the ipsilateral side of the metastasis we couldn't portray the MFB. The patient however wasn't depressive and didn't need any treatment in this direction later on. This can be due to the presence of a good developed MFB on the contralateral side which is able to take over the task alone. **Figures 3**, **4** can show the fibers without being compromised by a lesion. Here we can see precisely the size of the ROI and their location. **Figure 5** describes the case in which fibers of the MFB can differ in volume in one and the same patient without being compromised by a lesion. These differences can appear between the right and the left MFB in the same patient or there can be interindividual differences without any presence of special symptoms. The latter case can be seen if we compare **Figure 6** with **Figure 7**. In **Figure 8** we recognize the edema which is surrounding the tumor, in this case a metastasis. We can deduce that a lesion like edema can hinder the depiction of WMT by means of DTI. In **Figure 2** there

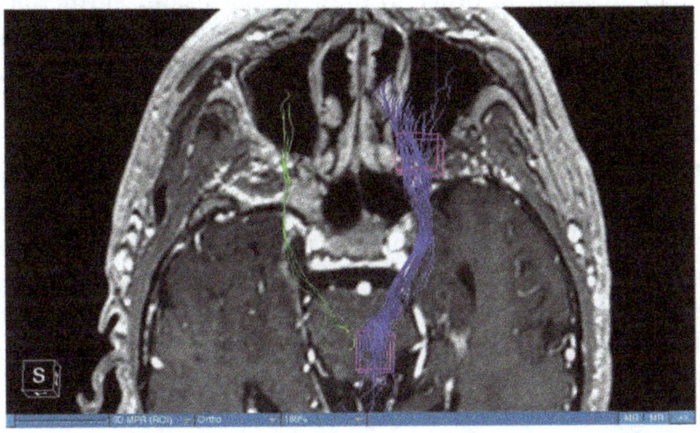

FIGURE 5 | MRI axial view, T1, DBS, blue: right MFB, green: left MFB.

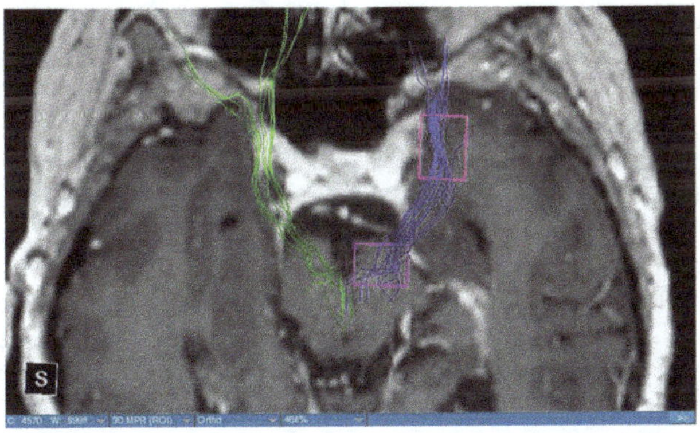

FIGURE 6 | MRI axial view, T1, DBS, blue: right MFB, green: left MFB.

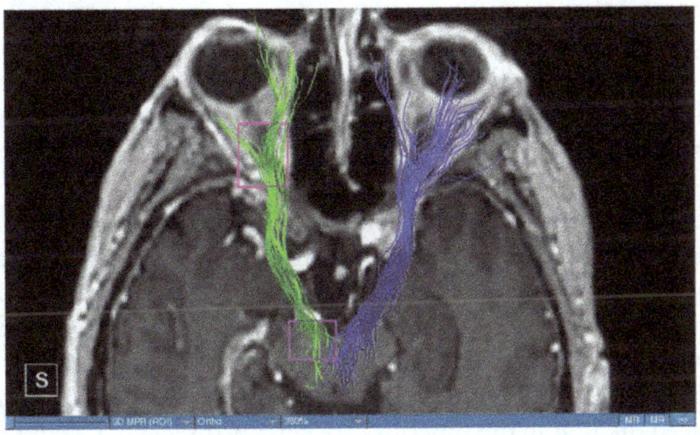

FIGURE 7 | MRI axial view, T1, DBS, blue: right MFB, green: left MFB.

was a lesion without edema which hindered the portrayal of the MFB. In this case we have the presence of the two. We didn't remark any differences in our patients concerning the fractional anisotropy. We have to say that none of our patients sufferend from a MD. Based on the Hamilton scale for depression no one from our patients fulfilled the criteria for MD. We have to admit however that when you announce to a patient a diagnosis like

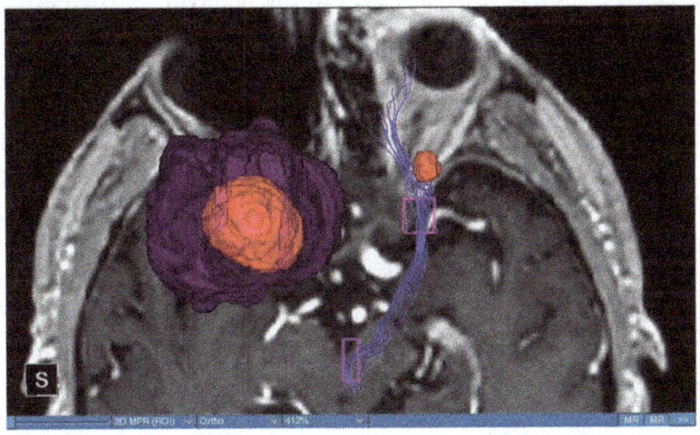

FIGURE 8 | MRI axial view, T1, red: Metastasis, purple: edema, blue: right MFB, left MFB is missing.

brain cancer, he might feel hopeless or sad but this is only one of the criteria in this scale and it is something expected. None of our patients needed a psychiatric surveillance and they were stable during their whole stay in the hospital.

DISCUSSION

The MFB is a WMT of the forebrain which has been keeping physicians occupied since the second half of the Nineteenth century. It was first described by Ganser in 1882 and later on other physicians tried to enlighten this WMT (Nieuwenhuys et al., 1982). The importance of the MFB becomes more evident when we know about its role as a key structure of the reward system (Bracht et al., 2014). The reward circuit is very important for developing motivated behaviors (Haber and Knutson, 2010). Significant components of this network are the anterior cingulated cortex, the orbital prefrontal cortex, the ventral striatum, the ventral pallidum, the dopamine neurons in the midbrain, NAC, and the VTA (Haber and Knutson, 2010). Neuroimaging studies like functional magnetic resonance imaging, positron emission tomography or DTI have been used to elucidate these areas more precisely (Wacker et al., 2009). DTI is used by physicians to depict WMT in healthy and non-healthy patients *in vivo* among others the MFB (Mesulam, 2005; Stadlbauer et al., 2006; Ciccarelli et al., 2008). This WMT has been identified in rodents and humans with partially big differences. Whereas in humans this WMT is described as a bipartite structure, in rodents this tract is located mainly in the lateral wall of the hypothalamus as a steak-like structure (Coenen et al., 2009a, 2012). However, despite these differences this tract connects the VTA with the lateral hypothalamus in all species. Our results confirm furthermore that this WMT borders various important structures of the brain like the hypothalamus, or the STN. These results correspond with the findings of other groups (Coenen et al., 2009a, 2012). Alteration of WMT who are responsible for the reward system might be responsible for MD (Coenen et al., 2009b). These alterations might be caused by inflammatory diseases or by different cerebral lesions. Tumors or edema might compromise the FA-values. In the same time they might be responsible for changes in the behavior of the patients. In our patient with a giant meningioma the first symptoms had predominantly a behavioral character. Her temper changed from absolutely calm to autoaggression. In her case we couldn't portray the MFB on the ipsilateral side of the tumor. In all our patients we didn't remark any special FA-reductions (**Figures 1, 2, 8**). Especially FA-reductions in the slMFB have been associated with anhedonia in patients with acute depression (Bracht et al., 2015b). Lower FA-values in the slMFB seem to be associated with melancholic depression also (Bracht et al., 2015a). However, there is a negative correlation between the hedonic capacity and the mean FA of the slMFB for patients in remission or for those who were never depressive (Bracht et al., 2015a). Lower FA in the left slMFB seems to be associated with more pronounced capacity to derive pleasure in patients who were never depressive or in patients in remission (Bracht et al., 2015a). Alterations have been found also in other structures which incorporate the slMFB (Bracht et al., 2015a): Reduction in FA-values has been found in melancholic patients too in VTA-orbitofrontal cortex connections too (Bracht et al., 2014). Besides that these authors found out that the higher the depression the lower the FA in melancholic patients (Bracht et al., 2014). These alterations seem to concern the slMFB. Alterations in this area of the brain might contribute to the severity of the disease (Bracht et al., 2014). Keeping in mind that tumors don't respect borders or WMT, we have to say that in their presence we might find the same alterations. Other neurodegenerative diseases might reveal the same results. In those cases we have to try to find out how big is the influence of the MD and how big that of the other illness. However, the authors found no correlation between hedonic tone and imMFB (Bracht et al., 2015a). This might lead to the assumption that slMFB is more important in cases of hedonia or anhedonia than the imMFB. The importance of the slMFB for patients with depression has been highlighted in another study. According to them, this part of the MFB is a very important station of reward and mood (Schoene-Bake et al., 2010). Another group came also to the conclusion that stimulating the slMFB might be advantageous in patients with depression (Schlaepfer et al., 2013). In a study using deterministic methods to identify the slMFB they saw positive results in the treatment of patients with MD by means of bilateral DBS in slMFB (Schlaepfer et al., 2013). We have to say that our patients weren't depressive and only the patient in **Figure 1** needed antidepressive medication in his follow-up. So according to these findings a reduction of the FA wasn't expected and ultimately wasn't present. The authors describe furthermore no changes in the mean FA of the slMFB in patients with remission and those who never were depressive (Bracht et al., 2015a,b). These changes are no markers however they seem to be state-dependent as they disappear when the patients are in remission (Bracht et al., 2015a). If there is no cerebral lesion we might tend to attribute these changes in FA to the MD but in the presence of a tumor or edema FA-value might be compromised too. In that case it might be difficult for physicians to attribute certain changes to MD, to the tumor, or to the edema. A comparison between patients without MD but with a tumor and those with MD but without a tumor would be necessary to see how the FA-value is influenced due to a certain situation in order to draw a conclusion. Furthermore, the MFB is confirmed as the central pathway of the reward system (Bracht et al., 2015a). Coenen et al. have portrayed two different branches of the MFB in humans. One of them is the medial branch which connects the lateral hypothalamus with the reticular formation of the brain stem and the lateral branch which projects to several centers of the brain like the subcoeruleus nucleus or the substantia nigra pars compacta (Coenen et al., 2009a). Both branches form a "W" shape in the coronal image according a study which was published recently, whereby the imMFB presents the middle portion of the "W," and the lateral portions of the "W" consist of the slMFB (Cho et al., 2015). Although the findings of this study were mostly comparable with the results of other physicians there was however a new insight in the relation between the anterior thalamic radiation (ATR) and the slMFB. The authors describe the position of the ATR superior to the slMFB lateral of this branch when entering the ALIC although it is situated medially before its entry (Cho et al., 2015). This knowledge might be of substantial importance for neurosurgeons who perform DBS in patients with MD. Stimulation of the slMFB might be beneficiary in patients with depression (Coenen et al., 2009a), whereas stimulation of the ATR is thought to have an opposing effect (Cho et al., 2015), therefore it is important for physicians to know the exact location of these tracts in order to avoid stimulation of the wrong WMT as well as to avoid a co-stimulation of both tracts. These results were obtained using a 7-Tesla-MRI and most of them were consistent with the results obtained by other authors before who were using a 3-Tesla-MRI (Coenen et al., 2012). One of the reasons for the discrepancy might be the fact that DTI has difficulties portraying kissing or crossing fibers in a satisfactory way (Wakana et al., 2004). For the depiction of the MFB there exist many possibilities which have lead to more or less the same results. Therefore, one group used for the portrayal of the MFB two ROI which were placed in the following way: one in the ventral midbrain and the second one included the NAC and the lateral hypothalamus (Coenen et al., 2009a). The lateral hypothalamus is an important part in the rodents MFB and corresponds more or less with the human imMFB. In another study the group around Coenen identified the MFB by using only one ROI which was placed in the VTA (Coenen et al., 2012). There was no difference found in the course of the MFB in comparison of the two different tracking methods. Another more recent study describes the identification of the MFB by using three ROI in patients who underwent DBS. This group placed the ROI in the superior cerebellar peduncle, VTA, and the dorsal raphe nucleus which present stations in the course of the MFB (Anthofer et al., 2015). slMFB was consistently depicted by their method whereas the imMFB could only be inconsistently portrayed (Anthofer et al., 2015). They depicted the MFB in 20 out of 22 hemispheres. In the remaining two they couldn't depict it. In our group we weren't able to portray the MFB in three hemispheres. These hemispheres were invaded by a lesion. In all our DBS patient we were able to portray the MFB on both sides. However, there aren't yet standardized parameters for the portrayal of the MFB. Thus, studies described here are performed on a small group of patients. This fact should be taken into account. DTI sequences with a higher resolution might be more helpful in this case.

Limitations concerning the visualization of WMT by means of DTI consist in the depiction of branched or merged fibers (Zhang et al., 2013). It seems to be very difficult to portray WMT like the MFB in regions which are invaded by cerebral lesion, particularly when these lesions are surrounded by a cerebral peritumoral edema (Zhang et al., 2013). In our group of patients we didn't experience any troubles in portraying the MFB in patients who were planned for a DBS (patients without cerebral lesions), however, we weren't able to portray this WMT in patients with cerebral lesions, which were 2 meningiomas and 1 metastasis. On one hand one can argue the MFB was damaged by the lesion, in these cases by the meningiomas or the metastasis, on the other hand the absence of the MFB on the side of the lesion might be attributed to the difficulties of DTI in depicting this tract in the presence of cerebral lesions. In our glioblastoma patient of **Figure 1** we were able to portray the MFB bilaterally but we have to keep in mind that there might be other fibers which weren't identified due to the lesion. If we compare **Figure 1** with **Figure 7** we remark a great interindividual difference between the two. The size and the volume of the fibers in **Figure 7** is much bigger than in **Figure 1**. In **Figures 2**, **8** the tract wasn't portrayed on the ipsilateral side of the brain tumor. When the depiction of a tract fails, it may not always mean that there is no tract at all (Hana et al., 2015). Cerebral lesions might affect WMT in different ways by invading, displacing, or disrupting them (Abdullah et al., 2013). In the case of the MFB they might compromise the mood of patients. In our DBS-patients we didn'experience any kind of a tendency to depression, however, in our glioblastoma patient there was the necessity of prescribing antidepressive medication as part of the further follow-up. In his case the tumor was localized between the two MFB and it concerned both frontal lobes (**Figure 1**). We should keep in mind that such medication might be necessary in many tumor patients and one might say one case is not very specific however when the MFB is concerned this might be a starting point. As the DTI doesn't say anything about the function of WMT we can't say that the fibers we are watching do perform their task correctly. Thus, a patient may have symptoms despite the MFB being identified. We might be allowed to say however that when the tract is damaged and the patients show symptoms which may be attributed to the functions of the tract that our imagery findings correspond with the clinics. Another case is that of a patient which was operated from a giant frontal meningioma. The MFB wasn't visible on the side of the tumor. This might be on one hand due to a limitation of the DTI or because the tumor destroyed the WMT. However, one of the main symptoms was the lack of enthusiasm. Again this might occur in many tumors but here it coincides with a non-visualization of the MFB. The presence of a cerebral lesion doesn't compulsorily mean that the depiction of the WMT won't be successful. We were able to depict the MFB on both sides e.g., in a patient with glioblastoma (**Figure 1**). Furthermore, DTI can't inform the physicians about the starting or the ending point of the WMT (Hana et al., 2015) which might lead to artifacts. Another important limitation of DTI which consist in the brain shift during surgery is an important issue we need to deal with (Abdullah et al., 2013). After opening the dura mater and after manipulation in the brain e.g., by removing a lesion or by putting an electrode inside the brain we don't have the same conditions we used to have before surgery. One can argue that for the resection of tumors in non-eloquent areas the results might be satisfactory but we have to keep in mind that one or two millimeters next to the MFB might be destructive for this WMT during tumor surgery. During DBS this distance might mean another WMT or another target point. By a localization of the MFB medially to the STN that would mean a stimulation of the STN instead of the MFB and vice-versa. In this case we might expect side-effects in our patients. This risk of costimulating the slMFB during DBS of the STN was described by Coenen et al. in another work (Coenen et al., 2009a). They presumed that acute hypomania during STN DBS might occur due to a unilateral and left sided activation of the imMFB (Coenen et al., 2009a). This part of the MFB is more associated with wanting while the slMFB is associated with liking (Coenen et al., 2009a). As our results furthermore show, the slMFB is situated in the ALIC. If we stimulate this part of the brain we might have an eventual unwanted motoric involvement in our patients. Other structures which might be affected during surgery in patients with DBS include the red nucleus or parts of the hypothalamus. In our results both parts of the MFB were localized superiorly to the visual pathway. Coenen et al. have reported that quality of life in patients with PD might be negatively influenced by depression during DBS of the STN. This seemed to happen when the electrode was located anteriorly, inferiorly and medially (Coenen et al., 2009b). As the MFB seems to be situated anteriorly and medially of the STN this seems to be obvious, however, it seems not to be clear why we have this influence inferiorly. As it is a part of the reward circuitry we already mentioned above, this WMT might be eventually used for DBS in patients suffering from MD. Keeping in mind all the important cerebral structures we mentioned above which we should avoid to stimulate, there seems to be no consensus as which part of the MFB is the best target point in patients suffering from MD. There have been many suggestions of target points which are partly connected by the MFB like the NAC, cingulate cortex, or the ventral internal capsule (Döbrössy et al., 2015). In animal models there have been studies observing DBS in STN or the NAC. The bilateral stimulation of these targets reduced addiction (Döbrössy et al., 2015). A recent study has shown that a stimulation of the MFB but not a stimulation of the Cg25 interacts with the reward system in rats (Edemann-Callesen et al., 2015). Another important issue is to know how many fibers need to be stimulated in order to achieve satisfactory results. Even if we stimulate the right structure, we might have disappointing results because of the lack of a sufficient volume of fibers wasn't stimulated. Concerning depression, different physicians have used different target points with different scores which makes it more difficult to draw a conclusion. Some of the target points include the NAC, the subcallosal cingulate gyrus, and experimentally the VTA (Döbrössy et al., 2015). All these structures have a common ground. Many of their afferent or efferent connections pass through the MFB (Döbrössy et al., 2015). The stimulation of these targets seems to reduce depression at a certain extent (Döbrössy et al., 2015). These results contradict old stimulation studies observed in rats that showed MFB stimulation was detrimental to the animals' health (Olds, 1963). Up to date it is very little known about the reaction of individuals when stimulating the MFB directly. Although there are differences between the studies conducted then and now, this shows however that a certain risk is always present. Before patients are approved for DBS e.g., in PD there has to be a reliability that they aren't going to commit suicide. All these facts need to be taken into account before operating on such a patient. This risk concerns however all patients who undergo the procedure of a DBS and not only those who suffer from depression. Schlaepfer et al. confirm the positive effect of DBS in patients with depression in targets like NAC but on a recent study with seven patients which was conducted by them, they obtained faster results, within days, by stimulating the slMFB bilaterally (Schlaepfer et al., 2013). Bilateral stimulation of the slMFB seems to be mandatory for positive results. On the other hand the ATR seems to mediate distress and sadness in humans (Coenen et al., 2012). This WMT runs in the proximity of the MFB and seems to be its counterpart. A balance between these two WMT seems to be mandatory for the well-being of a person. During DBS surgery, physicians should try to avoid this tract. And therefore the correct knowledge of its localization is mandatory in order to avoid unnecessary side effects. Satisfactory results are to be achieved when we portray the MFB and ATR by means of DTI in the same time. The use of DTI allows the depiction of the MFB and other WMTs in patients with cerebral lesions as well as in patients who will undergo a DBS. Its portrayal is easy and feasible for everyday routine. Nevertheless, a neurosurgeon needs to keep in mind the anatomy of the MFB and that of other structures in the surrounding for a successful surgery. The limitations of DTI however shouldn't be neglected. Based on our findings of this small group we have to say that depiction of the MFB is often compromised when other lesions are in the proximity of this tract but the identification of the MFB is still possible for every day routine. Tracts might be missing like in three of our patients or they can be influenced in other forms like invasion, infiltration, or displacement. However, patients don't seem to have symptoms when only one of the MFB is absent (**Figures 2, 8**). In this case the MFB of the other side might take over the task. The need for antidepressive medication might become necessary in the follow-up of patients with unilateral portrayal of the MFB (**Figure 1**). However, this can be an effect of the disease also. MFB can differ in its volume in one patient between the two hemispheres or it can be different between two different people without being influenced by some other lesion. Patients with cerebral lesions tend to have a less developed MFB than those without lesions. This doesn't mean that symptoms in such cases are present automatically. DTI is a tool that gives further insight in this tract but we should keep in mind that there are limitations which must be taken into account.

REFERENCES

Abdullah, K. G., Lubelski, D., Nucifora, P. G., and Brem, S. (2013). Use of diffusion tensor imaging in glioma resection. *Neurosurg. Focus.* 34:E1. doi: 10.3171/2013.1.FOCUS12412

Anthofer, J. M., Steib, K., Fellner, C., Lange, M., Brawanski, A., and Schlaier, J. (2015). DTI-based deterministic fibre tracking of the medial forebrain bundle. *Acta Neurochir (Wien).* 157, 469–477. doi: 10.1007/s00701-014-2335-y

Awan, N. R., Lozano, A., and Hamani, C. (2009). Deep brain stimulation: current and future perspectives. *Neurosurg. Focus.* 27:E2. doi: 10.3171/2009.4.FOCUS0982

Basser, P. J., Mattiello, J., and LeBihan, D. (1994). MR diffusion tensor spectroscopy and imaging. *Biophys. J.* 66, 259–267. doi: 10.1016/S0006-3495(94)80775-1

Berton, O., and Nestler, E. J. (2006). New approaches to antidepressant drug discovery: beyond monoamines. *Nat. Rev. Neurosci.* 7, 137–151. doi: 10.1038/nrn1846

Bracht, T., Doidge, A. N., Keedwell, P. A., and Jones, D. K. (2015a). Hedonic tone is associated with left supero-lateral medial forebrain bundle microstructure. *Psychol. Med.* 45, 865–874. doi: 10.1017/S0033291714001949

Bracht, T., Horn, H., Strik, W., Federspiel, A., Schnell, S., Höfle, O., et al. (2014). White matter microstructure alterations of the medial forebrain bundle in melancholic depression. *J. Affect. Disord.* 155, 186–193. doi: 10.1016/j.jad.2013.10.048

Bracht, T., Jones, D. K., Müller, T. J., Wiest, R., and Walther, S. (2015b). Limbic white matter microstructure plasticity reflects recovery from depression. *J. Affect. Disord.* 170, 143–149. doi: 10.1016/j.jad.2014.08.031

Chen, X. Z., Yin, X. M., Ai, L., Chen, Q., Li, S. W., and Dai, J. P. (2012). Differentiation between brain glioblastoma multiforme and solitary metastasis: qualitative and quantitative analysis based on routine MR imaging. *Am. J. Neuroradiol.* 33, 1907–1912. doi: 10.3174/ajnr.A3106

Cho, Z. H., Law, M., Chi, J. G., Choi, S. H., Park, S. Y., Kammen, A., et al. (2015). An anatomic review of thalamolimbic fiber tractography: ultra-high resolution direct visualization of thalamolimbic fibers anterior thalamic radiation, superolateral and inferomedial medial forebrain bundles, and newly identified septum pellucidum tract. *World Neurosurg.* 83, 54–61. doi: 10.1016/j.wneu.2013.08.022

Ciccarelli, O., Catani, M., Johansen-Berg, H., Clark, C., and Thompson, A. (2008). Diffusion-based tractography in neurological disorders: concepts, applications, and future developments. *Lancet Neurol.* 7, 715–727. doi: 10.1016/S1474-4422(08)70163-7

Coenen, V. A., Honey, C. R., Hurwitz, T., Rahman, A. A., McMaster, J., and Bürgel, U. (2009a). Medial forebrain bundle stimulation as a pathophysiological mechanism for hypomania in subthalamic nucleus deep brain stimulation for Parkinson's disease. *Neurosurgery* 64, 1106–1114. doi: 10.1227/01.NEU.0000345631.54446.06

Coenen, V. A., Hurwitz, T., Panksepp, J., Mädler, B., and Honey, C. R. (2009b). Medial forebrain bundle stimulation elicits psychotropic side effects in subthalamic nucleus deep brain stimulation for PD – new insights through diffusion tensor imaging. *Akt Neurol.* 36, P749. doi: 10.1055/s-0029-1238842

Coenen, V. A., Panksepp, J., Hurwitz, T. A., Urbach, H., and Mädler, B. (2012). Human medial forebrain bundle (MFB) and anterior thalamic radiation (ATR): imaging of two major subcortical pathways and the dynamic balance of opposite affects in understanding depression. *J. Neuropsychiatry Clin. Neurosci.* 24, 223–236. doi: 10.1176/appi.neuropsych.11080180

Coenen, V. A., Schlaepfer, T. E., Maedler, B., and Panksepp, J. (2011). Cross-species affective functions of the medial forebrain bundle-implications for the treatment of affective pain and depression in humans. *Neurosci. Biobehav. Rev.* 35, 1971–1981. doi: 10.1016/j.neubiorev.2010.12.009

Cohen, M. H., Shen, Y. L., Keegan, P., and Pazdur, R. (2009). FDA drug approval summary: bevacizumab (Avastin) as treatment of recurrent glioblastoma multiforme *Oncologist* 14, 1131–1138. doi: 10.1634/theoncologist.2009-0121

Curry, W. T. Jr., Cosgrove, G. R., Hochberg, F. H., Loeffler, J., and Zervas, N. T. (2005). Stereotactic interstitial radiosurgery for cerebral metastases. *J. Neurosurg.* 103, 630–635. doi: 10.3171/jns.2005.103.4.0630

Döbrössy, M. D., Furlanetti, L. L., and Coenen, V. A. (2015). Electrical stimulation of the medial forebrain bundle in pre-clinical studies of psychiatric disorders. *Neurosci. Biobehav. Rev.* 49, 32–42. doi: 10.1016/j.neubiorev.2014.11.018

Edemann-Callesen, H., Voget, M., Empl, L., Vogel, M., Wieske, F., Rummel, J., et al. (2015). Medial forebrain bundle deep brain stimulation has symptom-specific anti-depressant effects in rats and as opposed to ventromedial prefrontal cortex stimulation interacts with the reward system. *Brain Stimul.* 8, 714–723. doi: 10.1016/j.brs.2015.02.009

Furlanetti, L. L., Döbrössy, M. D., Aranda, I. A., and Coenen, V. A. (2015). Feasibility and safety of continuous and chronic bilateral deep brain stimulation of the medial forebrain bundle in the naïve sprague-dawley rat. *Behav. Neurol.* 2015:256196. doi: 10.1155/2015/256196

Gálvez, J. F., Keser, Z., Mwangi, B., Ghouse, A. A., Fenoy, A. J., Schulz, P. E., et al. (2015). The medial forebrain bundle as a deep brain stimulation target for treatment resistant depression: a review of published data. *Prog. Neuropsychopharmacol. Biol. Psychiatry.* 58C, 59–70. doi: 10.1016/j.pnpbp.2014.12.003

Greenberg, B. D., Askland, K. D., and Carpenter, L. L. (2008). The evolution of deep brain stimulation for neuropsychiatric disorders. *Front. Biosci.* 13:4638–4648. doi: 10.2741/3029

Haber, S. N., and Knutson, B. (2010). The reward circuit: linking primate anatomy and human imaging. *Neuropsychopharmacology* 35, 4–26. doi: 10.1038/npp.2009.129

Hana, A., Dooms, G., Boecher-Schwarz, H., and Hertel, F. (2015). Diffusion tensor imaging - Arcuate fasciculus and the importance for the neurosurgeon. *Clin. Neurol. Neurosurg.* 132, 61–67. doi: 10.1016/j.clineuro.2015.03.001

Hana, A., Husch, A., Gunness, V. R., Berthold, C., Hana, A., Dooms, G., et al. (2014). DTI of the visual pathway - white matter tracts and cerebral lesions. *J. Vis. Exp.* doi: 10.3791/51946

Karas, P. J., Mikell, C. B., Christian, E., Liker, M. A., and Sheth, S. A. (2013). Deep brain stimulation: a mechanistic and clinical update. *Neurosurg. Focus* 35, E1. doi: 10.3171/2013.9.FOCUS13383

Kinoshita, M., Yamada, K., Hashimoto, N., Kato, A., Izumoto, S., Baba, T., et al. (2005). Fiber-tracking does not accurately estimate size of fiber bundle in pathological condition: initial neurosurgical experience using neuronavigation and subcortical white matter stimulation. *Neuroimage* 25, 424–429. doi: 10.1016/j.neuroimage.2004.07.076

Kupfer, D. J., Frank, E., and Phillips, M. L. (2012). Major depressive disorder: new clinical, neurobiological, and treatment perspectives. *Lancet* 379, 1045–1055. doi: 10.1016/S0140-6736(11)60602-8

Le Bihan, D., Poupon, C., Amadon, A., and Lethimonnier, F. (2006). Artifacts and pitfalls in diffusion MRI. *J. Magn. Reson. Imaging* 3, 478–488. doi: 10.1002/jmri.20683

Mädler, B., and Coenen, V. A. (2012). Explaining clinical effects of deep brain stimulation through simplified target-specific modeling of the volume of activated tissue. *Am. J. Neuroradiol.* 33, 1072–1080. doi: 10.3174/ajnr.A2906

Mayberg, H. S. (1997). Limbic-cortical dysregulation: a proposed model of depression. *J. Neuropsychiatry Clin. Neurosci.* 9, 471–481. doi: 10.1176/jnp.9.3.471

Mesulam, M. (2005). Imaging connectivity in the human cerebral cortex: the next frontier? *Ann. Neurol.* 57, 5–7. doi: 10.1002/ana.20368

Morishita, T., Fayad, S. M., Higuchi, M. A., Nestor, K. A., and Foote, K. D. (2014). Deep brain stimulation for treatment-resistant depression: systematic review of clinical outcomes. *Neurotherapeutics* 11, 475–484. doi: 10.1007/s13311-014-0282-1

Nieuwenhuys, R., Geeraedts, L. M., and Veening, J. G. (1982). The medial forebrain bundle of the rat. I. General introduction. *J. Comp. Neurol.* 206, 49–81. doi: 10.1002/cne.902060106

Norden, A. D., Drappatz, J., and Wen, P. Y. (2009). Antiangiogenic therapies for high-grade glioma. *Nat. Rev. Neurol.* 5, 610–620. doi: 10.1038/nrneurol.2009.159

Olds, J. (1963). Self-stimulation experiments. *Science* 140, 218–220. doi: 10.1126/science.140.3563.218

Perlmutter, J. S., and Mink, J. W. (2006). Deep brain stimulation. *Annu. Rev. Neurosci.* 29, 229–257. doi: 10.1146/annurev.neuro.29.051605.112824

Rea, E., Rummel, J., Schmidt, T. T., Hadar, R., Heinz, A., Mathé, A. A., et al. (2014). Anti-anhedonic effect of deep brain stimulation of the prefrontal cortex and the dopaminergic reward system in a genetic rat model of depression: an intracranial self-stimulation paradigm study. *Brain Stimul.* 7, 21–28. doi: 10.1016/j.brs.2013.09.002

Schlaepfer, T. E., Bewernick, B. H., Kayser, S., Mädler, B., and Coenen, V. A. (2013). Rapid effects of deep brain stimulation for treatment-resistant major depression. *Biol. Psychiatry* 73, 1204–1212. doi: 10.1016/j.biopsych.2013.01.034

Schoene-Bake, J. C., Parpaley, Y., Weber, B., Panksepp, J., Hurwitz, T. A., and Coenen, V. A. (2010). Tractographic analysis of historical lesion surgery for depression. *Neuropsychopharmacology* 35, 2553–2563. doi: 10.1038/npp.2010.132

Stadlbauer, A., Nimsky, C., Buslei, R., Salomonowitz, E., Hammen, T., Buchfelder, M., et al. (2006). Diffusion tensor imaging and optimized fiber tracking in glioma patients: histopathologic evaluation of tumor-invaded white matter structures. *Neuroimage* 34, 949–956. doi: 10.1016/j.neuroimage.2006.08.051

Taghva, A. S., Malone, D. A., and Rezai, A. R. (2013). Deep brain stimulation for treatment-resistant depression. *World Neurosurg.* 80, S27.e17–24. doi: 10.1016/j.wneu.2012.10.068

Wacker, J., Dillon, D. G., Pizzagalli, D. A. (2009). The role of the nucleus accumbens and rostral anterior cingulate cortex in anhedonia: integration of resting EEG, fMRI, and volumetric techniques. *Neuroimage* 46, 327–337. doi: 10.1016/j.neuroimage.2009.01.058

Wakana, S., Jiang, H., Nagae-Poetscher, L. M., van Zijl, P. C., and Mori, S. (2004). Fiber tract-based atlas of human white matter anatomy. *Radiology* 230, 77–87. doi: 10.1148/radiol.2301021640

Wang, Y., Wang, Q., Haldar, J. P., Yeh, F. C., Xie, M., Sun, P., et al. (2011). Quantification of increased cellularity during inflammatory demyelination. *Brain* 134(Pt 12), 3590–3601. doi: 10.1093/brain/awr307

Zhang, H., Wang, Y., Lu, T., Qiu, B., Tang, Y., Ou, S., et al. (2013). Differences between generalized q-sampling imaging and diffusion tensor imaging in the preoperative visualization of the nerve fiber tracts within peritumoral edema in brain. *Neurosurgery* 73, 1044–1053. doi: 10.1227/NEU.0000000000000146

4

Feasibility of Diffusion Tractography for the Reconstruction of Intra-Thalamic and Cerebello-Thalamic Targets for Functional Neurosurgery: A Multi-Vendor Pilot Study in Four Subjects

András Jakab[1,2], Beat Werner[1], Marco Piccirelli[3], Kázmér Kovács[4], Ernst Martin[1], John S. Thornton[5], Tarek Yousry[5], Gabor Szekely[6] and Ruth O'Gorman Tuura[1]*

[1] Center for Magnetic Resonance Imaging Research, University Children's Hospital, Zürich, Switzerland, [2] Computational Imaging Research Lab, Department of Biomedical Imaging and Image-Guided Therapy, Medical University of Vienna, Vienna, Austria, [3] Department of Neuroradiology, University Hospital Zürich, Zürich, Switzerland, [4] Department of Biomedical Imaging and Laboratory Science, University of Debrecen, Debrecen, Hungary, [5] University College London Institute of Neurology, London, UK, [6] Computer Vision Laboratory, ETH Zürich, Zürich, Switzerland

****Correspondence:***
András Jakab
andras.jakab@kispi.uzh.ch

Functional stereotactic neurosurgery by means of deep brain stimulation or ablation provides an effective treatment for movement disorders, but the outcome of surgical interventions depends on the accuracy by which the target structures are reached. The purpose of this pilot study was to evaluate the feasibility of diffusion tensor imaging (DTI) based probabilistic tractography of deep brain structures that are commonly used for pre- and perioperative targeting for functional neurosurgery. Three targets were reconstructed based on their significance as intervention sites or as a no-go area to avoid adverse side effects: the connections propagating from the thalamus to (1) primary and supplementary motor areas, (2) to somatosensory areas and the cerebello-thalamic tract (CTT). We evaluated the overlap of the reconstructed connectivity based targets with corresponding atlas based data, and tested the inter-subject and inter-scanner variability by acquiring repeated DTI from four volunteers, and on three MRI scanners with similar sequence parameters. Compared to a 3D histological atlas of the human thalamus, moderate overlaps of 35-50% were measured between connectivity- and atlas based volumes, while the minimal distance between the centerpoints of atlas and connectivity targets was 2.5 mm. The variability caused by the MRI scanner was similar to the inter-subject variability, except for connections with the postcentral gyrus where it was higher. While CTT resolved the anatomically correct trajectory of the tract individually, high volumetric variability was found across subjects and between scanners. DTI can be applied in the clinical, preoperative setting to reconstruct the CTT and to localize subdivisions within the lateral thalamus. In our pilot study, such subdivisions moderately matched the borders of the ventrolateral-posteroventral (VL_{pv}) nucleus and the ventral-posterolateral (VPL) nucleus. Limitations of the currently used standard DTI protocols were exacerbated by large scanner-to-scanner variability of the connectivity-based targets.

Keywords: diffusion MRI, diffusion tensor imaging, brain connectivity, cerebello-thalamic tract, functional neurosurgery

INTRODUCTION

Functional stereotactic neurosurgery by means of deep brain stimulation or ablation provides an effective treatment for movement disorders including Parkinson's disease (Benabid et al., 1996; Ohye, 2009), essential tremor and dystonia (Baizabal-Carvallo et al., 2014). Since the brain and in particular the thalamic and subthalamic regions frequently targeted for functional stereotactic neurosurgery are tightly packed with neuronal circuits, the outcome of surgical interventions depends critically on the accuracy by which the target structures are reached (Hariz, 2002; Lanotte et al., 2002). Errors in targeting can compromise the efficacy of the treatment and lead to adverse side effects such as motor deficits (Baizabal-Carvallo and Jankovic, 2016), hypomania (Chopra et al., 2012), impulse control disorders (Amami et al., 2015), hemi-neglect, and dysarthria (Tripoliti et al., 2011). Therefore, novel and improved targeting approaches are required to provide optimal image guidance for tailored and personalized therapy.

Localization of the target structures can be performed either directly from MRI or indirectly from atlas coordinates and predefined anatomical landmarks (Lemaire et al., 2007). Given the inter-subject variability in anatomical position of the target nuclei (Morel et al., 1997), direct targeting is arguably more accurate, but this approach is limited by the low contrast and relatively low visibility of the target structures on MRI. This low visibility represents a particular challenge for neurosurgical targeting in the thalamus, which contains important target structures for stereotactic surgical interventions by means of ablative therapies such as centrolateral thalamotomy for pain, or deep-brain stimulation of the nucleus Vim (Benabid et al., 1996; Gallay et al., 2008; Martin et al., 2009).

In the clinical setting, while the relaxation properties depicted by T1- or T2-weighted MRI offer limited insight into the anatomy of the thalamus, recently, diffusion MRI based techniques have been suggested as a way to visualize various subdivisions representing possible target locations within the thalamus (Behrens et al., 2003a; Wiegell et al., 2003; Johansen-Berg et al., 2005; Traynor et al., 2010). Diffusion MRI and DTI can be used to estimate the intra-voxel incoherent diffusion driven motion of water molecules (Le Bihan and Johansen-Berg, 2012). The local orientation of diffusion correlates with the direction of axonal fibers within an image voxel, providing the basis for various tractography techniques that enable the macroscopic reconstruction of white matter structures, as well as the connectional anatomy of subcortical structures (Jonasson et al., 2007; Zhang et al., 2010; O'Muircheartaigh et al., 2011). While the most common way of using tractography is done by charting the white matter trajectories emerging from a "seed" area, the back-propagation of remote connections to a seed region allows the parcellation of cortical and subcortical areas based on their in- and outgoing connectivity (Behrens et al., 2003a; Johansen-Berg et al., 2004; Draganski et al., 2008). Furthermore, tractography can be used to directly reconstruct fiber pathways emerging from the thalamus, as potential white matter targets for functional neurosurgery (Kwon et al., 2011).

The direct mapping of the thalamic nuclei, such as the Vim through diffusion tractography is not possible, since the lateral thalamus acts as a relay station with specific and somatotopically organized cortico-thalamic connections (Kievit and Kuypers, 1977). However, the subdivision of the thalamus based on its remote connectivity is possible (connectivity-based segmentation: Johansen-Berg et al., 2005). Thalamic mapping utilizing various tractography and connectivity-based segmentation techniques has been suggested for preoperative prediction of target location for functional neurosurgery (Pouratian et al., 2011; Hyam et al., 2012; Lujan et al., 2012; Hunsche et al., 2013; Sudhyadhom et al., 2013; Anthofer et al., 2014; Torres et al., 2014; Avecillas-Chasin et al., 2016). Some previous studies have used connectivity-based segmentation methods to localize the intra-thalamic representation of motor and premotor connections to find the most probable location of the Vim target for functional neurosurgery (Pouratian et al., 2011; Hyam et al., 2012), while other studies investigated the link between the outcome of neurosurgery and the anatomical configuration of adjacent fiber tracts predicted by tractography (Butson et al., 2006; Anthofer et al., 2014). However, connectivity-based methods can also localize regions adjacent to the possible target areas with strong somatosensory connections, such as connections to the postcentral gyrus, providing a means to define safety margins around possible target areas to avoid adverse treatment effects. The definition of such "no-go" areas is particularly important for approaches such as MRI-guided high intensity focused ultrasound ablation, which relies heavily on the preoperative definition of possible target sites, as the intraoperative monitoring of adverse clinical symptoms is limited without intraoperative physiological monitoring.

In addition to the thalamic nuclei, other structures including the dentato-rubro-thalamic or CTT encompass fibers that act to coordinate the initiation, planning and timing of movement, and accordingly have also been proposed as a putative target for the alleviation of symptoms in various motor disorders

Abbreviations: AC, anterior commissure; CBT, connectivity based target; CTT, cerebello-thalamic tract; DTI, diffusion tensor imaging; DWI, diffusion weighted imaging; MNI, Montreal Neurological Institute; MRI, magnetic resonance imaging; PC, posterior commissure; Vim, nucleus ventralisintermedius; VL_{pv}, nucleus ventrolateralis part posteroventralis; VPL_p, nucleus ventralisposterolateralis posterior part.

(Ohye et al., 1993; Gallay et al., 2008; Schlaier et al., 2015). Diffusion tractography has been used successfully to reconstruct this structure in the clinical setting (Coenen et al., 2011a; Kwon et al., 2011; Schlaier et al., 2015), and has also been used to correlate outcome with the adjacency of this tract. However, studies investigating the link between outcome and the adjacency of the CTT have reported mixed accuracy, calling for a more precise evaluation of the reproducibility of the localization of this tract with tractography (Schlaier et al., 2015). A further challenge is to evaluate the correspondence of the tractography based target sites to the intra-operatively determined optimal stimulation site (Avecillas-Chasin et al., 2015; Coenen et al., 2016) or to compare the imaging based targets to boundaries based on the evaluation of histological samples, which are typically accepted as ground truth for neurosurgical target volumes.

The purpose of our pilot study was to evaluate the technical feasibility of DTI based probabilistic tractography for localizing target areas that are commonly used during functional neurosurgery. Three targets were selected for this evaluation based either on their importance as a primary location targeted for the alleviation of the symptoms of movement disorders (Vim or VL_{pv} nucleus), or as a putative white matter target for ablative therapy (cerebello-thalamic or dentate-rubro-thalamic tract), and lastly, a possible "no-go" area to avoid adverse effects during deep brain stimulation or ablative therapy (VPL nucleus with somatosensory connections). We aimed to test the feasibility of tractography using the following criteria. First, to demonstrate the correspondence to the histologically defined anatomical structures for the targets that have digitized 3D atlas data (VL_{pv} and VPL nucleus of the thalamus) in common neuroimaging space. Secondly, since various aspects of reproducibility represent a predictor of the expected accuracy of targeting during neurosurgery, we set out to quantify the reproducibility of tractography from the observed variability in target position across subjects and the corresponding reproducibility within a subject but on different MRI scanners.

MATERIALS AND METHODS

Study Population and Image Acquisition

Four volunteers with no neurological disorders participated in the study, and for each subject (ages: 28, 37, 40, and 52 years, gender: three males and one female) repeated scans were acquired on clinical MRI scanners of different manufacturers resulting in 10 different acquisitions. Diffusion weighted magnetic resonance imaging (DWI) sessions were carried out on three different 3.0T MRI systems: Siemens Skyra (Siemens Healthcare, Erlangen, Germany), GE Discovery MR750 (GE Healthcare, Milwaukee, WI, USA) and Phillips Ingenia (Phillips Healthcare, Best, The Netherlands), using spin echo echo-planar imaging sequences. The DWI acquisition details are summarized in **Table 1**. We will further refer to the scanners as Scanners 1, 2, and 3, not respecting the order of manufacturers in any depictions or tables. Reconstructed images were stored in DICOM format and were transferred to external workstations for image-processing.

TABLE 1 | Diffusion tensor imaging acquisition parameters used in the study.

	Scanner 1	Scanner 2	Scanner 3
Number of diffusion weighting directions	32*	32*	32*
Sequence type	2D EPI	2D EPI	2D EPI
B-factor	1000	1000	1000
Image matrix	128 * 128, 1.875 * 1.875 mm	112 * 112, 2 * 2 mm	96 * 96, 2 * 2 mm
Slice spacing	4 mm	2 mm	3.6 mm
TE/TR	95/4300 ms	92/10242 ms	80/6000 ms
NEX	1	1	1
Flip angle	90	90	90

**Protocol based on the study by Jones et al. (1999).*

MRI scans were carried out with ethical approval and informed consent was obtained for all subjects.

Image Processing

The following image processing steps were performed on the DWI data: (1) estimating symmetric tensors in each voxel of the diffusion data and using the tensor's eigenvalues to calculate secondary to generate DTI data, parametric maps, such as the fractional anisotropy images, (2) spatial standardization of DWI data to a standard neuroimaging template space, (3) estimation of intra-voxel distribution of multiple fiber populations. We carried out the DTI processing steps with the FMRIB Diffusion Toolbox in the FSL software package (Jenkinson et al., 2012). Fractional anisotropy images (maps characterizing the directionality or "orderedness" of diffusion) were calculated using an established approach described elsewhere (Basser and Pierpaoli, 1996; Basser et al., 2000). We performed non-linear spatial standardization to enable inter-subject comparison of anatomy, and quantitative evaluations are reported in standard neuroanatomical space throughout the manuscript. For each subject, fractional anisotropy images were used to determine a deformation field which transforms the images to a common reference space, the FMRIB58 fractional anisotropy template (identical to MNI-152 space), by means of the FNIRT non-linear registration algorithm available in the FSL package. The characterization of fiber distributions was carried out using a Bayesian procedure (Behrens et al., 2003b) which searches for two fiber populations in each image voxel in such a way that the possible orientations of diffusion displacements best fit the observed DWI data.

Mapping Connectivity-Based Targets within the Thalamus

Following the methods reported in the literature (Behrens et al., 2003a; Johansen-Berg et al., 2004, 2005; Klein et al., 2010; O'Muircheartaigh et al., 2011; Pouratian et al., 2011), thalamic connectivity-based subdivisions were defined by running probabilistic tractography from the thalamus volume to predefined cortical regions. Probabilistic fiber tracking was performed in DTI space to avoid interpolation of data; only the seed masks and the results were transferred to the standard space. The connection strength between each seed voxel and every remote brain voxel in the target regions was estimated as the probability of a tract reaching the target through a trajectory guided by the model of local diffusion characteristics. For each thalamic voxel, a counter variable increased when the emitted tracing samples entered any of the cortical masks, consequently resulting in back-projected connectivity probability maps corresponding to cortical territories delineated by using the Harvard-Oxford Atlas (Desikan et al., 2006). For each image voxel in standard space, 5000 tracing samples were used; loops and recursions were not allowed during fiber tracking. The images were divided by the total number of tracing particles that reached their destination (="waytotal" count).

Based on post mortem neuroanatomical data and previous *in vivo* studies on the cortico-thalamic system (Kievit and Kuypers, 1977; Yeterian and Pandya, 1988; Behrens et al., 2003a; Gallay et al., 2008), we considered the following cortical targets to best determine the connectivity-based subdivisions within the lateral thalamus. For fiber tracking, it was necessary to define a seed and remote target region. Since the VL_{pv} or Vim nucleus is known to project to primary motor and premotor regions and also to the cerebellum (Hyam et al., 2012), the seed region was defined as the entire thalamus volume and the target regions were determined in two steps. First, the precentral gyrus in the Harvard-Oxford Atlas was selected as the target for mapping the thalamocortical connectivity of the primary motor cortex. Then, the targets were extended to include the interconnections of the VL_{pv} nucleus, such that the remote tractography targets included the entire cerebellar volume, supplementary motor cortex and primary motor cortex (precentral gyrus) in the relevant standard atlases (Desikan et al., 2006). The VPL_a and VPL_p nuclei are known to be connected to somatosensory cortical areas and therefore the remote target was defined by using the postcentral gyrus volume in the Harvard-Oxford Atlas.

Anatomical Landmarks: Definition Using a Statistical Shape Model Based 3D Atlas of the Human Thalamus

Throughout the manuscript the nomenclature and anatomical definitions for the nuclei of the thalamus are based on the descriptions of Morel et al. (1997). Our study exploits the results of a recent study, which constructed a digitized 3D mean atlas using the histologically derived thalamic nucleus volumes by Morel et al. (1997), Niemann et al. (2000), and Krauth et al. (2010). Based on this atlas and the non-linear alignment described in a previous work (Jakab et al., 2012), high-resolution meshes of the thalamic nuclei were transformed to the standard MNI152 space. The individual nuclei volumes from the atlas were then re-sampled to an isotropic 1 mm image grid and image labels were constructed from the meshes. The transformation was based on a statistical shape model procedure (Blanc et al., 2009; Jakab et al., 2012), in which the predictor of intra-thalamic geometry was the thalamus outline, as derived from the manual segmentation of the thalamus in the T1-weighted image template in MNI space. While the original shape model atlas was constructed from seven histologically defined samples and hence incorporates population variability, for our study, the mean 3D volume of this dataset was used. The following structures were used from the atlas: VL_{pv}: ventro-lateral nucleus posteroventral part (analogous to the Vim nucleus), VPL_p: ventral-posterolateral nucleus posterior part and the whole-thalamus volume for visualization purposes. The MNI-transformed thalamus atlas and the atlas based targets used in our study are illustrated in **Supplementary Figure S1**. For illustration purposes, we used the histology based reconstructions provided by the Big Brain Atlas. This representation was based on the optically balanced non-linear matching of histological sections to a standard neuroimaging space (Amunts et al., 2013).

Tracking the Cerebello-Thalamic Tract

Probabilistic fiber tracking by means of Probtrackx in the FSL software was used to map the CTT in the study population using identical tracking settings to those utilized for the thalamus connectivity maps. Our method was based on the description by Kwon et al. (2011) who reported initial results on the feasibility of DTI in reconstructing this fiber pathway. Using a cerebellar atlas in standard neuroimaging space (Diedrichsen et al., 2009), the seed region to initiate the tractography was the dentate nucleus contralateral to the thalamus, while the final target was the entire thalamus volume. Fibers were kept if they passed through the following way-point targets in the given order: first, the contralateral superior cerebellar peduncle and then the ipsilateral red nucleus region dilated by four voxels. Regions used for reconstructing the tract are depicted in **Supplementary Figure S2**.

Quantitative Evaluations

Since the calculated connectivity-based targets (CBT) were extracted from probabilistic maps, their borders must be defined using arbitrary probability thresholds. The threshold choice will inherently affect the size of the target volume and its overlap percentage with the atlas based nuclei, e.g., a lower connectivity threshold will result in higher overlap between subjects, but the volume will be less specific to the targeted anatomical location. To achieve identical criteria for the threshold ranges across the study subjects, we used a range of percentile values of all non-zero voxel intensities to cut-off the connectivity values from the 50th to the 100th percentile, thereby selecting the voxels with the highest probability of connection to the cortical target regions. In practice, 50th percentile threshold meant that a large volume of the CBT is kept including regions of low probability of being interconnected to the relevant cortical region, while a 100th percentile threshold corresponded to the point which had the largest probability of connection to its target. All overlap and distance metrics were iteratively determined over this entire range of values. The dependency of the overlap with anatomical landmarks and the reproducibility was tested by using the following quantitative metrics:

1. Euclidian distance (mm) between the center-of-gravity (mid-point) point of the CBT and the relevant atlas targets. The coordinates for the center-of-gravity points of the

thresholded connectivity maps and the atlas targets were calculated using the *fslstats* tool in the FSL software package.
2. Volumetric overlap between the CBT and atlas targets, determined by the Dice overlap (0–1), The Dice overlap coefficient D was defined as:

$$D = \frac{2|X \cap Y|}{|X| + |Y|}$$

where X and Y are the two volume sets to be compared.

The first metric assumes that we use point-like targets, either determined by connectivity or a 3D atlas model, the latter assumes that the targets consist of volumetric label maps relevant for surgical localization. Quantitative evaluations of the connectivity maps and 3D voxelised atlas volumes and the visualizations were carried out with Matlab R2010a for Windows (The Mathworks Inc., Nattick, MA, USA) using in-house developed algorithms.

RESULTS

Correspondence of Thalamic Connectivity-Based Subdivisions to Atlas-Based Landmarks

The center-of-gravity points of the connectivity maps were located inside the atlas based targets in all cases and all scans. Center-of-gravity points are organized according to somatotopy along the lateral border of the thalamus, such that the connections to precentral gyrus are more anterior than the postcentral gyrus connections. In the present study, we described the correspondence of the VL_{pv} nucleus to two CBTs: the CBT using the precentral gyrus as target ("precentral connections") and the CBT using a more extended *a priori* target list of the VL_{pv} nucleus ("VL_{pv} connections").

While there was a good agreement of the volumes along the antero-posterior axis of the most lateral parts of the thalamus, the connectivity patterns did not overlap with the medial parts of the VL_{pv} or VPL nucleus, and only partially overlap with more medially located thalamic nuclei with known motor connectivity, such as the centro-median (CM) nucleus. In the midline, the VL_{pv} was oriented more anteriorly, while the CBT defined this nucleus differently: the connectivity-based segment appeared wedge-shaped (**Figures 1** and **2**), with the tip oriented toward the center of the thalamus.

The mid-point distances between CBT and the anatomical target for the VL_{pv} nucleus were lowest on the population level when the connectivity maps were thresholded at the 65–70th percentile (left side) and between the 80th and 90th percentile (right side), and remained below 2.5 mm if the threshold was set to lower than the 85th percentile on the left side and 92nd percentile on the right side (**Figure 1D**). The VL_{pv} nucleus overlapped modestly with the CBT, demonstrating greater overlap in the lateral thalamus regions (**Figure 1C**). While the lateral segments were correctly matched visually to the VL_{pv} nucleus, the maximum value of the Dice coefficient was modest, median $D = 0.32$ (right side, threshold: 87th percentile) and median $D = 0.30$ (left side, threshold: 90th percentile). While the calculations were carried out in MNI152 standard and symmetrical template space, and the thalamic seed volumes were also symmetric, we noted an apparent left–right difference between the CBT volumes (**Figures 1A,B**). Regarding other nuclei that showed minimal overlap with the CBT of the VL_{pv}: the CM nucleus showed no consistent overlap with the CBT volume (neither using VL_{pv}, nor the precentral targets), and only moderate overlap was observed in the most medial regions of the CBTs.

The precentral connections also showed moderate overlap with the atlas based VL_{pv} volume (**Figure 2**): the CBT calculated using a single precentral target region overlapped slightly more with the atlas target compared to the CBT defined with additional (cerebellar, supplementary motor and primary motor) targets, and no interhemispheric asymmetry was observed (**Figure 2B**). Using a threshold at the 89th percentile (left side) and 88th percentile (right side), a median Dice overlap of 0.34 and 0.31 was measured on the left and right sides, respectively (**Figure 2C**). The pointwise distances from the atlas based targets were in the range of 2.2–3 mm in the connectivity range between the 70th and 86th percentiles (**Figure 2D**).

In comparison with the previous two targets, the overlap between the postcentral gyrus connections and the atlas based VPL_p (and VPL_a) was larger (**Figure 3**). The mid-point distances between CBT and anatomical target for the VPL nucleus were lowest on the population level when the connectivity maps were thresholded at the 90th percentile, with median distances of 2.1 mm for the left and 2.4 mm for the right side (**Figure 3C**). The volumetric overlap between the CBT and the ABT for the VPL nucleus was generally higher than in the other examined thalamic nuclei. Consistent with results from the other nuclei, the maximum overlap was achieved by thresholding around the 90th percentile of the connectivity values (**Figure 3D**).

Selecting the Optimal Connectivity Threshold for Connectivity-Based Targets

Our results suggest that while the agreement with the atlas targets is higher if the connectivity threshold is increased (for example, a maximum is seen in **Figure 3C** at the 90th percentile threshold), the inter-subject reproducibility was decreased at larger connectivity thresholds. Therefore, it was necessary to determine a consensual cut-off value which represents a trade-off between the two feasibility metrics. First, we investigated the effect of connectivity probability thresholding on the expected reproducibility of CBT maps. The lower the connectivity threshold, the higher the inter-subject overlap (**Figure 4A**). This means, however, that the CBTs become less specific for the given neurosurgical target: as the connectivity threshold values converge to zero, almost the entire thalamus is included as a potential target volume, which is anatomically incorrect. In order to find the optimal connectivity-based threshold, representing a compromise between larger inter-subject reproducibility and larger overlap with the atlas target, we multiplied the two overlap metrics and located the maximum value of this combined metric (**Figure 4**). To provide a consensual value, we multiplied the median values of population-overlaps and the median values of

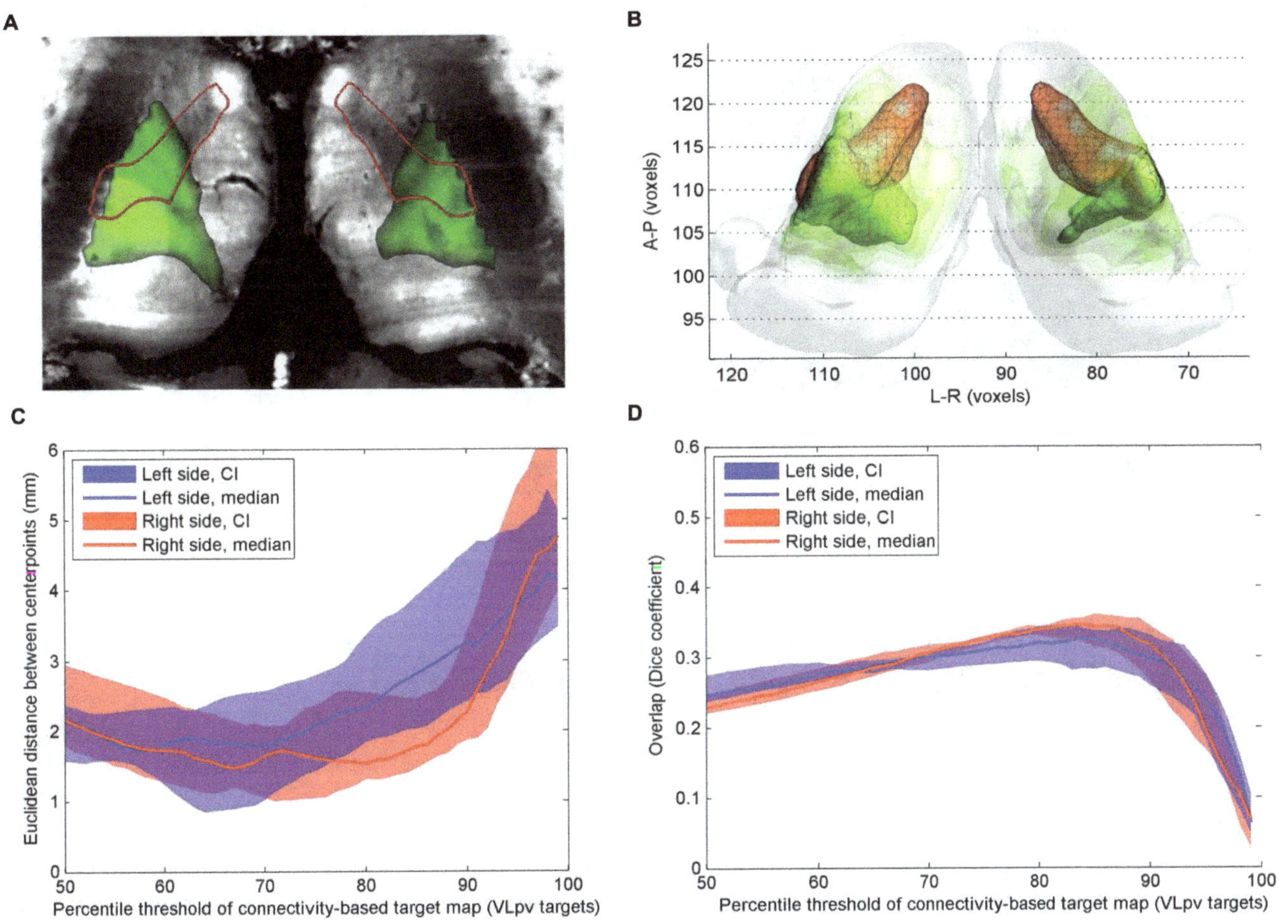

FIGURE 1 | Comparison of atlas and CBTs of the VL_{pv} nucleus. (A) Cross-sectional image derived from histological sections, in standard space (Big Brain Atlas, Amunts et al., 2013) with VL_{pv} overlaid (red outlines) and the CBT (green color scale); **(B)** 3D visualization of the CBT and atlas targets: connectivity-based targets were visualized in green color with different opacities reflecting to the summed probability across the study population (50–95th percentile range) while the VL_{pv} was depicted in red 3D mesh; **(C)** Euclidian distance of the center-of-gravity of the CBT to the atlas based target: dependency on the applied threshold values; **(D)** volumetric overlap with atlas based targets: dependency on the applied threshold.

the correspondence to the anatomical atlas. In a similar manner as for the overlap with the anatomical target (**Figure 4B**), the consensus metric also had a maximum, which was used to determine the optimal cut-off value (**Figure 4C**).

The optimal connectivity threshold values were the following. VL_{pv} left: 80th percentile; VL_{pv} right: 76th percentile; precentral CBT left: 90th percentile; precentral CBT right: 84th percentile; postcentral CBT left: 89th percentile; postcentral CBT right: 89th percentile. Throughout the study, these optimized cut-off values are used for visualization and further evaluation of reproducibility.

Reconstruction of the Cerebello-Thalamic Tract: Tractography-Based Anatomy

The CTT was reconstructed for each of the 10 datasets of the four participants. The typical trajectory of the DTI based reconstruction was the following. The tract emerged from the ipsilateral dentate nucleus, crossed to the opposite hemisphere at the level of superior cerebellar peduncle, and then passes medially and across the red nucleus. Cross-sectional images with annotations of the thalamic nuclei and major anatomical landmarks are shown in **Figure 5A**. The intra-thalamic terminations of the CTT overlapped with the VL_{pv} nucleus, but due to the technical limitations of DTI tractography, the CTT fibers appeared outside the thalamus and subthalamus, and continued to a diverse set of supratentorial areas. In order to provide plausible visualizations of the tract, we limited the field of view to the subthalamus and thalamus. A notable left–right asymmetry was detected on the population level, in which the right CTT (originating from left cerebellum) was found to be more strongly connected to its pathway targets. Compared to the intra-thalamic targets, the CTT reconstruction showed significantly larger variability across the population. In some cases, the pathway was split and alternative routes were taken, possibly due to errors in the estimation of crossing fibers. In some cases, zero or a very low inter-subject overlap was reported using

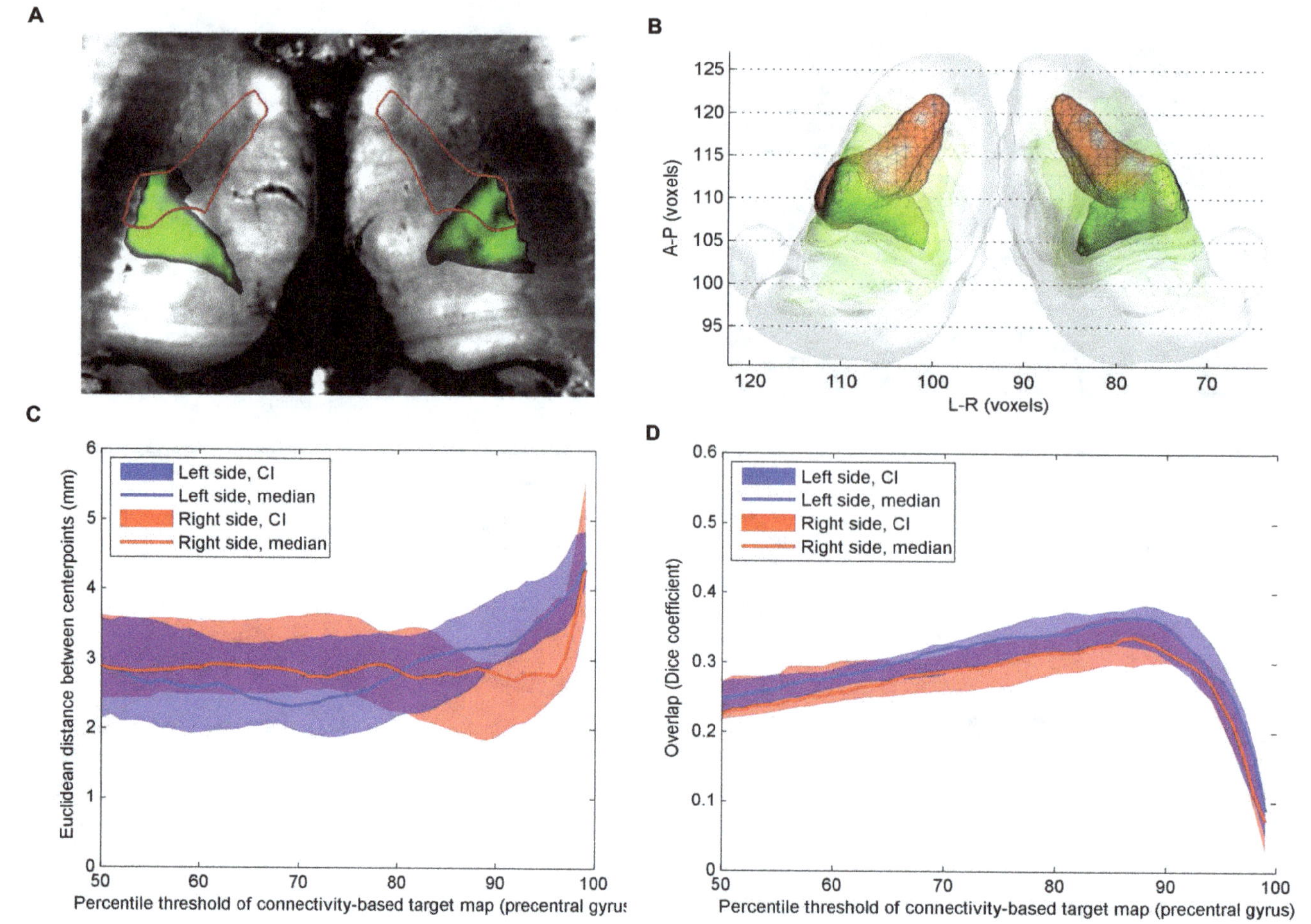

FIGURE 2 | Comparison of atlas based VL_{pv} nucleus and CBT using precentral gyrus connections. (A) Cross-sectional image derived from histological sections, in standard space (Big Brain Atlas, Amunts et al., 2013) with VL_{pv} overlaid (red outlines) and the CBT from the precentral gyrus (green color scale); **(B)** 3D visualization of the CBT and atlas targets: connectivity-based targets were visualized in green color with different opacities reflecting to the summed probability across the study population (50–95th percentile range) while the VL_{pv} was depicted in red 3D mesh; **(C)** Euclidian distance of the center-of-gravity of the CBT to the atlas based target: dependency on the applied threshold values; **(D)** volumetric overlap with atlas based targets: dependency on the applied threshold.

the 95th percentile of connectivity values, possibly due to splitting of the pathway into alternative routes, or due to the diminished sensitivity of locating the fibers at a single connectivity threshold. As observed for the intra-thalamic CBTs, the inter-scanner variability was similar to the inter-subject variability (**Table 2**).

Reproducibility of Connectivity-Based Targets

While the pre- and postcentral gyrus CBT were largely reproducible across different scanners (**Figures 6A,B,E,F**), the VL_{pv} CBT showed considerable variability (**Figures 6C,D**), as well as a larger volume and a modest interhemispheric asymmetry. We investigated the inter-scanner reproducibility of the CBT structures by comparing both the volumetric overlaps and the center-point distances. The maximum of the volumetric overlap was observed at similar connectivity percentiles as in the previous experiments; however, the center-point distances measured showed considerable differences between scanners of different vendors. The results obtained from Scanner 1 were found to match better the center-points of the ABTs, and the minimum Euclidean distances were below 2 mm when the CBT was thresholded at the 75th percentile. A similar effect was not observed using the data from the other two scanners. The volumetric overlaps for each of the 3 CBTs showed similar curves with maximum peaks at 90–95th percentiles. As summarized in **Table 2**, the overlap between CBTs across all subjects and scans was between 58 and 69% for the thalamic targets. When decoupling the variability into inter-subject within-scanner and intra-subject inter-scanner variability, we observed that for most of the structures, the inter-subject overlap was similar to the inter-scanner variability. Only in the case of the postcentral gyrus connections were the inter-scanner variability significantly higher (**Table 2**), meaning that the vendor type (Scanners 1–3) caused more variability than the anatomical differences between individuals after non-linear standardization.

While the thalamic CBTs were defined by setting a cut-off value of connection probability based on the optimization step

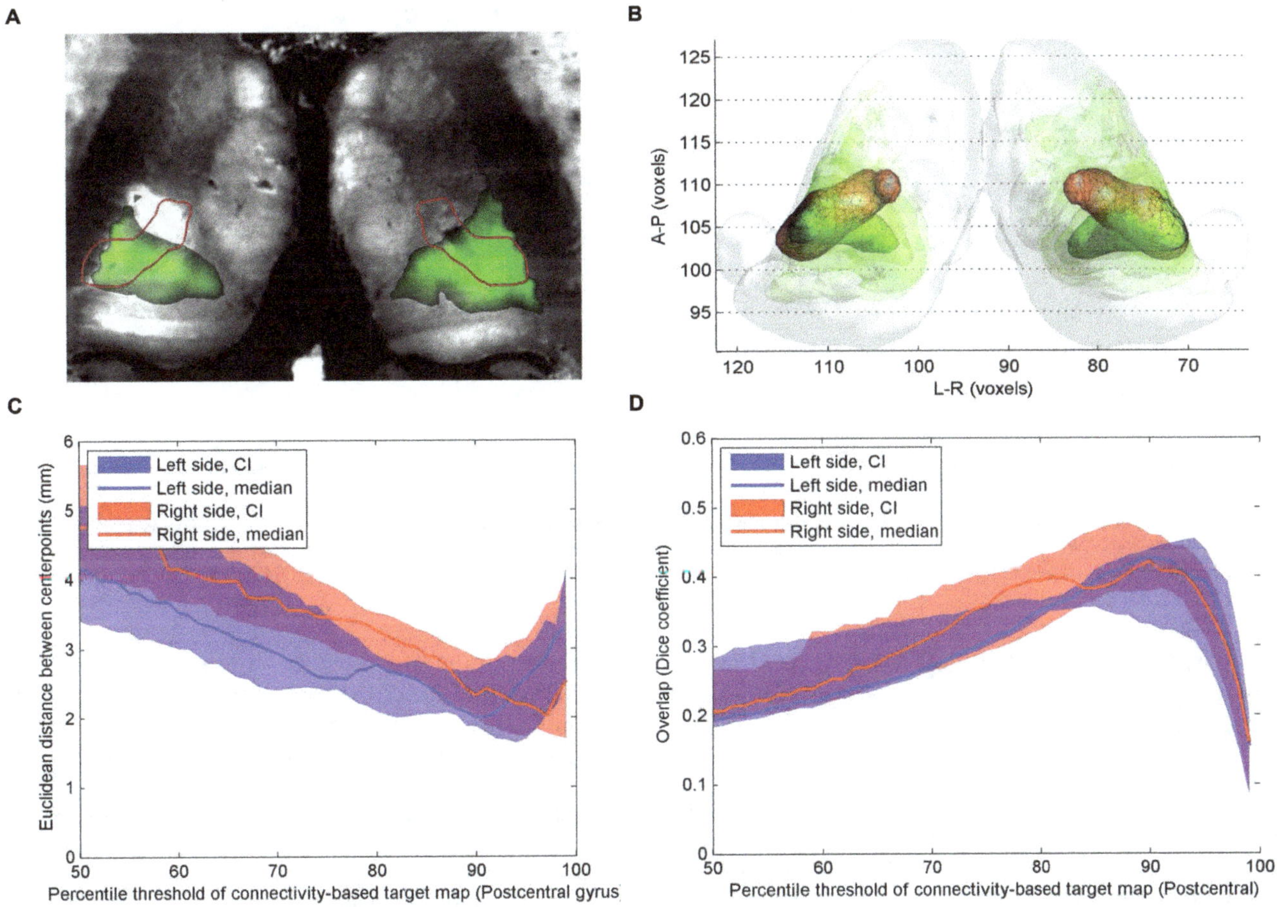

FIGURE 3 | Comparison of atlas based VPL_p nucleus and CBT using postcentral gyrus connections. (A) Cross-sectional image derived from histological sections, in standard space (Big Brain Atlas, Amunts et al., 2013) with VPL_p overlaid (red outlines) and the CBT from the postcentral gyrus (green color scale); **(B)** 3D visualization of the CBT and atlas targets: connectivity-based targets were visualized in green color with different opacities reflecting to the summed probability across the study population (50–95th percentile range) while the VPL_p was depicted in red 3D mesh; **(C)** Euclidian distance of the center-of-gravity of the CBT to the atlas based target: dependency on the applied threshold values; **(D)** volumetric overlap with atlas based targets: dependency on the applied threshold.

described above, we were not able to perform this optimization step for the CTT due to its specific shape and configuration. Since the CTT showed less variability in the sub-thalamic region, we decided to calculate the variability measures after restricting the volume of the tract to a 40 mm subvolume symmetrically around the AC-PC plane, which is most commonly used for neurosurgical targeting (20 mm ventral and 20 mm dorsal). After limiting to this volume and setting the connectivity value to the top 90th percentile of connections, a low overlap was observed for the CTT (**Table 2**). The CTT was significantly more reproducible across subjects on the right side (D = 37.4%) than on the left (20.7%), and the left CTT showed a similar phenomenon to the intrathalamic targets in that the inter-scanner variability exceeded the inter-subject variability.

DISCUSSION

The use of DTI based tractography of thalamocortical connections and the CTT for visualization of neurosurgical targets must be preceded by validation efforts that evaluate the technical feasibility in the clinical setting. By reconstructing various subdivisions of the thalamus in volunteers, we were able to quantify the overlap and pointwise distances to atlas-based anatomical targets. A particularly challenging aspect is to capture the population variability and scanner dependency of such reconstructions, and to the best of our knowledge, no previous study has tested the scanner dependency of these neurosurgically relevant thalamic and subthalamic structures. During this step, we optimized threshold values that delineated the connectivity based intrathalamic maps to obtain a volume: while the population variability was lower when lower thresholds were applied, the correspondence to the anatomical target was higher when applying higher connection thresholds. This effect appeared to have a maximum and therefore an optimal connection threshold could be determined. The same procedure was not possible for the CTT, as we do not have digitized 3D atlas data for this structure.

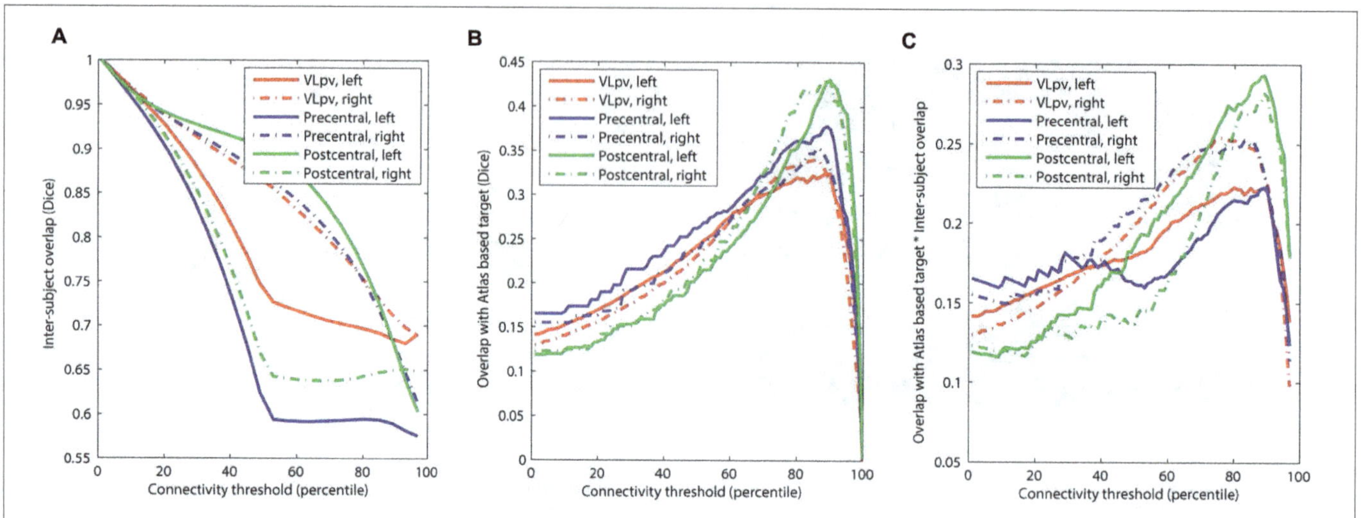

FIGURE 4 | Optimization of the connectivity threshold applied to connectivity based intrathalamic targets. (A) Inter-subject overlap as a function of the applied connectivity threshold; **(B)** overlap with anatomical atlas as a function of the applied connectivity threshold; **(C)** determining the population-level optimal threshold value as a maximum point of the function.

Functional Neurosurgical Targets in the Thalamus: Feasibility of the Tractography Based Approach

For reconstructing the fiber pathways that are interconnected with the thalamus, we chose to use probabilistic diffusion tractography. The first reports have confirmed that this technique is capable of resolving the complex within-voxel orientations of fibers within the gray-matter rich thalamus (Behrens et al., 2003a; Johansen-Berg et al., 2005), and that probabilistic tractography yields major advantages over deterministic approaches despite the much higher computational load (Descoteaux et al., 2009). For example, when estimating the orientation density function (i.e., the distribution of possible fiber direction within an image pixel), the deterministic approach only takes the most probable diffusion orientation, while the probabilistic framework models more complex fiber geometries, such as fanning, crossing or splaying. On the other hand, probabilistic tractography suffers from connectivity values that decrease with the distance from the initial seed point due to the fanning of fiber bundles (Descoteaux et al., 2009).

The reported overlap of the atlas volumes and the CBTs inside the thalamus was consistently lower than 50%, which can be explained by the known anatomical structure of the thalamus: while the lateral, especially ventrolateral parts of the thalamus have point-to-point interconnections with the cortex, the more medial zones have diffuse connectivity, such as the CM or centrolateral nucleus (Kievit and Kuypers, 1977; Morel et al., 1997). It is likely that diffusion based techniques are only able to resolve the anisotropically organized axons within the thalamus, which do not form well circumscribed subdomains, but rather show a gradient of connections on the antero-posterior axis. These anisotropic structures mix with the afferent fibers of the thalamus, which are located more ventrally. This error presumably also stemmed from the fact that diffusion tractography cannot distinguish between afferent and efferent connectivity and hence the projections of the thalamus in the two directions (i.e., the cortex and spinal cord) cannot be separated. Compared to the connectivity based volumes, the VL_{pv} nucleus appears larger and extends more dorsomedially in the reconstruction in **Figures 1** and **2**. However, it has been shown by microelectrode recordings in tremor that the associated rhythmic burst was found in a restricted area of the ventrointermedius nucleus, and only the lateral and ventrocaudal part of each nucleus, which was defined as the kinesthetic zone, was involved (Ohye et al., 1993).

Our results indicate that the Euclidian distance to the centerpoint of the atlas volume can be kept below 2.5 mm by applying optimized threshold values. This distance was considerably larger than the reported distances to experimentally defined target locations during surgery; for example, Pouratian et al. (2011) found DTI derived connections to be 0.36 mm away from the optimal stimulation sites. It is likely, however, that the centerpoints of the atlas based targets do not represent the optimal stimulation sites and therefore our results may underestimate the accuracy obtained with tractography. The localization of effective tremor treatment sites, therefore, might be better reflected in the thalamocortical connectivity patterns than the exact borders of the cytoarchitecturally determined areas. This is also supported by studies that compared the adjacency of the target site to reconstructed fibers (Owen et al., 2008; Coenen et al., 2011b; Hunsche et al., 2013; Torres et al., 2014), and by studies that evaluated the network emerging from the stimulation sites (Klein et al., 2012).

In most previous studies, the CBTs were defined using a single target region of interest within the cortex, although there is experimental support from imaging studies that the Vim or VL_{pv} nucleus has dominant connections beyond those of the primary motor cortex. For example, Hyam et al. (2012) showed that the Vim has high connection densities to the cerebellum, as well as to

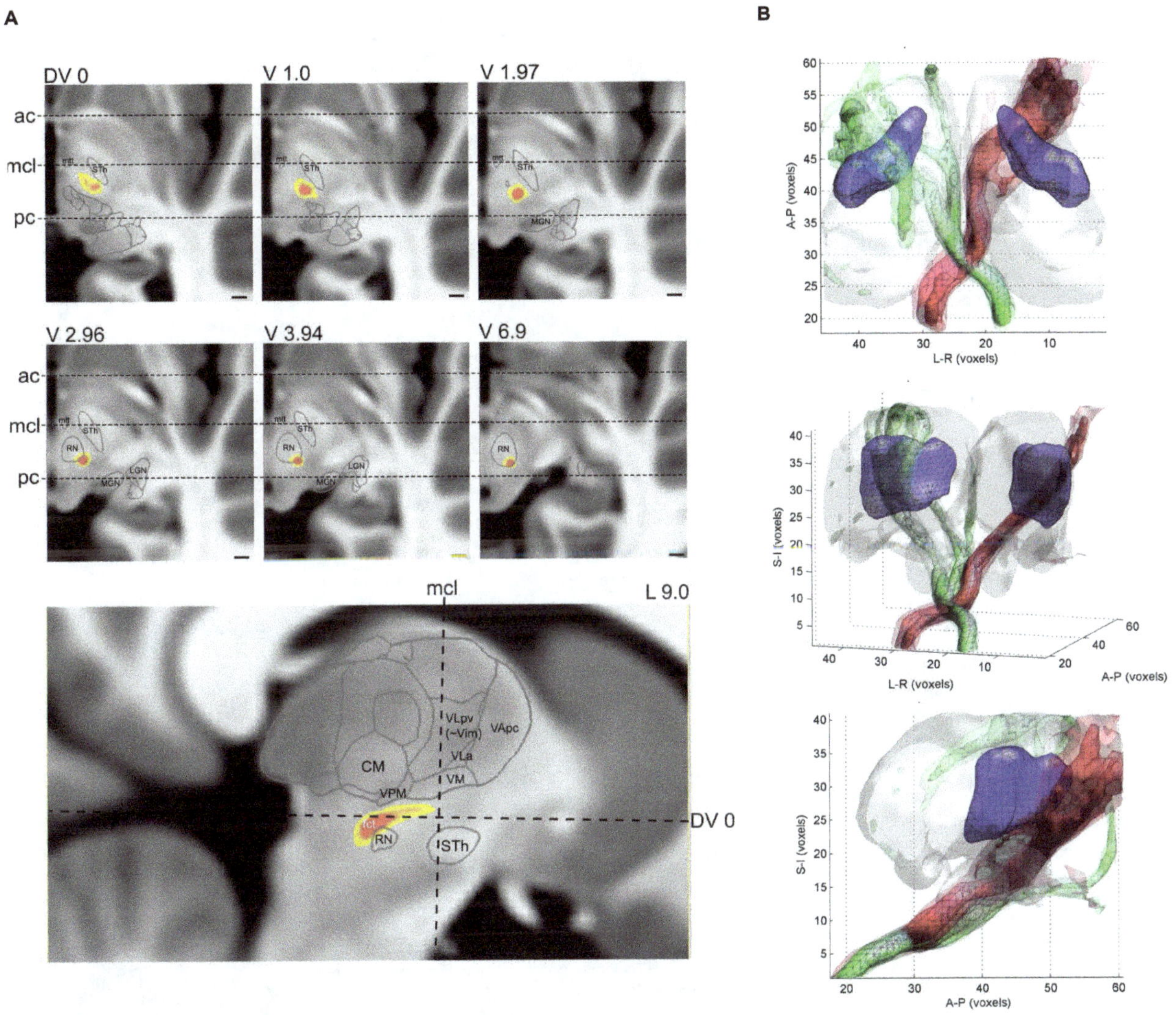

FIGURE 5 | Reconstruction of the CTT with diffusion tractography. (A) population-averaged connectivity map (yellow-red color) overlaid onto a cross-sectional image (T1-weighted MRI). Slice levels are relative to the AC-PC plane, and three major anatomical landmarks have been annotated, ac, anterior commissure, mcl, mid-commissural line, pc, posterior commissure. **(B)** 3D visualization of the population-averaged CTT. Different opacities correspond to the population probability from 50th percentile to 90th percentile.

the premotor and dorsolateral prefrontal cortex. This observation motivated us to use a more extended list of targets when back-projecting the connections into the thalamus: namely, in addition to the precentral gyrus, the cerebellum and premotor region were added. We observed that these additional target regions did decrease the center-point distance to the atlas-based target (**Figure 1**), but did not increase the overall reproducibility of the CBT. Furthermore, we observed interhemispheric asymmetry in the VL_{pv} CBT reconstruction, which was not the case when using only the precentral gyrus as remote connection target.

While a general good inter-patient reproducibility was found for the thalamic connectivity-based segmentations (Traynor et al., 2010; O'Muircheartaigh et al., 2011), especially for the lateral thalamus, little information is known about the dependency of scanner and sequence parameters. Interestingly, our study revealed that small differences in sequence settings and vendor-specific, underlying MR technology can contribute significant variability to the observed connectivity structure. In fact, the variability caused by scanner differences appeared to be similar or larger than the inter-subject variability within one scanner (precentral connections: 57–60% overlap between repeated scans on different scanners, 63-65% overlap between subjects on the same scanners, see **Table 2**). The non-linear matching used to normalize images to MNI space should reduce the inter-subject variability, but the uncertainty of the registration algorithm cannot be separated easily from the other apparent sources of variability, and significant inter-scanner variability remained even after normalization. The exact source of this inter-scanner variability is unknown, but may arise from a number of different hardware and software factors.

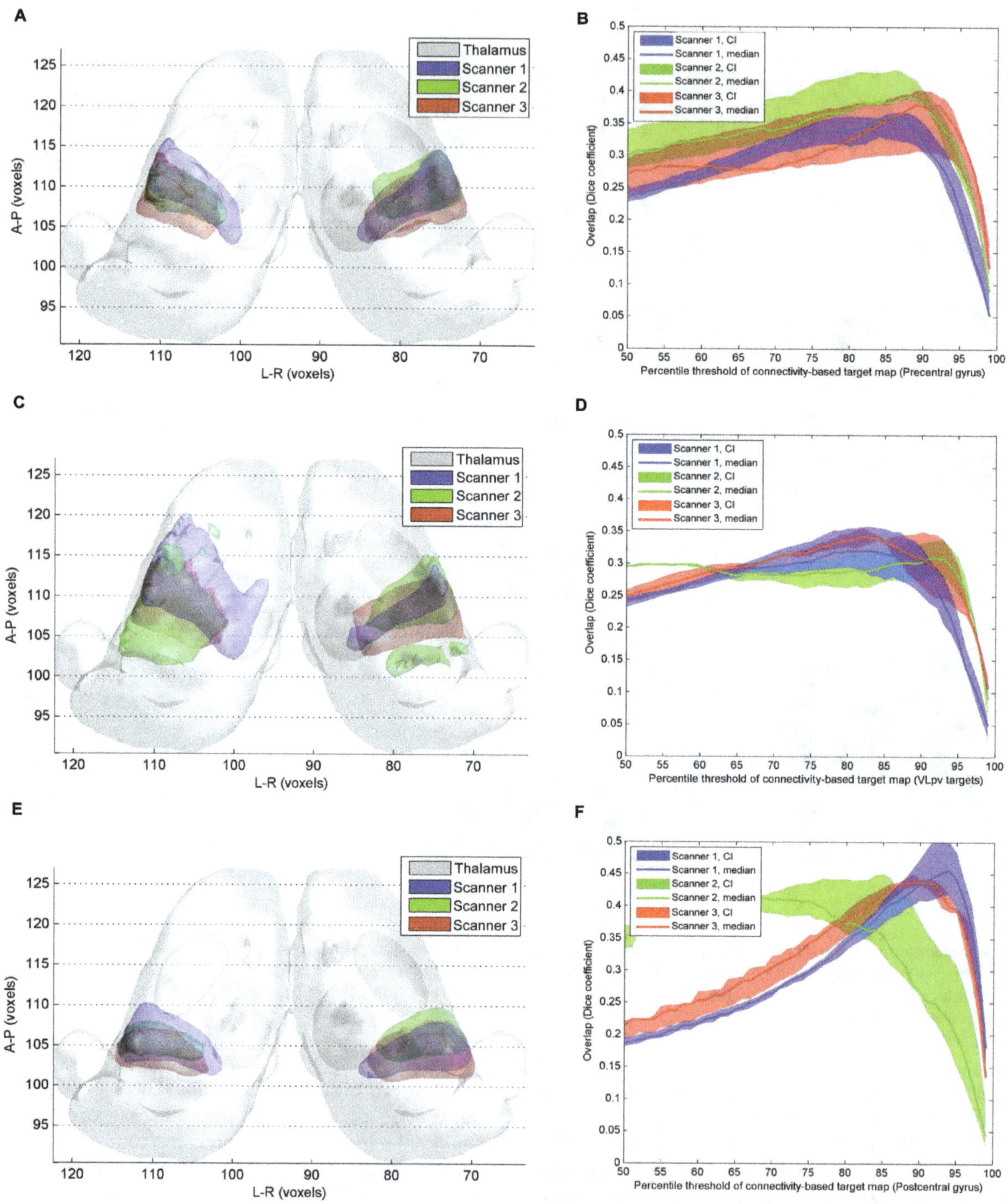

FIGURE 6 | Inter-scanner reproducibility of connectivity based intrathalamic targets. (A) 3D visualization of the inter-scanner variability of precentral CBT over the study population; **(C)** 3D visualization of the inter-scanner variability of VLpv CBT over the study population; **(E)** 3D visualization of the inter-scanner variability of VPLp CBT over the study population; **(B)** dependency of the inter-scanner variability of the precentral CBT volume on the applied connectivity threshold; **(D)** dependency of the inter-scanner variability of the VLpv CBT volume on the applied connectivity threshold; **(F)** dependency of the inter-scanner variability of the VPLp CBT volume on the applied connectivity threshold.

While some vendors use a spectrospatial (water excitation) pulse for fat suppression, others use fat saturation methods, resulting in different limitations on the minimum slice thickness allowed. Differences in these excitation pulses, coupled with differences in gradient design, geometric distortion, and the use of wide vs. narrow bore systems may contribute to the

TABLE 2 | Reproducibility measures of the CBTs: inter-subject and inter-scanner variability.

Thalamic nucleus, CBT	Within-subject, inter-scanner overlap (Dice, mean ± *SD*)	Inter-subject, within-scanner overlap (Dice, mean ± *SD*)	Difference between inter-scanner and inter-subject variability (*p*-value)	Overall overlap (Dice, mean ± *SD*)
Left VL_{pv}-proper	0.651 ± 0.112	0.720 ± 0.123	$p = 0.195$	0.662 ± 0.129
Right VL_{pv}-proper	0.703 ± 0.065	0.712 ± 0.095	$p = 0.806$	0693 ± 0.084
Left VL_{pv}-precentral	0.567 ± 0.141	0.631 ± 0.069	$p = 0.235$	0.580 ± 0.119
Right VL_{pv}-precentral	0.603 ± 0.082	0.651 ± 0.087	$p = 0.209$	0.587 ± 0.121
Left VPL_{p}-postcentral	0.745 ± 0.059	0.583 ± 0.159	$p = 0.0166$*	0.637 ± 0.136
Right VPL_{p}-postcentral	0.429 ± 0.103	0.331 ± 0.09	$p = 0.0325$*	0.641 ± 0.109
Left CTT	0.263 ± 0.369	0.213 ± 0.223	$p = 0.728$	0.239 ± 0.253
Right CTT	0.240 ± 0.364	0.328 ± 0.358	$p = 0.586$	0.261 ± 0.296

**Significant result, $p \leq 0.05$.*

observed inter-scanner variability, but future studies would be needed to elucidate further the sources of this observed variability. This inter-scanner variability further underscores the sensitivity of DTI and connectivity derived measures to sequence parameters and hardware parameters (Pfefferbaum et al., 2003; Takao et al., 2011, 2012; Bonilha et al., 2015; Kuhn et al., 2015).

Targeting the Cerebello-Thalamic Tract Using Tractography

Using the seed and target list known from the literature (Kwon et al., 2011), we were able to reconstruct the 3D trajectory of the CTT (**Figure 5**) using current standard clinical DTI protocols. The trajectory is similar to what we know about the anatomy of this tract, especially in the subthalamic region: after crossing to the contralateral hemisphere, the tract projects into the thalamus by passing near the red nucleus and sending collaterals to it, and the tract is generally located posterior to the mid-commissural line around the AC-PC plane (Gallay et al., 2008; Kwon et al., 2011). This observation is in line with observations from studies that aimed to reconstruct the dentate-rubro-thalamic connections in clinical datasets. We were unable to compare the CTT volume to atlas derived data, and to the best of our knowledge, no such studies have yet been performed, although many authors aimed to correlate the effective treatment site location to the reconstructed DTI-based target. For example, Coenen and colleagues showed the feasibility of the CTT mapping in tremor alleviation in case reports (Coenen et al., 2011a,b), and in a group of 11 patients (Coenen et al., 2014). In their study, effective contacts were located in proximity to the DRT; in moderate tremor reduction, the target fields were centered on its anterior border while in good and excellent tremor reduction, the target fields focused on its center. While Schlaier et al. (2015) were able to reconstruct the CTT in 90% of their subjects, they concluded that contacts closer to the tract did not provide better clinical effects than distant contacts. In our study, a low reproducibility was found for the tract, even after limiting the field of interest to a limited supero-inferior range near the AC-PC plane. This further highlights the challenge of using routine clinical DTI scans to reconstruct this tract, and indicates that further tests of reproducibility and sequence dependency are needed. We assume that by using high angular imaging, the complex white matter anatomy of the subthalamic region can better be reconstructed.

Study Limitations

Our study is limited by the small number of volunteers for whom we were able to acquire repeated DTI scans. This particularly limits our capability to test inter-subject variability and to decouple the variability caused by anatomical differences from the repeatability of imaging, uncertainty of fiber tracking and errors of image co-registration.

A major limitation in our study is the lack of ground truth information on thalamic fibers and the lack of population-wide histology-based atlases of white matter structures. This limits the generalisability of our validation: although we used a shape model that incorporated variability (Krauth et al., 2010; Jakab et al., 2012), it remains questionable if the mean volume in standard neuroimaging space is acceptable as a reference. It is particularly challenging to relate the diffusion tractography based structures to histological atlas. To achieve this goal, pre- or post mortem diffusion imaging with feasible image quality is needed, ideally with manual delineation of stained sections and a histological work-up identical to those in the classical atlases. Therefore, despite the technical feasibility of the tractography method, the present results do not encourage any changes to current practice in functional neurosurgery, rather they indicate that more comparative studies between MR and gold-standard anatomical or histopathological imaging are required.

While our study aimed to evaluate clinically feasible imaging protocols, such as the widely used 32-direction DTI, we assume that higher angular resolution diffusion datasets will reduce the variability associated with imaging, and will also allow us to resolve the challenging fiber anatomy of the thalamic and subthalamic region more accurately. For this, more sophisticated diffusion models and the resolution of multiple crossing fiber populations are necessary (Behrens et al., 2007).

Our study is further limited by its exploratory nature, and specifically the small participant group size. The widespread usage of probabilistic diffusion tractography for defining intra-thalamic and cerebello-thalamic targets must be preceded by large, preferably multi-centric validation efforts that test the technique during interventions and compare the results to those of the standard target localization methods. Furthermore, the inter-surgeon variability should also be evaluated, which can be a critical point when applying localization approaches that rely heavily on image processing with complex parameter settings.

CONCLUSION

In this pilot study, we demonstrated the reproducibility of DTI based tractography to map targets with relevance to preoperative planning. The accuracy with regard to the center-points of atlas-based targets was around 2.5 mm, and a relatively low volumetric overlap of 35–40% was observed. We conclude that the connectivity based subdivisions can only predict the lateral and ventral segments of the Vim or VL_{pv} nucleus and the postcentral connections emerging from the VPL nucleus. The applicability of connectivity-based segmentation methods with the current clinical sequence parameters is further limited by large scanner-to-scanner variability of the CBTs. Further investigations using higher angular resolution DTI are needed to elucidate the sources of this variability and to assess the precise contribution of subject-to-subject anatomical variability.

AUTHOR CONTRIBUTION

AJ, BW, EM, JT, TY, GS, and RT designed the study. AJ has written the manuscript, performed the analysis and created figures. KK has performed the analysis and contributed to the manuscript. RT has acquired data and contributed to the manuscript. EM has written the manuscript and provided expert consultation. MP has acquired data and provided expert consultation. All authors have read and edited the manuscript.

ACKNOWLEDGMENTS

AJ is supported by the European Union FP7 Marie Curie IEF Research grant FABRIC – , exploring the "Formation and Adaptation of the Brain Connectome," grant no. 2012-PIEF-GA-33003. This project was also supported from a UCL/ZNZ Collaboration grant, awarded to RT and TY.

SUPPLEMENTARY MATERIAL

FIGURE S1 | The statistical shape model based atlas of the human thalamus used in our study.

FIGURE S2 | Reconstruction of the CTT using diffusion tractography. 3D visualization of the seed and waypoint target regions used during fiber tracking.

REFERENCES

Amami, P., Dekker, I., Piacentini, S., Ferre, F., Romito, L. M., Franzini, A., et al. (2015). Impulse control behaviours in patients with parkinson's disease after subthalamic deep brain stimulation: de novo cases and 3-year follow-up. *J. Neurol. Neurosurg. Psychiatry* 86, 562–564. doi: 10.1136/jnnp-2013-307214

Amunts, K., Lepage, C., Borgeat, L., Mohlberg, H., Dickscheid, T., Rousseau, M. E., et al. (2013). BigBrain: an ultrahigh-resolution 3D human brain model. *Science* 340, 1472–1475. doi: 10.1126/science.1235381

Anthofer, J., Steib, K., Fellner, C., Lange, M., Brawanski, A., and Schlaier, J. (2014). The variability of atlas-based targets in relation to surrounding major fibre tracts in thalamic deep brain stimulation. *Acta Neurochir. (Wien)* 156, 1497–1504; discussion 1504. doi: 10.1007/s00701-014-2103-z

Avecillas-Chasin, J. M., Alonso-Frech, F., Parras, O., Del Prado, N., and Barcia, J. A. (2015). Assessment of a method to determine deep brain stimulation targets using deterministic tractography in a navigation system. *Neurosurg. Rev.* 38, 739–750; discussion 751. doi: 10.1007/s10143-015-0643-1

Avecillas-Chasin, J. M., Rascon-Ramirez, F., and Barcia, J. A. (2016). Tractographical model of the cortico-basal ganglia and corticothalamic connections: improving our understanding of deep brain stimulation. *Clin. Anat.* 29, 481–492. doi: 10.1002/ca.22689

Baizabal-Carvallo, J. F., and Jankovic, J. (2016). Movement disorders induced by deep brain stimulation. *Parkinsonism Relat. Disord.* 25, 1–9. doi: 10.1016/j.parkreldis.2016.01.014

Baizabal-Carvallo, J. F., Kagnoff, M. N., Jimenez-Shahed, J., Fekete, R., and Jankovic, J. (2014). The safety and efficacy of thalamic deep brain stimulation in essential tremor: 10 years and beyond. *J. Neurol. Neurosurg. Psychiatry* 85, 567–572. doi: 10.1136/jnnp-2013-304943

Basser, P. J., Pajevic, S., Pierpaoli, C., Duda, J., and Aldroubi, A. (2000). In vivo fiber tractography using DT-MRI data. *Magn. Reson. Med.* 44, 625–632. doi: 10.1002/1522-2594(200010)44:4<625::AID-MRM17>3.0.CO;2-O

Basser, P. J., and Pierpaoli, C. (1996). Microstructural and physiological features of tissues elucidated by quantitative-diffusion-tensor MRI. *J. Magn. Reson. Ser. B* 111, 209–219. doi: 10.1006/jmrb.1996.0086

Behrens, T. E. J., Berg, H. J., Jbabdi, S., Rushworth, M. F. S., and Woolrich, M. W. (2007). Probabilistic diffusion tractography with multiple fibre orientations: what can we gain? *Neuroimage* 34, 144–155. doi: 10.1016/j.neuroimage.2006.09.018

Behrens, T. E. J., Johansen-Berg, H., Woolrich, M. W., Smith, S. M., Wheeler-Kingshott, C., Boulby, P. A., et al. (2003a). Non-invasive mapping of connections between human thalamus and cortex using diffusion imaging. *Nat. Neurosci.* 6, 750–757. doi: 10.1038/nn1075 r

Behrens, T. E. J., Woolrich, M. W., Jenkinson, M., Johansen-Berg, H., Nunes, R. G., Clare, S., et al. (2003b). Characterization and propagation of uncertainty in diffusion-weighted MR imaging. *Magn. Reson. Med.* 50, 1077–1088. doi: 10.1002/mrm.10609

Benabid, A. L., Pollak, P., Gao, D., Hoffmann, D., Limousin, P., Gay, E., et al. (1996). Chronic electrical stimulation of the ventralis intermedius nucleus of the thalamus as a treatment of movement disorders. *J. Neurosurg.* 84, 203–214. doi: 10.3171/jns.1996.84.2.0203

Blanc, R., Reyes, M., Seiler, C., and Szekely, G. (2009). Conditional variability of statistical shape models based on surrogate variables. *Med. Image Comput. Comput. Assist. Interv.* 12, 84–91.

Bonilha, L., Gleichgerrcht, E., Fridriksson, J., Rorden, C., Breedlove, J. L., Nesland, T., et al. (2015). Reproducibility of the structural brain connectome derived from diffusion tensor imaging. *PLoS ONE* 10:e0135247. doi: 10.1371/journal.pone.0135247

Butson, C. R., Cooper, S. E., Henderson, J. M., and McIntyre, C. C. (2006). Predicting the effects of deep brain stimulation with diffusion tensor based electric field models. *Med. Image Comput. Comput. Assist. Interv.* 9, 429–437.

Chopra, A., Tye, S. J., Lee, K. H., Sampson, S., Matsumoto, J., Adams, A., et al. (2012). Underlying neurobiology and clinical correlates of mania status after subthalamic nucleus deep brain stimulation in parkinson's disease: a review of the literature. *J. Neuropsychiatry Clin. Neurosci.* 24, 102–110. doi: 10.1176/appi.neuropsych.10070109

Coenen, V. A., Allert, N., and Madler, B. (2011a). A role of diffusion tensor imaging fiber tracking in deep brain stimulation surgery: DBS of the dentato-rubro-thalamic tract (drt) for the treatment of therapy-refractory tremor. *Acta Neurochir. (Wien)* 153, 1579–1585. doi: 10.1007/s00701-011-1036-z discussion 1585,

Coenen, V. A., Allert, N., Paus, S., Kronenburger, M., Urbach, H., and Madler, B. (2014). Modulation of the cerebello-thalamo-cortical network in thalamic deep brain stimulation for tremor: a diffusion tensor imaging study. *Neurosurgery* 75, 657–669. doi: 10.1227/NEU.0000000000000540 discussion 669–670,

Coenen, V. A., Jenkner, C., Honey, C. R., and Madler, B. (2016). Electrophysiologic validation of diffusion tensor imaging tractography during deep brain stimulation surgery. *AJNR Am. J. Neuroradiol.* doi: 10.3174/ajnr.A4753 [Epub ahead of print]

Coenen, V. A., Madler, B., Schiffbauer, H., Urbach, H., and Allert, N. (2011b). Individual fiber anatomy of the subthalamic region revealed with diffusion tensor imaging: a concept to identify the deep brain stimulation target for tremor suppression. *Neurosurgery* 68, 1069–1075; discussion 1075–1076. doi: 10.1227/NEU.0b013e31820a1a20

Descoteaux, M., Deriche, R., Knosche, T. R., and Anwander, A. (2009). Deterministic and probabilistic tractography based on complex fibre orientation distributions. *IEEE Trans. Med. Imaging* 28, 269–286. doi: 10.1109/TMI.2008.2004424

Desikan, R. S., Ségonne, F., Fischl, B., Quinn, B. T., Dickerson, B. C., Blacker, D., et al. (2006). An automated labeling system for subdividing the human cerebral cortex on MRI scans into gyral based regions of interest. *Neuroimage* 31, 968–980. doi: 10.1016/j.neuroimage.2006.01.021

Diedrichsen, J., Balsters, J. H., Flavell, J., Cussans, E., and Ramnani, N. (2009). A probabilistic MR atlas of the human cerebellum. *Neuroimage* 46, 39–46. doi: 10.1016/j.neuroimage.2009.01.045

Draganski, B., Kherif, F., Kloppel, S., Cook, P. A., Alexander, D. C., Parker, G. J. M., et al. (2008). Evidence for segregated and integrative connectivity patterns in the human basal ganglia. *J. Neurosci.* 28, 7143–7152. doi: 10.1523/JNEUROSCI.1486-08.2008

Gallay, M., Jeanmonod, D., Liu, J., and Morel, A. (2008). Human pallidothalamic and cerebellothalamic tracts: anatomical basis for functional stereotactic neurosurgery. *Brain Struct. Funct.* 212, 443–463. doi: 10.1007/s00429-007-0170-0

Hariz, M. I. (2002). Safety and risk of microelectrode recording in surgery for movement disorders. *Stereotact. Funct. Neurosurg.* 78, 146–157. doi: 10.1159/000068960

Hunsche, S., Sauner, D., Runge, M. J., Lenartz, D., El Majdoub, F., Treuer, H., et al. (2013). Tractography-guided stimulation of somatosensory fibers for thalamic pain relief. *Stereotact. Funct. Neurosurg.* 91, 328–334. doi: 10.1159/000350024

Hyam, J. A., Owen, S. L., Kringelbach, M. L., Jenkinson, N., Stein, J. F., Green, A. L., et al. (2012). Contrasting connectivity of the ventralis intermedius and ventralis oralis posterior nuclei of the motor thalamus demonstrated by probabilistic tractography. *Neurosurgery* 70, 162–169; discussion 169. doi: 10.1227/NEU.0b013e3182262c9a

Jakab, A., Blanc, R., Berenyi, E. L., and Szekely, G. (2012). Generation of individualized thalamus target maps by using statistical shape models and thalamocortical tractography. *AJNR Am. J. Neuroradiol.* 33, 2110–2116. doi: 10.3174/ajnr.A3140

Jenkinson, M., Beckmann, C. F., Behrens, T. E., Woolrich, M. W., and Smith, S. M. (2012). FSL. *Neuroimage* 62, 782–790. doi: 10.1016/j.neuroimage.2011.09.015

Johansen-Berg, H., Behrens, T. E., Sillery, E., Ciccarelli, O., Thompson, A. J., Smith, S. M., et al. (2005). Functional-anatomical validation and individual variation of diffusion tractography-based segmentation of the human thalamus. *Cereb. Cortex* 15, 31–39. doi: 10.1093/cercor/bhh105

Johansen-Berg, H., Behrens, T. E. J., Robson, M. D., Drobnjak, I., Rushworth, M. F. S., Brady, J. M., et al. (2004). Changes in connectivity profiles define functionally distinct regions in human medial frontal cortex. *Proc. Natl. Acad. Sci. U.S.A.* 101, 13335–13340. doi: 10.1073/pnas.0403743101

Jonasson, L., Hagmann, P., Pollo, C., Bresson, X., Richero Wilson, C., Meuli, R., et al. (2007). A level set method for segmentation of the thalamus and its nuclei in DT-MRI. *Signal Process.* 87, 309–321. doi: 10.1016/j.sigpro.2005.12.017

Jones, D. K., Horsfield, M. A., and Simmons, A. (1999). Optimal strategies for measuring diffusion in anisotropic systems by magnetic resonance imaging. *Magn. Reson. Med.* 42, 515–525. doi: 10.1002/(SICI)1522-2594(199909)42:3<515::AID-MRM14>3.0.CO;2-Q

Kievit, J., and Kuypers, H. (1977). Organization of the thalamo-cortical connexions to the frontal lobe in the rhesus monkey. *Exp. Brain Res.* 29, 299–322.

Klein, J. C., Barbe, M. T., Seifried, C., Baudrexel, S., Runge, M., Maarouf, M., et al. (2012). The tremor network targeted by successful VIM deep brain stimulation in humans. *Neurology* 78, 787–795. doi: 10.1212/WNL.0b013e318249f702

Klein, J. C., Rushworth, M. F. S., Behrens, T. E. J., Mackay, C. E., de Crespigny, A. J., D'Arceuil, H., et al. (2010). Topography of connections between human prefrontal cortex and mediodorsal thalamus studied with diffusion tractography. *Neuroimage* 51, 555–564. doi: 10.1016/j.neuroimage.2010.02.062

Krauth, A., Blanc, R., Poveda, A., Jeanmonod, D., Morel, A., and Székely, G. (2010). A mean three-dimensional atlas of the human thalamus: generation from multiple histological data. *Neuroimage* 49, 2053–2062. doi: 10.1016/j.neuroimage.2009.10.042

Kuhn, T., Gullett, J. M., Nguyen, P., Boutzoukas, A. E., Ford, A., Colon-Perez, L. M., et al. (2015). Test-retest reliability of high angular resolution diffusion imaging acquisition within medial temporal lobe connections assessed via tract based spatial statistics, probabilistic tractography and a novel graph theory metric. *Brain Imaging Behav.* 10, 533–547. doi: 10.1007/s11682-015-9425-1

Kwon, H., Hong, J., Hong, C., Lee, D., Ahn, S., and Jang, S. (2011). Dentatorubrothalamic tract in human brain: diffusion tensor tractography study. *Neuroradiology* 53, 787–791. doi: 10.1007/s00234-011-0858-y

Lanotte, M. M., Rizzone, M., Bergamasco, B., Faccani, G., Melcarne, A., and Lopiano, L. (2002). Deep brain stimulation of the subthalamic nucleus: anatomical, neurophysiological, and outcome correlations with the effects of stimulation. *J. Neurol. Neurosurg. Psychiatry* 72, 53–58. doi: 10.1136/jnnp.72.1.53

Le Bihan, D., and Johansen-Berg, H. (2012). Diffusion MRI at 25: exploring brain tissue structure and function. *Neuroimage* 61, 324–341. doi: 10.1016/j.neuroimage.2011.11.006

Lemaire, J., Coste, J., Ouchchane, L., Caire, F., Nuti, C., Derost, P., et al. (2007). Brain mapping in stereotactic surgery: a brief overview from the probabilistic targeting to the patient-based anatomic mapping. *Neuroimage* 37, S109–S115. doi: 10.1016/j.neuroimage.2007.05.055

Lujan, J. L., Chaturvedi, A., Malone, D. A., Rezai, A. R., Machado, A. G., and McIntyre, C. C. (2012). Axonal pathways linked to therapeutic and nontherapeutic outcomes during psychiatric deep brain stimulation. *Hum. Brain Mapp.* 33, 958–968. doi: 10.1002/hbm.21262

Martin, E., Jeanmonod, D., Morel, A., Zadicario, E., and Werner, B. (2009). High-intensity focused ultrasound for noninvasive functional neurosurgery. *Ann. Neurol.* 66, 858–861. doi: 10.1002/ana.21801

Morel, A., Magnin, M., and Jeanmonod, D. (1997). Multiarchitectonic and stereotactic atlas of the human thalamus. *J. Comp. Neurol.* 387, 588–630. doi: 10.1002/(SICI)1096-9861(19971103)387:4<588::AID-CNE8>3.0.CO;2-Z

Niemann, K., Mennicken, V. R., Jeanmonod, D., and Morel, A. (2000). The morel stereotactic atlas of the human thalamus: Atlas-to-MR registration of internally consistent canonical model. *Neuroimage* 12, 601–616. doi: 10.1006/nimg.2000.0650

Ohye, C. (2009). "Selective thalamotomy," in *Practical Handbook of Neurosurgery*, ed. M. Sindou (Vienna: Springer), 1310–1328.

Ohye, C., Shibazaki, T., Hirai, T., Kawashima, Y., Hirato, M., and Matsumura, M. (1993). Tremor-mediating thalamic zone studied in humans and in monkeys. *Stereotact. Funct. Neurosurg.* 60, 136–145. doi: 10.1159/000100600

O'Muircheartaigh, J., Vollmar, C., Traynor, C., Barker, G. J., Kumari, V., Symms, M. R., et al. (2011). Clustering probabilistic tractograms using independent component analysis applied to the thalamus. *Neuroimage* 54, 2020–2032. doi: 10.1016/j.neuroimage.2010.09.054

Owen, S. L., Heath, J., Kringelbach, M., Green, A. L., Pereira, E. A., Jenkinson, N., et al. (2008). Pre-operative DTI and probabilisitic tractography in four patients with deep brain stimulation for chronic pain. *J. Clin. Neurosci.* 15, 801–805. doi: 10.1016/j.jocn.2007.06.010

Pfefferbaum, A., Adalsteinsson, E., and Sullivan, E. V. (2003). Replicability of diffusion tensor imaging measurements of fractional anisotropy and trace in brain. *J. Magn. Reson. Imaging* 18, 427–433. doi: 10.1002/jmri.10377

Pouratian, N., Zheng, Z., Bari, A. A., Behnke, E., Elias, W. J., and Desalles, A. A. (2011). Multi-institutional evaluation of deep brain stimulation targeting using probabilistic connectivity-based thalamic segmentation. *J. Neurosurg.* 115, 995–1004. doi: 10.3171/2011.7.JNS11250

Schlaier, J., Anthofer, J., Steib, K., Fellner, C., Rothenfusser, E., Brawanski, A., et al. (2015). Deep brain stimulation for essential tremor: targeting the dentato-rubro-thalamic tract? *Neuromodulation* 18, 105–112. doi: 10.1111/ner.12238

Sudhyadhom, A., McGregor, K., Okun, M. S., Foote, K. D., Trinastic, J., Crosson, B., et al. (2013). Delineation of motor and somatosensory thalamic subregions utilizing probabilistic diffusion tractography and electrophysiology. *J. Magn. Reson. Imaging* 37, 600–609. doi: 10.1002/jmri.23861

Takao, H., Hayashi, N., Kabasawa, H., and Ohtomo, K. (2012). Effect of scanner in longitudinal diffusion tensor imaging studies. *Hum. Brain Mapp.* 33, 466–477. doi: 10.1002/hbm.21225

Takao, H., Hayashi, N., and Ohtomo, K. (2011). Effect of scanner in asymmetry studies using diffusion tensor imaging. *Neuroimage* 54, 1053–1062. doi: 10.1016/j.neuroimage.2010.09.023

Torres, C. V., Manzanares, R., and Sola, R. G. (2014). Integrating diffusion tensor imaging-based tractography into deep brain stimulation surgery: a review of the literature. *Stereotact. Funct. Neurosurg.* 92, 282–290. doi: 10.1159/000362937

Traynor, C., Heckemann, R. A., Hammers, A., O'Muircheartaigh, J., Crum, W. R., Barker, G. J., et al. (2010). Reproducibility of thalamic segmentation based on probabilistic tractography. *Neuroimage* 52, 69–85. doi: 10.1016/j.neuroimage.2010.04.024

Tripoliti, E., Strong, L., Hickey, F., Foltynie, T., Zrinzo, L., Candelario, J., et al. (2011). Treatment of dysarthria following subthalamic nucleus deep brain stimulation for parkinson's disease. *Mov. Disord.* 26, 2434–2436. doi: 10.1002/mds.23887

Wiegell, M. R., Tuch, D. S., Larsson, H. B. W., and Wedeen, V. J. (2003). Automatic segmentation of thalamic nuclei from diffusion tensor magnetic resonance imaging. *Neuroimage* 19, 391–401. doi: 10.1016/S1053-8119(03)00044-2

Yeterian, E. H., and Pandya, D. N. (1988). Corticothalamic connections of paralimbic regions in the rhesus monkey. *J. Comp. Neurol.* 269, 130–146. doi: 10.1002/cne.902690111

Zhang, D., Snyder, A. Z., Shimony, J. S., Fox, M. D., and Raichle, M. E. (2010). Noninvasive functional and structural connectivity mapping of the human thalamocortical system. *Cereb. Cortex* 20, 1187–1194. doi: 10.1093/cercor/bhp182

5

Merged Group Tractography Evaluation with Selective Automated Group Integrated Tractography

David Q. Chen*[1]*, Jidan Zhong*[2]*, David J. Hayes*[2]*, Brendan Behan*[2]*, Matthew Walker*[1]*, Peter S.-P. Hung*[1] *and Mojgan Hodaie*[1,2,3,4]*

[1] Institute of Medical Science, Faculty of Medicine, University of Toronto, Toronto, ON, Canada, [2] Krembil Research Institute, University Health Network, Toronto, ON, Canada, [3] Division of Neurosurgery, Toronto Western Hospital and University of Toronto, Toronto, ON, Canada, [4] Joint Department of Medical Imaging, University Health Network, Toronto, ON, Canada

***Correspondence:**
Mojgan Hodaie
mojgan.hodaie@uhn.ca

Introduction: Tractography analysis in group-based studies across large populations has been difficult to implement. We propose Selective Automated Group Integrated Tractography (SAGIT), an automated group tractography software platform that incorporates multiple diffusion magnetic resonance imaging (dMRI) practices which will allow great accessibility to group-wise dMRI. We use a merged tractography approach that permits evaluation of tractography datasets at the group level. We also introduce an image normalized overlap score (NOS) that measures the quality of the group tractography results. We deploy SAGIT to evaluate deterministic and probabilistic constrained spherical deconvolution (CST_{det}, CST_{prob}) tractography, eXtended Streamline Tractography (XST), and diffusion tensor tractography (DTT) in their ability to delineate different neuroanatomy, as well as validating NOS across these different brain regions.

Materials and methods: Magnetic resonance sequences were acquired from 42 healthy adults. Anatomical and group registrations were performed using Automated Normalization Tools. Cortical segmentation was performed using FreeSurfer. Four tractography algorithms were used to delineate six sets of neuroanatomy: fornix, facial/vestibular-cochlear cranial nerve complex, vagus nerve, rubral–cerebellar decussation, optic radiation, and auditory radiation. The tracts were generated both with and without region of interest filters. The generated visual reports were then evaluated by five neuroscientists.

Results: At a group level, merged tractography demonstrated that different methods have different fiber distribution characteristics. CST_{prob} is prone to false-positives, and thereby suitable in anatomy with strong priors. CST_{det} and XST are more conservative, but have greater difficulty resolving hemispherical decussation and distant crossing projections. DTT consistently shows the worst reproducibility across the anatomies. Linear regression of rater scores against NOS shows significant ($p < 0.05$) correlation of the two sets of scores in filtered tractography. However, correlations are not significant ($p > 0.05$) for unfiltered tractography.

Conclusion: The tractography results demonstrated reliable and consistent performance of SAGIT across multiple subjects and techniques. Through SAGIT, we quantifiably demonstrated that different algorithms showed different strengths and weaknesses at a group level. While no single algorithm seems to be suitable for all anatomical tasks, it is useful to consider the use of a mix of algorithms for different anatomical segments. SAGIT appears to be a promising group-wise tractography analysis approach for this purpose.

Keywords: tractography, group-wise tractography, merged tractography, diffusion imaging, pipeline, multi-tensor, HARDI

INTRODUCTION

Diffusion magnetic resonance imaging (dMRI) tractography is an imaging analysis technique that permits non-invasive visualization of white matter anatomy *in vivo* (Basser et al., 2000). It is based on the observation that the Brownian motion of water molecules within white matter fibers is constrained by the axonal bundles, and therefore such anisotropic water diffusion can be used to probe tissue microstructure (Bihan et al., 2001). By scanning in multiple angular directions using diffusion weighted imaging (DWI) sequence, a model of diffusion can be estimated for each voxel of the scanned image volume.

In the classic single-tensor dMRI (also known as diffusion tensor image; DTI) model (Basser and Jones, 2002), a single tensor is constructed at each voxel based on Gaussian model of diffusion, which describes the dominant diffusion direction. Using the tensor information, tractography algorithms (Mori and van Zijl, 2002) can be used to trace out structures within the DTI volume. The limitation of DTI is that there is insufficient information to resolve areas with crossing fibers with one tensor per voxel. Improvements over the limits of the DTI model, particularly in increasing angular resolution to improve crossing fibers resolution has been a subject of great interest (Tuch et al., 2002; Fritzsche et al., 2010; Jeurissen et al., 2012).

To improve the crossing fiber information per voxel, significant changes in DWI acquisition strategies are required. These methods include diffusion spectrum imaging (DSI; Wedeen et al., 2005, 2008) which samples the Q-space in a Cartesian grid, and Q-ball imaging that is based on the Funk–Radon transform (Descoteaux et al., 2007; Cho et al., 2008) that samples the Q-space in a spherical shell. These approaches, as well as more complex multi-shell sampling strategies, aim to construct and sharpen an orientation distribution function (ODF) in order to provide better approximate of the underlying diffusion. These methods require complex and long DWI acquisitions that are often unsuitable for clinical applications. Alternatively, methods based on spherical deconvolution (SD) can be used on high angular resolution diffusion imaging (HARDI) scans of lesser angular resolution. The approach is to model the HARDI signal as a convolution of the fiber orientations. The resulting deconvoluted fiber orientation distribution (FOD) shows better discrimination of fiber directions compared to Q-ball under similar scanning parameters, but is susceptible to image noise (Tournier et al., 2004; Anderson, 2005; Dell'Acqua et al., 2007). Alternatively, multi-tensor model-based approaches estimate the fiber configuration with the assumption that there are no more than two or three crossings in a given voxel. These include eXtended Streamline Tractography (XST), which can delineate lateral projections of the corticospinal tract in the motor cortex, in DWI scans with 50 gradient directions (Qazi et al., 2009). Other tractography algorithm include stochastically resolving tract propagation based on established white matter prior probability (probabilistic tractography; Behrens et al., 2007). Probabilistic approaches, however, are predominantly image-based, and result in a visitation volume image that needs to be visualized volumetrically.

There is increasing recognition in the field on the value of incorporating dMRI tractography into group-based studies in large populations. However, group tractography analysis has a number of challenges. The dMRI-derived geometries are difficult to register due to the large dimensionality of variables and low spatial resolution. Direct linear and non-linear deformations of either the tensor/ODF field can also confound diffusion metrics. Inter-subject anatomical variability also poses challenges for direct tractography geometric clustering and registration, making tract bundle identifications difficult. Specific anatomical selection also needs to be considered. TRACULA (TRActs Constrained by Underlying Anatomy) (Yendiki et al., 2011), for example, is able to perform group tractography analysis on pre-defined major white matter bundles based on ball-and-stick probabilistic tractography template, however, there are no solutions available for fully customizable anatomy that incorporates new advances in dMRI tractography. Recently there are efforts to evaluate tractography algorithms with synthetic datasets such as Tractometer (Côté et al., 2012, 2013), as well as attempts to generate synthetic data from individuals (Wilkins et al., 2015). From these comparative studies, there is evidence that no single tractography algorithm is superior for the reconstruction of all white matter tracts. There are no detailed studies that have attempted to compare tractography algorithms across larger populations to determine their relative suitability for different white matter tract identification.

In the clinical setting, the anatomy of interest is often specific, and needs to be put in a context of high individual variability, therefore manual targeting of regions of interest (ROIs) are unavoidable. Across a population, manual ROI delineation is at the risk of high ROI placement variations due to operator bias. The complexity of tractography data across a population increases dramatically when iterative tuning of tractography parameters is considered. Therefore, a combined and automated approach to group tractography in neuroimaging is highly desirable.

There is a lack of well-organized diffusion tractography software framework that bridges the gap between group image registration, diffusion image processing, large-scale tractography delineations, and tractography evaluation. We propose an automated tractography software platform that incorporates existing and proven dMRI techniques, in order for group-wise dMRI to be more accessible to researchers. Selective Automated Group Integrated Tractography (SAGIT[1]) is a configurable and fully automated tractography generation and comparison pipeline. Its key contributions are: (a) automated preprocessing, registration and tractography across an arbitrary number of subjects; (b) flexibility in ROI definitions that allows high customizability for anatomical targeting; (c) expressive ROI query that works with pre-defined segmentation masks such as FreeSurfer; (d) compatibility with a number of popular tractography software that allows parameter iterations for consistent results. SAGIT enables researchers to examine the result of different tractography algorithms at the group level. We also introduce an image-based score (normalized overlap score, NOS) that can quantify the quality of the group tractography results across different tractography algorithms to further assist decision making for researchers.

Finally, we deploy our system to the evaluation of various tractography methods in their ability to delineate neuroanatomy that are highly specific but difficult to image. These include supra and infratentorial structures such as small white matter bundles in heavy crossing fibers (cranial nerves), pontine decussation (rubrocerebellar pathway), and curved central pathways (fornix, visual, and auditory radiations). We recruited five neuroanatomists to evaluate and rate the resulting visual reports generated by SAGIT. We then compared the results of NOSs and the human raters to assess the automated NOS as a tractography reproducibility metric.

MATERIALS AND METHODS

MRI Acquisitions

Magnetic resonance (MR) images were acquired using GE Signa HDx 3 Tesla scanner with an eight-channel head-coil. MR sequences were acquired from 42 healthy adults (mean age 30.4 ± 8.1 years). Ethics approval was granted by the University Health Network Research Ethics Board (Toronto, Canada), MR images were acquired at the Toronto Western Hospital, and all subjects gave their informed written consent. DWI were acquired with 1 B0 scan, 60 gradient directions, 3 mm slice thickness and in-plane resolution of 0.9375 × 0.9375 mm, $b = 1000$ s/mm^2, echo time (TE) = 86.4 ms, repetition time (TR) = 17,000 ms, flip angle = 90°, field of view (FOV) = 240 mm, and matrix = 256 × 256. T1 fast spoiled gradient echo (FSPGR) anatomical scans were acquired with 1 mm slice thickness and in-plane resolution of 0.9375 × 0.9375 mm, slice spacing = 1 mm, TE = 5.052 ms, TR = 11.956 ms, flip angle = 20°, FOV = 240 mm, and matrix = 256 × 256.

Preprocessing

In order to automate the generation of tractography using multiple methods and minimize user-bias, the SAGIT framework is created (**Figure 1**). DWI sequences were corrected for eddy-current and motion distortions with appropriate rotational corrections to gradient vectors (Leemans and Jones, 2009). Fractional anisotropy (FA), axial diffusivity (AD), and radial diffusivity (RD) maps were generated from the DWI. A group-specific average anatomical template was created with subject T1 image, and intra-subject T1 to DWI space was obtained using symmetric diffeomorphic registration (SyN) with Automated Normalization Tools (ANTs; Avants et al., 2008). Cortical and subcortical segmentations based on the T1 images were obtained with FreeSurfer segmentation software (Fischl et al., 2002).

Tractography Delineation

The tractography methods attempted to reconstruct the bilateral white matter anatomy of the fornix, facial/vestibular-cochlear cranial nerve complex (CN VII/VIII), vagus nerve (CN X), red nucleus pontine decussation (RN), lateral geniculate visual pathway (LGN) and medial geniculate auditory pathway (MGN). Seeding ROIs were defined on the group template, and projected to the individual DWI space.

Tractography filters were defined using a custom query expression to generate gray matter/white matter boundary inclusion and exclusion filter masks based on the FreeSurfer segmentations (see Supplementary Material Data Sheet 1). No filtering rules were applied for the fornix. The fornix is used as a control group to judge rating bias. The unfiltered (filtering rules were not applied) versions of each anatomy were also generated for evaluation.

Single-tensor diffusion tensor tractography (DTT) using 3D Slicer version 3 (Tuch et al., 2000; Pieper et al., 2006), two-tensor tractography using XST (Qazi et al., 2009), constrained SD-based deterministic streamline tractography (CST_{det}; Tournier et al., 2012) and constrained SD-based probabilistic tractography (CST_{prob}; Tournier et al., 2010) using MRtrix version 3 were evaluated (see Supplementary Material Data Sheet 2 for parameters).

FA, AD, and RD scalars were sampled and embedded into the tractography models using tri-linear interpolation from the corresponding image volumes in native DWI space. The affine and non-linear image registration transforms were applied to deform the native tracts from the DWI space to the template space; all corresponding tracts of the same anatomy in template space were then merged into one single tractography model, to obtain the merged group tractography geometry.

The individual tractography models were also converted to binary spatial images, and the resulting images were transformed to the template space. Multiple binary images were stacked together to form the conjunction percentage overlap image. The overlaps were then visualized using concentric isosurfaces created from step-wise (10%) thresholds of the underlying overlap volume using the MayaVI data visualization library (Ramachandran and Varoquaux, 2011). A color lookup table with even visual brightness falloff (van der Walt and Smith, 2015) was chosen to avoid visual judgment biases from the color presentation. Different viewpoints (axial, coronal, sagittal, and perspective) were created for each

[1]https://github.com/sinkpoint/sagit

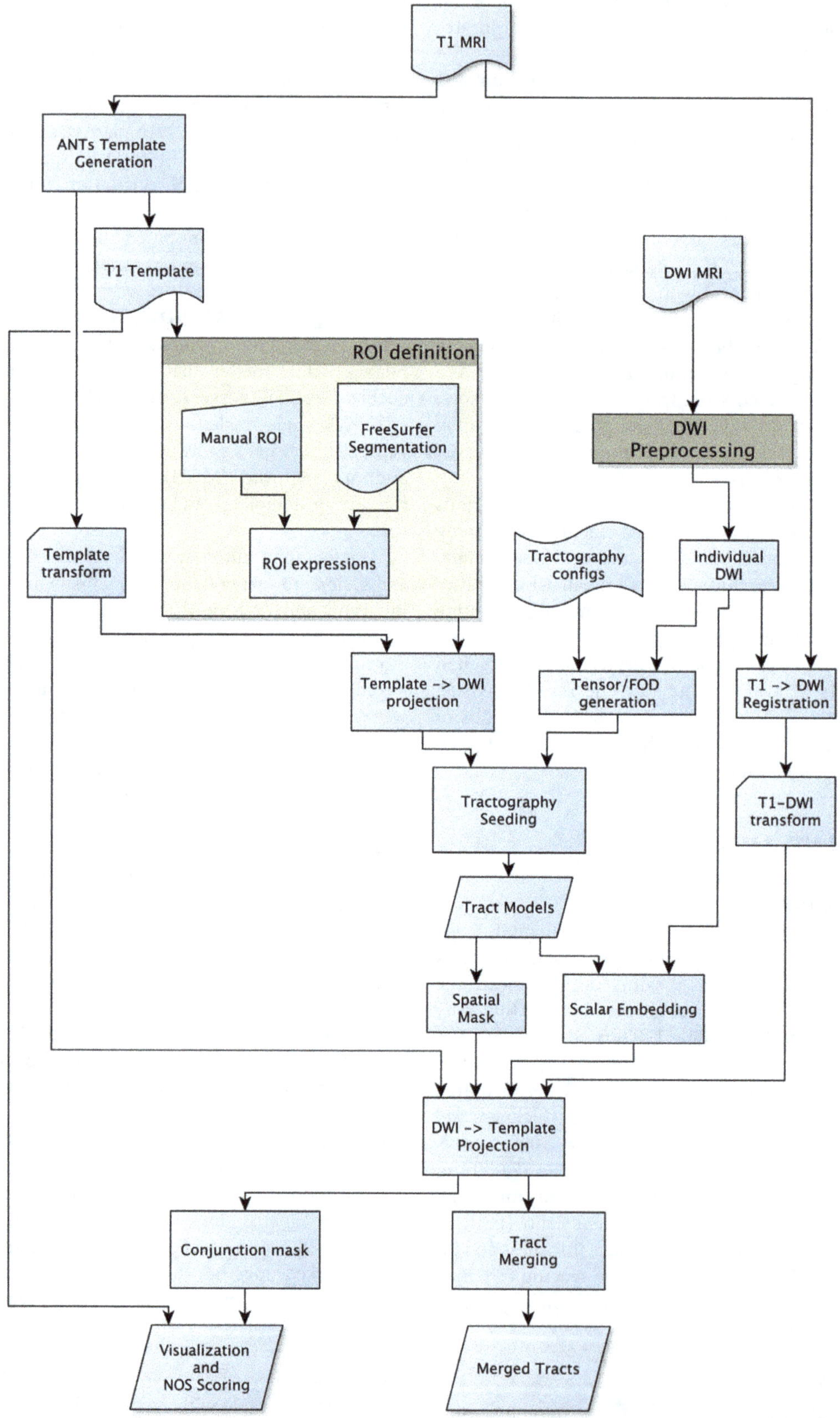

FIGURE 1 | Flow diagram of the SAGIT group tractography framework. The SAGIT framework is designed to be fully configurable and extensible.

visualization, and then composed together to create the visual report.

Tractography Evaluation

The generated visual reports were then evaluated by five neuroscientists in a blinded study using a set of rating criteria (see Supplementary Material Table 1). The conjunction images were at the same time used to generate NOSs. The NOS quantified the conjunction image generated by overlapping tractography masks to meaningfully determine the spatial agreement independent of anatomy. The assumption was that given a conjunction image, where its voxel value s denotes a range of overlap percentages between 0 and 100%, and value *1* denotes the 100% overlap value, we formalize it as $s \in [0, 1]$, and define NOS as:

$$n^{-1} \sum_{i=0}^{n-1} \frac{\ln(\nu_i)}{\ln(\nu_0)}$$

where n was the number of bins; v_0 was the number of voxels where $s > 0$; v_i was the number of voxels with $0 < s \geq \frac{i}{n}$; this study used $n = 10$. Examples of NOS behavior are available in **Figure 2** for the left red nucleus projections.

The rater scores were then normalized to each anatomy, and the normalized rater scores were linearly regressed against the NOSs for correlations. Linear regression of rater scores against NOS was performed using the R-statistics library (R Development Core Team, 2012).

RESULTS

The fornix was shown to be consistent across the different algorithms. The visual report (**Figure 3**; the complete visual report can be found in Supplementary Material Data Sheet 3) suggested that the subregions of the fornix were consistently delineated. The merged fornix tracts (**Figure 4**) showed different patterns of streamline distributions. CST_{prob} and XST both showed wide spread streamline dispersions, while CST_{det} and particularly DTT were limited to the region of the fornix. The fornix ratings (**Figure 5**) showed essentially no variability between raters. The fornix NOSs (**Figure 6**) similarly were consistent across the algorithms with little variability. Both filtered and unfiltered ratings were identical.

For the CN VII/VIII, CST_{prob}, CST_{det}, and XST were all able to delineate the cranial as well as brainstem segments of the nerve (**Figure 3**). CST_{prob}, however, also delineated much of the cerebellum. DTT by Slicer was not able to delineate the brainstem portions of the fiber and therefore was scored lower than the other methods. These differences in delineation can be more clearly seen in the merged tracts (**Figure 4**), where the XST also showed further lateral delineations of CN VII/VIII. In unfiltered tractography, there was much more inter-rater variability for all except CST_{prob} (**Figure 5**). CST_{det} and XST also showed lower average rating when unfiltered. The NOS showed similar trend where DTT resulted in the lowest score (**Figure 6**). The NOS also showed higher score for CST_{det} when comparing to XST. There were no notable changes in NOSs in unfiltered tractography.

For CN X, CST_{prob} was rated the highest with no inter-rater variability. CST_{det} and XST resulted in more rating variability and a lower average score (**Figure 5**). CST_{prob} visually showed delineations that extended into the ipsilateral higher brain regions even with filters (**Figures 3** and **4**). DTT showed the worst reproducibility, although its anatomy was recognizable in a small number of individuals. In unfiltered tractography, CST_{det} and XST showed reduced variability, and visually showed delineations of ascending and brainstem projects. DTT also showed improved ratings when unfiltered (**Figure 5**). NOSs (**Figure 6**) for both filtered and unfiltered CN X tractography similarly showed an overall increase in score with unfiltered tractography.

For the red nucleus projections, visually CST_{prob} showed the most consistent reproducibility of the decussation (**Figures 3** and **4**), with XST showing higher reproducibility over CST_{det}. DTT failed to delineate the pathway and instead delineated an erroneous path that decussated at the corpus callosum. CST_{prob}, CST_{det}, and XST resulted similar ratings, with unfiltered tracts showing lower rating and higher variability. DTT had the lowest rating, and very high variability (**Figure 5**). NOS of the red nucleus projections highlighted the stronger performance of the CST_{prob} over the other algorithms, and XST result was scored higher than CST_{det} (**Figure 6**). The NOSs of unfiltered tracts were notably higher for all algorithms, as the resulting tracts seemed to delineate much of the cortical spinal projections.

The optic radiation showed the greatest reproducibility with CST_{prob}, where the Meyer's loop could be seen in the result (**Figures 3** and **4**). CST_{det} and XST showed low reproducibility of less than 20%, and DTT failed to delineate any structure on the right side (see Supplementary Material Data Sheet 3). The ratings reflected the observation (**Figure 5**), with CST_{prob} having the full rating. CST_{det} was rated higher in filtered tractography, while XST was rated higher when unfiltered. DTT also showed higher ratings when unfiltered. NOS characterized the drop-off in reproducibility in filtered tractography for the deterministic methods (**Figure 6**), and the trend of rating under filtered tractography matched well with the ratings. NOS for unfiltered tractography, however, showed little match with ratings.

The auditory radiation was the least reproducible region. In filtered tractography, although CST_{prob} showed high reproducibility in tractography (**Figures 3** and **4**), it was not clear if its delineation was correct. Visually there were wide spread area of false positives toward the occipital and anterior temporal lobe. The deterministic methods all showed poor ability to reach the Heschl's gyrus. DTT was completely unable to produce any structures at all. For filtered ratings, CST_{prob} was the highest, and with XST rated higher than CST_{det} (**Figure 5**). DTT scored 0 due to the lack of delineated structures. When unfiltered, all algorithms showed widespread false positives in the hemispheres. Unfiltered ratings were over all higher than filtered ratings. NOSs trends for filtered tractography matched well with ratings, but also highlighted the large differences in reproducibility (**Figure 6**). While NOSs under unfiltered tractography did not correlate with ratings.

Linear regression of rater scores against NOS (**Figure 7**) showed significant ($p < 0.05$) correlation of the two sets of scores in filtered tractography. However, correlations were not

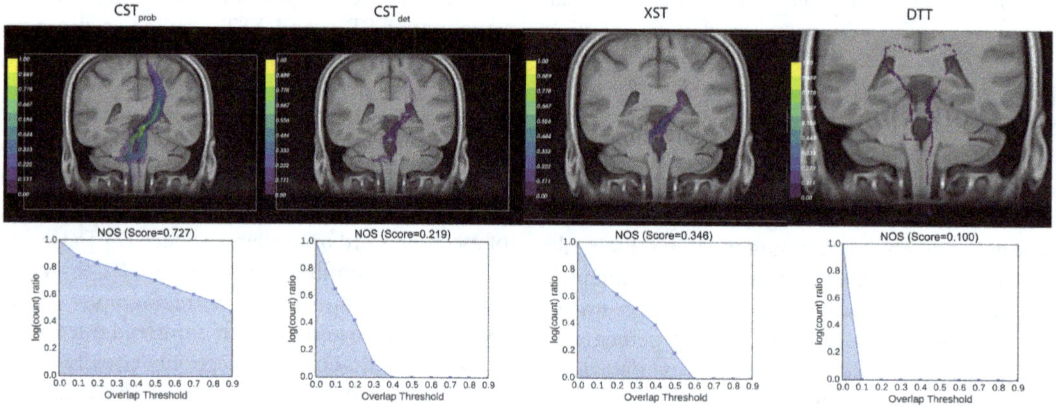

FIGURE 2 | Examples of NOSs of different conjunction images: the figure shows the coronal view of the left red nucleus tractography projections, as produced by different algorithms. The NOS correlates closely with the visual color scale. It can also resolve visually similar comparisons, such as the rating between XST and CST_{det} results.

significant ($p > 0.05$) for unfiltered tractography. It can be observed that NOS in unfiltered tractography agrees well with visual intuition, however, rater variability and anatomical reports suggested greater false positives when presented with unfiltered results.

DISCUSSION

The present study performed automated group tractography generation and collation report on six sets of neuroanatomy in 42 subjects using four different types of tractography algorithms. The proposed automation pipeline performed with great reliability. We have designed the automated pipeline to offer the ability to generate and collate tractography on a large scale. The key benefit of this approach is the vastly improved inter-subject tract reproducibility as a result of ROI filtering, and speed for tractography data generation. The method offers flexibility for researchers in ROI placements and parameter control for these tractography algorithms. The merged tractography permits additional analysis of the group-based anatomical reconstructions, and the auto-generated visual reports also reduce data confusion and improve research efficiency.

The most critical component of the pipeline is the reliability of image registrations. For this purpose, we picked ANTs since it is state-of-the-art and widely tested and deployed in numerous neuroimaging studies (Klein et al., 2009; Avants et al., 2011). For T1 to DWI co-registration, we used mean DWI (MDWI) as the registration intermediate. MDWI appears to be a reliable T1–DWI co-registration intermediate in the absence of reverse-blip DWI acquisitions (Chen et al., 2015a). Future studies can also potentially improve T1–DWI co-registration, for example, with the possible use of anisotropic power image (Dell'Acqua et al., 2014).

We have deployed the pipeline to the task of delineating six sets of neuroanatomy from clinical DWI data. The anatomies were chosen to test the limits of the SAGIT pipeline as well as the tractography algorithms. These anatomies are often shown in an existing atlas, and contain curving projections that are difficult to delineate, but are nevertheless well defined and contain clear anatomical landmarks for ease of judgment. In total, we included two sets of cranial nerves (CN VII/VIII and CN X) for their small but precise anatomy; rubrocerebellar projections of the red nucleus, due to the difficulty of imaging the pontine decussation; optical radiation for its well defined landmarks and the Meyer's loop, which is difficult to image; auditory radiation, which is particularly difficult due to its course, that passes through a three-way crossing in temporal lobe. The fornix serves as the control anatomical structure. We have previously studied fornix subregion anatomies extensively (Chen et al., 2015b), and it is a popular anatomy to showcase the ability of new tractography algorithms due to the curvature of the forniceal crura (Garyfallidis et al., 2014).

It can be observed that results of averaged tractography image conjunction across a group are visually similar to probabilistic tractography in an individual, and that the group junction image seems to stabilize as the number of subject increase. It can be argued that the conjunction image captures the probable volume across a sampled population for a particular neuroanatomy in the template space. Their exact similarity and differences from probabilistic tractography at a group level should be explored in future studies. Additionally, the fidelity of the merged anatomy is often higher than what would be available from an individual. The result supports the validity of this technical approach. It is possible that the resulting average delineations can be used to generate population-specific anatomy atlases. It is also possible to use fiber density images rather than binary mask for conjunction. However, the result of an average fiber density image is difficult to interpret, and therefore should be explored in future studies.

When attempting to judge tractography delineation quality, human experts often are able to assess a particular delineation by visually identifying known anatomical priors. Direct tracto-graphy visualizations suggest that wide streamline dispersions often obscure anatomical details in visualizations,

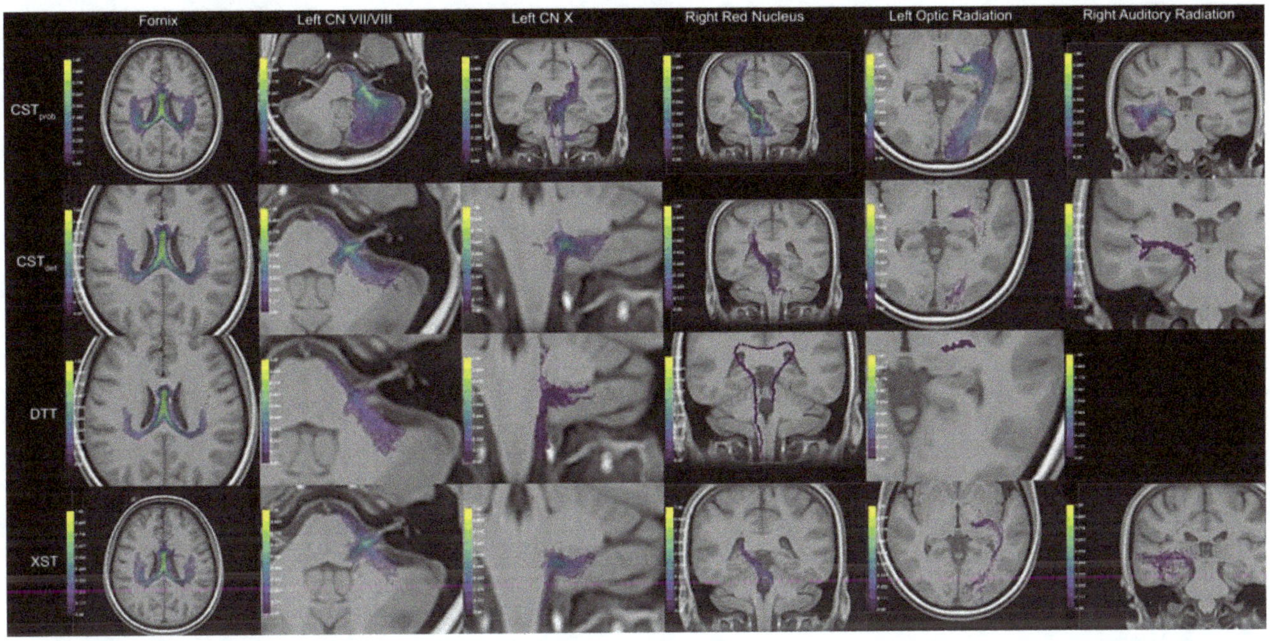

FIGURE 3 | Example of the auto-generated visual panels. The panels that best represent the resulting anatomy are compiled. For anatomical reference, the best representative anatomy image slice is composed with the tract conjunction map. The color scale of the conjunction image represents the percentage reproducible for each region, where 1 = 100%. For each algorithm (rows), different visual perspectives are created. Together six different anatomies were delineated (columns). To see the full visual reports generated, please see Supplementary Material Data Sheet 3.

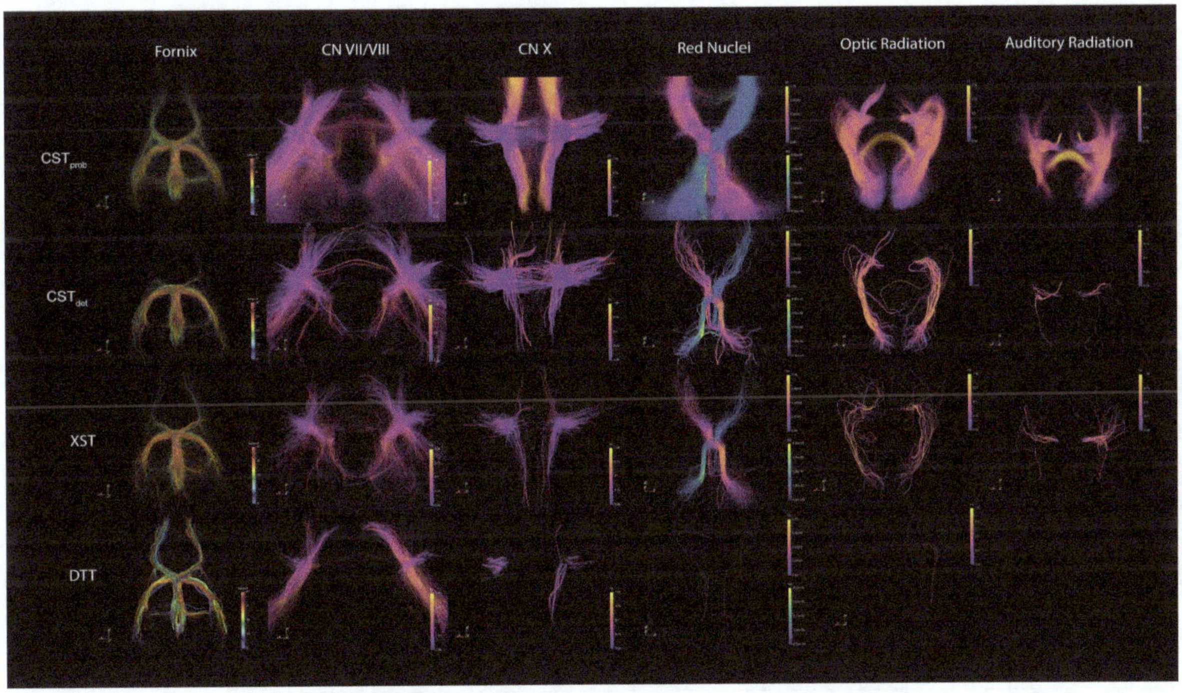

FIGURE 4 | Example of merged tractography models for each of the techniques and anatomies. The fornix is colored to distinguish tracts from each of the 42 subjects, in order to demonstrate the effect of combining the group data. The other anatomies are colored by FA intensity. The specific FA measures from each point were sampled from their native DWI space before tractography deformation. The grouping of the similar FA measures across the subjects show that the registrations were accurate. The red nuclei show different metrics (FA and AD) depending on lateralization, in order to highlight the pontine decussation.

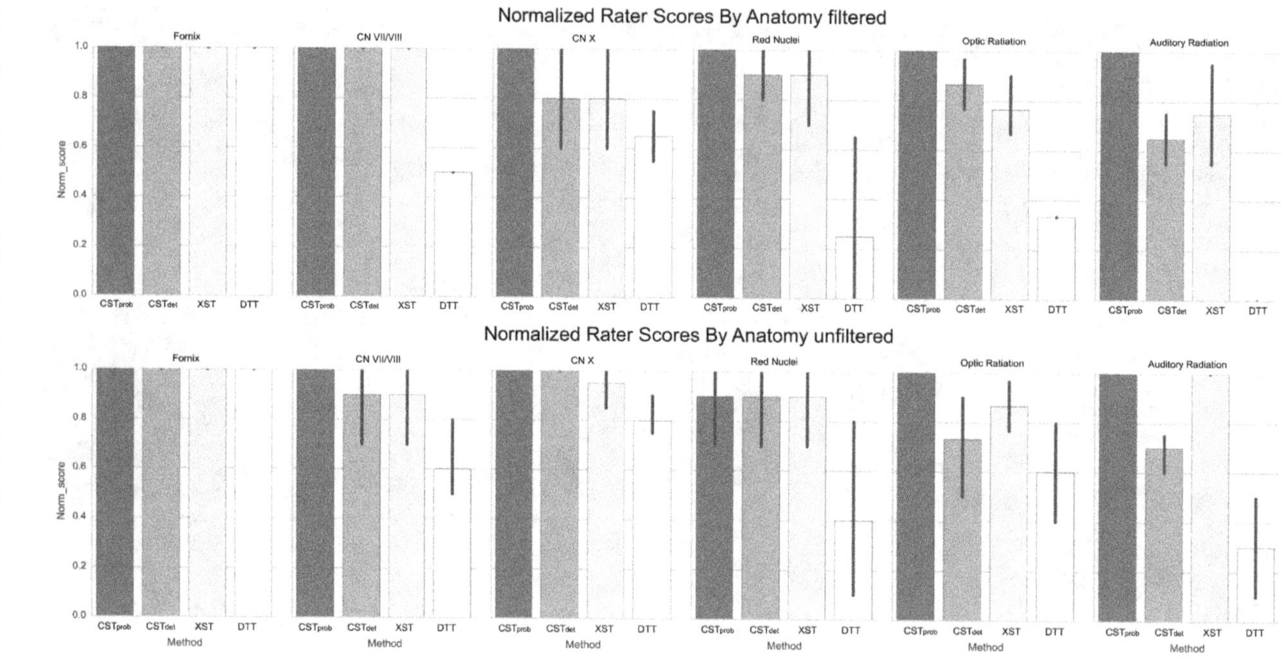

FIGURE 5 | Normalized anatomical scores as rated by experts. The error bars denote standard deviations of the ratings. The fornix serves as the control anatomy, therefore the represented filtered and unfiltered image are identical. It can be observed that unfiltered anatomy increases rater variability in some and decrease in others.

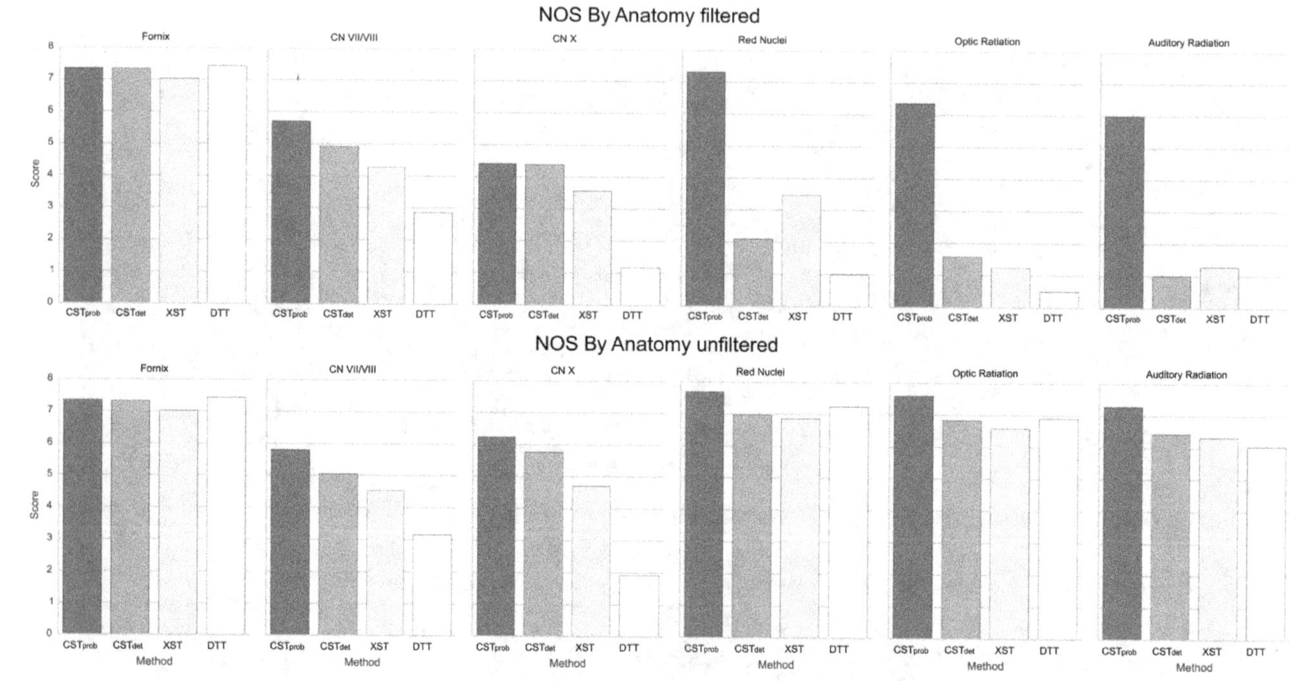

FIGURE 6 | NOSs for each anatomy. It can be noted that having ROI filters severely reduces reproducibility in deterministic methods.

making anatomical assessment difficult (**Figure 4**). Therefore, image conjunctions offer better ability to assess reproducibility than direct tractography renderings alone. We aimed to develop an automated assessment of tractography reproducibility, since (a) researchers are often prone to judgment bias when exposed to large number of tractography results, and that subtle differences in results are often hard to distinguish, and (b) in an automated pipeline, the assessment score is necessary to allow iteratively fine

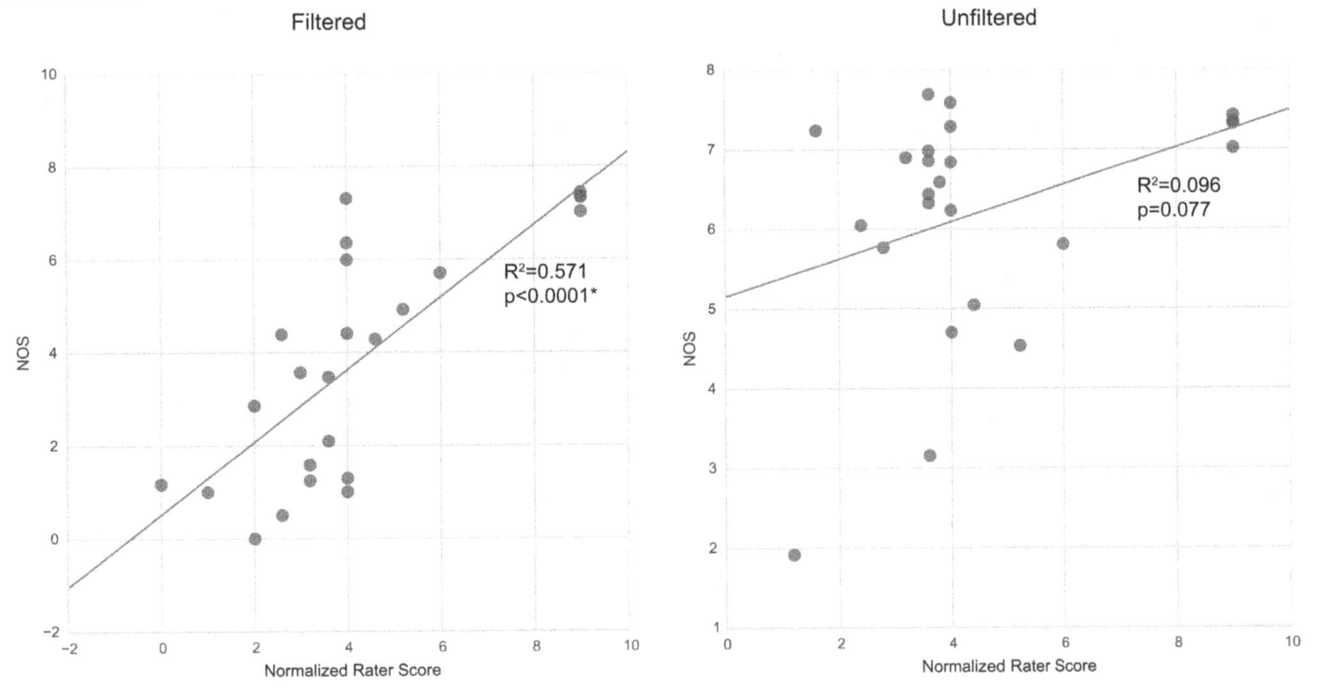

FIGURE 7 | Correlation between rating scores and NOS. Filtered tractography NOS is significantly ($p < 0.05$) correlated with ratings. However, unfiltered tractography show no significance.

tuning of tractography parameters. Since current neuroimaging techniques are not yet able to reliably classify neuroanatomy from tractography or image-based morphology, it is desirable for a computing pipeline to optimize and present the most reproducible tractography delineating across a population based on a particular set of ROIs as a first step. Subsequent anatomical assessment can then be made by a human expert, and the appropriate changes in ROI filter strategy can be made. This approach allows researchers with strong neuroanatomy backgrounds, but are less technically inclined, to make better judgments when performing group tractography.

The NOS and rater scores correlated significantly in filtered tractography. There was, however, little correlation in the case when tractography were unfiltered. The NOSs are closely related to the change in visual scale of the averaged result; thus, suggesting that human ratings assessments of filtered tractography are well encapsulated by the NOS, whereas the human decision factors for unfiltered tractography are more complex. Since the rating questionnaire is based on yes/no decisions on subanatomy identification, it is possible that the raters preferred to err more on false-positives than risking false-negatives, and this is what contributes to the differences in unfiltered tractography ratings. This means that human rating can become unpredictably biased with different filtering parameters and a more stable rating metric such as NOS may be more desirable.

For the specific tractography algorithms, CST_{prob} produces the highest ratings, and performs particularly well in the optical radiation. It also results in more false-positives. This is most evident in CN VII/VIII and CN X results. In these cases the cranial nerve anatomies are very specific and local, and yet CST_{prob} produces more false-positive projections to distant regions. In the fornix there are also erroneous tract extensions into the corpus callosum. Deterministic methods in comparison are more conservative and therefore result in lower scores. They perform well when the anatomy is regional and has finer features. Both CST_{det} and XST performed well with cranial nerves. XST is able to image the rubrocerebellar pontine decussation with more reliability than CST_{det}. While CST_{prob} decussation delineation shows the highest reproducibility, it also produces wider projection coverage that is harder to interpret. The low DTT score is not surprising, as the single-tensor's inability to resolve crossing-fibers is well known. Based on the result of the study, we recommend the use of CST_{prob} for tasks in which the target anatomy is well defined and false positively can be easily recognized, or when interhemispheric and long projection distances are desired. For exploratory tractography, where filtering locations are not well defined, or when the anatomy features are close together, deterministic methods are recommended. When comparing CST_{det} and XST, it appears that XST is more conservative and thereby results in less false-positives. It also has better ability in resolving hemispherical decussations, as evident by the results of the rubrocerebellar projections. In practice, the two methods are very close in performance. Note, however, that the comparison is not exhaustive of the possible parameter combinations on either method, and therefore automated tuning of the parameters can answer this question more definitively.

It is evident from this study that there is no single tractography algorithm that is superior in all aspects. The recent Tractometer challenge (Neher et al., 2015), which compared a wide range of tractography algorithms, including DTT and CST on a high resolution DWI phantom, has come to the same observation. It is clear that algorithm choice is highly task-dependent. Given that vast number of neuropathologies are not well understood, there is often no available ground truth of neuroanatomical measure in the clinical environment from which to form priors regarding algorithm performance. Automatic tuning of tractography parameters in order to maximize anatomy and population-specific reproducibility, and thereby allowing task-specific tractography algorithm recommendations is a highly desirable future direction. The SAGIT platform and NOS are a first step toward this goal.

Limitations

For this study the DWI images were acquired at 0.94 × 0.94 × 3 mm^3 voxel resolution. The dataset was acquired for the purpose of cranial nerve visualization on a 3 T GE HDx MRI with eight-channels head coil, and is therefore incapable of less than 2.6 mm isovoxel DWI resolution at a clinically acceptable scanning time. For example, the average trigeminal nerve, one of the larger cranial nerves, has a diameter of about 2 mm, as of such we compromised on an anisotropic voxel resolution to gain in-plane resolution. We believe our findings are novel for the application of clinical tractography delineations in less than ideal conditions.

The limit of the NOS is closely tied to the performance of its associated tractography algorithm. An algorithm and its associated parameters may consistently produce the wrong result in all subjects and produce a high NOS, or it may produce no results, and result in a NOS of 0. Both of these cases are regular occurrences in single-subject tractography analysis. With merged tractography, it is easier to recognize such faults. This is because in practice, incorrect tract paths are often the result of imaging anomalies or algorithm limit, and are unstable across a population. This can be observed as a general trend in **Figure 3**, for example, where DTI delineation of the rubrocerebellar tract is clearly incorrect, and results in low NOS. Therefore, NOS is capable of characterizing the uncertainty as a result of low algorithmic performance. In the case of false positives that are highly consistent, SAGIT can help researchers make more informed judgment.

CONCLUSION

In this study, the SAGIT platform was created as an automated group tractography software platform that incorporated existing and proven dMRI practices, in order for group-wise dMRI to be more accessible to researchers. The tractography results demonstrated reliable and consistent performance of SAGIT across multiple subjects and techniques. By deploying SAGIT on 42 subjects, we quantifiably demonstrated that merged tractography is able to demonstrate algorithmic differences at a group-level. CST_{prob} is prone to false-positives, and thereby is suitable when the targeted anatomy is well known. CST_{det} and XST are more conservative, but have more trouble resolving hemispherical decussation and distant crossing projections. The NOS shows significant correlation with rater score for filtered tractography. Therefore it may be used for automated ratings of group tract results. As no single algorithm seems to be suitable for all anatomical tasks, it would be useful to consider using a mix of algorithms for different anatomical segments. Finally, we have demonstrated that merged tractography is a promising group-wise tractography analysis approach.

AUTHOR CONTRIBUTIONS

DC is the first author responsible for the original research and write up. JZ, DH, BB, MW, and PH contributed to the on going research design, and write up. MH is the principal investigator.

REFERENCES

Anderson, A. W. (2005). Measurement of fiber orientation distributions using high angular resolution diffusion imaging. *Magn. Reson. Med.* 54, 1194–1206. doi: 10.1002/mrm.20667

Avants, B. B., Epstein, C. L., Grossman, M., and Gee, J. C. (2008). Symmetric diffeomorphic image registration with cross-correlation: evaluating automated labeling of elderly and neurodegenerative brain. *Med. Image Anal.* 12, 26–41. doi: 10.1016/j.media.2007.06.004

Avants, B. B., Tustison, N. J., Song, G., Cook, P. A., Klein, A., and Gee, J. C. (2011). A reproducible evaluation of ANTs similarity metric performance in brain image registration. *Neuroimage* 54, 2033–2044. doi: 10.1016/j.neuroimage.2010.09.025

Basser, P. J., and Jones, D. K. (2002). Diffusion-tensor MRI: theory, experimental design and data analysis - a technical review. *NMR Biomed.* 15, 456–467. doi: 10.1002/nbm.783

Basser, P. J., Pajevic, S., Pierpaoli, C., Duda, J., and Aldroubi, A. (2000). In vivo fiber tractography using DT-MRI data. *Magn. Reson. Med.* 44, 625–632. doi: 10.1002/1522-2594(200010)44:4<625::AID-MRM17>3.0.CO;2-O

Behrens, T. E. J., Berg, H. J., Jbabdi, S., Rushworth, M. F. S., and Woolrich, M. W. (2007). Probabilistic diffusion tractography with multiple fibre orientations: what can we gain? *Neuroimage* 34, 144–155. doi: 10.1016/j.neuroimage.2006.09.018

Bihan, D., Le Poupon, C., Clark, C. A., Pappata, S., Molko, N., and Chabriat, H. (2001). Diffusion tensor imaging: concepts and applications. *J. Magn. Reson. Imaging* 546, 534–546. doi: 10.1002/jmri.1076

Chen, D. Q., Hayes, D., Davis, K., and Hodaie, M. (2015a). "Correcting diffusion weight image distortions using anisotropy power maps, a comparative study," in *Poster at the Annual Meeting of the Organization for Human Brain Mapping*, Honolulu, HI.

Chen, D. Q., Strauss, I., Hayes, D. J., Davis, K. D., and Hodaie, M. (2015b). Age-related changes in diffusion tensor imaging metrics of fornix subregions in healthy humans. *Stereotact. Funct. Neurosurg.* 93, 151–159. doi: 10.1159/000368442

Cho, K.-H., Yeh, C.-H., Tournier, J.-D., Chao, Y.-P., Chen, J.-H., and Lin, C.-P. (2008). Evaluation of the accuracy and angular resolution of q-ball imaging. *Neuroimage* 42, 262–271. doi: 10.1016/j.neuroimage.2008.03.053

Côté, M.-A., Boré, A., Girard, G., Houde, J.-C., and Descoteaux, M. (2012). Tractometer: online evaluation system for tractography. *Med. Image Comput. Comput. Assist. Interv.* 15, 699–706.

Côté, M.-A., Girard, G., Boré, A., Garyfallidis, E., Houde, J.-C., and Descoteaux, M. (2013). Tractometer: towards validation of tractography pipelines. *Med. Image Anal.* 17, 844–857. doi: 10.1016/j.media.2013.03.009

Dell'Acqua, F., Lacerda, L., Catani, M., and Simmons, A. (2014). "Anisotropic power maps: a diffusion contrast to reveal low anisotropy tissues from HARDI data," in *Proceedings of the International Society for Magnetic Resonance in Medicine*, Milan.

Dell'Acqua, F., Rizzo, G., Scifo, P., Clarke, R. A., Scotti, G., and Fazio, F. (2007). A model-based deconvolution approach to solve fiber crossing in diffusion-weighted MR imaging. *IEEE Trans. Biomed. Eng.* 54, 462–472. doi: 10.1109/TBME.2006.888830

Descoteaux, M., Angelino, E., Fitzgibbons, S., and Deriche, R. (2007). Regularized, fast, and robust analytical Q-ball imaging. *Magn. Reson. Med.* 58, 497–510. doi: 10.1002/mrm.21277

Fischl, B., Salat, D. H., Busa, E., Albert, M., Dieterich, M., Haselgrove, C., et al. (2002). Whole brain segmentation: automated labeling of neuroanatomical structures in the human brain. *Neuron* 33, 341–355. doi: 10.1016/S0896-6273(02)00569-X

Fritzsche, K. H., Laun, F. B., Meinzer, H.-P., and Stieltjes, B. (2010). Opportunities and pitfalls in the quantification of fiber integrity: what can we gain from Q-ball imaging? *Neuroimage* 51, 242–251. doi: 10.1016/j.neuroimage.2010.02.007

Garyfallidis, E., Brett, M., Amirbekian, B., Rokem, A., van der Walt, S., Descoteaux, M., et al. (2014). Dipy, a library for the analysis of diffusion MRI data. *Front Neuroinform* 8:8. doi: 10.3389/fninf.2014.00008

Jeurissen, B., Leemans, A., Tournier, J.-D., Jones, D. K., and Sijbers, J. (2012). Investigating the prevalence of complex fiber configurations in white matter tissue with diffusion magnetic resonance imaging. *Hum. Brain Mapp.* 34, 2747–2766. doi: 10.1002/hbm.22099

Klein, A., Andersson, J., Ardekani, B. A., Ashburner, J., Avants, B., Chiang, M. C., et al. (2009). Evaluation of 14 nonlinear deformation algorithms applied to human brain MRI registration. *Neuroimage* 46, 786–802. doi: 10.1016/j.neuroimage.2008.12.037

Leemans, A., and Jones, D. K. (2009). The B-matrix must be rotated when correcting for subject motion in DTI data. *Magn. Reson. Med.* 61, 1336–1349. doi: 10.1002/mrm.21890

Mori, S., and van Zijl, P. C. M. (2002). Fiber tracking: principles and strategies - a technical review. *NMR Biomed.* 15, 468–480. doi: 10.1002/nbm.781

Neher, P. F., Descoteaux, M., Houde, J.-C., Stieltjes, B., and Maier-Hein, K. H. (2015). Strengths and weaknesses of state of the art fiber tractography pipelines – a comprehensive in-vivo and phantom evaluation study using tractometer. *Med. Image Anal.* 26, 287–305. doi: 10.1016/j.media.2015.10.011

Pieper, S., Lorensen, B., Schroeder, W., and Kikinis, R. (2006). "The NA-MIC Kit: ITK, VTK, pipelines, grids and 3D slicer as an open platform for the medical image computing community," in *Proceedings of the 3rd IEEE International Symposium on Biomedical Imaging: Macro to Nano*, (Arlington, VA: IEEE), 698–701.

Qazi, A. A., Radmanesh, A., O'Donnell, L., Kindlmann, G., Peled, S., Whalen, S., et al. (2009). Resolving crossings in the corticospinal tract by two-tensor streamline tractography: method and clinical assessment using fMRI. *Neuroimage* 47(Suppl. 2), T98–T106. doi: 10.1016/j.neuroimage.2008.06.034

R Development Core Team (2012). *R: A Language and Environment for Statistical Computing*. Vienna: R Foundation for Statistical Computing.

Ramachandran, P., and Varoquaux, G. (2011). Mayavi: 3D visualization of scientific data. *Comput. Sci. Eng.* 13, 40–51. doi: 10.1109/MCSE.2011.35

Tournier, J.-D., Calamante, F., and Connelly, A. (2010). Improved probabilistic streamlines tractography by 2 nd order integration over fibre orientation distributions. *Ismrm* 88, 2010.

Tournier, J.-D., Calamante, F., and Connelly, A. (2012). MRtrix: diffusion tractography in crossing fiber regions. *Int. J. Imaging Syst. Technol.* 22, 53–66. doi: 10.1002/ima.22005

Tournier, J.-D., Calamante, F., Gadian, D. G., and Connelly, A. (2004). Direct estimation of the fiber orientation density function from diffusion-weighted MRI data using spherical deconvolution. *Neuroimage* 23, 1176–1185. doi: 10.1016/j.neuroimage.2004.07.037

Tuch, D. S., Reese, T. G., Wiegell, M. R., Makris, N., Belliveau, J. W., and Wedeen, V. J. (2002). High angular resolution diffusion imaging reveals intravoxel white matter fiber heterogeneity. *Magn. Reson. Med.* 48, 577–582. doi: 10.1002/mrm.10268

Tuch, D. S. D., Belliveau, J. J. W., and Wedeen, V. V. J. V. (2000). "A path integral approach to white matter tractography," in *Proceedings of 8th Annual Meeting of ISMRM*, Denver, CO.

van der Walt, S., and Smith, N. (2015). *A Better Default Colormap for Matplotlib. Python in Science (SciPy) Conference.* Available at: https://bids.github.io/colormap/

Wedeen, V. J., Hagmann, P., Tseng, W.-Y. I., Reese, T. G., and Weisskoff, R. M. (2005). Mapping complex tissue architecture with diffusion spectrum magnetic resonance imaging. *Magn. Reson. Med.* 54, 1377–1386. doi: 10.1002/mrm.20642

Wedeen, V. J., Wang, R. P., Schmahmann, J. D., Benner, T., Tseng, W. Y. I., Dai, G., et al. (2008). Diffusion spectrum magnetic resonance imaging (DSI) tractography of crossing fibers. *Neuroimage* 41, 1267–1277. doi: 10.1016/j.neuroimage.2008.03.036

Wilkins, B., Lee, N., Gajawelli, N., Law, M., and Leporé, N. (2015). Fiber estimation and tractography in diffusion MRI: development of simulated brain images and comparison of multi-fiber analysis methods at clinical b-values. *Neuroimage* 109, 341–356. doi: 10.1016/j.neuroimage.2014.12.060

Yendiki, A., Panneck, P., Srinivasan, P., Stevens, A., Zöllei, L., Augustinack, J., et al. (2011). Automated probabilistic reconstruction of white-matter pathways in health and disease using an atlas of the underlying anatomy. *Front. Neuroinform.* 5:23. doi: 10.3389/fninf.2011.00023

6

Affective Circuitry Alterations in Patients with Trigeminal Neuralgia

Dave J. Hayes[1,2], David Q. Chen[2], Jidan Zhong[2], Ariel Lin[1], Brendan Behan[2], Matthew Walker[2] and Mojgan Hodaie[2*]

[1] Psychology Department and Neuroscience Program, Union College, Schenectady, NY, United States, [2] Division of Brain, Imaging and Behaviour Systems Neuroscience and Division of Neurosurgery, Department of Surgery, Toronto Western Hospital, Krembil Research Institute, University Health Network, University of Toronto, Toronto, ON, Canada

***Correspondence:**
Mojgan Hodaie
mojgan.hodaie@uhn.ca;
dave.hayes@utoronto.ca

Trigeminal neuralgia (TN) is a severe chronic neuropathic facial pain disorder. Affect-related behavioral and structural brain changes have been noted across chronic pain disorders, but have not been well-studied in TN. We examined the potential impact of TN (37 patients: 23 with right-sided TN, 14 with left-sided TN), compared to age- and sex-matched healthy controls, on three major white matter tracts responsible for carrying affect-related signals—i.e., cingulum, fornix, and medial forebrain bundle. Diffusion magnetic resonance imaging (dMRI), deterministic multi-tensor tractography for tract modeling, and a model-driven region-of-interest approach was used. We also used volumetric gray matter analysis on key targets of these pathways (i.e., hippocampus, cingulate cortex subregions, nucleus accumbens, and ventral diencephalon). Hypotheses included: (1) successful modeling of tracts; (2) altered white matter microstructure of the cingulum and medial forebrain bundle (via changes in dMRI metrics such as fractional anisotropy, and mean, axial, and radial diffusivities) compared to controls; (3) no alterations in the control region of the fornix; (4) corresponding decreases in gray matter volumes. Results showed (1) all 325 tracts were successfully modeled, although 11 were partially complete; (2) The cingulum and medial forebrain bundle (MFB) were altered in those with TN, with dMRI metric changes in the middle ($p = 0.001$) and posterior cingulum ($p < 0.0001$), and the MFB near the ventral tegmental area (MFB-VTA) ($p = 0.001$). The posterior cingulum and MFB-VTA also showed unilateral differences between right- and left-sided TN patients; (3) No differences were noted at any fornix subdivision; (4) decreased volumes were noted for the hippocampus, posterior cingulate, nucleus accumbens, and ventral diencephalon. Together, these results support the notion of selectively altered affective circuits in patients with TN, which may be related to the experience of negative affect and the increased comorbidity of mood and anxiety disorders in this population.

Keywords: DTI, dMRI, diffusion magnetic resonance, chronic neuropathic pain, gray matter, MRI, emotion, structural neuroimaging

---

Abbreviations: AD, axial diffusivity; dMRI, diffusion magnetic resonance imaging; FA, fractional anisotropy; GM, gray matter; Hipp, hippocampus; MD, mean diffusivity; MFB, medial forebrain bundle; NAc, nucleus accumbens; PCC, posterior cingulate; PFC, prefrontal cortex; RD, radial diffusivity; ROI, region of interest; TN, trigeminal neuralgia; VD, ventral diencephalon; VTA, ventral tegmental area; WM, white matter.

INTRODUCTION

Trigeminal neuralgia (TN) is the most common chronic neuropathic facial pain disorder, characterized by the sudden onset of intermittent, intense, shock-like pain in distributions of the trigeminal nerve branches (Elias and Burchiel, 2002). Typically described as the worst pain imaginable, it is associated with high levels of negative affect and continued stress (Carlson, 2007; Vachon-presseau et al., 2013). Recently, diffusion magnetic resonance imaging (dMRI) was used to provide *in vivo* evidence of brain white matter alterations in TN patients, showing decreased fractional anisotropy (FA) and increased mean (MD), axial (AD), and radial (RD) diffusivities in affected trigeminal nerves (DeSouza et al., 2014). These dMRI metrics reflect the diffusivity of water along white matter tracts and support the presence of nerve alterations consistent with compression (Lutz et al., 2015). However, the neurovascular compression of the trigeminal nerve does not fully explain the disorder's presence, intensity, or clinical outcomes (Hilton et al., 1994; Miller et al., 2009; Hodaie and Coello, 2013; Ko et al., 2015). Moreover, changes in gray matter (GM) volumes and cortical thickness have been noted for clusters of voxels located within the anterior cingulate, thalamus, PAG, basal ganglia, insula, and orbitofrontal cortex (Desouza et al., 2013). Pharmacological treatments are not effective in many patients (Moulin et al., 2014) and, although neurosurgical treatments are capable of eliminating TN entirely in some cases, 20–30% of patients do not show improvement 1-year post-surgery (Hodaie and Coello, 2013). A better understanding of factors beyond nerve compression are needed to advance therapeutic decision making and improve prognostication. One promising avenue of inquiry focuses on classical affective or "limbic" circuitry as these are known to be involved in the regulation of states related to negative affect, pain, and stress. However, it is currently unclear if alterations in affective circuitry are related to the pathology of TN.

Human and animal studies have underscored altered psychological processing and affective circuitry in chronic neuropathic pain (Simons et al., 2013; Papini et al., 2015). For instance, an fMRI study showed that patients transitioning from acute to chronic back pain over a 1-year period had corresponding shifts in brain activity from classical pain-related (e.g., anterior cingulate cortex, anterior insula, thalamus) to more affect-related activations, involving the prefrontal cortex (PFC), amygdala, and nucleus accumbens/ventral striatum (NAc) (Hashmi et al., 2013; Vachon-Presseau et al., 2016). Patients with postherpetic neuralgia also showed altered affective circuit activations, including within the NAc and ventral tegmental area (VTA) (Geha et al., 2007), and those with fibromyalgia appear to show abnormal VTA responding to affective stimuli (Loggia et al., 2014). These are mirrored in animal studies which have identified changes in many cortical (e.g., cingulate, insula, hippocampus) and subcortical (e.g., NAc and VTA) regions (Yalcin et al., 2014). For instance, lesions of the rat cingulate cortex can reduce the aversiveness of neuropathic pain without impacting sensation, reward-related responding, or memory (Qu et al., 2011), while VTA disruptions caused by the upregulation of glial cells may be related to the persistence of chronic pain (Taylor et al., 2015).

Prior work from our group using a whole-brain, voxel-wise, analysis of white matter revealed lowered FA and higher MD in the middle cingulum, along with alterations in the corpus callosum, posterior corona radiata, and superior longitudinal fasciculus (DeSouza et al., 2014). Many neuroimaging studies have identified the cingulum in the processing of pain and negative affect (Hayes and Northoff, 2011, 2012; Shackman et al., 2011), and cingulotomy procedures in animals and humans can successfully reduce the unpleasantness of chronic pain (Yen et al., 2005; Qu et al., 2011). The use of whole-brain voxel-wise analytical programs has improved the objectivity of dMRI data at the group level, however, steps involving smoothing, registration, and masking significantly reduce the sensitivity of such analyses to uncover targeted abnormalities across subjects (for an in-depth discussion, including concerns related to white matter analysis using the widely-used software tract-based spatial statistics, see Bach et al., 2014). In the present work, we used an *a priori* neuroanatomical approach, which was highly sensitive to individual differences across subjects, to test the broad hypothesis that two major, well-defined, affective white matter tracts—the cingulum and medial forebrain bundle (MFB)—and their immediately targeted GM structures (i.e., cingulate cortex subregions, nucleus accumbens, and ventral diencephalon) would be altered in patients with TN compared to healthy controls.

Deterministic multi-tensor tractography was used to model three major affective white matter tracts (i.e., fornix, cingulum, MFB), followed by model-driven region-of-interest (ROI) analyses. The multi-tensor was chosen over a single-tensor approach as it has been shown to improve the modeling of tracts that are dense, highly crossing or angled, and travel over relatively long distances (Descoteaux et al., 2009; Qazi et al., 2009; Khalsa et al., 2014). The ROI approach avoided the problems that arise with the smoothing, registration, and masking required in many programs, such as tract-based spatial statistics, and allowed for a targeted subregional tract analysis at the individual level, in native space, which was analysable at the group level. With this combined approach, we tested the specific hypotheses that: (1) the fornix, cingulum, and MFB will be successfully modeled in TN patients, as well as healthy controls, using multi-tensor tractography; (2) ROI analysis from major subregions of the cingulum (i.e., anterior, middle, and posterior) and MFB (i.e., at the levels of the PFC, NAc, and VTA) will reveal differences in dMRI metrics (i.e., changes in FA, MD, AD, and RD) from controls consistent with the notion of altered affective circuitry in those with TN; (3) there will be no alterations in the fornix which will serve as a control region—as it has not been associated with chronic pain throughout the literature; (4) GM regions which are immediately innervated by the cingulum and MFB (i.e., cingulate cortex, nucleus accumbens, and ventral diencephalon) will show a decreased volume, reflecting the chronic impact of neuropathic pain.

MATERIALS AND METHODS

Participants

Retrospective analyses of dMRI data were carried out in 37 TN patients with unilateral pain (23 with right-sided, R-TN, and 14 with left-sided, L-TN, pain) and 28 healthy controls. All patients and volunteers were previously scanned at Toronto Western Hospital, and approval was granted by the University Health Network Research Ethics Board (Toronto, Canada). All healthy control volunteers gave written consent, while the UHN REB does not require this for retrospective analyses of patient data. Patient data was obtained through chart review, and the inclusion criteria were extreme unilateral pain consistent with a clinical diagnosis of TN, and not another disorder, as well as no prior brain surgeries. These patients were candidates for neurosurgery and, as such, were all treatment-resistant and reported the most intense subjective pain levels (e.g., a 9 or 10 on a 10-point scale) during clinical examinations. Patient demographic data can be seen in **Table 1**. R-TN (8 male; average age 47 ± 12; range 23–67 years) and L-TN (5 male; average age 55 ± 10; range 36–70 years) subjects were analyzed against sex- and age-matched healthy controls. The average ages and ranges for healthy controls of R-TN and L-TN patients, were 47 ± 12, range 23–65 and 53 ± 10, range 34–67, respectively. For optimal age- and sex-matching, 9 control subjects were used for both R-TN and L-TN analyses.

TABLE 1 | Patient demographic data.

Patient code	Side	Sex	Age (years)	Pain duration (years)	Medication (At time of surgery)
1	L	M	67	7	Carbamazepine
2	L	M	49	0.5	Carbamazepine
3	L	F	65	7	Gabapentin, Lamotrigine, Oxcarbazepine
4	L	M	63	3	Duloxetine, Baclofen
5	L	F	70	–	None
6	L	F	53	8	Gabapentin
7	L	M	48	4	Carbamazepine
8	L	F	55	–	Pregabalin
9	L	F	50	2	Carbamazepine, Gabapentin
10	L	M	36	9	Carbamazepine
11	L	F	54	3	Carbamazepine, Ketorolac
12	L	F	42	3	Gabapentin, Nortriptyline
13	R	M	46	8	Ibuprofen
14	R	F	52	10	Duloxetine, Topiramate
15	R	M	43	2	Carbamazepine, Diazepam
16	R	F	61	4	Carbamazepine, Gabapentin
17	R	F	40	8	Baclofen, Gabapentin
18	R	F	33	5	Gabapentin
19	R	F	38	6	Carbamazepine
20	R	M	52	6	Carbamazepine, Hydromorphone
21	R	F	59	4	Carbamazepine, Pregabalin
22	R	F	38	5	Carbamazepine, Pregabalin
23	R	F	67	1	Gabapentin, Hydromorphone
24	R	F	63	7	Carbamazepine
25	L	F	64	2	Gabapentin
26	R	M	61	2	Pregabalin
27	L	F	49	–	Carbamazepine
28	R	F	45	4	None
29	R	F	47	2	Carbamazepine, Gabapentin
30	R	F	53	2	Carbamazepine
31	R	M	38	1	Carbamazepine, Pregabalin
32	R	M	23	–	Carbamazepine
33	R	F	52	–	None
34	R	F	52	5	Carbamazepine
35	R	M	24	–	Carbamazepine, Nortriptyline
36	R	F	63	12	Pregabalin
37	R	M	38	2	Carbamazepine

MR Acquisition and Processing of Diffusion-Weighted and Anatomical Images

MR images were acquired on a GE Signa HDxt 3-tesla scanner (GE Healthcare, WI, USA) using an 8-channel phased-array head coil. Diffusion-weighted images were acquired over 12 min using 60 non-collinear directions with a dual-spin echo planar sequence to reduce eddy-current distortions. We used the Array Spatial Sensitivity Encoding Technique, or ASSET, with a factor of 2 and the following parameters: 0.94 × 0.94 × 3.0 mm voxels, 128 × 128 matrix, FOV = 24 cm, TE = 86.4 ms, TR = 12 s, b = 1,000 s/mm^2. Images were processed using 3D Slicer v 4.3.1 (MA-MIC©, http://www.slicer.org) (Pieper et al., 2004) and FSL v 5.0 (FMRIB Software Library, http://www.fmrib.ox.ac.uk/fsl/) (Smith et al., 2004) in a Linux environment. Diffusion-weighted scans were corrected for motion and eddy-current in FSL, and the b-matrices were corrected by averaging the rotational component of the gradient affine transforms and applying these to the original matrices (Leemans and Jones, 2009). 3D Slicer was used for visualization of diffusion magnetic resonance images (dMRI), seed and ROI drawing, tensor estimation, and the creation of scalar maps for fractional anisotropy (FA), and mean (MD), axial (AD), and radial (RD) diffusivities at the individual level. Anatomical T1-weighted axial images were acquired with a 3D Fast Spoiled Gradient Echo sequence, (0.9 × 0.9 × 1.0 mm^3 voxels from a 256 × 256 matrix with a 5 ms echo time, 12 ms repetition time, and a 300 ms inversion time.

Multi-Tensor Tractography Modeling

The fornix, and left and right cingula and MFB tracts were modeled from a single seed using the eXtended Streamline Tractography, or XST, deterministic multi-tensor tractographic algorithm (Qazi et al., 2009) (**Figure 1**). We chose a deterministic algorithm as Khalsa et al. (2014) showed that probabilistic is inferior to deterministic multi-tensor tractography in reconstructing longer brain pathways such as the ones described here (Khalsa et al., 2014). This resulted in the creation of 325 tractographic models across all subjects—65 midline forniceal models, 130 bilateral MFB, and 130 bilateral cingula models. Seeds to generate each tract were drawn in 3D Slicer using the FA map as a guide. Seed parameters were kept constant within tracts

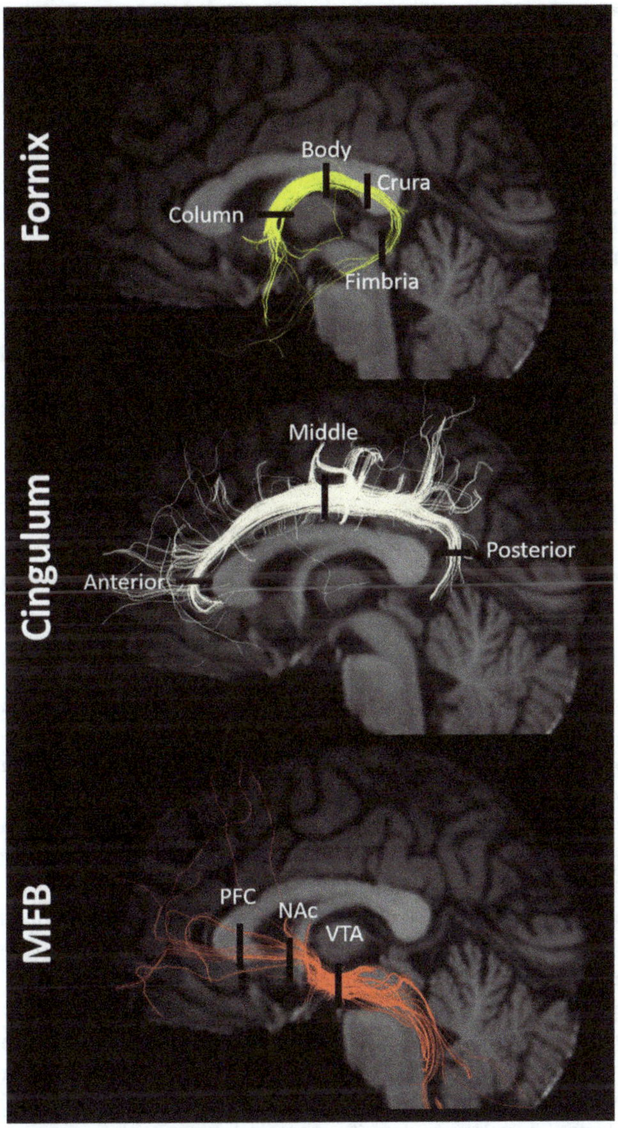

FIGURE 1 | Tracts and ROIs. Example of fornix, cingulum, and MFB multi-tensor tractography models in a single subject with regions-of-interest (ROIs) indicated by black lines. NAc, nucleus accumbens/ventral striatum; PFC, prefrontal cortex; VTA, ventral tegmental area.

and across subjects: fornix seeded at body (height x width: 2 × 10 voxels in coronal plane; volume: 53 mm^3), middle cingulum (2 × 8 voxels coronal; 42 mm^3), MFB near VTA (2 × 5 voxels coronal; 26 mm^3). The following multi-tensor tractography parameters were used: seeding point spacing of 0.25 mm, or 64 points/voxel, and streamline propagations initiated at fractional anisotropy > 0.2, tensor fractional = 0.1, curve radius = 0.8 radians, minimal path length = 10 mm, step size = 1 mm. In the few cases where the tract was incompletely modeled (see Results section below), we shifted the original seed in the most appropriate way (e.g., if the left fimbria was not complete, we shifted the original seed one voxel to the left) and remodeled until a complete tract was modeled (or could not be generated).

Model-Driven Region-of-Interest (ROI) White Matter Tract Analysis

A ROI approach was used to investigate potential differences in dMRI metrics (FA, MD, AD, RD) across major anatomical subregions of the fornix, cingulum, and MFB (**Figure 1**). Six ROIs were drawn for each tract, resulting in 18 ROIs per subject, and placement was guided by the multi-tensor tractography model as described below. ROIs were drawn directly in native space (instead of using an inverse transformation from standard space) because using anatomical landmarks in conjunction with the tractography model allowed for the unbiased, individualized, placement of the ROIs. In other words, this model-driven approach allowed for a comparative analysis across patient and control groups based on highly individualized ROIs—similar to an approach that could be adopted in future for clinical use.

The inclusion criteria for ROI creation was as follows: (1) ROIs were anatomically bounded, meaning that the tractographic models and color-by-orientation FA maps were used to ensure that ROIs included voxels in biologically relevant areas (e.g., did not contain irrelevant/low FA voxels which could bias the diffusivity measures); (2) selected voxels were coextensive, meaning that only neighboring voxels around the points of highest density in the model were chosen; (3) ROIs were drawn in 2 adjacent slices (four slices for all fimbria ROIs in an attempt to account for the thinness of this tract); (4) selected voxels included at least three streamlines in the coronal plane or two streamlines in the axial plane, to account for the greater surface area of the coronal plane.

ROIs were chosen based on prior studies of the main anatomical divisions of the fornix (Chen et al., 2015), cingulum (Jones et al., 2013), and MFB (Coenen et al., 2011, 2012a). Descriptive anatomical localizations of each ROI were as follows (**Figure 1**). For the fornix: column (midline structure with vertical course superior to the anterior commissure), body (midline structure following the roof of the third ventricle), crura (identified as the caudal bifurcation of the body—ROIs were drawn at the first instance of clear separation in the coronal plane), and fimbria (ROIs were drawn in the first four coronal slices anterior to the inflection point of the crura-to-fimbria curve). For the Cingulum: anterior (Ant-Cing; at the curve of the genu in the axial plane), middle (Mid-Cing; near the middle point between the anterior and posterior ROIs in the coronal plane), and posterior (Post-Cing; at the curve of the splenium in the axial plane) ROIs were drawn. For the MFB: anterior (PFC-MFB; at the level of the prefrontal cortex, PFC, dorsolateral to the corpus callosum genu), middle (NAc-MFB; at the level of the nucleus accumbens, Nac, using the first two coronal slices anterior to the anterior commissure), and posterior (MFB-VTA; just anterior to the ventral tegmental area, VTA) ROIs were drawn.

First (i.e., Level 1) and second (i.e., Levels 2a or 2b)-level analyses were performed where appropriate (see **Figure 2** for an illustration). A Bonferroni correction for multiple comparisons (i.e., mixed ANOVAs across 6 ROIs × 3 tracts) resulted in an alpha threshold of $p < 0.002$. Statistically significant results from Level 1 led to second-level analyses. Level 1 compared each patient group against their respective control group, i.e., patients

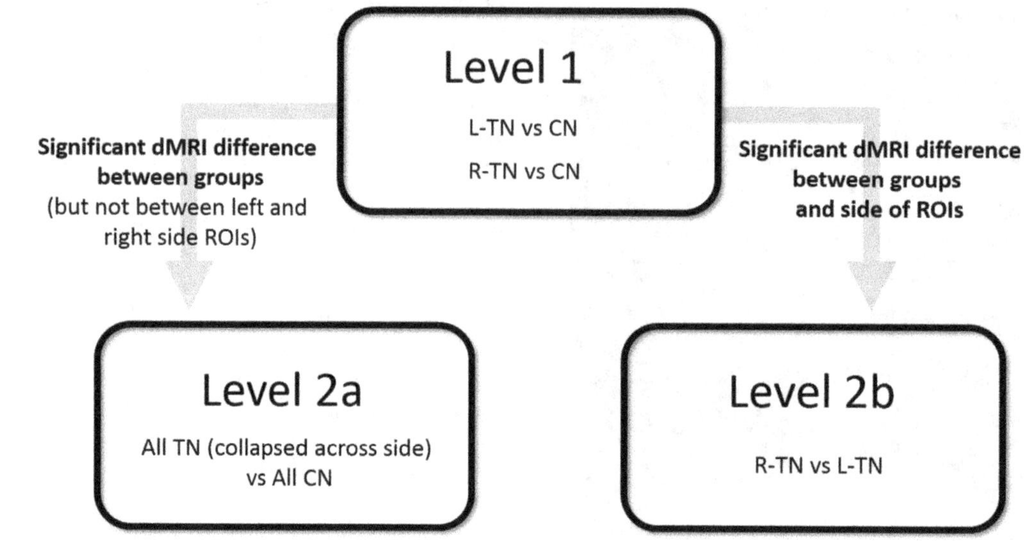

FIGURE 2 | Illustration of statistical design. CN, control subjects; ROI, region of interest; R- and L-TN, trigeminal neuralgia patients with right- and left-sided pain, respectively.

with right-sided TN pain (R-TN vs. R-CN) or left-sided pain (L-TN vs. L-CN) vs. controls. Level 2a compared all TN vs. CN when findings from Level 1 indicated that it was appropriate to pool the data from both R-TN and L-TN. Specifically, second-level analysis in Level 2a was used when Level 1 indicated a significant patient vs. control difference in dMRI values but not between the left- and right-sided ROIs in at least one TN group, supporting the notion that the dMRI differences were not specific to one side of the brain. Level 2b directly compared R-TN vs. L-TN when findings from Level 1 indicated that these groups were distinct from both controls as well as each other. Second-level analysis in Level 2b was used when the results from Level 1 indicated an interaction of dMRI metrics and side of ROI or when there were main effects of both dMRI metrics and side of ROI. Repeated measures ANOVAs (2 sides × 4 dMRI metrics) were used to test within- and between-group differences at each pair of ROIs. For Level 1, this resulted in three ANOVAs performed for each of the MFB and cingula, and four ANOVAS for the fornix. Main (sides × dMRI metrics × group) and subordinate interaction terms were considered (i.e., side × dMRI; side × group; dMRI × group). Significant interaction results were followed with appropriate *post-hoc t*-tests. All statistical analyses were performed in SPSS 17.0 (Chicago, IL, USA).

Gray Matter (GM) Volumetric ROI Analysis

GM volumetric analysis was performed using FreeSurfer software (version 5.3.0; http://surfer.nmr.mgh.harvard.edu/). Briefly, the pipeline includes motion correction, removal of the skull, intensity normalization, transformation to a common Talairach space, and an automated segmentation of cortical and subcortical structures. Further details are discussed elsewhere (e.g., Fischl et al., 2002; Fischl, 2012). For a complete reference of how Freesurfer segments the brain, see Destrieux et al. (2010). Upon completion, each segmented brain was manually inspected, slice by slice, for possible abnormalities and corrected for inaccuracies in the automated tracing algorithm using manually placed control editing points and the auto-reconstruction procedure (McCarthy et al., 2015).

We looked at the volumes of areas immediately innervated by the cingulum (i.e., anterior cingulate, middle cingulate, posterior cingulate, and isthmus), MFB (i.e., nucleus accumbens and ventral diencephalon, which primarily consists of the VTA, substantia nigra, hypothalamus, and mammillary bodies), and fornix (i.e., hippocampus), and which are automatically segmented using Freesurfer. It is worth noting that there is overlapping innervation between many structures, including the MFB and fornix both innervating regions of the ventral diencephalon while the MFB and cingulum both innervate the anterior cingulate cortex. To control for variations in size, all analyses were performed using a ratio of the structure's volume divided by the total intracranial volume of each participant. Each ROI was analyzed using a repeated measures ANOVA (group × side), followed by appropriate *post-hoc* testing ($p < 0.05$). First-stage analysis compared each patient group (those with right-sided, R-TN, or left-sided, L-TN pain) to their respective control group, and this was followed with R-TN vs. L-TN ANOVAs if the first-stage analyses were significant. A Bonferroni correction for multiple comparisons (i.e., mixed ANOVAs across 7 ROIs) resulted in an alpha threshold of $p < 0.007$.

RESULTS

Multi-Tensor Tractography Modeling

All 325 tracts were successfully modeled in every subject (see **Figure 1** for a typical example at the individual level). However, 19 model tracts were not complete—meaning that they had streamlines which appeared anatomically accurate, but did not allow for the creation of ROIs based on the criteria outlined above. In almost all cases, too few streamlines per voxel precluded ROI drawing. Eight of these were adequately reconstructed following the re-seeding strategy noted above, leaving a final number of 11 incomplete tracts following several re-modeling attempts. These included the following: the fimbria of the fornix was not complete for 3 R-TN patients (2 on right side, 1 on left side), 1 L-TN patient (left side), and 3 healthy controls (right side); one right-sided posterior cingulum model was not complete for a R-TN patient; and 3 left-sided MFB models were not complete at the level of the prefrontal cortex in 3 R-TN patients. ROIs were not drawn in incomplete areas (see above for ROI-drawing criteria), but were successfully drawn for all other sites (i.e., 11 ROIs could not be drawn).

Model-Driven White Matter Tract ROI Analysis

Mean values and standard errors of the mean (SEM) for dMRI metrics extracted from each ROI across groups are displayed in **Table 2**. The dMRI metrics are fractional anisotropy (FA), and mean (MD), axial (AD), and radial (RD) diffusivities. Values of parametric statistical significance between patient and control groups are indicated in black. For specific significance, see **Table 3**. Note that the MD, AD, and RD have been scaled up by a factor of 1,000 for interpretive ease.

The results from significant statistical analyses can be found in **Table 3**. The main FA findings are illustrated using scatterplots (Weissgerber et al., 2015) in **Figure 3**, and all correspond to changes in MD and also changes in either AD, RD, or both. Briefly, no significance (NS) was seen for any forniceal ROIs. For the cingula, both the middle and posterior ROIs were significantly different. The middle ROI showed a difference for L-TN vs. L-CN for the dMRI × group interaction (dxg: $p = 0.03$), but not for the R-TN vs. R-CN (dxg: $p = 0.07$), while comparing all TN patients vs. controls revealed a significant bilateral decrease in FA (see **Figure 3**) and increases in MD and RD ($p = 0.001$). The posterior ROI showed interactions between each patient group and their respective control groups which was significant for the side of ROI. Level 2b analysis confirmed this R-TN vs. L-TN difference showing particularly that FA and AD were significantly different between these groups on the left side of the brain ($p < 0.0001$). Finally, the MFB showed differences at the level of the VTA in L-TN and R-TN patients compared to their control groups ($p = 0.001$; **Figure 3**)—revealing that MD and RD are lower in the right-side of L-TN, when compared to R-TN, patients. See Supplementary Table 1 for results from all non-significant findings.

Gray Matter ROI Analysis

All statistically significant results are noted in **Table 4** and illustrated in **Figure 4**. In brief, we investigated the volumes of all four major subregions of the cingulate cortex, the NAc, VD, and the hippocampus. We noted significant bilateral volumetric decreases in the posterior cingulate, NAc, VD, and hippocampus in both TN groups compared to healthy controls. Alternately, no differences were noted in the rostral ACC, middle ACC, or isthmus.

TABLE 2 | Mean dMRI values by ROI.

Tract	ROI	dMRI metric ± SEM																															
		R-CN								L-CN								R-TN								L-TN							
		FA	±	MD	±	AD	±	RD	±	FA	±	MD	±	AD	±	RD	±	FA	±	MD	±	AD	±	RD	±	FA	±	MD	±	AD	±	RD	±
Fornix	Column	0.436	0.012	1.482	0.047	2.153	0.051	1.146	0.046	0.435	0.015	1.476	0.059	2.145	0.063	1.141	0.057	0.436	0.017	1.451	0.053	2.128	0.058	1.112	0.053	0.427	0.023	1.482	0.073	2.148	0.077	1.150	0.075
	Body	0.326	0.009	1.487	0.065	2.026	0.089	1.217	0.054	0.324	0.012	1.519	0.084	2.064	0.113	1.247	0.072	0.321	0.009	1.527	0.097	2.084	0.138	1.248	0.078	0.330	0.008	1.645	0.096	2.275	0.140	1.329	0.076
	L_Crus	0.277	0.008	1.749	0.086	2.268	0.112	1.489	0.074	0.256	0.008	1.856	0.117	2.369	0.149	1.600	0.102	0.266	0.010	1.716	0.102	2.206	0.121	1.470	0.093	0.272	0.011	1.737	0.115	2.258	0.147	1.476	0.101
	R_Crus	0.279	0.009	1.632	0.080	2.111	0.097	1.392	0.073	0.275	0.013	1.779	0.105	2.298	0.120	1.519	0.100	0.263	0.009	1.538	0.121	1.967	0.143	1.323	0.110	0.265	0.012	1.627	0.123	2.085	0.143	1.399	0.114
	L_Fimbria	0.526	0.025	0.925	0.034	1.527	0.037	0.624	0.039	0.492	0.030	0.971	0.051	1.543	0.057	0.685	0.054	0.500	0.026	0.933	0.032	1.502	0.045	0.649	0.039	0.466	0.022	0.957	0.027	1.502	0.043	0.684	0.027
	R_Fimbria	0.556	0.022	0.891	0.029	1.517	0.044	0.579	0.026	0.538	0.028	0.956	0.042	1.594	0.038	0.636	0.048	0.532	0.022	0.953	0.06[illegible]	1.550	0.065	0.654	0.062	0.545	0.021	0.932	0.032	1.562	0.030	0.617	0.035
Cingulum	L_Anterior	0.501	0.017	0.899	0.022	1.459	0.033	0.619	0.023	0.499	0.019	0.897	0.020	1.450	0.030	0.621	0.023	0.477	0.018	0.922	0.016	1.458	0.022	0.654	0.024	0.496	0.018	0.915	0.014	1.474	0.018	0.635	0.022
	R_Anterior	0.466	0.014	0.878	0.017	1.369	0.023	0.632	0.020	0.471	0.017	0.881	0.023	1.390	0.033	0.627	0.024	0.459	0.013	0.897	0.013	1.390	0.019	0.650	0.016	0.455	0.012	0.930	0.014	1.433	0.022	0.678	0.016
	L_Middle	**0.481**	**0.011**	**0.795**	**0.012**	1.265	0.017	**0.560**	**0.014**	**0.483**	**0.013**	**0.789**	**0.018**	1.259	0.025	**0.554**	**0.019**	**0.460**	**0.012**	**0.829**	**0.012**	1.289	0.012	**0.600**	**0.017**	**0.451**	**0.015**	**0.820**	**0.011**	1.256	0.019	**0.602**	**0.014**
	R_Middle	**0.439**	**0.013**	**0.789**	**0.014**	1.193	0.016	**0.587**	**0.016**	**0.453**	**0.014**	**0.777**	**0.021**	1.195	0.028	**0.569**	**0.022**	**0.411**	**0.009**	**0.840**	**0.015**	1.235	0.020	**0.643**	**0.015**	**0.422**	**0.011**	**0.829**	**0.011**	1.231	0.019	**0.628**	**0.012**
	L_Posterior	**0.513**	**0.017**	0.737	0.010	**1.213**	**0.020**	0.499	0.015	**0.520**	**0.022**	0.738	0.010	**1.222**	**0.019**	0.496	0.019	**0.482**	**0.014**	0.791	0.010	**1.263**	**0.015**	0.555	0.014	**0.432**	**0.017**	0.779	0.015	**1.180**	**0.027**	0.578	0.017
	R_Posterior	0.580	0.021	0.719	0.007	1.267	0.031	0.445	0.014	0.532	0.024	0.726	0.007	1.221	0.036	0.478	0.015	0.455	0.017	0.765	0.013	1.193	0.029	0.551	0.013	0.470	0.020	0.763	0.013	1.204	0.036	0.542	0.009
MFB	L_PFC	0.490	0.019	0.792	0.023	1.266	0.026	0.554	0.027	0.513	0.020	0.770	0.017	1.263	0.028	0.523	0.020	0.531	0.026	0.796	0.019	1.328	0.028	0.530	0.025	0.469	0.030	0.774	0.022	1.221	0.045	0.550	0.026
	R_PFC	0.449	0.022	0.789	0.016	1.222	0.034	0.573	0.017	0.474	0.024	0.791	0.019	1.258	0.044	0.558	0.019	0.490	0.019	0.840	0.026	1.348	0.033	0.586	0.029	0.475	0.021	0.801	0.023	1.263	0.034	0.570	0.025
	L_NAc	0.548	0.016	0.802	0.020	1.343	0.022	0.532	0.022	0.588	0.024	0.771	0.015	1.353	0.027	0.480	0.024	0.549	0.018	0.817	0.020	1.383	0.030	0.535	0.022	0.517	0.025	0.853	0.035	1.393	0.048	0.584	0.035
	R_NAc	0.526	0.013	0.808	0.016	1.329	0.027	0.548	0.016	0.542	0.015	0.796	0.016	1.340	0.031	0.524	0.017	0.531	0.015	0.873	0.020	1.458	0.032	0.581	0.020	0.522	0.016	0.865	0.018	1.417	0.029	0.589	0.020
	L_VTA	0.468	0.009	0.861	0.020	1.332	0.036	0.626	0.016	0.454	0.013	0.862	0.030	1.313	0.054	0.636	0.023	0.440	0.010	0.950	0.025	1.426	0.037	0.712	0.023	0.437	0.011	0.918	0.023	1.390	0.037	0.683	0.019
	R_VTA	0.481	0.011	**0.943**	**0.033**	1.465	0.047	**0.682**	**0.029**	0.488	0.014	**0.972**	**0.051**	1.526	0.077	**0.695**	**0.040**	0.459	0.012	**0.968**	**0.029**	1.473	0.037	**0.716**	**0.028**	0.491	0.014	**0.879**	**0.017**	1.392	0.028	**0.622**	**0.017**

All means dMRI values (FA, MD, AD, RD), and SEM, for each ROI across subject groups. Bolded numbers indicate significant findings described in ***Table 3****. AD, (axial diffusivity); FA, (fractional anisotropy); L-CN, (control group for L-TN); R-CN, (control group for R-TN); MD, (mean diffusivity); RD, (radial diffusivity). MD, AD, and RD were scaled up by 1000x.*

TABLE 3 | White matter ROI statistical analyses summary.

Tract	ROI	Level 1								Level 2a				Level 2b			
			R-TN vs. CN				L-TN vs. CN				All TN vs. CN				L-TN vs. R-TN		
		Interaction	F-value	P-value	Post-hoc tests	Interaction	F-value	P-value	Post-hoc tests	Interaction	F-value	P-value	Post-hoc tests	Interaction	F-value	P-value	Post-hoc tests
Fornix	Column	NS	–	–	–	NS	–	–	–	–	–	–	–	–	–	–	–
	Body	NS	–	–	–	NS	–	–	–	–	–	–	–	–	–	–	–
	Crura	NS	–	–	–	NS	–	–	–	–	–	–	–	–	–	–	–
	Fimbria	NS	–	–	–	NS	–	–	–	–	–	–	–	–	–	–	–
Cingulum	Anterior	NS	–	–	–	NS	–	–	–	–	–	–	–	–	–	–	–
	Middle	NS, but dxg	$F_{(3,132)} = 2.409$	0.070	Incr MD/RD	dxg sxd	$F_{(3,78)} = 3.137$ $F_{(3,78)} = 10.23$	0.030 <0.0001	Right: Inc MD/RD	dxg	$F_{(3,189)} =$ 5.52	0.001	Bilateral: Dec FA, Inc MD/RD	–	–	–	–
	Posterior	sxdxg	$F_{(3,129)} = 9.138$	<0.0001	Right: Dec FA, Inc MD/RD Left: Inc MD/RD/AD	dxg	$F_{(3,78)} = 9.823$	<0.0001	Right: Inc R MD/RD Left: Dec FA, Inc MD/RD	–	–	–	–	sxdxg	$F_{(3,99)} =$ 6.61	<0.0001	L FA: L-TN < R-TN L AD: L-TN > R-TN
MFB	PFC	sxd	$F_{(3,123)} = 3.50$	0.018	Right: Inc AD	NS	–	–	–	–	–	–	–	–	–	–	–
	NAc	NS	–	–	–	dxg	$F_{(3,78)} = 3.50$	0.019	Inc MD/RD	NS	$F_{(3,189)} =$ 0.85	0.5	–	–	–	–	–
	VTA	dxg NS, but sxd	$F_{(3,132)} = 5.92$ $F_{(3,132)} = 2.50$	0.001 0.063	Left: Dec FA, Inc MD/RD	NS sxdxg sxd	$F_{(3,78)} = 0.96$ $F_{(3,78)} = 16.58$	0.42 <0.0001	–	–	–	–	–	sxdxg	$F_{(3,105)} =$ 5.6	0.001	R MD/RD: L-TN < R-TN

Significant findings following repeated measures ANOVAs (group x dMRI values x side: g x d x s; group x side: g x s; dMRI x group: d x g), and results from post-hoc tests identifying increases (Inc) or decreases (Dec) in dMRI values compared to controls (Levels 1 & 2a) or between patient groups (Level 2b). NS = non-significant for both sxdxg and dxg with reported statistics for sxdxg. Alpha threshold corrected for multiple comparisons is $p < 0.002$.

DISCUSSION

This is the first study to investigate the potential relationship between the structure of major affective brain circuits (**Figure 1**) in those with TN (**Table 1**). In line with our first hypothesis, all 325 tracts across TN patients and healthy controls were successfully modeled, with only 11/1170 unusable ROIs (due to partially incomplete tracts). Of the three affect-related tracts, the cingula and MFB revealed alterations in those with TN (**Tables 2, 3**). Alterations in dMRI metrics of the middle and posterior cingulum, and the MFB near the VTA, along with decreased gray matter (GM) volumes in the posterior cingulate (PCC), nucleus accumbens (NAc), and ventral diencephalon (VD), further suggest that chronic neuropathic pain associated with TN is related to changes in the microstructure of these circuits (**Figures 3, 4, Table 4**). Unexpectedly, no clear differences were noted for the anterior cingulum, PFC-MFB, or NAc-MFB white matter ROIs (**Tables 2, 3**) or for the rostral ACC, middle ACC, or isthmus GM ROIs (**Table 4**). As anticipated, the fornix—along the four major subdivisions (Chen et al., 2015) studied here—did not demonstrate any alterations, further suggesting that affective circuitry is not indiscriminately altered in those with TN. Finally, decreased bilateral hippocampal volumes in TN are consistent with changes seen in other pain- and stress-related disorders, however we were unable to compare most of the associated fimbria in this region due to limitations of the tractography modeling.

Taken together, these results support the notion of selectively altered affective circuits in patients with TN which may be related to their experience of negative affect and the comorbidity of mood and anxiety disorders seen in this population. Moreover, these findings should be considered in the design of future studies aimed at elucidating how changes in white and gray matter structures—which are neuroanatomically remote from the trigeminal nerve—can help to further characterize patients with TN.

Affective Circuit Disruptions in TN: Mid-Cingulum, Post-Cingulum and PCC, and MFB-VTA and VD

The middle and posterior sections of the cingulate cortex have been associated with the processing of the affective, sensory, and perceptual dimensions of pain as well as cognitive-attentional control (Shackman et al., 2011; Leech and Sharp, 2014). The cingulum is the major white matter tract running along the cingulate cortices, providing broad direct connectivity between the prefrontal and posterior cingulate cortices, and the midcingulum also sends local projections upward to the sensorimotor, frontal, and parietal cortices (Jones et al., 2013; Heilbronner and Haber, 2014). Here, we replicated prior findings from our group (DeSouza et al., 2014) showing alterations in dMRI metrics for TN patients compared to healthy controls, i.e., decreased FA and increased MD and RD, in the bilateral midcingula (**Figure 3**, **Table 3**). These were found using the multi-tensor tractography model-driven ROI approach, while

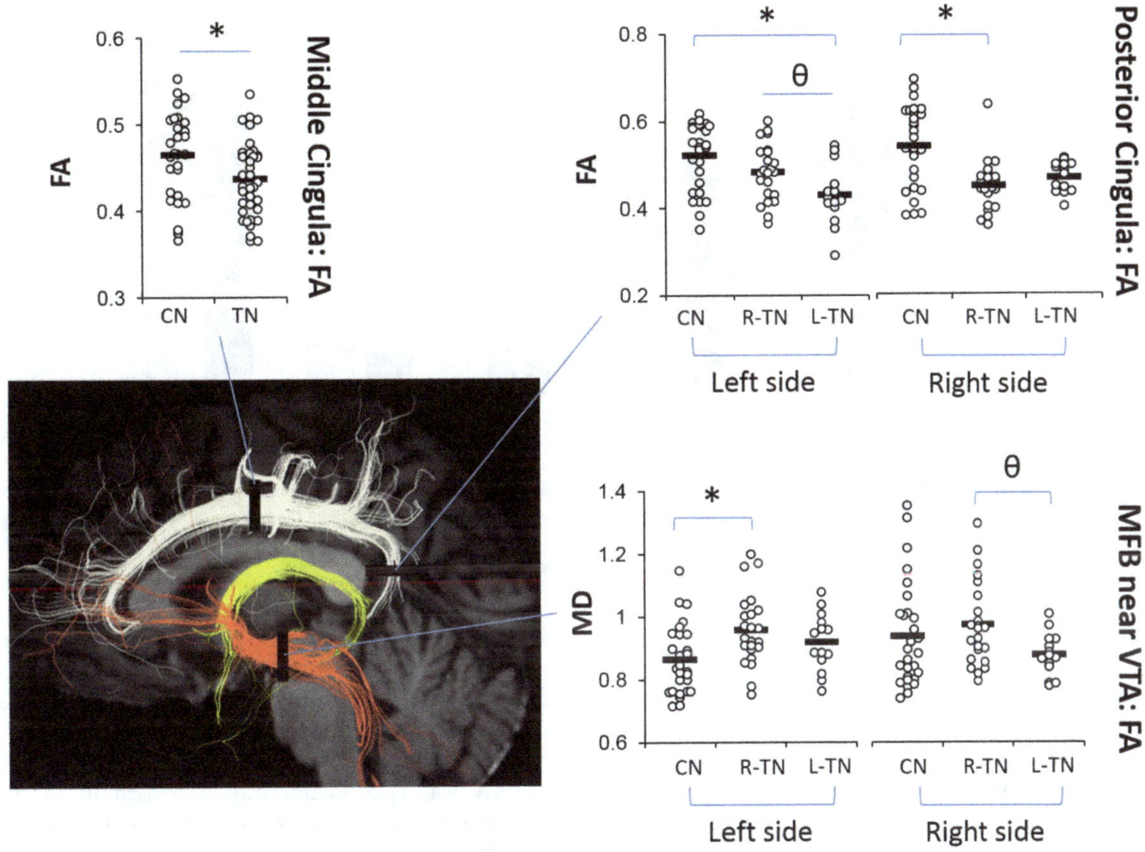

FIGURE 3 | Main dMRI findings in cingula (FA) and MFB-VTA (MD). Scatterplots showing ROIs where fractional anisotropy (FA) for the middle and posterior cingula, and mean diffusivity (MD) for the MFB-VTA, is different from controls (*) or between patient groups (θ), indicated by *post-hoc* tests ($p < 0.05$) following repeated measures ANOVA. MD was scaled up by 1000x. Corresponding changes in other dMRI metrics for these regions are indicated in **Table 3**.

TABLE 4 | Gray matter ROI statistical analyses summary.

Associated Tract	ROI	R-TN vs. CN				L-TN vs. CN			
		Interaction	***F*-value**	***P*-value**	***Post-hoc* tests**	**Interaction**	***F*-value**	***P*-value**	***Post-hoc* tests**
Fornix	Hippocampus	g sxg	19.33 2.0	<0.0001 0.16	TN < CN bilaterally	g sxg	12.76 12.72	0.001 0.003	TN < CN bilaterally
Cingulate	Anterior	NS (after MC)	–	–	–	NS (after MC)	–	–	–
	Middle	NS (after MC)	–	–	–	NS (after MC)	–	–	–
	Posterior	g sxg	16.05 1.43	0.0002 0.24	TN < CN bilaterally	g sxg (NS)	15.04 0.165	0.001 0.7	TN < CN bilaterally
	Isthmus	NS (after MC)	–	–	–	NS	–	–	–
MFB	NAc	g sxg	17.09 11.41	0.0001 0.002	TN < CN bilaterally, but only CN show L-NAc < R-NAc	g sxg	13.27 8.56	0.001 0.007	TN < CN bilaterally, but only CN show L-NAc < R-NAc
	Ventral diencephalon (including midbrain and hypothalamus)	g sxg	22.67 3.62	<0.0001 0.06	TN < CN bilaterally	g sxg	13.73 2.5	0.001 0.13	TN < CN bilaterally

Significant findings for repeated measures ANOVAs (group: g; group x side: g x s), and results from post-hoc tests identifying changes in gray matter volumes (mm^3) in TN patients vs. healthy controls (CN). Alpha threshold corrected for multiple comparisons (MC) is $p < 0.007$.

prior findings were uncovered using a whole-brain voxel-wise approach, i.e., FSL's TBSS. The identified role of the midcingulate region as a hub involved in the affective dimension of pain has been well-established by the abundant translational evidence (Hayes and Northoff, 2012), although how precisely it is involved in the integration of processing related to affect,

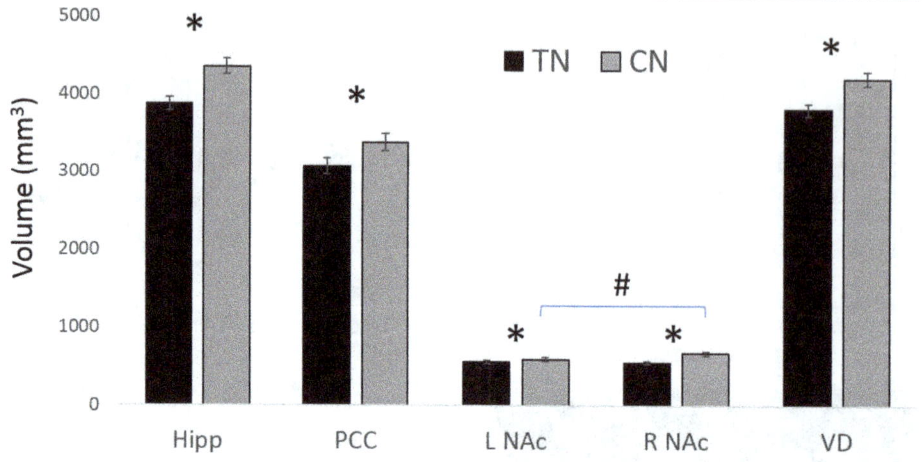

FIGURE 4 | Main GM findings. The main results showing gray matter (GM) decreases in patients with TN compared to healthy controls (CN). * = significant between groups; # L NAc is smaller than R NAc in CN; all results are significant at $p < 0.05$ following ANOVA with corrections for multiple comparisons. Hipp, (Hippocampus); NAc, (nucleus accumbens); PCC, (posterior cingulate cortex); VD, (ventral diencephalon). See **Table 4** for corresponding statistics.

salience, and pain requires further study (Shackman et al., 2011).

We also extended upon prior findings by showing changes in the posterior cingulum and PCC which were significant across all groups, i.e., bilateral decreases in PCC volume along with decreased FA on the patient's affected side, and increased MD and RD bilaterally in both R-TN and L-TN patients (**Tables 3, 4**). This is consistent with nearby changes to the posterior corona radiata, posterior superior longitudinal fasciculus, and posterior corpus callosum identified previously (DeSouza et al., 2014) as these nearby regions share overlapping innervation. In fact, given the smoothing and registration steps involved in whole-brain voxel-wise analyses used previously, and the proximity of these other tracts to the cingulum, it is possible that some of the nearby changes identified previously are actually alterations of the cingulum (Bach et al., 2014)—however, we did not test this explicitly here as it would require the independent reconstruction of these more complex highly-crossing tracts. TN-related alterations of the posterior cingulum—which connects the nearby posterior cingulate, precuneus, retrosplenial/isthmus, and parietal cortices to frontal, temporal, and subcortical sites (Jones et al., 2013; Heilbronner and Haber, 2014)—was anticipated, as the posterior cingulate-precuneus has been identified as a functionally relevant area in previous chronic pain neuroimaging studies. In particular, the posterior cingulate is a key structure of the default mode network, and altered structural-functional connectivity within this network and sensorimotor regions has been identified in patients with fibromyalgia (Cifre et al., 2012; Flodin et al., 2014), temporomandibular disorder (Weissman-Fogel et al., 2011; Kucyi et al., 2014), and chronic back pain (Kregel et al., 2015).

The current inclusion of an L-TN group, unlike prior studies which included only patients with R-TN, allowed for the investigation of potential differences between these patient groups—this is also why our first stage of analysis considered each R-TN and L-TN group separately. Identification of unilateral differences in FA, however, was unexpected. This finding suggests that those suffering from right-sided TN pain may show greater alterations in their right-sided posterior cingulum, and vice versa for L-TN patients (although right-side FA was also significantly decreased in L-TN patients), when compared to healthy controls as well as when compared between patient groups (**Figure 3**). Although unexpected, a few reports are in line with such unilateral findings, as patients with fibromyalgia show altered processing in posterior cingulate cortex and, ipsilateral to a painful stimulus, secondary somatosensory cortex (Gracely, 2004). Also, those with complex regional pain syndrome show increased activation of the posterior cingulate during stimulation of their symptomatic hand (Freund et al., 2010). Further study is required to fully understand the significance of this unilateral difference, especially since only bilateral and not unilateral decreases in PCC volume were noted here.

Interestingly, our results suggest that the left-sided MFB, just anterior to the VTA region, may be different in patients compared to controls. We noted dMRI changes (i.e., decreased FA, increased MD and RD) in R-TN patients in the left MFB-VTA when compared to healthy controls (**Figure 3**, **Table 3**; however, the L-TN group showed no dMRI changes, which may be due to the latter group's smaller size). These results are also consistent with the decreased volumes of the VD (consisting mainly of the VTA, substantia nigra, hypothalamus, and mammillary bodies) seen here (**Figure 4**), although this decrease was bilateral in both R-TN and L-TN groups. Although few studies have considered laterality differences for the MFB or VTA, one recent study showed the left MFB FA correlated with the ability to experience pleasure (Bracht et al., 2015). The MFB connects the VTA, NAc, and PFC, and has been successfully reconstructed by others using tractographic models (Coenen et al., 2012b; Hana et al., 2015). It is strongly implicated in the processing of appetitive and aversive stimuli (Hayes et al., 2014), and the VTA is important in human pain processing (Fairhurst et al., 2007; Hayes and Northoff, 2012). Animal studies have identified a host of neurochemical factors involved in regulating the nociceptive response within the VTA, including a complex involvement of orexin, opioids, and dopamine (Yazdi-Ravandi et al., 2014; Hipolito et al., 2015). Increased VTA microglial activation is associated with chronic neuropathic pain (Taylor et al., 2015), and is one possible explanation for the altered dMRI metrics in the present study, as increased microglial activation reflects local inflammation which may lead to disruptions in water diffusivity, decreased FA, and increased MD and RD (Alexander et al., 2007; Po et al., 2012).

Interestingly, previous animal studies have described asymmetrical structure and function within the mesocorticolimbic system with a general bias for left-sided aversive, and right-sided appetitive, processing found in some studies (Rosen et al., 1984; Besson and Louilot, 1995). This makes our second-level finding of lower MD and RD values in L-TN compared with R-TN patients intriguing—however, at this point, the relevance of this finding is unclear and is not further supported by the GM findings. Taken together, these results suggest that the alterations in the left-sided MFB-VTA tract and bilateral decreases in the VD seen in our study may reflect altered aversion-related processing, broadly consistent with the experience of chronic neuropathic pain and persistent negative affect.

Disruptions Are Not Evenly Distributed: Ant-Cingulum, PFC-MFB, NAc-MFB, and Fornix

The present study included the fornix as a tract involved in affective processing, but which has not been consistently identified as a structure impacted in chronic neuropathic pain. In fact, only one study links chronic pain to changes in the fornix, finding higher FA in the whole fornix of patients with irritable bowel syndrome (Chen et al., 2011). However, these findings should be considered cautiously as there were only 10 patients analyzed compared to controls ($p = 0.014$) using whole-brain voxel-wise analysis (Bach et al., 2014; and see discussion above). Consistent with our hypothesis, we found no forniceal differences in the present study between TN patients and controls—across ROIs which were chosen based on previously identified anatomical subdivisions (i.e., column, body, crura, and fimbria) (Chen et al., 2015). However, a major GM target of the fornix, the hippocampus, did show decreased volumes bilaterally in TN patients. This is consistent with prior evidence showing decreased hippocampal volumes in response to chronic pain and stress (although see Smallwood et al., 2013 for evidence that the right hippocampus might actually be larger in some cases) and may also correspond to decreases in anterior fimbria FA values—although tractographic modeling prevented us from investigating this in the present study (see limitations below for further discussion).

Contrary to our original hypotheses, however, we found no changes within the anterior cingulum (Ant-Cing), or along the MFB at the levels of the PFC or NAc/ventral striatum (Supplementary Table 1). Projections from both the Ant-Cing and PFC-MFB enter the medial prefrontal cortex, a region involved in the processing and contextualization of healthy affective responses (Roy et al., 2012; Hayes et al., 2014), and which has shown decreased gray matter volume and altered FA in other studies of chronic neuropathic pain (Moayedi et al., 2012; Ivo et al., 2013; Lin, 2014). Nonetheless, our current findings are in line with prior studies in TN showing white matter changes primarily in middle and posterior tracts (Gustin et al., 2012; Moayedi et al., 2012; DeSouza et al., 2014). Importantly, the absence of findings here does not preclude the involvement of the prefrontal cortex in TN, as other studies have shown it to predict painful responsivity and exposure to childhood stressors despite not showing direct intraregional functional or structural changes (Hayes et al., 2013; Duncan et al., 2015). The splayed nature of the PFC-MFB tract also resulted in a greater variability in ROI placement compared to all other ROIs, which were relatively anatomically confined, and it is possible that this variability may have prevented the identification of clear changes in this region.

Perhaps the most unexpected negative finding was the absence of changes in NAc-MFB microstructure, despite the fact that the MFB was well-modeled at this level in all subjects (**Figure 1**). This was not expected given prior findings in both rats (Chang et al., 2014) and humans (Baliki et al., 2010; Hashmi et al., 2013) of NAc functional changes and the role of PFC-NAc connectivity in subjects with chronic neuropathic pain (Baliki et al., 2012; Lee et al., 2015). Alternately, the finding of decreased NAc volumes (**Figure 4**, **Table 4**) in TN patients is consistent with the role of this structure in pain and affective processing and is in agreement with prior pain studies (Geha et al., 2008; Gustin et al., 2011). Although our NAc-MFB ROIs were selected using clear anatomical landmarks (Lucas-Neto et al., 2014), it remains the case that fibers from the MFB are intertwined with the fibers of the anterior limb of the internal capsule at this level (Coenen et al., 2012a,b; Hana et al., 2015), and so selected voxels will likely contain many non-MFB fibers in this region compared to the MFB-VTA.

Limitations and Future Directions

This study investigated the hypothesis that chronic pain and associated negative affect associated with TN would correspond to changes in major limbic circuits, as seen in altered white and gray matter. The patients were candidates for neurosurgery and, as such, were treatment-resistant and reported the most intense pain imaginable on standard scales. As is typical in these patients, all reported the highest levels of subjective pain (a 9 or 10 on a 10-point scale), and many reported subjective changes in anxiety or mood over time. Unfortunately, there was not enough variability to look for correlations related to subjective pain reports, and no standard measures of mood or anxiety were taken during clinical visits. We intend to include such measures in future.

Psychosocial comorbidities are known to play a significant role in the risk of developing, and progression of, chronic neuropathic pain syndromes (Turk et al., 2010; Simons et al.,

2013). The TN patients in the present study were screened as potential surgical candidates and were included here because there were no obvious psychiatric or psychological disorders present. It should be noted, however, that this is not assessed through formal psychiatric screening, but by standard neurological and neurosurgical clinical assessments. Nearly all patients were on some form of medication (**Table 1**)—typically antiepileptics whose effects on dMRI metrics have not been studied. Although the effects of these drugs have not been well-studied in this regard, there is evidence that the long-term use of antiepileptics (such as carbamazepine, the main pharmacological treatment used in our sample) in those with temporal lobe epilepsy results in alterations in the hippocampus, posterior cingulate, and thalamus (Haneef et al., 2015). In particular, the authors found reduced betweenness centrality (a measure of connectivity, or "hubness," used in graph theory) in the hippocampus and increased betweenness centrality in the cingulate—and particularly in the posterior cingulate. This raises the possibility that our findings, particularly for the posterior cingulate, may be related in part to the long-term use of these compounds. Further research is needed to disentangle these effects.

The three tracts were chosen for their role as major affective pathways, as well as their relatively low-variability across subjects. Nonetheless, a primary limitation of the current approach is the increased variability in some subregions (e.g., PFC-MFB) over others as well as the inability to explore all anatomical subregions in detail. For instance, although we saw no fornix changes in the present analysis, there could be subtler changes in the finer projections of the pre- and post-commissural fornix, as these project to highly relevant affective regions such as the accumbens and hypothalamus, or in the anterior portion of the fimbria. Indeed, although white and gray matter changes do not necessarily occur in unison, the extent to which the hippocampal volumes are decreased here raises the possibility that the fimbria may also be altered. The anterior portion of the fimbria is especially interesting given that many human and animal studies related to chronic stress or pain have shown appreciable changes in hippocampal volumes (Bremner, 2006; Smallwood et al., 2013; Vachon-presseau et al., 2013; Vachon-Presseau et al., 2016).

CONCLUSION

This is the first study to use an *a priori* investigation of the impact of TN on affective circuits, finding white matter alterations in the middle and posterior cingulum and near the MFB-VTA, and corresponding gray matter changes in the PCC and VD as well as decreased NAc volumes. Based on these promising findings, we are currently undertaking studies to determine if these abnormalities are linked directly with other functional brain differences and affective behavioral measures. We will also look at whether post-surgical outcomes of patients who received neurosurgical interventions, have reversals of such alterations following successful surgeries. Further studies should also look at whether these findings can be used to help more accurately tailor clinical and surgical approaches to individuals, as there are numerous surgical approaches available for which it is currently challenging to predict favorable outcomes.

AUTHOR CONTRIBUTIONS

DH, DC, BB, MW, JZ, AL, and MH contributed to the experimental design and analysis. DC and MH collected the data. DH and MH wrote the paper.

ACKNOWLEDGMENTS

The authors would like to thank Ms. Tessa Burkholder for her assistance in acquiring clinical information.

REFERENCES

Alexander, A. L., Lee, J. E., Lazar, M., and Field, A. S. (2007). Diffusion tensor imaging of the brain. *Neurotherapeutics* 4, 316–329. doi: 10.1016/j.nurt.2007.05.011

Bach, M., Laun, F. B., Leemans, A., Tax, C. M. W., Biessels, G. J., Stieltjes, B., et al. (2014). Methodological considerations on tract-based spatial statistics (TBSS). *Neuroimage* 100, 358–369. doi: 10.1016/j.neuroimage.2014.06.021

Baliki, M. N., Geha, P. Y., Fields, H. L., and Apkarian, A. V. (2010). Predicting value of pain and analgesia: nucleus accumbens response to noxious stimuli changes in the presence of chronic pain. *Neuron* 66, 149–160. doi: 10.1016/j.neuron.2010.03.002

Baliki, M. N., Petre, B., Torbey, S., Herrmann, K. M., Huang, L., Schnitzer, T. J., et al. (2012). Corticostriatal functional connectivity predicts transition to chronic back pain. *Nat. Neurosci.* 15, 1117–1119. doi: 10.1038/nn.3153

Besson, C., and Louilot, A. (1995). Asymmetrical involvement of mesolimbic dopaminergic neurons in affective perception. *Neuroscience* 68, 963–968.

Bracht, T., Doidge, A. N., Keedwell, P. A., and Jones, D. K. (2015). Hedonic tone is associated with left supero-lateral medial forebrain bundle microstructure. *Psychol. Med.* 45, 865–874. doi: 10.1017/S0033291714001949

Bremner, J. D. (2006). Traumatic stress: effects on the brain. *Dialogues Clin. Neurosci.* 8, 445–461.

Carlson, C. R. (2007). Psychological factors associated with orofacial pains. *Dent. Clin. North Am.* 51, 145–160. doi: 10.1016/j.cden.2006.09.001

Chang, P.-C., Pollema-Mays, S. L., Centeno, M. V., Procissi, D., Contini, M., Baria, A. T., et al. (2014). Role of nucleus accumbens in neuropathic pain: linked multi-scale evidence in the rat transitioning to neuropathic pain. *Pain* 155, 1128–1139. doi: 10.1016/j.pain.2014.02.019

Chen, D. Q., Strauss, I., Hayes, D. J., Davis, K. D., and Hodaie, M. (2015). Age-related changes in diffusion tensor imaging metrics of fornix subregions in healthy humans. *Stereotact. Funct. Neurosurg.* 93, 151–159. doi: 10.1159/000368442

Chen, J. Y.-W., Blankstein, U., Diamant, N. E., and Davis, K. D. (2011). White matter abnormalities in irritable bowel syndrome and relation to individual factors. *Brain Res.* 1392, 121–131. doi: 10.1016/j.brainres.2011.03.069

Cifre, I., Sitges, C., Fraiman, D., Munoz, M. A., Balenzuela, P., Gonzalez-Roldan, A., et al. (2012). Disrupted Functional connectivity of the pain network in fibromyalgia. *Psychosom. Med.* 74, 55–62. doi: 10.1097/PSY.0b013e3182408f04

Coenen, V. A., Panksepp, J., Hurwitz, T. A., Urbach, H., and Mädler, B. (2012a).

Human medial forebrain bundle (MFB) and anterior thalamic radiation (ATR): imaging of two major subcortical pathways and the dynamic balance of opposite affects in understanding depression. *J. Neuropsychiatry Clin. Neurosci.* 24, 223–236. doi: 10.1176/appi.neuropsych.11080180

Coenen, V. A., Schlaepfer, T. E., Allert, N., and Mädler, B. (2012b). Diffusion tensor imaging and neuromodulation: DTI as key technology for deep brain stimulation. *Int. Rev. Neurobiol.* 107, 207–234. doi: 10.1016/B978-0-12-404706-8.00011-5

Coenen, V. A., Schlaepfer, T. E., Maedler, B., and Panksepp, J. (2011). Cross-species affective functions of the medial forebrain bundle-Implications for the treatment of affective pain and depression in humans. *Neurosci. Biobehav. Rev.* 35, 1971–1981. doi: 10.1016/j.neubiorev.2010.12.009

Descoteaux, M., Deriche, R., Knösche, T. R., and Anwander, A. (2009). Deterministic and probabilistic tractography based on complex fibre orientation distributions. *IEEE Trans. Med. Imaging* 28, 269–286. doi: 10.1109/TMI.2008.2004424

DeSouza, D. D., Hodaie, M., and Davis, K. D. (2014). Abnormal trigeminal nerve microstructure and brain white matter in idiopathic trigeminal neuralgia. *Pain* 155, 37–44. doi: 10.1016/j.pain.2013.08.029

Desouza, D. D., Moayedi, M., Chen, D. Q., Davis, K. D., and Hodaie, M. (2013). Sensorimotor and pain modulation brain abnormalities in trigeminal neuralgia: a paroxysmal, sensory-triggered neuropathic pain. *PLoS ONE* 8:e66340. doi: 10.1371/journal.pone.0066340

Destrieux, C., Fischl, B., Dale, A., and Halgren, E. (2010). Automatic parcellation of human cortical gyri and sulci using standard anatomical nomenclature. *Neuroimage* 53, 1–15. doi: 10.1016/j.neuroimage.2010.06.010

Duncan, N., Hayes, D., Wiebking, C., Tiret, B., Pietruska, K., Chen, D. Q., et al. (2015). Negative childhood experiences alter a prefrontal-insular-motor cortical network in healthy adults: A preliminary multimodal rsfMRI-fMRI-MRS-dMRI study. *Hum. Brain Mapp.* 36, 4622–4637. doi: 10.1002/hbm.22941

Elias, W. J., and Burchiel, K. J. (2002). Trigeminal neuralgia and other neuropathic pain syndromes of the head and face. *Curr.Pain Headache Rep.* 6, 115–124.

Fairhurst, M., Wiech, K., Dunckley, P., and Tracey, I. (2007). Anticipatory brainstem activity predicts neural processing of pain in humans. *Pain* 128, 101–110. doi: 10.1016/j.pain.2006.09.001

Fischl, B. (2012). NeuroImage *FreeSurfer* 62, 774–781. doi: 10.1016/j.neuroimage.2012.01.021

Fischl, B., Salat, D. H., Busa, E., Albert, M., Dieterich, M., Haselgrove, C., et al. (2002). Whole brain segmentation: automated labeling of neuroanatomical structures in the human brain. *Neuron* 33, 341–355.

Flodin, P. D., Martinsen, S., Löfgren, M., Bileviciute-Ljungar, I., Kosek, E., and Fransson, P. (2014). Fibromyalgia is associated with decreased connectivity between pain- and sensorimotor brain areas. *Brain Connect.* 62:2545. doi: 10.1089/brain.2014.0274

Freund, W., Wunderlich, A. P., Stuber, G., Mayer, F., Steffen, P., Mentzel, M., et al. (2010). Different activation of opercular and posterior cingulate cortex (PCC) in patients with complex regional pain syndrome (CRPS I) compared with healthy controls during perception of electrically induced pain: a functional MRI study. *Clin. J. Pain* 26, 339–347. doi: 10.1097/AJP.0b013e3181cb4055

Geha, P. Y., Baliki, M. N., Harden, R. N., Bauer, W. R., Parrish, T. B., and Apkarian, A. V. (2008). The brain in chronic CRPS pain: abnormal gray-white matter interactions in emotional and autonomic regions. *Neuron* 60, 570–581. doi: 10.1016/j.neuron.2008.08.022

Geha, P., Baliki, M., Chialvo, D., and Harden, R. (2007). Brain activity for spontaneous pain of postherpetic neuralgia and its modulation by lidocaine patch therapy. *Pain* 128, 88–100. doi: 10.1016/j.pain.2006.09.014

Gracely, R. H. (2004). Pain catastrophizing and neural responses to pain among persons with fibromyalgia. *Brain* 127, 835–843. doi: 10.1093/brain/awh098

Gustin, S. M., Peck, C. C., Cheney, L. B., Macey, P. M., Murray, G. M., and Henderson, L. A. (2012). Pain and plasticity: is chronic pain always associated with somatosensory cortex activity and reorganization? *J. Neurosci.* 32, 14874–14884. doi: 10.1523/JNEUROSCI.1733-12.2012

Gustin, S. M., Peck, C. C., Wilcox, S. L., Nash, P. G., Murray, G. M., and Henderson, L. A. (2011). Different pain, different brain: thalamic anatomy in neuropathic and non-neuropathic chronic pain syndromes. *J. Neurosci.* 31, 5956–5964. doi: 10.1523/JNEUROSCI.5980-10.2011

Hana, A., Hana, A., Dooms, G., Boecher-Schwarz, H., and Hertel, F. (2015). Visualization of the medial forebrain bundle using diffusion tensor imaging. *Front. Neuroanat.* 9:139. doi: 10.3389/fnana.2015.00139

Haneef, Z., Levin, H. S., and Chiang, S. (2015). Brain graph topology changes associated with anti-epileptic drug use. *Brain Connect.* 5, 284–291. doi: 10.1089/brain.2014.0304

Hashmi, J. A., Baliki, M. N., Huang, L., Baria, A. T., Torbey, S., Hermann, K. M., et al. (2013). Shape shifting pain: chronification of back pain shifts brain representation from nociceptive to emotional circuits. *Brain* 136, 2751–2768. doi: 10.1093/brain/awt211

Hayes, D. J., and Northoff, G. (2011). Identifying a network of brain regions involved in aversion-related processing: a cross-species translational investigation. *Front. Integr. Neurosci.* 5:49. doi: 10.3389/fnint.2011.00049

Hayes, D. J., and Northoff, G. (2012). Common brain activations for painful and non-painful aversive stimuli. *BMC Neurosci.* 13:60. doi: 10.1186/1471-2202-13-60

Hayes, D. J., Duncan, N. W., Wiebking, C., Pietruska, K., Qin, P., Lang, S., et al. (2013). GABAA receptors predict aversion-related brain responses: an fMRI-PET investigation in healthy humans. *Neuropsychopharmacology* 38, 1438–1450. doi: 10.1038/npp.2013.40

Hayes, D. J., Duncan, N. W., Xu, J., and Northoff, G. (2014). A comparison of neural responses to appetitive and aversive stimuli in humans and other mammals. *Neurosci. Biobehav. Rev.* 45, 350–368. doi: 10.1016/j.neubiorev.2014.06.018

Heilbronner, S. R., and Haber, S. N. (2014). Frontal cortical and subcortical projections provide a basis for segmenting the cingulum bundle: implications for neuroimaging and psychiatric disorders. *J. Neurosci.* 34, 10041–10054. doi: 10.1523/JNEUROSCI.5459-13.2014

Hilton, D., Love, S., Gradidge, T., and Coakham, H. (1994). Pathological findings associated with trigeminal neuralgia caused by vascular compressionTitle. *Neurosurgery* 35, 299–303.

Hipolito, L., Wilson-Poe, A., Campos-Jurado, Y., Zhong, E., Gonzalez-Romero, J., Virag, L., et al. (2015). Inflammatory pain promotes increased opioid self-administration: role of dysregulated ventral tegmental area opioid receptors. *J. Neurosci.* 35, 12217–12231. doi: 10.1523/JNEUROSCI.1053-15.2015

Hodaie, M., and Coello, A. F. (2013). Advances in the management of trigeminal neuralgia. *J. Neurosurg. Sci.* 57, 13–21.

Ivo, R., Nicklas, A., Dargel, J., Sobottke, R., Delank, K.-S., Eysel, P., et al. (2013). Brain structural and psychometric alterations in chronic low back pain. *Eur. Spine J.* 22, 1958–1964. doi: 10.1007/s00586-013-2692-x

Jones, D. K., Christiansen, K. F., Chapman, R. J., and Aggleton, J. P. (2013). Distinct subdivisions of the cingulum bundle revealed by diffusion MRI fibre tracking: implications for neuropsychological investigations. *Neuropsychologia* 51, 67–78. doi: 10.1016/j.neuropsychologia.2012.11.018

Khalsa, S., Mayhew, S. D., Chechlacz, M., Bagary, M., and Bagshaw, A. P. (2014). The structural and functional connectivity of the posterior cingulate cortex: comparison between deterministic and probabilistic tractography for the investigation of structure-function relationships. *Neuroimage* 102, 118–127. doi: 10.1016/j.neuroimage.2013.12.022

Ko, A. L., Lee, A., Raslan, A. M., Ozpinar, A., McCartney, S., and Burchiel, K. J. (2015). Trigeminal neuralgia without neurovascular compression presents earlier than trigeminal neuralgia with neurovascular compression. *J. Neurosurg.* 123, 1519–1527. doi: 10.3171/2014.11.JNS141741

Kregel, J., Meeus, M., Malfliet, A., Dolphens, M., Danneels, L., Nijs, J., et al. (2015). Structural and functional brain abnormalities in chronic low back pain: a systematic review. *Semin. Arthritis Rheum.* 45, 229–237. doi: 10.1016/j.semarthrit.2015.05.002

Kucyi, A., Moayedi, M., Weissman-Fogel, I., Goldberg, M. B., Freeman, B. V., Tenenbaum, H. C., et al. (2014). Enhanced medial prefrontal-default mode network functional connectivity in chronic pain and its association with pain rumination. *J. Neurosci.* 34, 3969–3975. doi: 10.1523/JNEUROSCI.5055-13.2014

Lee, M., Manders, T. R., Eberle, S. E., Su, C., D'amour, J., Yang, R., et al. (2015). Activation of corticostriatal circuitry relieves chronic neuropathic pain. *J. Neurosci.* 35, 5247–5259. doi: 10.1523/JNEUROSCI.3494-14.2015

Leech, R., and Sharp, D. J. (2014). The role of the posterior cingulate cortex in cognition and disease. *Brain* 137, 12–32. doi: 10.1093/brain/awt162

Leemans, A., and Jones, D. K. (2009). The B-matrix must be rotated when correcting for subject motion in DTI data. *Magn. Reson. Med.* 61, 1336–1349. doi: 10.1002/mrm.21890

Lin, C.-S. (2014). Brain signature of chronic orofacial pain: a systematic review and meta-analysis on neuroimaging research of trigeminal neuropathic pain and temporomandibular joint disorders. *PLoS ONE* 9:e94300. doi: 10.1371/journal.pone.0094300

Loggia, M. L., Berna, C., Kim, J., Cahalan, C. M., Gollub, R. L., Wasan, A. D., et al. (2014). Disrupted brain circuitry for pain-related reward/punishment in fibromyalgia. *Arthritis Rheumatol.* 66, 203–212. doi: 10.1002/art.38191

Lucas-Neto, L., Mourato, B., Neto, D., Oliveira, E., Martins, H., Correia, F., et al. (2014). The nucleus accumbens beyond the anterior commissure: implications for psychosurgery. *Stereotact. Funct. Neurosurg.* 92, 291–299. doi: 10.1159/000365115

Lutz, J., Thon, N., Stahl, R., Lummel, N., Tonn, J., Linn, J., et al. (2015). Microstructural alterations in trigeminal neuralgia determined by diffusion tensor imaging are independent of symptom duration, severity, and type of neurovascular conflict. *J. Neurosurg.* 124, 823–830. doi: 10.3171/2015.2.JNS142587

McCarthy, C. S., Ramprashad, A., Thompson, C., Botti, J. A., Coman, I. L., and Kates, W. R. (2015). A comparison of FreeSurfer-generated data with and without manual intervention. *Front. Neurosci.* 9:379. doi: 10.3389/fnins.2015.00379

Miller, J., Acar, F., and Burchiel, K. J. (2009). Classification of trigeminal neuralgia: clinical, therapeutic, and prognostic implications in a series of 144 patients undergoing microvascular decompression. *J. Neurosurg.* 111, 1231–1234. doi: 10.3171/2008.6.17604

Moayedi, M., Weissman-Fogel, I., Salomons, T. V., Crawley, A. P., Goldberg, M. B., Freeman, B. V., et al. (2012). White matter brain and trigeminal nerve abnormalities in temporomandibular disorder. *Pain* 153, 1467–1477. doi: 10.1016/j.pain.2012.04.003

Moulin, D. E., Boulanger, A., Clark, A. J., Clarke, H., Dmd, T. D., and Finley, G. A. (2014). Pharmacological management of chronic neuropathic pain : revised consensus statement from the Canadian Pain Society. *Pain Res. Manag.* 19, 328–335.

Papini, M. R., Fuchs, P. N., and Torres, C. (2015). Behavioral neuroscience of psychological pain. *Neurosci. Biobehav. Rev.* 48, 53–69. doi: 10.1016/j.neubiorev.2014.11.012

Pieper, S., Halle, M., and Kikinis, R. (2004). "3D Slicer," in *Proc. 1st IEEE Int. Symp. Biomed. Imaging From Nano to Macro* Vol. 1, (Arlington, VA), 632–635.

Po, C., Kalthoff, D., Kim, Y. B., Nelles, M., and Hoehn, M. (2012). White matter reorganization and functional response after focal cerebral ischemia in the rat. *PLoS ONE* 7:e45629. doi: 10.1371/journal.pone.0045629

Qazi, A. A., Radmanesh, A., O'Donnell, L., Kindlmann, G., Peled, S., Whalen, S., et al. (2009). Resolving crossings in the corticospinal tract by two-tensor streamline tractography: method and clinical assessment using fMRI. *Neuroimage* 47(Suppl. 2), T98–T106. doi: 10.1016/j.neuroimage.2008.06.034

Qu, C., King, T., Okun, A., Lai, J., Fields, H. L., and Porreca, F. (2011). Lesion of the rostral anterior cingulate cortex eliminates the aversiveness of spontaneous neuropathic pain following partial or complete axotomy. *Pain* 152, 1641–1648. doi: 10.1016/j.pain.2011.03.002

Rosen, G. D., Finklestein, S., Stoll, A., Yutzey, D., and Denenberg, V. H. (1984). Neurochemical asymmetries in the albino rat's cortex, striatum, and nucleus accumbens. *Life Sci.* 34, 1143–1148.

Roy, M., Shohamy, D., and Wager, T. D. (2012). Ventromedial prefrontal-subcortical systems and the generation of affective meaning. *Trends Cogn. Sci.* 16, 147–156. doi: 10.1016/j.tics.2012.01.005

Shackman, A. J., Salomons, T. V., Slagter, H. A., Fox, A. S., Winter, J. J., and Davidson, R. J. (2011). The integration of negative affect, pain and cognitive control in the cingulate cortex. *Nat. Rev. Neurosci.* 12, 154–167. doi: 10.1038/nrn2994

Simons, L., Elman, I., and Borsook, D. (2013). Psychological processing in chronic pain: a neural systems approach. *Neurosci. Biobehav. Rev.* 39, 61–78. doi: 10.1016/j.neubiorev.2013.12.006

Smallwood, R. F., Laird, A. R., Ramage, A. E., Parkinson, A. L., Lewis, J., Clauw, D. J., et al. (2013). Structural brain anomalies and chronic pain: a quantitative meta-analysis of gray matter volume. *J. Pain* 14, 663–675. doi: 10.1016/j.jpain.2013.03.001

Smith, S. M., Jenkinson, M., Woolrich, M. W., Beckmann, C. F., Behrens, T. E. J., Johansen-Berg, H., et al. (2004). Advances in functional and structural MR image analysis and implementation as FSL. *Neuroimage* 23(Suppl. 1), S208–S219. doi: 10.1016/j.neuroimage.2004.07.051

Taylor, A. M. W., Castonguay, A., Taylor, A. J., Murphy, N. P., Ghogha, A., Cook, C., et al. (2015). Microglia disrupt mesolimbic reward circuitry in chronic pain. *J. Neurosci.* 35, 8442–8450. doi: 10.1523/JNEUROSCI.4036-14.2015

Turk, D. C., Audette, J., Levy, R. M., Mackey, S. C., and Stanos, S. (2010). Assessment and treatment of psychosocial comorbidities in patients with neuropathic pain. *Mayo Clin. Proc.* 85, S42–50. doi: 10.4065/mcp.2009.0648

Vachon-presseau, E., Roy, M., Martel, M., Caron, E., Plante, I., Sullivan, M. J., et al. (2013). The stress model of chronic pain : evidence from basal cortisol and hippocampal structure and function in humans. *Brain* 36(Pt 3), 815–827. doi: 10.1093/brain/aws371

Vachon-Presseau, E., Tétreault, P., Petre, B., Huang, L., Berger, S. E., Torbey, S., et al. (2016). Corticolimbic anatomical characteristics predetermine risk for chronic pain. *Brain* 139, 1958–1970. doi: 10.1093/brain/aww100

Weissgerber, T. L., Milic, N. M., Winham, S. J., and Garovic, V. D. (2015). Beyond bar and line graphs: time for a new data presentation paradigm. *PLoS Biol.* 13:e1002128. doi: 10.1371/journal.pbio.1002128

Weissman-Fogel, I., Moayedi, M., Tenenbaum, H. C., Goldberg, M. B., Freeman, B. V., and Davis, K. D. (2011). Abnormal cortical activity in patients with temporomandibular disorder evoked by cognitive and emotional tasks. *Pain* 152, 384–396. doi: 10.1016/j.pain.2010.10.046

Yalcin, I., Barthas, F., and Barrot, M. (2014). Emotional consequences of neuropathic pain: insight from preclinical studies. *Neurosci. Biobehav. Rev.* 47C, 154–164. doi: 10.1016/j.neubiorev.2014.08.002

Yazdi-Ravandi, S., Razavi, Y., Haghparast, A., Goudarzvand, M., and Haghparast, A. (2014). Orexin A induced antinociception in the ventral tegmental area involves D1 and D2 receptors in the nucleus accumbens. *Pharmacol. Biochem. Behav.* 126, 1–6. doi: 10.1016/j.pbb.2014.08.009

Yen, C. P., Kung, S. S., Su, Y. F., Lin, W. C., Howng, S. L., and Kwan, A. L. (2005). Stereotactic bilateral anterior cingulotomy for intractable pain. *J. Clin. Neurosci.* 12, 886–890. doi: 10.1016/j.jocn.2004.11.018

7

Structural Magnetic Resonance Imaging can Identify Trigeminal System Abnormalities in Classical Trigeminal Neuralgia

Danielle D. DeSouza[1], *Mojgan Hodaie*[2,3,4†] *and Karen D. Davis*[2,3,4*†]

[1] Department of Neurology and Neurological Sciences, Stanford University, Stanford, CA, USA, [2] Division of Brain, Imaging and Behavior-Systems Neuroscience, Krembil Research Institute, University Health Network, Toronto, ON, Canada, [3] Institute of Medical Science, University of Toronto, Toronto, ON, Canada, [4] Division of Neurosurgery, Toronto Western Hospital and Department of Surgery, University of Toronto, Toronto, ON, Canada

***Correspondence:**
Karen D. Davis
kdavis@uhnres.utoronto.ca

†Drs. Hodaie and Davis are co-senior authors who contributed equally to the manuscript.

Classical trigeminal neuralgia (TN) is a chronic pain disorder that has been described as one of the most severe pains one can suffer. The most prevalent theory of TN etiology is that the trigeminal nerve is compressed at the root entry zone (REZ) by blood vessels. However, there is significant evidence showing a lack of neurovascular compression (NVC) for many cases of classical TN. Furthermore, a considerable number of patients who are asymptomatic have MR evidence of NVC. Since there is no validated animal model that reproduces the clinical features of TN, our understanding of TN pathology mainly comes from biopsy studies that have limitations. Sophisticated structural MRI techniques including diffusion tensor imaging provide new opportunities to assess the trigeminal nerves and CNS to provide insight into TN etiology and pathogenesis. Specifically, studies have used high-resolution structural MRI methods to visualize patterns of trigeminal nerve-vessel relationships and to detect subtle pathological features at the trigeminal REZ. Structural MRI has also identified CNS abnormalities in cortical and subcortical gray matter and white matter and demonstrated that effective neurosurgical treatment for TN is associated with a reversal of specific nerve and brain abnormalities. In conclusion, this review highlights the advanced structural neuroimaging methods that are valuable tools to assess the trigeminal system in TN and may inform our current understanding of TN pathology. These methods may in the future have clinical utility for the development of neuroimaging-based biomarkers of TN.

Keywords: trigeminal neuralgia, structural MRI, DTI, plasticity, pain

Trigeminal neuralgia (TN), characterized by excruciating attacks of electric shock-like unilateral facial pain, has been described as one of the most severe pains one can experience. There are an estimated 15,000 new cases of TN diagnosed in the United States each year and with greater awareness and better diagnostic criteria, recent studies suggest that this is likely an underestimate (Pollock and Ecker, 2005; Hall et al., 2006). Each year, thousands of patients undergo surgery for TN in the United States, with estimated costs exceeding $100 million (Pollock and Ecker, 2005). These treatments result in excellent outcomes for many patients, but some patients do not experience any pain relief. As such, noninvasive measures to predict clinical outcomes from treatment are needed. Our understanding of TN has drastically grown over the past few centuries, but the etiology and pathophysiological mechanisms underlying TN are still not well understood. Recent studies using noninvasive neuroimaging methods, such as structural MRI, have provided new insight into our understanding of TN and mechanisms of treatment response. In this review, we will discuss theories of TN pathophysiology, how advanced neuroimaging methods contribute to our current understanding of TN, and future directions for clinical trials that may use these methods to inform treatment selection and response for TN patients based on brain and/or nerve biomarkers.

CENTRAL AND PERIPHERAL THEORIES OF TN ETIOLOGY AND PATHOPHYSIOLOGY

In the 1850s, some theorized that TN might involve a central etiology. For example, Trousseau observed that because the painful paroxysms experienced by TN patients resembled a convulsive seizure he termed "epileptiform neuralgia" (Trousseau, 1853), TN was due to paroxysmal activity in the trigeminal system similar to cerebral paroxysmal discharges experienced by epilepsy patients. Other evidence suggesting a CNS contribution to TN was that pain attacks were self-sustained once triggered, larger in magnitude than the stimulus, and were followed by a refractory period during which time another attack could not be triggered (Kugelberg and Lindblom, 1959). As such, the antiepileptic medication, carbamazepine was considered as a treatment for TN, and is still one of the most frequently prescribed medications for TN (Hall et al., 2006). Antiepileptic medications can effectively manage TN pain initially and not only act on the brain but also on peripheral nerves by slowing motor and sensory fiber conduction velocities (Traccis et al., 1983).

We now know that central sensitization or use-dependent synaptic plasticity can occur when there is the sustained or repetitive activation of primary afferent fibers including nociceptors (Woolf and Salter, 2000). CNS neurons (e.g., those in the dorsal horn of the spinal cord or in the spinal trigeminal nucleus of the brainstem) change the gain of their responsiveness to sensory input such that they have amplified responses to noxious and innocuous stimuli. This change is triggered by intracellular cascades, which lead to facilitated excitatory transmission and depressed inhibition (Woolf and Salter, 2000). When there is inflammation, neuropeptides and neurotrophic factors such as substance P and brain-derived neurotropic factor are released from the terminals of the primary afferents (Kidd and Urban, 2001). This activates intracellular cascades with the net result being facilitated excitatory transmission produced by an exaggerated response to stimuli, an expansion of the receptive field size such that there is a spread of sensitivity to regions outside of the injured tissue, and a reduction in the threshold for activation of afferent inputs so that central neurons are responsive to even innocuous inputs (Kilo et al., 1994; Woolf and Salter, 2000; Kidd and Urban, 2001). There is evidence suggesting that many of these changes are mediated by N-methyl-D-aspartate (NMDA) receptors. There are also NMDA receptor-independent mechanisms for facilitating excitatory synaptic transmission, primarily via mechanisms involving a subset of α-amino-3-hydroxy-5-methyl-4-isoxazolepropionic acid (AMPA) receptors (Gu et al., 1996). Furthermore, there can be a long-term depression of gamma-aminobutyric acid (GABA) and glycine dorsal horn neurons, which have inhibitory effects on afferent input (Sandkuhler and Gebhart, 1984; Woolf and Salter, 2000).

Central contributions in TN remain debatable, but ample evidence, primarily from surgical experience, suggests that the origin of TN and its pathogenesis involves the trigeminal nerve at the root entry zone (REZ; Nurmikko and Eldridge, 2001). The most common theory of classical TN etiology is a peripheral theory involving the compression of the trigeminal REZ by blood vessels (Nurmikko and Eldridge, 2001). This was first described by Dandy (1929), who observed that TN patients frequently had grooves or indentations in their trigeminal nerves made by offending vessels (**Figure 1**). Several lines of evidence have led to the proposition that over time this sustained static or pulsatile vascular compression leads to focal points of damage on the trigeminal nerve, resulting in the characteristic pain attacks in TN. Corroborating this, several studies have used ultrastructural and immunohistochemical techniques to demonstrate pathological changes, most notably demyelination of the trigeminal nerves in patients with TN (Kerr and Miller, 1966; Hilton et al., 1994; Rappaport et al., 1997; Love et al., 1998; Devor et al., 2002b; Marinković et al., 2009). Indeed, trigeminal root biopsies from patients with TN show that in regions with the most severe neurovascular compression (NVC) there are few axons remaining and that nearly all of these axons were demyelinated and in close apposition to each other (Rappaport et al., 1997; Devor et al., 2002b). Since we currently lack a validated animal model that reproduces the clinical features of TN, much of what we know about TN pathology comes from these biopsy studies, which limits our ability to test theories of TN pathophysiology.

Compressive syndromes that affect the spinal dorsal REZ (e.g., disc herniation, spinal stenosis and tumor growth) can also be a source of severe pain (Kobayashi et al., 2004). Anatomically, the spinal dorsal REZ not only includes proximal dorsal nerve rootlets, but also Lissauer's tract and the superficial dorsal horn laminae I-V (Bozkurt et al., 2012). Therefore, pain symptoms can vary depending on the location and extent of the compression in the spinal dorsal REZ. An example can be seen with patients who have spinal disc herniation. When compression affects the dorsal roots of the lumbar spine, radicular pain such as sciatica is common. Pain symptoms of sciatica are variable but like TN pain, it is typically unilateral and can be electric-shock like in quality (Freynhagen and Baron, 2009). However, unlike TN pain, sciatica pain is more frequently persistent and other sensory abnormalities such as numbness and paresthesias are often evident. A minority of TN patients have also reported sensory abnormalities and autonomic symptoms. In one study, 31% of patients reported ipsilateral autonomic

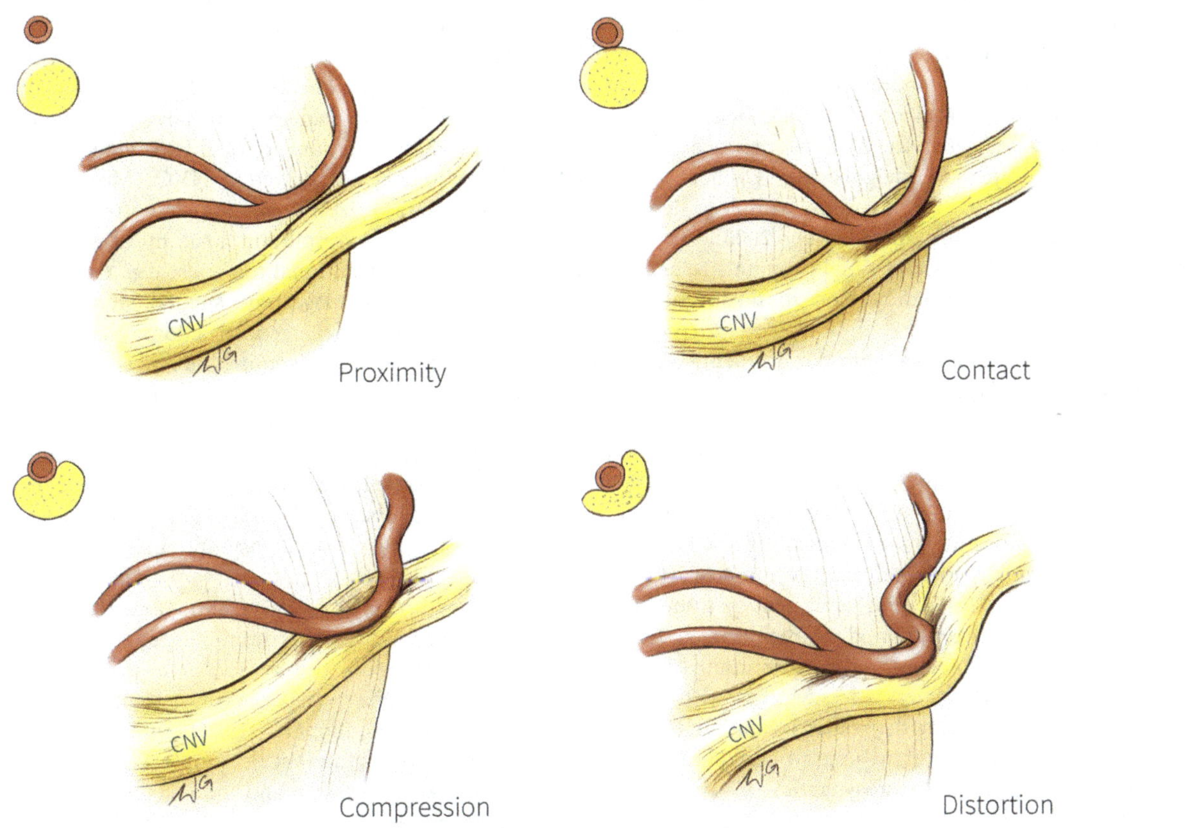

FIGURE 1 | Trigeminal nerve-vessel relationships. A schematic illustration depicting examples of trigeminal-nerve vessel relationships at the cerebellopontine angle, with corresponding cross-sections in the upper left corner of each panel. Proximity (upper left panel): vessel in close proximity to trigeminal nerve but without contact; Contact (upper right panel): simple contact of the trigeminal nerve by a vessel but without compression or distortion of the nerve; Compression (bottom left panel): vessel compressing the trigeminal nerve; Distortion (bottom right panel): compression severe enough to deform the trigeminal nerve. CN V, trigeminal nerve.

symptoms (e.g., conjunctival injection/tearing, running/clogged nose) during pain attacks and for 5% of these patients ($n = 8$), the symptoms occurred with every pain attack (Maarbjerg et al., 2014). These symptoms occurred more commonly in patients that had pain affecting the ophthalmic branch of the trigeminal nerve. In addition, three of these patients had a dual diagnosis of TN and either short-lasting unilateral neuralgiform headache attacks with cranial autonomic features (SUNA), short-lasting unilateral neuralgiform headache attacks with conjunctival injection and tearing (SUNCT), or cluster headache, which may have contributed to these autonomic symptoms.

One theory that has gained recognition for blending pathological findings associated with NVC of the trigeminal REZ and the unique symptoms of TN pain is the *ignition hypothesis* (Rappaport and Devor, 1994) which was more recently updated to account for advances made in our understanding of nerve pathophysiology (Devor et al., 2002a). This theory proposes that TN pain results from an abnormal generation of sensory impulses of trigeminal fibers generated from regions of demyelination, or other structural abnormalities, referred to as pacemaker sites. While damaged neurons can be spontaneously active following injury (Burchiel, 1980; Love and Coakham, 2001; Devor et al., 2002a), other neurons may be silent, but have hair-trigger thresholds such that a momentary stimulation can produce firing lasting several seconds. This phenomenon is referred to as *afterdischarge* (Devor et al., 2002a). Afterdischarge can recruit neighboring neurons via neuron-to-neuron coupling, which this hypothesis suggests may underlie the paroxysmal explosion of pain characteristic of TN. The ignition hypothesis also describes how the activation of the NVC-induced demyelinated fibers that primarily convey non-nociceptive sensory information may result in a TN pain attack. In cases where there is nerve damage such as demyelination, the axons of sensory neurons come in closer contact with each other at these sites, and when one neuron fires, it can now depolarize previously silent neighbors (Rappaport and Devor, 1994; Devor et al., 2002a). When this cross-excitation occurs between individual axon pairs that become electrically coupled, it is referred to as ephaptic crosstalk/transmission (Seltzer and Devor, 1979). In the TN literature, ephaptic crosstalk between fibers mediating light touch (Aβ fibers) and those involved in nociception

(Aδ and c fibers), has been considered to account for TN pain attacks that are triggered by brief stimuli such as light touch to the face (Love and Coakham, 2001; Nurmikko and Eldridge, 2001). Corroborating this, electrophysiological recordings in the rat dorsal root ganglion demonstrated that neuronal activity triggered in A-fibers produce a transient depolarization in passive neighboring C-fibers and that approximately 90% of the neurons sampled demonstrate cross-depolarization (Amir and Devor, 2000). The authors concluded that this crosstalk might augment neuropathic sensory abnormalities including pain in the event of nerve injury.

Despite the considerable evidence for TN being a peripheral disorder, some have argued that the NVC theory of TN cannot sufficiently explain the disorder because some individuals can develop TN in the absence of NVC, and some individuals with NVC never develop TN. Additionally, in TN cases where NVC is evident, the CNS may also contribute to TN pathophysiology, since it is well known that CNS plasticity can occur following peripheral nerve injury (Taylor et al., 2009; Davis et al., 2011). For example, peripheral nerve injury can result in the sustained or repetitive activation of primary afferent fibers and central sensitization. This change is triggered by intracellular cascades, which lead to facilitated excitatory transmission and depressed inhibition (Woolf and Salter, 2000). This can occur at one synapse (homosynaptic) or at multiple synapses (heterosynaptic). Classically, TN is characterized by paroxysmal pain with patients typically being pain-free between attacks. Over time, however, these attacks may occur more frequently, with less pain-free periods in between them. It is possible that the CNS changes that accompany peripheral nerve injury contribute to evolving TN symptoms. However, this relationship remains to be determined. While some of the mechanisms underlying TN pathophysiology remain controversial, neuroimaging methods and in particular, studies using MRI to examine trigeminal nerve and brain structure, have provided valuable insight into these mechanisms.

STRUCTURAL MRI: A NONINVASIVE MEANS TO STUDY PERIPHERAL THEORIES OF TN

Structural MRI is widely used in both clinical practice and research. However, MRI for research typically involves specialized protocols and post-processing techniques. Structural MRI for TN research uses *high-resolution anatomical imaging* (variations of T1- and T2-weighted images) to assess anatomical characteristics and patterns of NVC, brain gray matter volume and cortical thickness (CT) and *diffusion imaging* (diffusion tensor images (DTI)) to assess brain white matter and trigeminal nerve microstructure.

Structural MRI can be used to test whether NVC sufficiently explains TN etiology. Some have argued that NVC cannot be the only cause of TN because blood vessels are often seen in the vicinity of the trigeminal nerve on routine autopsy or even on conventional MRI scans of unaffected nerves or in asymptomatic individuals without any TN (Nurmikko and Eldridge, 2001; Miller et al., 2009; Satoh et al., 2009; Antonini et al., 2014). Still, surgical cases suggest approximately 80–90% of TN patients have NVC at their trigeminal nerves ipsilateral to their side of pain (Love and Coakham, 2001; Satoh et al., 2009). But, conventional two-dimensional imaging is not always reliable in detecting NVC (Meaney et al., 1995). To better characterize the anatomical patterns of NVC in patients with TN, high resolution anatomical scans, combined with other non-conventional methods (e.g., three-dimensional time-of-flight MR angiography, spoiled gradient-recalled imaging, nerve/vessel model reconstructions) have shown that NVC at the unaffected trigeminal nerve is typically not as severe as at the affected nerve, nor is it enough to produce nerve dislocation or distortion (Anderson et al., 2006; Lorenzoni et al., 2012). In contrast, nerve dislocation or distortion occurs frequently at the affected trigeminal nerve, suggesting that NVC associated with TN is more severe than at the unaffected nerve or in asymptomatic individuals (Lorenzoni et al., 2012).

Structural MR has also been used to categorize NVC into four categories based on the extent of nerve circumference in contact with the vessel as a proxy of severity: severe (NVC with the vessel covering >20% of the trigeminal nerve circumference); moderate (NVC with vessel covering <20% of the nerve circumference); simple (vessel contacts the nerve; **Figure 1**, top right) and none (vessel in proximity to the nerve; **Figure 1**, top left; Satoh et al., 2009). Moderate and severe NVC may result in compression or distortion of the trigeminal nerve (**Figure 1**, bottom panels). NVC of the affected trigeminal nerve tends to be severe in patients with TN, whereas NVC at the unaffected nerves of patients or in healthy individuals are mostly of the simple contact form (Satoh et al., 2009).

TN is also associated with atrophy of the affected trigeminal nerve (Erbay et al., 2006; Antonini et al., 2014; Leal et al., 2014). High-resolution MR has demonstrated that the mean diameter and cross-sectional area of the trigeminal nerve on the symptomatic side of TN patients is smaller compared to the asymptomatic side. It was proposed that atrophy is likely secondary to structural abnormalities of the trigeminal nerve, including axonal loss and demyelination that result from NVC (Erbay et al., 2006). Corroborating these findings, a recent study reported that trigeminal NVC as detected by MRI is likely to be symptomatic when it is accompanied by anatomical nerve changes including nerve atrophy (Antonini et al., 2014).

Peripheral theories of TN also emphasize the importance of the REZ in TN etiology and pathophysiology, with recent DTI studies providing support of this theory. Anatomically, myelinated axons at the REZ are primarily associated with CNS myelin produced by oligodendrocytes, which transitions to peripheral myelin produced by Schwann cells (Peker et al., 2006). Immunohistochemical studies have demonstrated NVC-induced focal demyelination that largely affects the CNS myelin at the trigeminal REZ (Marinković et al., 2009). In this study, trigeminal nerve roots of patients with trigeminal pain syndromes were obtained during autopsy. Of the patients with TN, 83% had neurovascular relationships at the transition zone between central and peripheral myelin. At this location, various changes in the central myelin were observed including deformation and demyelination. In contrast, segmental demyelination affected only a few individual nerve fibers in the regions adjacent to the NVC (Marinković et al., 2009). The notion that CNS myelin is primarily disrupted at the REZ of TN patients is consistent with peripheral myelin being significantly more resistant to compression and damage. Therefore, the REZ is likely a key region in TN pathophysiology. This provides the rationale for why vascular contact more distally along the trigeminal nerve can occur in individuals without any history of TN (Nurmikko and Eldridge, 2001).

Immunohistochemical studies rely on trigeminal nerve biopsy samples extracted during surgical procedures for TN or during autopsy. However, DTI provides a noninvasive means for examining trigeminal nerve microstructure *in vivo*. DTI involves fitting a tensor, which is an ellipsoid shaped mathematical model, at each brain voxel of a diffusion MR scan. The tensor is characterized by three orthogonal eigenvectors and their associated eigenvalues (λ_1, λ_2, λ_3). In general, the shape of the tensor carries information about the three-dimensional character of the water molecules' diffusion. There are several measures of tissue microstructure that can be derived from these eigenvalues, the most widely used being fractional anisotropy (FA; **Figure 2A**). FA ranges from zero (i.e., completely isotropic) to one (i.e., completely anisotropic). Diffusion varies for different tissue types because the structural barriers innate to certain tissues hinder diffusion. These variations are reflected by the shape of the tensor derived from a voxel of that tissue type. For example, the shape of a tensor derived from a voxel within the CSF would be roughly spherical in shape, indicating that diffusion is not hindered and molecules can flow equally in all directions. In this case, diffusion is said to be isotropic. In contrast, there are several barriers to diffusion in white matter bundles making diffusion along the length of the axis greater than across it. Diffusion is said to be anisotropic when this occurs and the shape of the tensor is less spherical.

This has motivated a handful of studies to examine structural abnormalities in the trigeminal nerves of patients with TN using FA as measure (Herweh et al., 2007; Fujiwara et al., 2011; Leal et al., 2011; Lutz et al., 2011). In these studies, FA was extracted from the trigeminal nerves of patients and healthy control participants, with the majority of the studies (Herweh et al., 2007; Leal et al., 2011; Lutz et al., 2011) focusing on

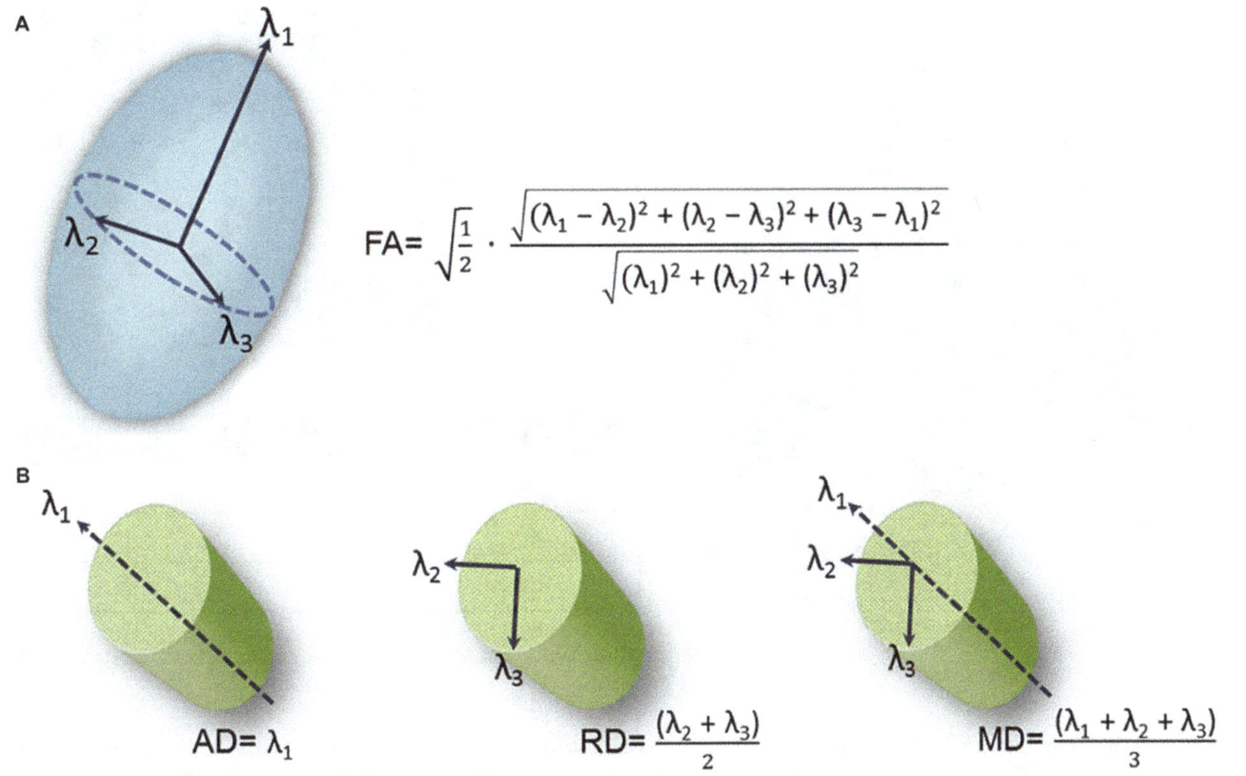

FIGURE 2 | Schematic representation of diffusion tensor images (DTI)-derived metrics. A schematic representation of the tensor model and formulas of four DTI-derived metrics: fractional anisotropy (FA; **A**) and axial diffusivity (AD; diffusion along the length of the axon (λ_1, left), radial diffusivity (RD; diffusion perpendicular to the length of the axon (average of λ_2 and λ_3, center) and mean diffusivity (MD; average diffusion regardless of direction (mean of λ_1, λ_2 and λ_3, right; **B**). Figure is adapted from DeSouza et al. (2014) with permission (Rightslink license number: 3823931416268).

trigeminal REZ values. The results indicated that FA was lower in the affected REZ of TN patients with NVC, consistent with there being disrupted nerve organization at this location. These studies demonstrated that a noninvasive *in vivo* measure of trigeminal nerve microstructure could be used to detect abnormalities in the trigeminal nerves of TN patients. However, the studies did have some limitations. First, the data were acquired using resolutions that may not have been sufficient to reveal all abnormalities. In DTI, multiple images are collected so that the signal can be sensitized to diffusion in different directions, building up multiple measurements for each voxel in the brain (Johansen-Berg and Rushworth, 2009). In these aforementioned studies, a relatively low number of diffusion gradient-directions were used (i.e., two of these studies collected diffusion data with only six directions; Herweh et al., 2007; Fujiwara et al., 2011), one study with 15 directions (Lutz et al., 2011), and the other with 32 directions (Leal et al., 2011). While only six noncollinear directions are required to estimate the diffusion tensor, many more images are usually required to boost the signal intensity-to-noise ratio (Mukherjee et al., 2008). The rationale for sampling more directions is that it reduces orientational dependence and increases the accuracy and precision of estimating tensor-derived parameters such as FA (Mukherjee et al., 2008). Second, many of these studies primarily assessed the DTI metric FA, that does not fully describe the tensor shape. Therefore, information important for a full interpretation of the findings was limited because other DTI metrics such as mean, radial and axial diffusivities (MD, RD, AD) were not collected. As shown in **Figure 2B**, AD corresponds to the main diffusion direction, or diffusion along the length of the axon (λ_1), RD corresponds to diffusion perpendicular to the main diffusion direction (average of λ_2 and λ_3), and MD measures the local magnitude of diffusion regardless of direction (average of λ_1, λ_2 and λ_3). These other measures of tissue microstructure have been linked to specific pathophysiological mechanisms such as demyelination, neuroinflammation and edema (Alexander et al., 2007), as diffusion is particularly sensitive to changes in the architecture of cellular membranes that can occur under certain pathological conditions. While reduced FA has been reported across a broad spectrum of disorders (Alexander et al., 2007), the direction of MD, RD and AD changes are more variable depending on the precise underlying pathophysiology and can provide useful information as to why FA is decreased in TN.

Recently, we assessed all four of these described diffusion metrics at the trigeminal REZ and demonstrated that TN patients not only have lower FA at their affected REZ, but

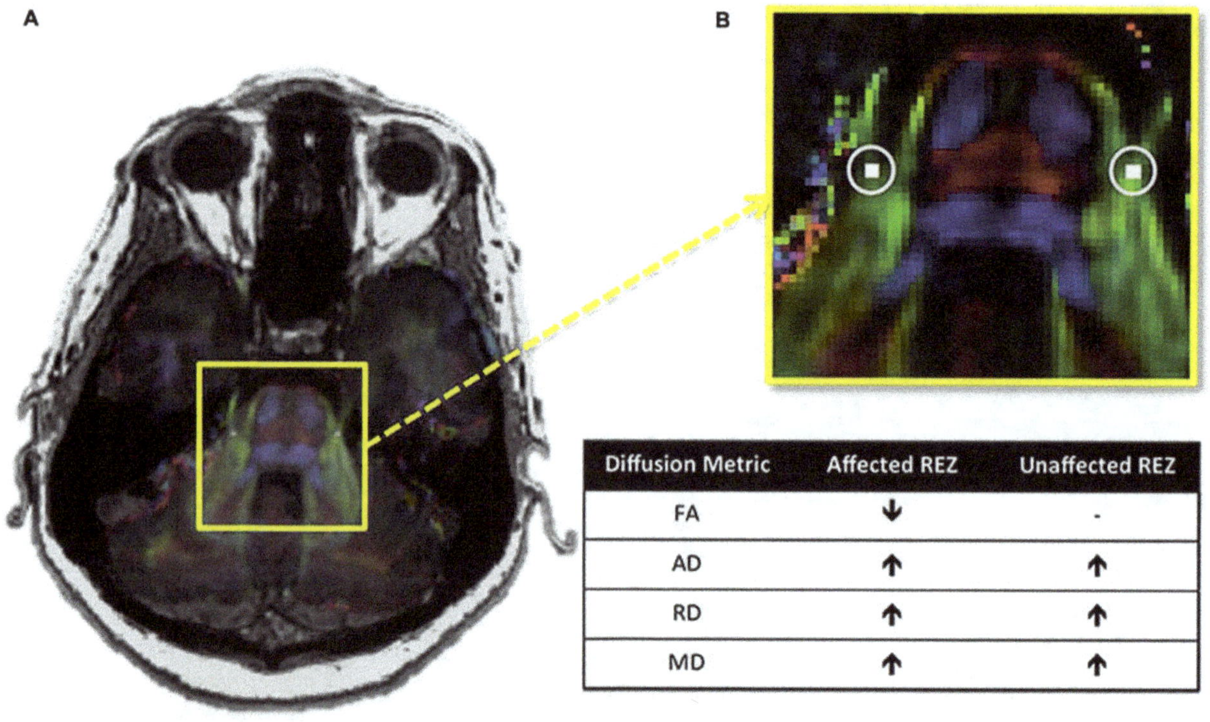

Diffusion Metric	Affected REZ	Unaffected REZ
FA	↓	-
AD	↑	↑
RD	↑	↑
MD	↑	↑

FIGURE 3 | Trigeminal root entry zone (REZ) abnormalities in trigeminal neuralgia (TN). (A) An axial T1-weighted MRI slice at the level of the pons is shown on the left, with a DTI image at the same level superimposed over it. The yellow box highlights the pons of the brainstem and the cisternal portions of the left and right trigeminal nerves. **(B)** A zoomed-in version of this box reveals the location of the REZ masks (white squares, highlighted with circles) used to extract each of the four examined DTI metrics in TN patients and controls. Between-group comparisons revealed that TN patients had abnormalities in all four metrics examined. The chart shows the direction of these abnormalities in patients relative to controls. Specifically, TN patients had lower FA at the affected trigeminal REZ, and higher AD, RD and MD bilaterally. DTI, diffusion tensor imaging; FA, fractional anisotropy; RD, radial diffusivity; MD, mean diffusivity; AD, axial diffusivity. – Signifies no significant difference. Panels **(A,B)** were adapted from DeSouza et al. (2014) with permission (RightsLink license number: 3823931416268).

also higher AD, RD and MD (DeSouza et al., 2014; **Figure 3**). Our finding of increased MD and RD may be linked to NVC-induced focal demyelination of the trigeminal REZ (Marinković et al., 2010), neuroinflammatory processes, and/or edema (Beaulieu, 2002) affecting the trigeminal system, since these increases were also observed at the unaffected REZ. Therefore, DTI can detect subtle pathological features at the trigeminal REZ supporting a role for this region's involvement in TN pathophysiology.

STRUCTURAL MRI REVEALS BRAIN ABNORMALITIES IN TN

Brain gray matter abnormalities have been identified in patients with chronic pain (Davis and Moayedi, 2013). The most common location of gray matter abnormalities include regions implicated in the multidimensional experience of pain such as the prefrontal cortex (PFC), insula, anterior and mid-cingulate cortices (ACC, MCC), thalamus, primary and secondary somatosensory cortices (S1, S2), basal ganglia, amygdala and brainstem (Davis and Moayedi, 2013). These abnormalities are commonly found for many types of chronic pain including those affecting the trigeminal system such as migraine (Rocca et al., 2006), trigeminal neuropathic pain (DaSilva et al., 2008; Gustin et al., 2011), and temporomandibular disorder (TMD; Moayedi et al., 2011). Since some abnormalities are common across most chronic pains (e.g., cortical thinning in the anterior insula, cingulate cortex and dorsolateral prefrontal cortices; Davis and Moayedi, 2013), these areas likely reflect pain chronicity in general, and may be associated with negative affect and changes in pain modulation (Wiech and Tracey, 2009) as opposed to a specific pain symptom. However, the direction of the gray matter abnormalities in other brain regions varies across patient populations. For example, S1 shows thickening in patients with TMD (Moayedi et al., 2011), but shows thinning in patients with trigeminal neuropathic pain compared to controls (Gustin et al., 2011). Differences in the direction of abnormality may reflect specific symptomology (e.g., hyper- vs. hypo-sensitivity), as it is following peripheral nerve injury (Taylor et al., 2009) and provide insight into disease mechanisms. For example, mechanisms pertaining to gray matter underlying MR-detectable differences in brain structure may include changes in neuronal size or number, synaptogenesis, dendritic branching, axon sprouting, synaptic pruning, neuronal cell death, alterations in vasculature and the size or numbers of glial cells (Blumenfeld-Katzir et al., 2011; Zatorre et al., 2012).

We recently employed high-resolution T1-weighted scans of patients with TN and examined subcortical and cortical brain gray matter using voxel-based morphometry and CT analyses, respectively (DeSouza et al., 2013). Compared to healthy controls, we identified widespread abnormalities in regions that contribute to sensory-discriminative and cognitive-affective dimensions of pain, pain modulation, and motor function. Specifically, TN patients had greater gray matter in the thalamus, contralateral S1 (putative face area), amygdala, frontal pole (FP), periaqueductal gray (PAG), primary motor cortex (M1) and basal ganglia, and cortical thinning in the orbitofrontal cortex (OFC), pregenual anterior cingulate cortex (pgACC) and insula (DeSouza et al., 2013; **Figures 4A,B**). These findings may reflect unique symptomatology because TN is characterized by paroxysmal pain triggered by innocuous stimuli or movements, and is without major sensory loss. The findings may be a consequence of the pain or be pre-existing and contribute to the development of TN (**Figure 4C**).

A handful of other studies have examined gray matter in patients with trigeminal pain syndromes including TN. Similar to our findings, less gray matter in the ACC, anterior insula, and OFC were reported in these patients compared to healthy controls (Gustin et al., 2011; Obermann et al., 2013; Li et al., 2016). However, in contrast to our findings, the patients also had decreased gray matter in the S1, thalamus (Gustin et al., 2011; Obermann et al., 2013) and caudate nucleus. The differences in these findings with our own may be due to the mixed trigeminal pain patient groups that were examined and the different methodology used to assess gray matter. For example, in one study, the patient group included those with either trigeminal neuropathic pain or TN (Gustin et al., 2011). In this study, the authors reported that only patients with trigeminal neuropathic pain (and not patients with TN) contributed to the decreased thalamic volume result in patients. In another study, patients with classical TN and TN with concomitant facial pain were compared to healthy controls (Obermann et al., 2013). While the authors report no differences between the two patient populations, the results reported derive from a mix of both types of trigeminal pain compared to controls. Additionally, the use of different methods to assess cortical gray matter may have contributed to the differences in results. The human cerebral cortex of humans is highly folded with its thickness varying across regions. CT analysis (as implemented by DeSouza et al., 2013) was developed to provide an automated means to accurately measure the thickness of the cerebral cortex with submillimeter accuracy. In contrast, voxel-based morphometry approaches (as implemented by Gustin et al., 2011; Obermann et al., 2013; Li et al., 2016) are less accurate or can be insufficient in detecting cortical differences (Fischl et al., 2004).

In addition to widespread gray matter abnormalities, several studies have reported abnormalities in the brain white matter of chronic pain patients, many of which interconnect gray matter regions involved in the multi-dimensional experience of pain. A popular method used to examine white matter abnormalities in chronic pain patients compared to healthy controls is Tract-Based Spatial Statistics, which makes whole-brain comparisons of white matter DTI metrics (Rocca et al., 2008; Moayedi et al., 2012; Szabó et al., 2012). White matter abnormalities in the form of lower FA have been reported in several chronic pain disorders including migraine (Szabó et al., 2012) and TMD (Moayedi et al., 2012). The location of these abnormalities is variable between chronic pains and may be related to factors such as disease duration or pain symptomology (Rocca et al., 2008). To determine if there is abnormal brain white matter in patients with TN, we compared brain FA between TN and healthy control groups using Tract-Based Spatial Statistics (DeSouza et al., 2014). We found that patients had widespread abnormalities characterized by lower FA

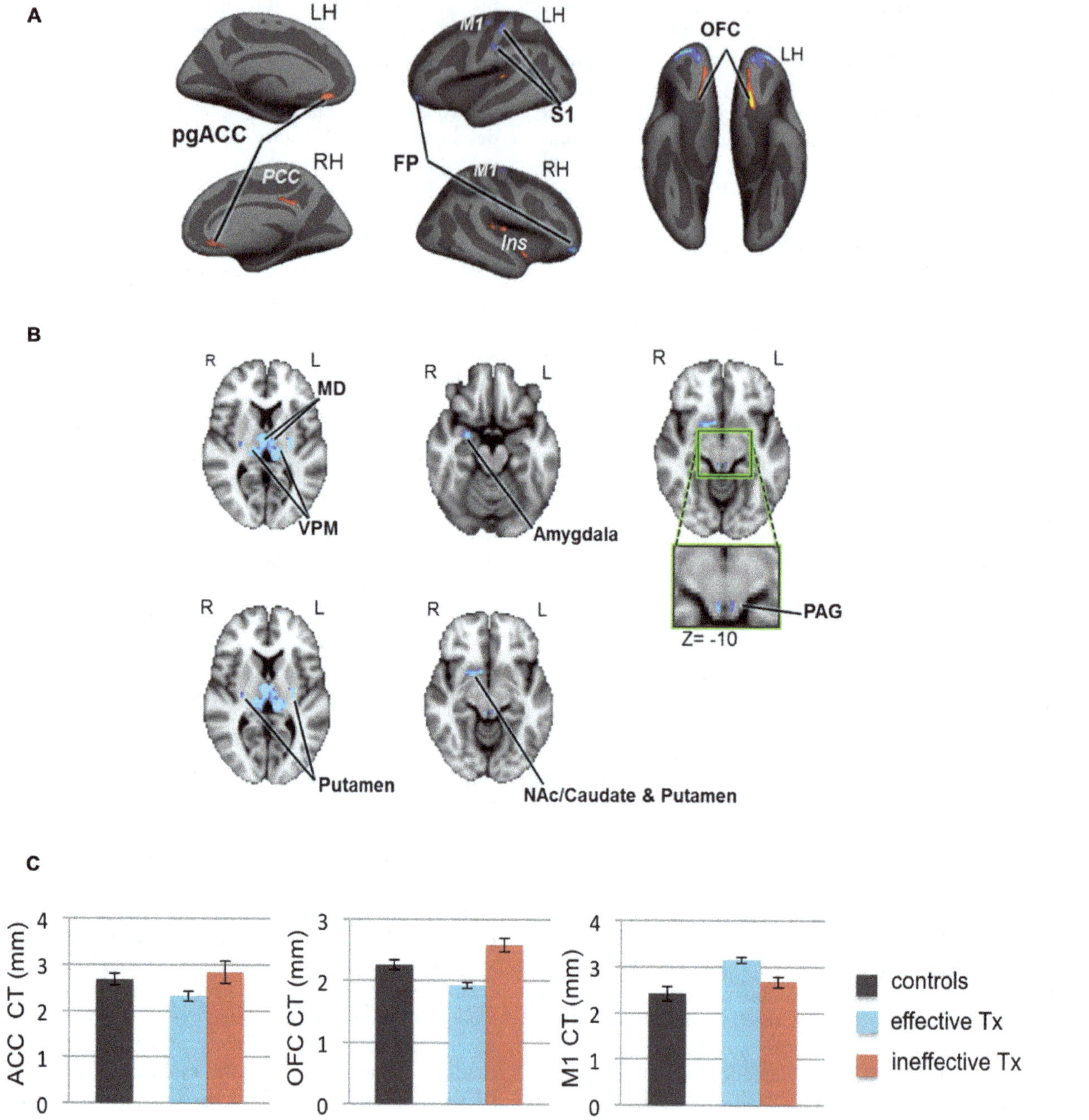

FIGURE 4 | Widespread gray matter abnormalities in patients with TN. (A) CT analysis revealed several cortical gray matter abnormalities in TN patients. Compared to controls, patients had thinner cortex (red clusters) in the pgACC bilaterally, the right ins including the dorsal posterior insula and the ventral anterior insula (vAI), and the ventral OFC bilaterally. TN patients had thicker cortex (blue clusters) in the bilateral FP and M1, and left S1 (putative face area, contralateral to their side of pain). **(B)** Patients also had several subcortical gray matter abnormalities as determined using voxel-based morphometry. Compared to controls, TN patient had larger volumes (blue clusters) in the sensory thalamus, including the MD and VPM thalamus bilaterally, the right amygdala, the posterior putamen bilaterally, PAG (green box shows magnified region), and regions of the right NAc, anterior putamen, and caudate. **(C)** Prior to surgery, CT abnormalities (compared to healthy controls) in the pgACC, the OFC and M1, were more pronounced in the TN patients who had significant pain relief after effective Tx (blue bars) compared to those in which treatment was ineffective (red bars). These pre-treatment baseline CT levels were significantly different between the groups of patients that achieved effective vs. ineffective effects of surgery. While it remains unknown as to whether these abnormalities are a consequence of the pain or are pre-existing and contribute to the development of TN, these preliminary data suggest that certain abnormalities may have predictive value to identify patients that will benefit from treatment. Abbreviations: LH, left hemisphere; RH, right hemisphere; R, right; L, left; pgACC, pregenual anterior cingulate cortex; PCC, posterior cingulate cortex; ins, insular cortex; OFC, orbitofrontal cortex; FP, frontal pole; M1, primary motor cortex; S1, primary somatosensory cortex. MD, medial dorsal nucleus (thalamus); VPM, ventral posterior medial nucleus (thalamus); NAc, nucleus accumbens; PAG, periaqueductal gray. CT, cortical thickness; Tx, treatment. Panels **(A,B)** have been reproduced from DeSouza et al. (2013), © 2013 DeSouza et al.

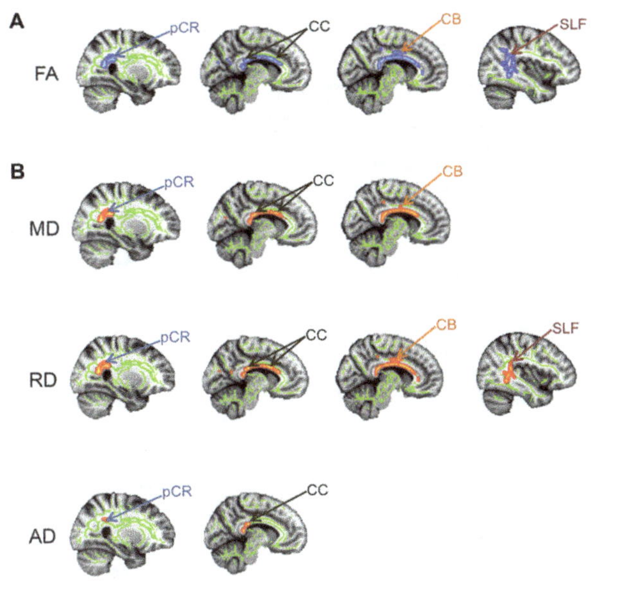

FIGURE 5 | Brain white matter abnormalities in TN. Tract-based spatial statistics results showing that TN patients have several regions of abnormal brain white matter, compared to controls. Specifically, TN patients had significantly lower FA (blues clusters; **A**) and higher MD, RD and AD (red clusters; **B**) in the white matter areas indicated by arrows**.** pCR, posterior corona radiata; CC, corpus callosum; CB, cingulum bundle; SLF, superior longitudinal fasciculus; FA, fractional anisotropy; RD, radial diffusivity; MD, mean diffusivity; AD, axial diffusivity. This figure has been reproduced from DeSouza et al. (2014) with permission (RightsLink license number: 3823931416268).

in the corpus callosum (CC), cingulum, posterior corona radiate (pCR) and superior longitudinal fasciculus (SLF) contralateral to their side of pain (**Figure 5A**). Within these regions of lower FA, we also determined that RD and MD were significantly higher in the CC and cingulum (with AD also being higher in the splenium of the CC), and that RD was higher in the SLF (**Figure 5B**). These tracts connect some gray matter regions involved in the multi-dimensional experience of pain, attention, and motor functions that we previously showed to be abnormal in TN. Therefore, while TN is known to involve dysfunction of the trigeminal nerve, patients also have several areas of abnormal brain white matter that may be contributing to the unique symptoms of TN pain and/or compensatory motor behaviors. In combination with the gray matter findings, these results suggest a role for the CNS in the development and/or maintenance of TN.

While in these cross-sectional studies it was not possible to confirm whether the observed brain abnormalities were pre-existing or occurred as a consequence of TN, studies examining how effective treatment impacts these abnormalities are starting to provide valuable insight.

TREATMENT EFFECTS ON MR-DETECTABLE ABNORMALITIES IN TN

A handful of studies have used structural MRI to demonstrate that some gray matter abnormalities in patients with chronic pain are reversible following effective treatment (Gwilym et al., 2010; Seminowicz et al., 2011; Rodriguez-Raecke et al., 2013). This suggests that they in part arise as a consequence of being in pain and do not necessarily cause the pain. There are currently several treatment approaches available for the management of TN. Although medications are always the first line of treatment (Zakrzewska and Akram, 2011), over time, pain attacks may be longer lasting, occur more frequently, and be less responsive to medications, leading patients to seek neurosurgical intervention for pain relief (Nurmikko and Eldridge, 2001). Surgical treatments for TN target the trigeminal nerve at different anatomical sites (**Figure 6**) with the goal of displacing the offending vessel at the trigeminal REZ, as in microvascular decompression (MVD) surgery, or partially injuring the trigeminal nerve distal to the REZ to reduce nociceptive signaling, as in Gamma Knife radiosurgery (GKRS; **Figure 6**; Zakrzewska and Akram, 2011). Both of these treatments result in a high proportion of patients with good or complete pain relief. As such, we recently examined how effective MVD surgery, and GKRS (as denoted by a 75% reduction in pre-treatment pain intensity scores) impact brain gray matter and trigeminal REZ abnormalities as measured by T1-weighted and DTI images, respectively

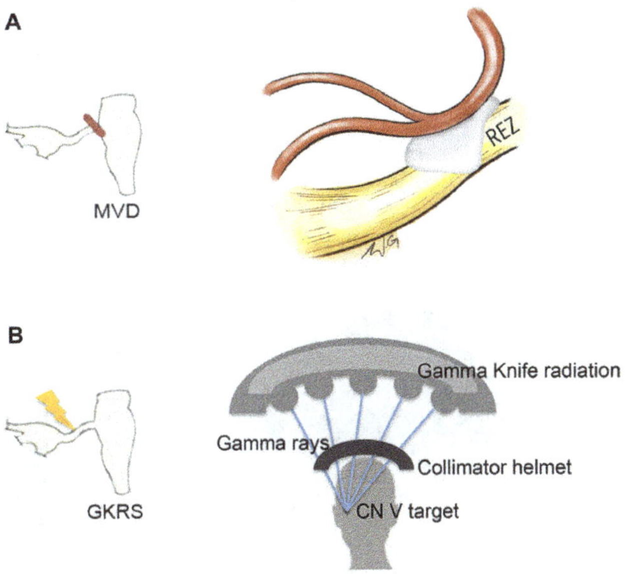

FIGURE 6 | Neurosurgical treatment options for TN. Two neurosurgical treatment options for TN include microvascular decompression (MVD) surgery, which aims to decompress the trigeminal nerve at the REZ **(A, left)** and Gamma Knife radiosurgery (GKRS), which targets the trigeminal nerve distal to the REZ **(B, left)**. MVD surgery uses a retrosigmoid craniotomy to remove a small piece of skull via a small incision behind the ear. The cerebellopontine angle is then approached, and using microscopic magnification, the location of the trigeminal nerve and offending vessel is identified. Nerve decompression is done by dissecting the arachnoid tissue surrounding the nerve and offending vessel and placing pieces of shredded Teflon© between them **(A, right)**. GKRS is a focal radiosurgery technique. Gamma rays are emitted from approximately 200 radioactive cobalt-60 sources precisely focused on the trigeminal nerve using a collimator helmet **(B, right)** and a stereotactic frame (not shown). Abbreviations: CN V, trigeminal nerve; REZ, root entry zone.

A

Effective	Pre-Tx		Post-Tx	
DTI Metric	Aff REZ	Unaff REZ	Aff REZ	Unaff REZ
FA	↓	-	-	-
AD	↑	↑	-	↑
RD	↑	↑	-	-
MD	↑	↑	-	-

Ineffective	Pre-Tx		Post-Tx	
DTI Metric	Aff REZ	Unaff REZ	Aff REZ	Unaff REZ
FA	↓	-	↓	-
AD	-	-	↑	-
RD	↑	-	↑	-
MD	↑	-	↑	-

B

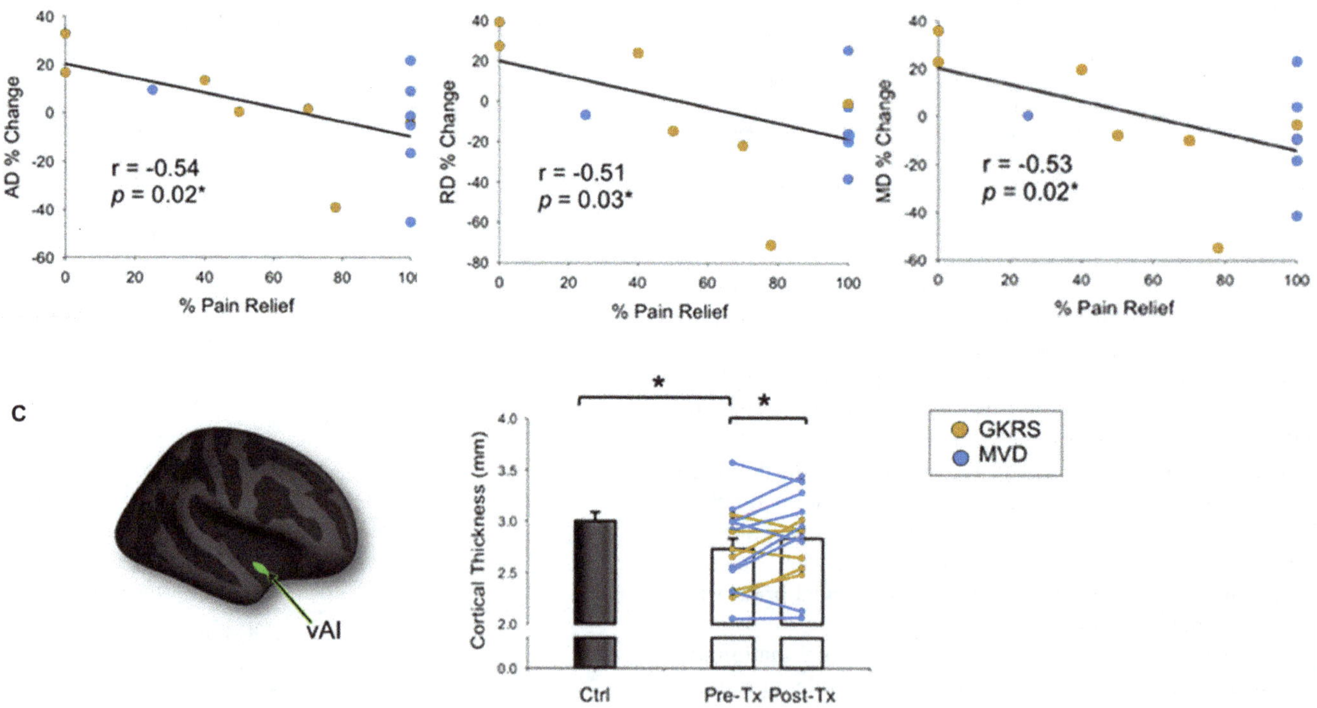

FIGURE 7 | Effects of neurosurgical treatment for TN on trigeminal REZ and brain abnormalities (A). Patients undergoing neurosurgical treatment for TN were deemed to have either effective or ineffective treatment based on a threshold of ≥75% reduction in baseline pain intensity ratings. Only patients that had effective treatment showed a reversal of pre-treatment trigeminal REZ abnormalities in FA, AD, RD and MD following treatment (green box). In contrast, pre-treatment REZ abnormalities persisted in patients that had ineffective treatment (green box). Arrows indicate direction of abnormalities relative to controls. **(B)** The degree of normalization of AD, RD and MD abnormalities only at the affected trigeminal REZ was associated with the degree of pain relief achieved by TN patients. **(C)** The vAI (green cluster on inflated brain) was the only gray matter region to normalize in patients following effective treatment only. Specifically, prior to treatment patients had significantly thinner vAI thickness compared to controls. Following treatment, vAI thickness significantly increased to become comparable to control vAI thickness. Bar graphs of mean CT values ± SEM (in mm) are shown for controls (black bars) and patients (white bars). Individual patient data are also shown pre- and post-treatment, with patients who received GKRS in orange, and MVD surgery in blue. Tx, treatment; Aff REZ, affected root entry zone; Unaff REZ, unaffected root entry zone; FA, fractional anisotropy; RD, radial diffusivity; MD, mean diffusivity; AD, axial diffusivity; Ctl, controls; vAI, ventral anterior insula; GKRS, Gamma Knife Radiosurgery; MVD, microvascular decompression. Panels **(B,C)** have been adapted from DeSouza et al. (2015) with permission (Rightslink license number: 3823931191470). Asterisks indicate significance at $p < 0.05$ level.

(DeSouza et al., 2015). Our results indicated that effective surgical treatment was associated with the resolution of trigeminal abnormalities at both the affected and unaffected REZ (**Figure 7A**). However, only the proportion of MD, RD and AD normalization at the affected REZ correlated with the degree of pain relief (DeSouza et al., 2015; **Figure 7B**). These DTI findings at the REZ support a peripheral theory of TN and corroborate the importance of the REZ in TN pathophysiology.

In addition to the REZ normalization, we also found that right ventral anterior insula (vAI) thinning normalized towards the level of healthy controls following effective neurosurgical treatment for TN (DeSouza et al., 2015; **Figure 7C**). The right-lateralization of this finding is consistent with other studies that have reported right-lateralized activations in the context of pain expectation and the emotional modulation of pain (Wiech and Tracey, 2009). Interestingly, vAI normalization was not associated with pain relief as shown in other chronic pain disorders (Seminowicz et al., 2011), suggesting that for TN patients, vAI normalization may have occurred secondarily to the resolution of the affected REZ abnormalities, which were associated with pain relief. Since most studies of chronic pain report thinning of the AI, cingulate, and prefrontal cortices, it is possible that these abnormalities reflect pain chronicity in general, or other aspects of pain perception such as negative affect (Wiech and Tracey, 2009; Kurth et al., 2010; Chang et al., 2013). Since effective treatment can reverse vAI thinning in TN, our study provided novel evidence that some central abnormalities occur as a consequence of TN pain and likely contribute to the maintenance of this disorder.

PREDICTING TN TREATMENT OUTCOMES: THE FUTURE OF IMAGING?

While many patients experience excellent outcomes from TN treatments, some experience minimal pain relief. That is, there is individual variability with regard to patient responsiveness to treatment. Since conventional clinical diagnostic measures cannot predict which patients will benefit from a given treatment approach for TN, neuroimaging may be an effective tool to noninvasively provide brain-based biomarkers to support the optimal treatment selection for individual TN patients. We previously established that TN is associated with subtle, yet widespread abnormalities in brain structure as measured by morphometric and microstructural measures of brain gray matter and white matter (DeSouza et al., 2013, 2014). Furthermore, our preliminary data suggest that some pre-treatment cortical abnormalities differ between patients that achieve good vs. poor treatment outcomes (**Figure 4C**). As such, future studies may determine which of these measures most accurately predict treatment outcome using a machine learning approach. The application of machine learning algorithms to pain neuroimaging has become a recent topic of interest (e.g., Woo et al., 2014; Chong et al., 2016; Lindquist et al., 2016; Tu et al., 2016), with clinical applications arguably having the greatest need for this type of prediction method (Rosa and Seymour, 2014).

Machine learning approaches based on neuroimaging data have been used to distinguish physical and social pain/rejection (Woo et al., 2014), differentiate migraine patients from controls, and decode subjective pain intensities (Wager et al., 2013; Tu et al., 2016). In general, neuroimaging data can be used to train a discriminative classifier, such as a support vector machine, to make predictions about new data. Clinically, it would be highly advantageous to have brain-based biomarkers that can predict outcomes in individual patients based on models that were trained on prior groups to make out-of-sample predictions (Lindquist et al., 2016). Knowing in advance which patients may better benefit from a certain treatment type (e.g., GKRS) would be enormously important for personalized and effective pain management, and it would reduce costs associated with unsuccessful treatment.

While the predictive accuracy of a classification algorithm based solely on morphological measures is cautioned (Labus et al., 2015), structural MRI measures in combination with functional connectivity measures may be highly informative for predicting treatment response. In one study, a combination of structural and resting-state functional MRI measures were shown to accurately predict treatment response in patients with social anxiety disorder (Whitfield-Gabrieli et al., 2015). It could also provide insight into the fundamental mechanisms underlying individuality of pain and its alleviation and complement patient self-reports.

SUMMARY

In this review, we have provided structural neuroimaging evidence to support peripheral theories of TN etiology and pathophysiology, showed a role for the CNS in TN pain, and discussed implications for the use of potential neuroimaging-based biomarkers to predict treatment response. It is becoming increasingly understood that TN pathophysiology is associated with both trigeminal nerve and brain abnormalities. While future studies are needed to assess the extent to which these abnormalities are the cause or consequence of TN, it is clear that structural MRI methods offer a valuable means to noninvasively examine the trigeminal system *in vivo* and inform our understanding of trigeminal nerve and brain abnormalities in TN.

AUTHOR CONTRIBUTIONS

DDD: concept and design for manuscript content; critical revision of the manuscript for important intellectual content. MH and KDD: concept and design for manuscript content; interpretation of findings; critical revision of the manuscript for important intellectual content; supervising.

ACKNOWLEDGMENTS

We thank Wendy Gu, MScBMC Candidate, University of Toronto, for **Figure 1** and her contribution to **Figure 6**. We thank the Canadian Institute of Health Research for grant support.

REFERENCES

Alexander, A. L., Lee, J. E., Lazar, M., and Field, A. S. (2007). Diffusion tensor imaging of the brain. *Neurotherapeutics* 4, 316–329. doi: 10.1016/j.nurt.2007.05.011

Amir, R., and Devor, M. (2000). Functional cross-excitation between afferent A- and C-neurons in dorsal root ganglia. *Neuroscience* 95, 189–195. doi: 10.1016/s0306-4522(99)00388-7

Anderson, V. C., Berryhill, P. C., Sandquist, M. A., Ciaverella, D. P., Nesbit, G. M., and Burchiel, K. J. (2006). High-resolution three-dimensional magnetic resonance angiography and three-dimensional spoiled gradient-recalled imaging in the evaluation of neurovascular compression in patients with trigeminal neuralgia: a double-blind pilot study. *Neurosurgery* 58, 666–673. doi: 10.1227/01.NEU.0000197117.34888.DE

Antonini, G., Di Pasquale, A., Cruccu, G., Truini, A., Morino, S., Saltelli, G., et al. (2014). Magnetic resonance imaging contribution for diagnosing symptomatic neurovascular contact in classical trigeminal neuralgia: a blinded case-control study and meta-analysis. *Pain* 155, 1464–1471. doi: 10.1016/j.pain.2014.04.020

Beaulieu, C. (2002). The basis of anisotropic water diffusion in the nervous system—a technical review. *NMR Biomed.* 15, 435–455. doi: 10.1002/nbm.782

Blumenfeld-Katzir, T., Pasternak, O., Dagan, M., and Assaf, Y. (2011). Diffusion MRI of structural brain plasticity induced by a learning and memory task. *PLoS One* 6:e20678. doi: 10.1371/journal.pone.0020678

Bozkurt, M., Canbay, S., Neves, G. F., Aktüre, E., Fidan, E., Salamat, M. S., et al. (2012). Microsurgical anatomy of the dorsal thoracic rootlets and dorsal root entry zones. *Acta Neurochir. (Wien)* 154, 1235–1239. doi: 10.1007/s00701-012-1395-0

Burchiel, K. J. (1980). Abnormal impulse generation in focally demyelinated trigeminal roots. *J. Neurosurg.* 53, 674–683. doi: 10.3171/jns.1980.53.5.0674

Chang, L. J., Yarkoni, T., Khaw, M. W., and Sanfey, A. G. (2013). Decoding the role of the insula in human cognition: functional parcellation and large-scale reverse inference. *Cereb. Cortex* 23, 739–749. doi: 10.1093/cercor/bhs065

Chong, C. D., Gaw, N., Fu, Y., Li, J., Wu, T., and Schwedt, T. J. (2016). Migraine classification using magnetic resonance imaging resting-state functional connectivity data. *Cephalalgia* doi: 10.1177/0333102416652091 [Epub ahead of print].

Dandy, W. E. (1929). An operation for the cure of tic douloureux: partial section of the sensory root at the pons. *Arch. Surg.* 18, 687–734. doi: 10.1001/archsurg.1929.04420030081005

DaSilva, A. F., Becerra, L., Pendse, G., Chizh, B., Tully, S., and Borsook, D. (2008). Colocalized structural and functional changes in the cortex of patients with trigeminal neuropathic pain. *PLoS One* 3:e3396. doi: 10.1371/journal.pone.0003396

Davis, K. D., and Moayedi, M. (2013). Central mechanisms of pain revealed through functional and structural MRI. *J. Neuroimmune Pharmacol.* 8, 518–534. doi: 10.1007/s11481-012-9386-8

Davis, K. D., Taylor, K. S., and Anastakis, D. J. (2011). Nerve injury triggers changes in the brain. *Neuroscientist* 17, 407–422. doi: 10.1177/1073858410389185

DeSouza, D. D., Davis, K. D., and Hodaie, M. (2015). Reversal of insular and microstructural nerve abnormalities following effective surgical treatment for trigeminal neuralgia. *Pain* 156, 1112–1123. doi: 10.1097/j.pain.0000000000000156

DeSouza, D. D., Hodaie, M., and Davis, K. D. (2014). Abnormal trigeminal nerve microstructure and brain white matter in idiopathic trigeminal neuralgia. *Pain* 155, 37–44. doi: 10.1016/j.pain.2013.08.029

DeSouza, D. D., Moayedi, M., Chen, D. Q., Davis, K. D., and Hodaie, M. (2013). Sensorimotor and pain modulation brain abnormalities in trigeminal neuralgia: a paroxysmal, sensory-triggered neuropathic pain. *PLoS One* 8:e66340. doi: 10.1371/journal.pone.0066340

Devor, M., Amir, R., and Rappaport, Z. H. (2002a). Pathophysiology of trigeminal neuralgia: the ignition hypothesis. *Clin. J. Pain* 18, 4–13. doi: 10.1097/00002508-200201000-00002

Devor, M., Govrin-Lippmann, R., and Rappaport, Z. H. (2002b). Mechanism of trigeminal neuralgia: an ultrastructural analysis of trigeminal root specimens obtained during microvascular decompression surgery. *J. Neurosurg.* 96, 532–543. doi: 10.3171/jns.2002.96.3.0532

Erbay, S. H., Bhadelia, R. A., O'Callaghan, M., Gupta, P., Riesenburger, R., Krackov, W., et al. (2006). Nerve atrophy in severe trigeminal neuralgia: noninvasive confirmation at MR imaging—initial experience. *Radiology* 238, 689–692. doi: 10.1148/radiol.2382042214

Fischl, B., van der Kouwe, A., Destrieux, C., Halgren, E., Ségonne, F., Salat, D. H., et al. (2004). Automatically parcellating the human cerebral cortex. *Cereb. Cortex* 14, 11–22. doi: 10.1093/cercor/bhg087

Freynhagen, R., and Baron, R. (2009). The evaluation of neuropathic components in low back pain. *Curr. Pain Headache Rep.* 13, 185–190. doi: 10.1007/s11916-009-0032-y

Fujiwara, S., Sasaki, M., Wada, T., Kudo, K., Hirooka, R., Ishigaki, D., et al. (2011). High-resolution diffusion tensor imaging for the detection of diffusion abnormalities in the trigeminal nerves of patients with trigeminal neuralgia caused by neurovascular compression. *J. Neuroimaging* 21, e102–e108. doi: 10.1111/j.1552-6569.2010.00508.x

Gu, J. G., Albuquerque, C., Lee, C. J., and MacDermott, A. B. (1996). Synaptic strengthening through activation of Ca^{2+}-permeable AMPA receptors. *Nature* 381, 793–796. doi: 10.1038/381793a0

Gustin, S. M., Peck, C. C., Wilcox, S. L., Nash, P. G., Murray, G. M., and Henderson, L. A. (2011). Different pain, different brain: thalamic anatomy in neuropathic and non-neuropathic chronic pain syndromes. *J. Neurosci.* 31, 5956–5964. doi: 10.1523/jneurosci.5980-10.2011

Gwilym, S. E., Filippini, N., Douaud, G., Carr, A. J., and Tracey, I. (2010). Thalamic atrophy associated with painful osteoarthritis of the hip is reversible after arthroplasty: a longitudinal voxel-based morphometric study. *Arthritis Rheum.* 62, 2930–2940. doi: 10.1002/art.27585

Hall, G. C., Carroll, D., Parry, D., and McQuay, H. J. (2006). Epidemiology and treatment of neuropathic pain: the UK primary care perspective. *Pain* 122, 156–162. doi: 10.1016/j.pain.2006.01.030

Herweh, C., Kress, B., Rasche, D., Tronnier, V., Tröger, J., Sartor, K., et al. (2007). Loss of anisotropy in trigeminal neuralgia revealed by diffusion tensor imaging. *Neurology* 68, 776–778. doi: 10.1212/01.wnl.0000256340.16766.1d

Hilton, D. A., Love, S., Gradidge, T., and Coakham, H. B. (1994). Pathological findings associated with trigeminal neuralgia caused by vascular compression. *Neurosurgery* 35, 299–303. doi: 10.1227/00006123-199408000-00017

Johansen-Berg, H., and Rushworth, M. F. (2009). Using diffusion imaging to study human connectional anatomy. *Annu. Rev. Neurosci.* 32, 75–94. doi: 10.1146/annurev.neuro.051508.135735

Kerr, F. W., and Miller, R. H. (1966). The pathology of trigeminal neuralgia. Electron microscopic studies. *Arch. Neurol.* 15, 308–319. doi: 10.1001/archneur.1966.00470150086014

Kidd, B. L., and Urban, L. A. (2001). Mechanisms of inflammatory pain. *Br. J. Anaesth.* 87, 3–11. doi: 10.1093/bja/87.1.3

Kilo, S., Schmelz, M., Koltzenburg, M., and Handwerker, H. O. (1994). Different patterns of hyperalgesia induced by experimental inflammation in human skin. *Brain* 117, 385–396. doi: 10.1093/brain/117.2.385

Kobayashi, S., Yoshizawa, H., and Yamada, S. (2004). Pathology of lumbar nerve root compression. Part 1: intraradicular inflammatory changes induced by mechanical compression. *J. Orthop. Res.* 22, 170–179. doi: 10.1016/s0736-0266(03)00131-1

Kugelberg, E., and Lindblom, U. (1959). The mechanism of the pain in trigeminal neuralgia. *J. Neurol. Neurosurg. Psychiatry* 22, 36–43. doi: 10.1136/jnnp.22.1.36

Kurth, F., Zilles, K., Fox, P. T., Laird, A. R., and Eickhoff, S. B. (2010). A link between the systems: functional differentiation and integration within the human insula revealed by meta-analysis. *Brain Struct. Funct.* 214, 519–534. doi: 10.1007/s00429-010-0255-z

Labus, J. S., Van Horn, J. D., Gupta, A., Alaverdyan, M., Torgerson, C., Ashe-McNalley, C., et al. (2015). Multivariate morphological brain signatures predict patients with chronic abdominal pain from healthy control subjects. *Pain* 156, 1545–1554. doi: 10.1097/j.pain.0000000000000196

Leal, P. R., Barbier, C., Hermier, M., Souza, M. A., Cristino-Filho, G., and Sindou, M. (2014). Atrophic changes in the trigeminal nerves of patients with trigeminal neuralgia due to neurovascular compression and their association with the severity of compression and clinical outcomes. *J. Neurosurg.* 120, 1484–1495. doi: 10.3171/2014.2.JNS131288

Leal, P. R., Roch, J. A., Hermier, M., Souza, M. A., Cristino-Filho, G., and Sindou, M. (2011). Structural abnormalities of the trigeminal root revealed by diffusion tensor imaging in patients with trigeminal neuralgia caused by neurovascular compression: a prospective, double-blind, controlled study. *Pain* 152, 2357–2364. doi: 10.1016/j.pain.2011.06.029

Li, M., Yan, J., Li, S., Wang, T., Zhan, W., Wen, H., et al. (2016). Reduced volume of gray matter in patients with trigeminal neuralgia. *Brain Imaging Behav.* doi: 10.1007/s11682-016-9529-2 [Epub ahead of print].

Lindquist, M. A., Krishnan, A., López-Solà, M., Jepma, M., Woo, C. W., Koban, L., et al. (2016). Group-regularized individual prediction: theory and application to pain. *Neuroimage* doi: 10.1016/j.neuroimage.2015.10.074 [Epub ahead of print].

Lorenzoni, J., David, P., and Levivier, M. (2012). Patterns of neurovascular compression in patients with classic trigeminal neuralgia: a high-resolution MRI-based study. *Eur. J. Radiol.* 81, 1851–1857. doi: 10.1016/j.ejrad.2009.09.017

Love, S., and Coakham, H. B. (2001). Trigeminal neuralgia: pathology and pathogenesis. *Brain* 124, 2347–2360. doi: 10.1093/brain/124.12.2347

Love, S., Hilton, D. A., and Coakham, H. B. (1998). Central demyelination of the Vth nerve root in trigeminal neuralgia associated with vascular compression. *Brain Pathol.* 8, 1–11; discussion 11–12. doi: 10.1111/j.1750-3639.1998.tb00126.x

Lutz, J., Linn, J., Mehrkens, J. H., Thon, N., Stahl, R., Seelos, K., et al. (2011). Trigeminal neuralgia due to neurovascular compression: high-spatial-resolution diffusion-tensor imaging reveals microstructural neural changes. *Radiology* 258, 524–530. doi: 10.1148/radiol.10100477

Maarbjerg, S., Gozalov, A., Olesen, J., and Bendtsen, L. (2014). Trigeminal neuralgia–a prospective systematic study of clinical characteristics in 158 patients. *Headache* 54, 1574–1582. doi: 10.1111/head.12441

Marinković, S., Çetković, M., Gibo, H., Todorović, V., Jancić, J., and Milisavljević, M. (2010). Immunohistochemistry of displaced sensory neurons in the trigeminal nerve root. *Cells Tissues Organs* 191, 326–335. doi: 10.1159/000258702

Marinković, S., Gibo, H., Todorović, V., Antić, B., Kovacević, D., Milisavljević, M., et al. (2009). Ultrastructure and immunohistochemistry of the trigeminal peripheral myelinated axons in patients with neuralgia. *Clin. Neurol. Neurosurg.* 111, 795–800. doi: 10.1016/j.clineuro.2009.07.020

Meaney, J. F., Eldridge, P. R., Dunn, L. T., Nixon, T. E., Whitehouse, G. H., and Miles, J. B. (1995). Demonstration of neurovascular compression in trigeminal neuralgia with magnetic resonance imaging. Comparison with surgical findings in 52 consecutive operative cases. *J. Neurosurg.* 83, 799–805. doi: 10.3171/jns.1995.83.5.0799

Miller, J. P., Acar, F., Hamilton, B. E., and Burchiel, K. J. (2009). Radiographic evaluation of trigeminal neurovascular compression in patients with and without trigeminal neuralgia. *J. Neurosurg.* 110, 627–632. doi: 10.3171/2008.6.17620

Moayedi, M., Weissman-Fogel, I., Crawley, A. P., Goldberg, M. B., Freeman, B. V., Tenenbaum, H. C., et al. (2011). Contribution of chronic pain and neuroticism to abnormal forebrain gray matter in patients with temporomandibular disorder. *Neuroimage* 55, 277–286. doi: 10.1016/j.neuroimage.2010.12.013

Moayedi, M., Weissman-Fogel, I., Salomons, T. V., Crawley, A. P., Goldberg, M. B., Freeman, B. V., et al. (2012). White matter brain and trigeminal nerve abnormalities in temporomandibular disorder. *Pain* 153, 1467–1477. doi: 10.1016/j.pain.2012.04.003

Mukherjee, P., Chung, S. W., Berman, J. I., Hess, C. P., and Henry, R. G. (2008). Diffusion tensor MR imaging and fiber tractography: technical considerations. *Am. J. Neuroradiol.* 29, 843–852. doi: 10.3174/ajnr.A1052

Nurmikko, T. J., and Eldridge, P. R. (2001). Trigeminal neuralgia—pathophysiology, diagnosis and current treatment. *Br. J. Anaesth.* 87, 117–132. doi: 10.1093/bja/87.1.117

Obermann, M., Rodriguez-Raecke, R., Naegel, S., Holle, D., Mueller, D., Yoon, M. S., et al. (2013). Gray matter volume reduction reflects chronic pain in trigeminal neuralgia. *Neuroimage* 74, 352–358. doi: 10.1016/j.neuroimage.2013.02.029

Peker, S., Kurtkaya, O., Uzün, I., and Pamir, M. N. (2006). Microanatomy of the central myelin-peripheral myelin transition zone of the trigeminal nerve. *Neurosurgery* 59, 354–359; discussion 354–359. doi: 10.1227/01.neu.0000223501.27220.69

Pollock, B. E., and Ecker, R. D. (2005). A prospective cost-effectiveness study of trigeminal neuralgia surgery. *Clin. J. Pain* 21, 317–322. doi: 10.1097/01.ajp.0000125267.40304.57

Rappaport, Z. H., and Devor, M. (1994). Trigeminal neuralgia: the role of self-sustaining discharge in the trigeminal ganglion. *Pain* 56, 127–138. doi: 10.1016/0304-3959(94)90086-8

Rappaport, Z. H., Govrin-Lippmann, R., and Devor, M. (1997). An electron-microscopic analysis of biopsy samples of the trigeminal root taken during microvascular decompressive surgery. *Stereotact Funct. Neurosurg.* 68, 182–186. doi: 10.1159/000099920

Rocca, M. A., Ceccarelli, A., Falini, A., Colombo, B., Tortorella, P., Bernasconi, L., et al. (2006). Brain gray matter changes in migraine patients with T2-visible lesions: a 3-T MRI study. *Stroke* 37, 1765–1770. doi: 10.1161/01.str.0000226589.00599.4d

Rocca, M. A., Pagani, E., Colombo, B., Tortorella, P., Falini, A., Comi, G., et al. (2008). Selective diffusion changes of the visual pathways in patients with migraine: a 3-T tractography study. *Cephalalgia* 28, 1061–1068. doi: 10.1111/j.1468-2982.2008.01655.x

Rodriguez-Raecke, R., Niemeier, A., Ihle, K., Ruether, W., and May, A. (2013). Structural brain changes in chronic pain reflect probably neither damage nor atrophy. *PLoS One* 8:e54475. doi: 10.1371/journal.pone.0054475

Rosa, M. J., and Seymour, B. (2014). Decoding the matrix: benefits and limitations of applying machine learning algorithms to pain neuroimaging. *Pain* 155, 864–867. doi: 10.1016/j.pain.2014.02.013

Sandkuhler, J., and Gebhart, G. F. (1984). Relative contributions of the nucleus raphe magnus and adjacent medullary reticular formation to the inhibition by stimulation in the periaqueductal gray of a spinal nociceptive reflex in the pentobarbital-anesthetized rat. *Brain Res.* 305, 77–87. doi: 10.1016/0006-8993(84)91121-1

Satoh, T., Omi, M., Nabeshima, M., Onoda, K., and Date, I. (2009). Severity analysis of neurovascular contact in patients with trigeminal neuralgia: assessment with the inner view of the 3D MR cisternogram and angiogram fusion imaging. *Am. J. Neuroradiol.* 30, 603–607. doi: 10.3174/ajnr.A1409

Seltzer, Z., and Devor, M. (1979). Ephaptic transmission in chronically damaged peripheral nerves. *Neurology* 29, 1061–1064. doi: 10.1212/wnl.29.7.1061

Seminowicz, D. A., Wideman, T. H., Naso, L., Hatami-Khoroushahi, Z., Fallatah, S., Ware, M. A., et al. (2011). Effective treatment of chronic low back pain in humans reverses abnormal brain anatomy and function. *J. Neurosci.* 31, 7540–7550. doi: 10.1523/JNEUROSCI.5280-10.2011

Szabó, N., Kincses, Z. T., Párdutz, A., Tajti, J., Szok, D., Tuka, B., et al. (2012). White matter microstructural alterations in migraine: a diffusion-weighted MRI study. *Pain* 153, 651–656. doi: 10.1016/j.pain.2011.11.029

Taylor, K. S., Anastakis, D. J., and Davis, K. D. (2009). Cutting your nerve changes your brain. *Brain* 132, 3122–3133. doi: 10.1093/brain/awp231

Traccis, S., Monaco, F., Sechi, G. P., Moglia, A., and Mutani, R. (1983). Long-term therapy with carbamazepine: effects on nerve conduction velocity. *Eur. Neurol.* 22, 410–416. doi: 10.1159/000115594

Trousseau, A. (1853). De la nevralgie epileptiforme. *Arch. Gen. Med.* 1, 33–44.

Tu, Y., Tan, A., Bai, Y., Hung, Y. S., and Zhang, Z. (2016). Decoding subjective intensity of nociceptive pain from pre-stimulus and post-stimulus brain activities. *Front. Comput. Neurosci.* 10:32. doi: 10.3389/fncom.2016.00032

Wager, T. D., Atlas, L. Y., Lindquist, M. A., Roy, M., Woo, C.-W., and Kross, E. (2013). An fMRI-based neurologic signature of physical pain. *N. Engl. J. Med.* 368, 1388–1397. doi: 10.1056/NEJMoa1204471

Whitfield-Gabrieli, S., Ghosh, S. S., Nieto-Castanon, A., Saygin, Z., Doehrmann, O., Chai, X. J., et al. (2015). Brain connectomics predict response to treatment in social anxiety disorder. *Mol. Psychiatry* 21, 680–685. doi: 10.1038/mp.2015.109

Wiech, K., and Tracey, I. (2009). The influence of negative emotions on pain: behavioral effects and neural mechanisms. *Neuroimage* 47, 987–994. doi: 10.1016/j.neuroimage.2009.05.059

Woo, C.-W., Koban, L., Kross, E., Lindquist, M. A., Banich, M. T., Ruzic, L., et al. (2014). Separate neural representations for physical pain and social rejection. *Nat. Commun.* 5:5380. doi: 10.1038/ncomms6380

Woolf, C. J., and Salter, M. W. (2000). Neuronal plasticity: increasing the gain in pain. *Science* 288, 1765–1769. doi: 10.1126/science.288.5472.1765

Zakrzewska, J. M., and Akram, H. (2011). Neurosurgical interventions for the treatment of classical trigeminal neuralgia. *Cochrane Database Syst. Rev.* 7:CD007312. doi: 10.1002/14651858.cd007312

Zatorre, R. J., Fields, R. D., and Johansen-Berg, H. (2012). Plasticity in gray and white: neuroimaging changes in brain structure during learning. *Nat. Neurosci.* 15, 528–536. doi: 10.1038/nn.3045

8

A Newly Identified Frontal Path from Fornix in Septum Pellucidum with 7.0T MRI Track Density Imaging (TDI) – The Septum Pellucidum Tract (SPT)

Zang-Hee Cho[1], *Je-Geun Chi*[1,2], *Sang-Han Choi*[1], *Se-Hong Oh*[1,3], *Sung-Yeon Park*[1], *Sun Ha Paek*[4], *Chan-Woong Park*[1], *Fernando Calamante*[5,6]* *and Young-Bo Kim*[1]

[1] *Neuroscience Research Institute, Gachon University of Medicine and Science, Incheon, South Korea,* [2] *Department of Pathology, Seoul National University College of Medicine, Seoul, South Korea,* [3] *Department of Radiology, School of Medicine, University of Pennsylvania, Philadelphia, PA, USA,* [4] *Departments of Neurosurgery, Seoul National University College of Medicine, Seoul, South Korea,* [5] *The Florey Institute of Neuroscience and Mental Health, Melbourne, VIC, Australia,* [6] *Department of Medicine, Austin Health and Northern Health, University of Melbourne, Melbourne, VIC, Australia*

***Correspondence:**
Fernando Calamante
fernando.calamante@florey.edu.au

The high anatomical contrast achieved with the newly emerging MRI tractographic technique of super-resolution track density imaging (TDI) encouraged us to search for a new fiber tract in the septum pellucidum. Although this septum pellucidum tract (SPT) has been observed previously, its connections were unclear due to ambiguity and limited resolution of conventional MRI images. It is now possible to identify detailed parts of SPT with the increased resolution of TDI, which involves diffusion MRI imaging, whole-brain tractography, and voxel subdivision using the track-count information. Four healthy male subjects were included in the study. The experiment was performed with 7.0T MRI, following the guidelines of the institute's institutional review board. Data were processed with the super-resolution TDI technique to generate a tractographic map with 0.18 mm isotropic resolution. The SPT was identified in all subjects. Based on additional seed tracking method with inter-axis correlation search, we have succeeded in identifying a new frontal lobe pathway in the SPT. We hypothesize that the tract is connected as a superior dorsal branch of the fornix that leads to the prefrontal cortex.

Keywords: 7.0T MRI, track density imaging, septum pellucidum tract, fornix, fiber tracking, tractography, diffusion MRI

INTRODUCTION

Despite substantial progress with diffusion tensor imaging (DTI; Basser et al., 1994) in MRI in the last two decades, its sensitivity to accurately image white matter tracts in the brain remains somewhat limited (Tournier et al., 2011). More recently, however, several new post processing imaging techniques have been introduced (Tournier et al., 2007; Calamante et al., 2010, 2011), including super-resolution track density imaging (TDI), which was shown to greatly increase the sensitivity for visualization of white matter structures (Calamante et al., 2010). Sensitivity is increased even further when these methods are combined with ultra-high field MRI (Calamante et al., 2012, 2013; Kurniawan et al., 2014; Richards et al., 2014; Cho et al., 2015a,b; Ullmann et al., 2015). These new methods therefore encouraged us to search for a fiber tract in the septum pellucidum, which is difficult to visualize *in vivo* due to the limited resolution, contrast and sensitivity of current DTI MRI images.

A set of anatomical images of brain structures with the fornix in the septum pellucidum is shown in **Figures 1** and **2**. These anatomical images are interesting because although some tissues or fibers seem visible in the septum pellucidum, no detail description has been paid to these fibers (see for example figure on page 24 of the Brain Atlas, by Hanaway et al., 1990). Similarly, another interesting clue toward this structure is given by the DTI atlas of Mori et al. (2005) and Oishi et al. (2010), in which they showed some indications that there may be fibers extending from the crus of the fornix to the anterior and dorsal aspect of the septum pellucidum. While some faint images of dorsal branches of the fornix are visible in these images, they are difficult to recognize, and there is in fact no mention of the existence of such a structure. Recently, there was a paper describing this fiber in the septum pellucidum (Cho et al., 2015b), but the connections from this fiber were still unclear. Based on data from additional subjects, and further analysis using a seed-based

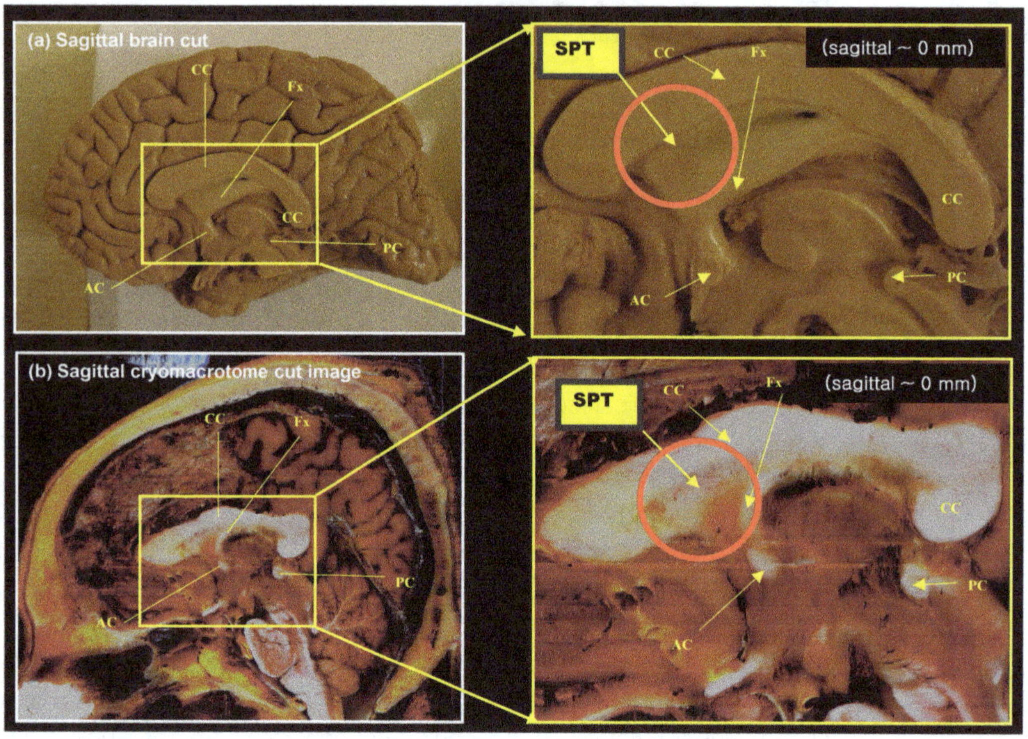

FIGURE 1 | Anatomy of the septum pellucidum area (red circle). (a) Mid-sagittal brain image (sagittal, 0 mm) with its extended region of interest (ROI) image (yellow box). **(b)** Middle sagittal cryomacrotome image with its extended ROI image (yellow box). Although the septum pellucidum tract (SPT) has been unknown until now, it does subtly appear in these images: the SPT can be seen as shown in **(a)**. It is also visible in **(b)** as a dorsal branch of the fornix in the frontal area of the septum pellucidum. AC, anterior commissure, CC, corpus callosum, Fx, fornix, PC, posterior commissure.

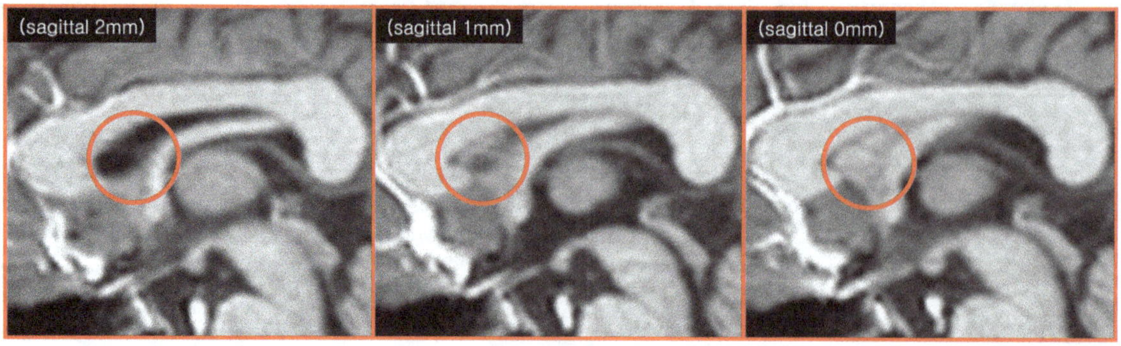

FIGURE 2 | Another indication of the SPT is seen in the anatomical images of modern MRI scanners (3T T1-weighted sagittal MRI images). The images at 1 and 0 mm show some faint structures in the septum pellucidum area (red circle), but not in the image at 2 mm.

tracking method, in this study we have identified and confirmed additional connections from this fiber (the septum pellucidum tract, SPT) to frontal areas. It is hypothesized that this new structure could be a potential new target for neurosurgery, such as for deep brain stimulation (DBS) where many emerging targets are being sought.

MATERIALS AND METHODS

The new STP fiber was identified by super-resolution TDI maps obtained from ultra-high field diffusion MRI data (e.g., see **Figure 3**), and was further confirmed by the seed-based tracking approach and an inter-axis correlation search (Cho et al., 2015b). The inter-axis correlation refers to a manual method for co-localizing structures seen on TDI maps using perpendicular lines placed on coronal, sagittal, and axial images; intersecting inter-axis lines are then manually and visually correlated between the orthogonal planes. Data acquisition and processing therefore consisted of four steps: diffusion weighted imaging (DWI) data acquisition, TDI data processing, seed-based tracking, and the inter-axis correlation search.

Diffusion weighted imaging data were obtained on a 7.0T MRI scanner (Magnetom 7.0T, Siemens, Erlangen, Germany), and the experiment was performed following the guidelines and with the approval of the institute's institutional review board and Korea food and drug administration. Four young healthy male subjects (age: 24–30 years) were recruited as volunteers, and no one had a record of any health related problems. DWI data were acquired using a single-shot diffusion-weighted echo planar imaging (EPI) sequence with the following parameters: TR/TE = 6,000/83 ms, matrix size = 128 × 128, field-of-view 230 mm × 230 mm, 45 slices, 1.8 mm isotropic resolution, 64 diffusion-weighted directions, b-value = 2,000 s/mm^2, one $b = 0$ image, GRAPPA with factor 3, bandwidth 1562 Hz/pixel, and three repeats, for a total acquisition time of 19 min 0.5 s.

Diffusion weighted imaging data were then processed to calculate super-resolution TDI maps, which involves constrained spherical deconvolution (Tournier et al., 2007) to calculate the fiber orientation distribution (FOD) in each voxel, whole brain probabilistic fiber-tracking, and track-count mapping with voxel sub-division (Calamante et al., 2010). The TDI analysis was carried out using the MRtrix software program (Brain Research Institute, Florey Neuroscience Institutes, Melbourne, Victoria, Australia, http://www.brain.org.au/software/mrtrix/index.html) (Tournier et al., 2012). Relevant tracking parameters were: tracking type = SD_PROB, track minimum length = 20 mm, step-size = 0.02 mm, curvature radius constraint = 0.04 mm, FOD cutoff for track termination = 0.3, and number of tracks = 6,000,000 (Tournier et al., 2012). The final TDI image was generated with a nominal isotropic resolution of 0.18 mm, i.e., corresponding to a voxel size 1/1000 smaller than the acquired DWI data. These TDI maps were color-coded according to the direction of the fibers (based on the mean color of all streamline segments within the voxel (Calamante et al., 2010), i.e., with red: left-right, green: anterior-posterior, and blue: inferior-superior), to generate the so-called directionally-encoded color (DEC) TDI maps.

We have also performed seed-based tracking analysis to further identify and characterize the SPT, particularly to identify the connection to forebrain areas. We selected a single voxel seed point or region of interest in the SPT, which lied in the medial part of sagittal view image (sagittal slice between −1 mm and +1 mm), as shown with yellow crosses in **Figure 4** (see Results section). Based on the SPT seed, the 'streamtrack' function in MRtrix was used for probabilistic seed-based tracking, with the following relevant parameters: tracking type (SD_PROB), track minimum length = 20 mm, step-size = 0.02 mm, curvature radius constraint = 0.08 mm, number of tracks = 1,000 (Tournier et al., 2012).

To further confirm the seed-based tracking results and to help with the identification of the SPT fiber, we performed an additional inter-axis correlation search (Cho et al., 2015b) in the sagittal and axial views.

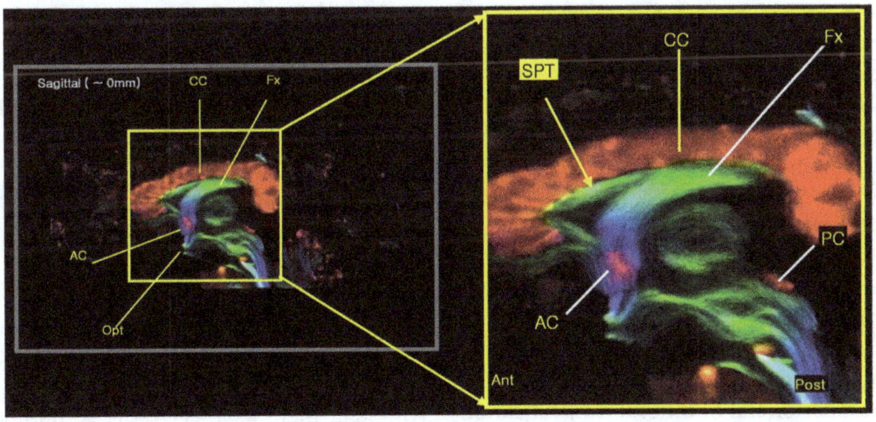

FIGURE 3 | The new 7.0T super-resolution DEC TDI began to clearly show the tract at the septum pellucidum area in a sagittal view image, especially with its expanded image at right side. The color-coding indicates the main local orientation (red: left–right, green: anterior–posterior, blue: inferior–superior).

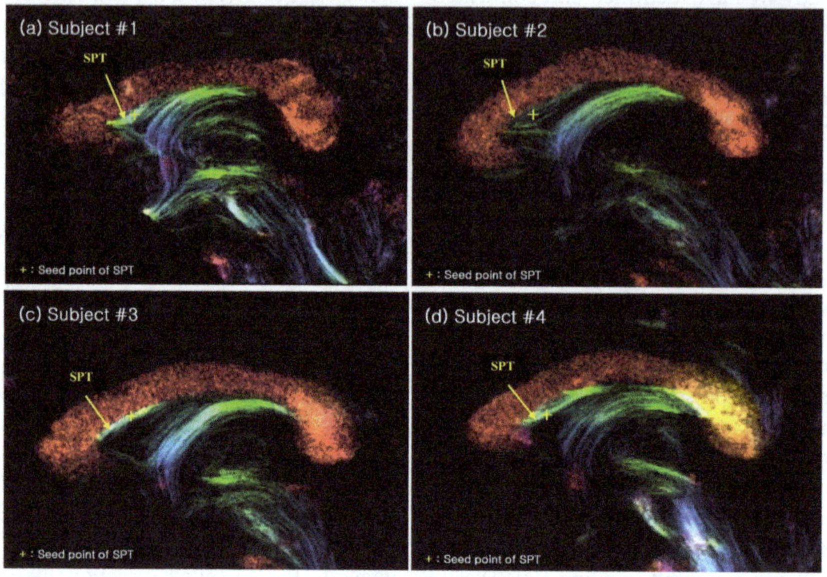

FIGURE 4 | The SPT on the super-resolution DEC TDI of four different subjects (labelled as (a), (b), (c) and (d), respectively). The SPTs are indicated by yellow arrows and yellow crosses. The latter are used as the seed points for the search of the SPTs and its connections (see **Figure 5**). The color-coding indicates the main local orientation (red: left–right, green: anterior–posterior, blue: inferior–superior).

RESULTS

We found several interesting features of the SPT based on the current study. First, the new fiber, which was observed clearly in all four subjects, appeared to be a dorsal branch of the fornix (**Figure 4**). SPT branches were clearly visible and differentiated from the main body of the fornix as well as from the corpus callosum (e.g., see expanded image in **Figure 3**, where the SPT can be seen as the green structure adjacent to the corpus callosum in a mid-brain sagittal slice); the distinction between the SPT and surrounding structures was greatly facilitated by the high resolution and high contrast of the DEC-TDI maps. In particular, in the sagittal view, the SPT appeared to originate from the caudal aspect or crus of the fornix and extend toward the genu of the corpus callosum, as if it were an anterior dorsal branch of the fornix at the septum pellucidum. The SPT is implicitly shown in **Figures 1** and **2**; however, no specific reference has ever been mentioned regarding this fiber (Hanaway et al., 1990; Mori et al., 2005; Oishi et al., 2010). Moreover, specific mention of the presence of additional fiber distribution in this area would have been extremely difficult to make solely based on anatomical images such as those shown in **Figures 1** and **2,** due to limited contrast and/or resolution.

Second, the SPT seems to be directed toward the prefrontal area from the frontal end of the septum pellucidum (**Figures 5A–D**). In the mid-sagittal view [**Figure 5A**(i)] in subject #1, as well as for the other subjects in **Figures 5A–D**, the SPT abruptly reaches the anterior end of the septum pellucidum or immediately behind the genu of the corpus callosum, splits laterally, and it is eventually directed toward prefrontal areas. SPT presents only in the midline of the septum pellucidum and more or less disappears as it leaves the midline or the septum pellucidum (only within −3 mm to +3 mm from the midline). We were able to trace the forwardly directed SPT tract as shown in **Figure 5** in the axial view images, and found that the SPT was split laterally at the genu or end of the anterior aspect of the SPT, and appears directed toward the prefrontal area, particularly toward the superior frontal area, by following the genu of the corpus callosum (Note: these projections toward the superior frontal area cannot be visualized in the specific planes shown in **Figure 5**). The SPT seems to circle around the corpus callosum and merge with the anterior limb of the internal capsule or minor forceps.

Third, the posterior part of the SPT is connected to the body or crus of fornix (**Figure 6**). To confirm the connection of the SPT to the main body of the fornix, we examined the area using an inter-axis correlation search (Cho et al., 2015b) with coronal view data at 1 mm (**Figure 6A**) and 19 mm (**Figure 6B**), respectively, with the midline sagittal view data at 0 mm. The SPT is separated from the superior dorsal branch of the fornix at the caudal aspect (**Figure 6A**) and the SPT distinguishes itself from the other part of the fornix in the anterior aspect, such as the pre-and post-commissural fornix as shown in **Figure 6B**.

DISCUSSION

Although there have been a large number of studies about the septum pellucidum, the fiber in the septum pellucidum has not been well described so far, and the connection from this area is at best unknown based on anatomical and tractography

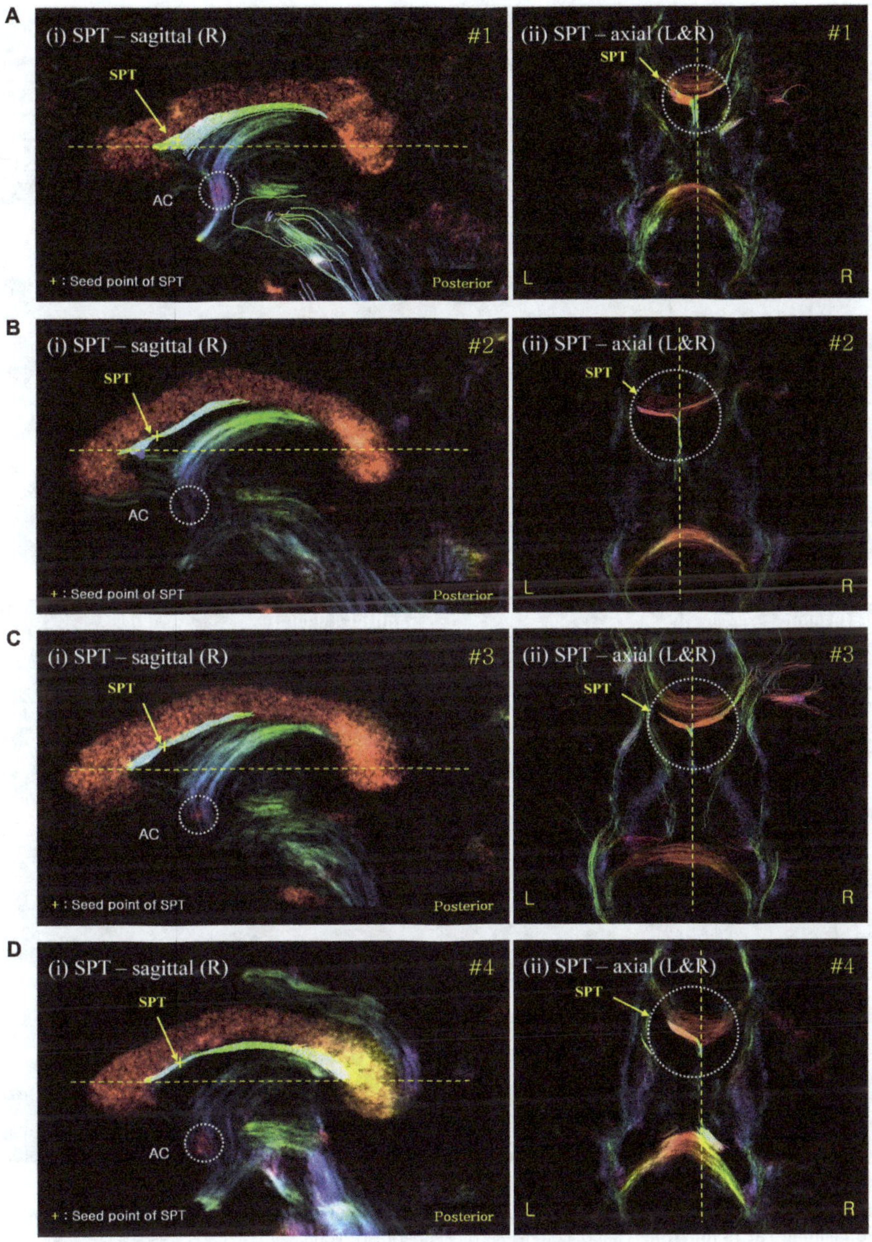

FIGURE 5 | Septum pellucidum tract seed-based tracking results shown with correlated sagittal and axial view images. (A) The SPT seed-based tracking result from subject #1; **(B–D)** equivalent results from subjects #2, #3, and #4, respectively. The left [also labeled (i)] and right (ii) columns show the seed-based tracking results in sagittal view images and their corresponding axial view images, respectively. The tracks displayed correspond to those within a 0.54 mm slab (i.e., also including the tracks in the surrounding slices) overlaid on the DEC-TDI map. The yellow cross on the SPT of the sagittal view images (left) indicates the seed point positions in each data-set. The color-coding of the background image indicates the main local orientation (red: left–right, green: anterior–posterior, blue: inferior–superior). AC, anterior commissure (as indicated by the dashed circle in the sagittal images). The dashed circle in the axial images highlights the area of the SPT at the anterior end of the septum pellucidum where it splits laterally.

approaches. The septum pellucidum is a thin vertical sheet of nervous tissue that is covered on either side by the ependyma. The ependyma forms a single layer of cuboidal or columnar cells that are different from the fiber (Richard, 2001). However, in some reports, the medial surface of the septum pellucidum is claimed to be some form of white matter structure (Swayam et al., 2006; Marinković et al., 2009). In this study, guided by the super-resolution TDI technique from ultra-high field 7T MRI, we have clearly observed the existence of the fiber in the septum pellucidum and identified its frontal connection, which were further confirmed using an inter-axis correlation search between coronal and sagittal view image data.

The fornix is one of the major fibers in the limbic system with numerous functional connections; however, no direct

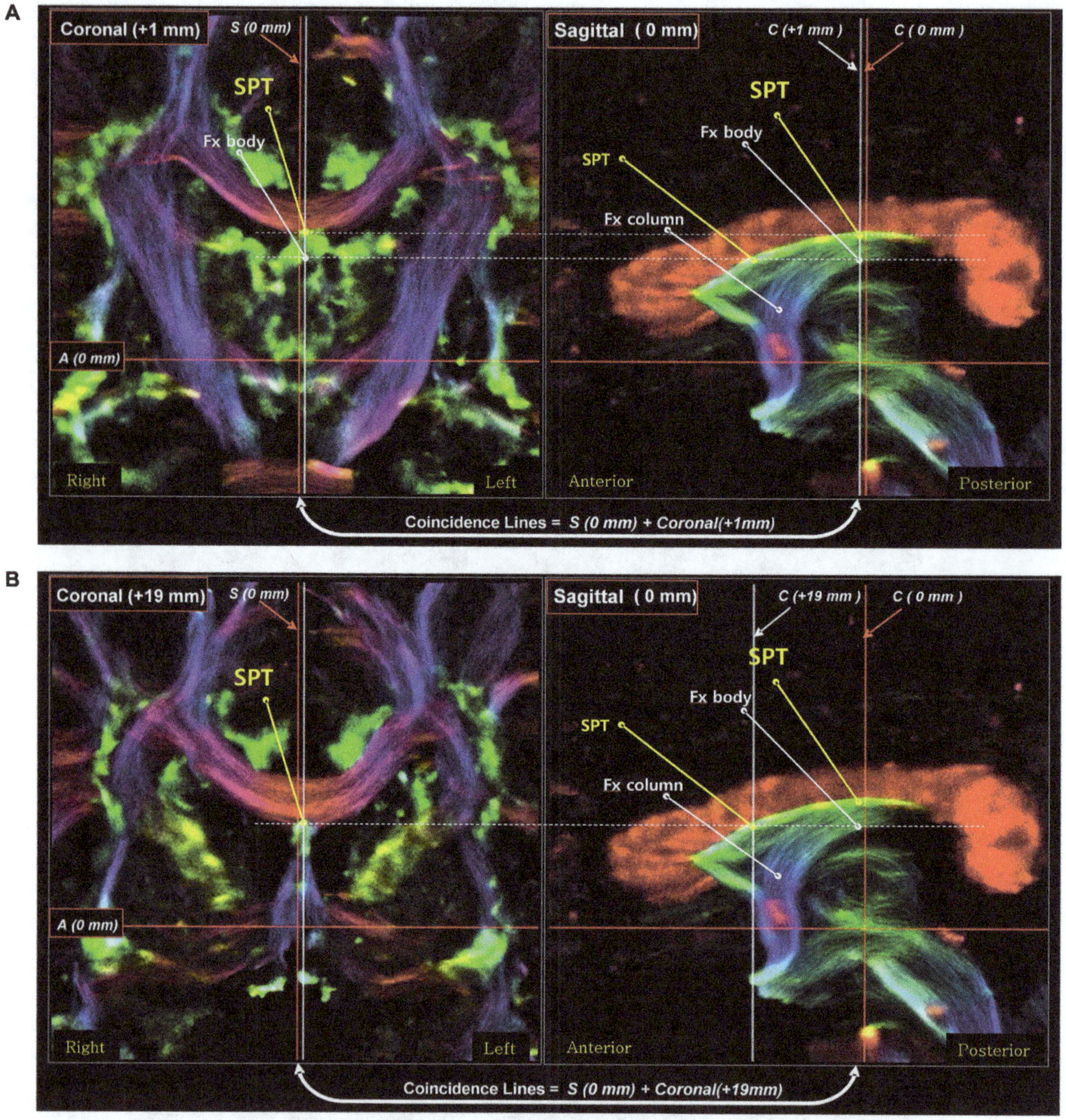

FIGURE 6 | An inter-axis correlation search for the corroboration of the SPT in a sagittal view image with two coronal view images on the left [coronal image at 1 mm (A) and coronal image at 19 mm (B)]. A set of coronal-sagittal super-resolution DEC TDI maps was selected, and an inter-axis correlation study was conducted. The SPT is clearly visible both in the coronal and sagittal views. The thick white lines are the coincidence lines where the values are the same in both images. The result of this correlation search suggests that the SPT is a new separate dorsal-anterior branch of the fornix (Fx), different from the main body of the fornix, the precommissural fornix. Part of this figure has been modified from a figure previously published in Cho et al. (2015b), with permission from Elsevier.

connections to prefrontal areas have been found other than the septal nucleus and the nucleus accumbens. Based on previous studies, the pre-commissural fornix is well known, both from human histological studies as well as *in vivo* MRI/DTI studies; however, little is known about the SPT and even its connections. This newly identified SPT appears as a dorsal branch of the fornix and connected to the prefrontal area. The SPT is not only connected to the fornix but also to the prefrontal cortex, as shown in **Figure 5**, where the two bifurcated branches of the SPT are connected toward the prefrontal cortex. We hypothesized that the SPT could be an important and unique route for the direct connection of the hippocampus or hippocampal complex, which consists of the para-hippocampal gyrus to entorhinal cortex, to the prefrontal cortex, which includes the dorsolateral prefrontal cortex and septal nuclei, through the fornix; a connection that has not been observed previously. Future studies are required to validate and further characterize this possible new connection. Until those studies are carried out, the exact extent of the apparent frontal connections identified in the current study should be considered as preliminary findings.

Importantly, considering the fact that the SPT is connected to the septal nuclei and possibly to the dorsolateral prefrontal cortex, it could play an important role in controlling the cognitive and attractive activity such as the sorrow and pleasure. We hypothesize that this structure could therefore be a new target for external intervention, such as by DBS, which has begun to be applied in treatment of major depressive disorders or other cognitive diseases, such as the Alzheimer's and obsessive and compulsive disorder, or even post-traumatic stress disorder (PTSD; Srejic et al., 2015). Future studies are required to test this hypothesis.

Interestingly, the SPT defined here was highlighted as a structure just above the fornix with lower fractional anisotropy (FA) in patients with Alzheimer's disease compared with cognitively normal individuals in a voxel-based analysis (see sagittal view of Figure 2A in Oishi et al., 2011). This provides further evidence of the potential important clinical significance of this newly identified structure.

Technical Issues

While ultra-high field MRI was used in the current study, other suitable studies at lower field strengths, such as 3T, should be also possible to visualize in principle the SPT given it is a relatively large structure; identification and visualization is facilitated now based on the results presented here, which have demonstrated that the structure exists and where it is located. For example, similar super-resolution DEC-TDI maps at 3T, or high-resolution DTI maps based on multi-shot acquisitions (Porter and Heidemann, 2009) should be suitable to identify the SPT at 3T. It should be noted, however, that the latter acquisition approach is typically associated with much longer acquisition times, and therefore might be less suited for clinical applications; this is in fact a benefit of the TDI method, where the extra time is spent on post-processing, without necessarily extending the acquisition time.

The choice of super-resolution level is a compromise between several factors, including processing time (the higher the resolution the more tracks are required), output file size and memory requirements (the DEC-TDI data sets shown here were >1 GB in size), and the size of the structure of interest (smaller structures require higher super-resolution). The 0.18 mm voxel dimension (corresponding to a 1/10 super-resolution in each orientation) was found to be a suitable compromise. As mentioned above, given the SPT is a relatively large structure, lower super-resolution levels are likely to have been sufficient for identification; however, as shown in Figure 1 of Calamante et al. (2010), the structure's conspicuity and sharpness would have been lower.

Finally, it should be noted that diffusion MRI fiber-tracking does not directly visualize the axonal fibers but rather infers an estimate of the location and orientation of white matter bundles based on the diffusion of water molecules. Diffusion MRI fiber-tracking is subject to a number of well-known limitations and possible sources of error, including the effect of 'kissing' and 'crossing fibers,' the effect of noise, partial volume, etc. (Tournier et al., 2011). To minimize these sources of error, we used here state-of-the art methods, including advanced models to characterize multiple fiber populations and a probabilistic fiber-tracking algorithm (see Materials and Methods section). It is important to emphasize, however, that validation of fiber-tracking methods remains an area of major challenge and great interest in the field of diffusion MRI, and results from fiber-tracking based methods should be considered with caution since they can be influenced by many technical issues.

AUTHOR CONTRIBUTIONS

1. Substantial contributions to the conception or design of the work (Z-HC, J-GC, S-HP, FC, Y-BK).
2. Substantial contributions to the acquisition of data (S-HC, S-HO, S-YP).
3. Substantial contributions to the analysis of data (Z-HC, J-GC, C-WP, FC).
4. Substantial contributions to the interpretation of data (Z-HC, J-GC, S-HP, C-WP, FC).
5. Drafting the work or revising it critically for important intellectual content (all authors: Z-HC, J-GC, S-HC, S-HO, S-YP, S-HP, C-WP, FC, Y-BK).
6. Final approval of the version to be published (all authors: Z-HC, J-GC, S-HC, S-HO, S-YP, S-HP, C-WP, FC, Y-BK).
7. Agreement to be accountable for all aspects of the work in ensuring that questions related to the accuracy or integrity of any part of the work are appropriately investigated and resolved (all authors: Z-HC, J-GC, S-HC, S-HO, S-YP, S-HP, C-WP, FC, Y-BK).

ACKNOWLEDGMENTS

This study was supported by the Korea National Research Foundation (NRF), the Ministry of Education, Science, and Technology (2008-2004159) and a Korea Science and Engineering Foundation grant (10200002134). FC is grateful to the National Health and Medical Research Council of Australia (APP628952), the Australian Research Council (FT110100726), and the Victorian Government's Operational Infrastructure Support Grant for their support. The Korea Institute of Planning & Evaluation for Technology in Food, Agriculture, Forestry, and Fisheries, Republic of Korea (311011-05-3-SB020), the Korea Healthcare Technology R&D Project (HI11C21100200) funded by Ministry of Health & Welfare, Republic of Korea, the Technology Innovation Program (10050154, Business Model Development for Personalized Medicine Based on Integrated Genome and Clinical Information) funded by the Ministry of Trade, Industry & Energy (MI, Korea), and the Bio & Medical Technology Development Program of the NRF funded by the Korean government, MSIP (2015M3C7A1028926).

REFERENCES

Basser, P. J., Mattiello, J., and LeBihan, D. (1994). MR diffusion tensor spectroscopy and imaging. *Biophys. J.* 66, 259–267. doi: 10.1016/S0006-3495(94)80775-1

Calamante, F., Oh, S. H., Tournier, J. D., Park, S. Y., Son, Y. D., Chung, J. Y., et al. (2013). Super-resolution track-density imaging of thalamic substructures: comparison with high-resolution anatomical magnetic resonance imaging at 7.0T. *Hum. Brain Mapp.* 34, 2538–2548. doi: 10.1002/hbm.22083

Calamante, F., Tournier, J. D., Heidemann, R. M., Anwander, A., Jackson, G. D., and Connelly, A. (2011). Track density imaging (TDI): validation of super-resolution property. *Neuroimage* 56, 1259–1266. doi: 10.1016/j.neuroimage.2011.02.059

Calamante, F., Tournier, J. D., Jackson, G. D., and Connelly, A. (2010). Track-density imaging (TDI): super-resolution white matter imaging using whole-brain track-density mapping. *Neuroimage* 53, 1233–1243. doi: 10.1016/j.neuroimage.2010.07.024

Calamante, F., Tournier, J. D., Kurniawan, N. D., Yang, Z., Gyengesi, E., Galloway, G. J., et al. (2012). Super-resolution track-density imaging studies of mouse brain: comparison to histology. *Neuroimage* 59, 286–296. doi: 10.1016/j.neuroimage.2011.07.014

Cho, Z. H., Calamante, F., and Chi, J. G. (2015a). *7.0 Tesla MRI Brain White Matter Atlas*, 2nd Edn. Berlin: Springer-Verlag. doi: 10.1007/978-3-642-54392-0

Cho, Z. H., Law, M., Chi, J. G., Choi, S. H., Park, S. Y., Kammen, A., et al. (2015b). An anatomical review of thalamo-limbic fiber tractography:ultra-high resolution direct visualization of thalamo-limbic fibers atr, slmfb, immfb, and newly identified septum pellucidum tract. *World Neurosurg.* 83, 54–61. doi: 10.1016/j.wneu.2013.08.022

Hanaway, J., Woolsey, T. A., and Gado, M. H. (1990). *Brain Atlas.* Bethesda, MD: Fitzgerald Science Press, Inc.

Kurniawan, N. D., Richards, K., Yang, Z., Shie, D., Ullmann, J. F. P., Moldrich, R. X., et al. (2014). Visualization of mouse barrel cortex using ex-vivo track density imaging. *Neuroimage* 87,465–475. doi: 10.1016/j.neuroimage.2013.09.030

Marinković, S., Gibo, H., Todorović, V., Antić, B., Kovacević, D., Milisavljević, M., et al. (2009). Ultrastructure and immunohistochemistry of the trigeminal peripheral myelinated axons in patients with neuralgia. *Clin. Neurol. Neurosurg.* 111, 795–800. doi: 10.1016/j.clineuro.2009.07.020

Mori, S., Wakana, S., Nagae-Poetscher, L., and van Zijl, P. C. M. (2005). *MRI Atlas of Human White Matter.* Armsterdam: Elsevier.

Oishi, K., Akhter, K., Mielke, M., Ceritoglu, C., Zhang, J., Jiang, H., et al. (2011). Multi-modal MRI analysis with disease-specific spatial filtering: initial testing to predict mild cognitive impairment patients who convert to Alzheimer's disease. *Front. Neurol.* 2:54. doi: 10.3389/fneur.2011.00054

Oishi, K., Faria, A., van Zijl, P. C. M., and Mori, S. (2010). *MRI Atlas of Human White Matter.* Armsterdam: Elsevier.

Porter, D. A., and Heidemann, R. M. (2009). High resolution diffusion-weighted imaging using readout-segmented echo-planar imaging, parallel imaging and a two-dimensional navigator-based reacquisition. *Magn. Reson. Med.* 62, 468–475. doi: 10.1002/mrm.22024

Richard, S. S. (2001). *Clinical Neuroanatomy.* Baltimore, MD: Lippincott Williams & Wilkins.

Richards, K., Calamante, F., Tournier, J. D., Kurniawan, N. D., Sadeghian, F., Retchford, A. R., et al. (2014). Mapping somatosensory connectivity in adult mice using diffusion MRI tractography and super-resolution track density imaging. *Neuroimage* 102(Pt 2), 381–392. doi: 10.1016/j.neuroimage.2014.07.048

Srejic, L. R., Prescott, I. A., Zhang, P., Strauss, I., Dostrovsky, J. O., Giacobbe, P., et al. (2015). Paired pulse depression in the subcallosal cingulate region of depression patients. *Biol. Psychiatry* 78:e3–e4. doi: 10.1016/j.biopsych.2014.09.018

Swayam, J. S., Sirisha, B., Sai, S. D., and Sree, L. D. (2006). Cavum septi pellucidi and setum pellucidi. *J. Anat. Soc. India* 58, 24–28.

Tournier, J. D., Calamante, F., and Connelly, A. (2007). Robust determination of the fibre orientation distribution in diffusion MRI: non-negativity constrained super-resolved spherical deconvolution. *Neuroimage* 35, 1459–1472. doi: 10.1016/j.neuroimage.2007.02.016

Tournier, J. D., Calamante, F., and Connelly, A. (2012). MRtrix: diffusion tractography in crossing fiber regions. *Int. J. Imag Syst. Tech.* 22, 53–66. doi: 10.1002/ima.22005

Tournier, J. D., Mori, S., and Leemans, A. (2011). Diffusion tensor imaging and beyond. *Magn. Reson. Med.* 65, 1532–1556. doi: 10.1002/mrm.22924

Ullmann, J. F. P., Calamante, F., Collin, S. P., Reutens, D. C., and Kurniawan, N. D. (2015). Enhanced characterization of the zebrafish brain as revealed by super resolution track-density imaging. *Brain Struct. Funct.* 220, 457–4 doi: 10.1007/s00429-013-0667-7

9

Widespread Volumetric Brain Changes following Tooth Loss in Female Mice

Limor Avivi-Arber[1,2], Ze'ev Seltzer[1,2,3,4,5], Miriam Friedel[6], Jason P. Lerch[6,7], Massieh Moayedi[1,2], Karen D. Davis[1,8,9,10] and Barry J. Sessle[1,2,3]*

[1] University of Toronto Centre for the Study of Pain, University of Toronto, Toronto, ON, Canada, [2] Faculty of Dentistry, University of Toronto, Toronto, ON, Canada, [3] Department of Physiology, Faculty of Medicine, University of Toronto, Toronto, ON, Canada, [4] Department of Anesthesiology, University Health Network, Toronto, ON, Canada, [5] Central Institute of Mental Health, University of Heidelberg, Mannheim, Germany, [6] Mouse Imaging Centre, Hospital for Sick Children, Toronto, ON, Canada, [7] Medical Biophysics, Faculty of Medicine, University of Toronto, Toronto, ON, Canada, [8] Department of Surgery, University of Toronto, Toronto, ON, Canada, [9] Institute of Medical Science, University of Toronto, Toronto, ON, Canada, [10] Division of Brain, Imaging and Behaviour - Systems Neuroscience, Krembil Research Institute, Toronto Western Hospital, University Health Network, Toronto, ON, Canada

***Correspondence:**
Limor Avivi-Arber
limor.avivi.arber@utoronto.ca

Tooth loss is associated with altered sensory, motor, cognitive and emotional functions. These changes vary highly in the population and are accompanied by structural and functional changes in brain regions mediating these functions. It is unclear to what extent this variability in behavior and function is caused by genetic and/or environmental determinants and which brain regions undergo structural plasticity that mediates these changes. Thus, the overall goal of our research program is to identify genetic variants that control structural and functional plasticity following tooth loss. As a step toward this goal, here our aim was to determine whether structural magnetic resonance imaging (sMRI) is sensitive to detect quantifiable volumetric differences in the brains of mice of different genetic background receiving tooth extraction or sham operation. We used 67 adult female mice of 7 strains, comprising the A/J (A) and C57BL/6J (B) strains and a randomly selected sample of 5 of the 23 AXB-BXA strains (AXB1, AXB4, AXB24, BXA14, BXA24) that were produced from the A and B parental mice by recombinations and inbreeding. This panel of 25 inbred strains of genetically diverse inbred strains of mice is used for mapping chromosomal intervals throughout the genome that harbor candidate genes controlling the phenotypic variance of any trait under study. Under general anesthesia, 39 mice received extraction of 3 right maxillary molar teeth and 28 mice received sham operation. On post-extraction day 21, *post-mortem* whole-brain high-resolution sMRI was used to quantify the volume of 160 brain regions. Compared to sham operation, tooth extraction was associated with a significantly reduced regional and voxel-wise volumes of cortical brain regions involved in processing somatosensory, motor, cognitive and emotional functions, and increased volumes in subcortical sensorimotor and temporal limbic forebrain regions including the amygdala. Additionally, comparison of the 10 BXA14 and 21 BXA24 mice revealed significant volumetric differences between the two strains in several brain regions. These findings highlight the utility of high-resolution sMRI for studying tooth loss-induced structural brain plasticity in mice, and provide a foundation for further phenotyping structural brain changes following tooth loss in the full AXB-BXA panel to facilitate mapping genes that control brain plasticity following orofacial injury.

Keywords: tooth loss, trigeminal nerve, sMRI, brain imaging (MRI), plasticity, neuroplasticity, genetic variation, animal model

INTRODUCTION

Loss of teeth remains a significant health problem worldwide. For example, 20% of senior adults in Western countries are considered "orally disabled," and tooth loss is associated with a compromised quality of life, manifesting as difficulties in chewing and speaking, pain or alterations in other oral sensations such as stereognosis and proprioception, as well as impaired memory, cognitive and emotional functions (for reviews see Feine and Carlsson, 2003; Crocombe et al., 2009; Avivi-Arber et al., 2011; Trulsson et al., 2012; Sessle et al., 2013; Klineberg et al., 2014; Cerutti-Kopplin et al., 2016). Since life expectancy is progressively increasing in most populations, tooth loss and the associated impairments represent an increasing societal burden (Avivi-Arber et al., 2011; Trulsson et al., 2012). However, these effects of tooth loss vary substantially across individuals (Haraldson et al., 1988; Zarb et al., 2013; Carr and Brown, 2015), both in terms of the type and severity of the outcomes, and also in the rate and quality of recovery. This suggests that while these traits are impacted by variable environmental factors, they may also be under genetic influences which are still unknown (Mishra et al., 2007; Seltzer and Mogil, 2008; Katz and Seltzer, 2009; Missitzi et al., 2013). Finding ways to prevent or treat tooth loss-induced impairments depends on knowledge of the involved genetic, cellular, molecular, structural, and functional brain mechanisms, which is currently largely lacking.

Structural magnetic resonance imaging (sMRI) as well as functional MRI (fMRI) have been used to study how the brain responds to changes in orofacial functions. For example, human studies have revealed that altered dentitional states including tooth loss and their restoration are accompanied by widespread structural and functional brain changes in regions involved in processing and controlling sensory, motor, cognitive and emotional functions (Yan et al., 2008; Ono et al., 2010; Luraschi et al., 2013; Ohkubo et al., 2013; Shoi et al., 2014). In addition, such changes also occur following training and learning of oral motor skills, as well as in chronic orofacial pain conditions (Momose et al., 1997; Onozuka et al., 2002; Jiang et al., 2010, 2015; Arima et al., 2011; Gerstner et al., 2011; Gustin et al., 2011; Moayedi et al., 2011; Weissman-Fogel et al., 2011; Desouza et al., 2013). However, the cellular, molecular, and genetic mechanisms underlying these structural and functional changes are unclear but can be elucidated by utilizing brain imaging techniques in animals along with other invasive techniques such as electrophysiology and immunohistochemistry.

We and others have already shown that tooth extraction in rodents can also induce functional and structural changes in both glial and neuronal cells within brain regions involved in processing orofacial sensory and motor functions as well as cognitive and emotional behaviors (Avivi-Arber et al., 2014, 2015; Varathan et al., 2014; Chen et al., 2015; Watase et al., 2016). High resolution sMRI in rodents can provide an excellent readout of anatomical brain changes in mice following nerve injury, housing in an enriched environment, or maze training and such changes are also associated with cellular and molecular changes (Seminowicz et al., 2009; Lerch et al., 2011b; Cahill et al., 2015; Scholz et al., 2015a). However, it is still unclear whether sMRI can be utilized in mice to reveal volumetric regional brain changes following tooth extraction, whether it can detect volumetric regional brain differences in mice of different genetic background, and whether it can be utilized as a phenotyping method to identify genetic sources for inter-individual differences in brain plasticity following tooth loss.

As a first step, here our aim was to determine whether sMRI is sensitive to detect quantifiable volumetric differences in the brain of mice of different genetic background that received tooth extraction or sham operation. We randomly selected 7 strains, comprising A/J ('A') and C57BL/6J ('B') and 5 of the 23 AXB-BXA strains that were produced from the A and B parental mice by recombinations and inbreeding (Marshall et al., 1992; Lu et al., 1994; Sampson et al., 1998; Seltzer et al., 2001; Bennett et al., 2003). This panel of 25 genetically unique inbred strains has already been genetically mapped and has been widely used for mapping chromosomal intervals throughout the genome that harbor candidate genes controlling various phenotypes including spontaneous and stimulus-evoked neuropathic pain following orofacial and lumbar nerve injuries (Seltzer et al., 2001; Zhang S. H. et al., 2006; Nissenbaum et al., 2010; Mashregi et al., 2011; Soleimannejad et al., 2012).

METHODS

All experimental procedures were approved by the University of Toronto Animal Care Committee, in accordance with the Canadian Council on Animal Care Guidelines and the regulations of The Ontario Animals for Research Act (R.S.O. 1990). All experimental procedures (i.e., tooth extraction and sham operation, perfusions and preparation for the sMRI) were completed by the same investigator (LAA), adhering to the same standard protocols to ensure consistency. The sMRI data were analyzed in a blinded manner by one investigator (MF). Although, single housing might induce stress that could affect treatment outcome, control mice that received the sham treatment as well as mice receiving tooth extraction were single-housed to minimize social effects that might mask treatment effects (Devor et al., 2007; Seminowicz et al., 2009). Mice were housed in the same temperature and humidity-controlled environmental conditions, maintained at a 12-h light/dark cycle (lights switched on at 07:00 and off at 19:00 h). Starting at 2 weeks prior to the intraoral manipulation, all mice received a diet of mashed chow and water *ad libitum* to avoid discomfort from biting on a hard chow and to ensure adequate food and drink intake.

Study Groups

We utilized young adult (11–18 weeks) female mice of the following 5 recombinant inbred AXB-BXA strains: AXB1-PgnJ (termed 'AXB1'; 5 extraction, 3 sham), AXB24-PgnJ (termed 'AXB1'; 5 extraction, 3 sham), AXB4-PgnJ (termed 'AXB4'; 3 extraction, 3 sham), BXA24-PgnJ (termed 'BXA24'; 12 extraction, 9 sham;), and BXA14-PgnJ (termed 'BXA14'; 7 extraction, 3 sham). These strains were randomly selected from the 23 AXB-BXA strain panel. In addition, we used 5 A (3 extraction, 2 sham) and 9 B mice (5 extraction, 4 sham). Breeding nuclei of all strains were originally purchased from Jax Labs (Bar Arbor, MI) and multiplied on demand in our animal facility. We used in this study female mice because the incidence of postoperative orofacial neuropathies is higher in women than in men (Macfarlane, 2014). A recent meta-analysis study suggests that utilization of female mice in studies such as the present does not require monitoring of the estrous cycle (Prendergast et al., 2014).

Mice were randomly allocated into Sham and Extraction groups and experiments were performed in a random sequence to reduce potential testing bias. For each strain, mice of the same age were assigned to undergo extraction or sham operation. Under general anesthesia, we extracted 3 right maxillary molar teeth in mice of the Extraction group ($n = 39$) (see procedure below), and mice in the Sham group ($n = 28$) received the same operation but without actual tooth extraction. Mice were monitored daily to assess food consumption, general behavior, and any postoperative complications such as bleeding or inflammation. Body weight was checked regularly to ensure a continuous gain of body weight. Mice demonstrated a slower rate of weight gain per day during the first 3–5 postoperative days but then resumed normal gain of body weight (0.5–1 g/d).

Consistent with our previously documented electrophysiological and immunohistochemical findings in rats and mice, demonstrating that changes in pain behavior and neuronal responses in the orofacial primary sensorimotor cortex are apparent on days 7–28 following orofacial injury (Zhang S. H. et al., 2006; Avivi-Arber et al., 2010a, 2015; Mashregi et al., 2011; Soleimannejad et al., 2012; Varathan et al., 2014; Hayashi et al., 2015), mice in the present study were killed humanely 21 days postoperatively. All mice were fixation-perfused transcardially and the brains were imaged as described below. Sixteen mice had to be excluded for technical reasons. The numbers of mice per strain listed above are the net included in the analysis.

Molar Tooth Extraction and Sham Operation

Extraction and sham operations were carried out under general anesthesia (Isoflurane), using standard aseptic surgical conditions. Pulse oximeter monitoring verified that the heart rate and oxygen saturation levels were within the physiological range (i.e., 333–430 beats/min, 90–100% O_2). A feedback-controlled heating pad maintained the mouse core temperature at 37–37.5°C. The mouth was kept open by pulling down the 2 mandibular incisors with a rubber band. In the Extraction group the 3 right maxillary molar teeth were luxated (Avivi-Arber et al., 2010b, 2015). Sham mice had the same general anesthesia and mouth opening but no actual tooth extraction. These procedures took up to 30 min. No analgesics or anti-inflammatory medications were administered postoperatively because of their possible confounding effect on the sMRI data.

Structural Magnetic Resonance Imaging

sMRI scanning and data analysis followed previously published standard protocols (Lerch et al., 2011a,b; Cahill et al., 2012) and are described below only briefly.

Sample Preparation

Under general anesthesia (Ketamine HCl, 150 mg/kg and Xylazine, 10 mg/kg; i.p.) mice were perfused on postoperative day 21 with 30 ml mixture of 0.1 M phosphate-buffered saline (PBS), 10 U/mL Heparin and 2 mM ProHance® (an sMRI contrast enhancing agent), followed by perfusion of 30 ml 4% paraformaldehyde (PFA) in PBS and 2 mM ProHance®. The maxilla and skull containing the brain were post-fixed in 4% PFA and 2 mM ProHance® at 4°C for 12 h, then transferred to 4% PBS, 0.02% sodium azide and 2 mM ProHance® and stored at 4°C until scanned.

sMRI Acquisition

A multi-channel 7.0 Tesla, 40 cm diameter bore magnet MRI scanner (Varian Inc. Palo Alto, CA) was used to acquire images of mouse brains. Brains were intact in their skulls and placed in Fluorinert, and 16 samples were scanned at one time in a 16-coil solenoid array. Parameters used were: a T2-weighted 3D fast spin-echo sequence, with TR = 2000 ms, echo train length = 6, TEeff = 42 ms, field-of-view = 25 × 28 × 14 mm, matrix size = 450 × 504 × 250, and voxel size = 56 × 56 × 56 μm (Lerch et al., 2011b; Cahill et al., 2012).

sMRI Analysis

In order to visualize and compare changes across mice, an automated image registration-based approach was used to align all brains and create a consensus average (i.e., "atlas"). Image registration involved linear alignment of all images through a series of rotations, translations, scales, and shears. This was followed by locally deforming each scan through an iterative non-linear alignment procedure, bringing all scans into exact correspondence in an unbiased fashion. This registration was assumed to bring all homologous anatomical points into alignment. Next, the total brain volume was calculated for every mouse.

Our analytic approach to assess the volume of discrete brain regions between tooth extraction and sham operation was the following: First, we calculated the group mean volume of known neuroanatomical brain regions. For this purpose, a segmented atlas dividing the brain into 160 separate regions was aligned onto the study-population-specific atlas (Dorr et al., 2008; Ullmann et al., 2013; Steadman et al., 2014). Then, a deformation field was calculated for each mouse that determined how much the individual mouse's anatomy had to be transformed to fit the final atlas space, also facilitating the assessment of the degree to which this deformation field differed across mice in the study (Nieman et al., 2006; Lerch et al., 2011b). The determinant of each deformation field, known as Jacobian Coefficient (JC), was calculated for each voxel in the brain of every mouse. This coefficient is a measure of the deformation of each voxel with respect to the atlas image. It can be thought of as the amount by which the volume of that voxel had to be multiplied to reach the consensus average. Thus, a $JC = 1$ indicates no change, while $JC > 1$ signifies expansion and <1 denotes shrinkage of that voxel volume with respect to the volume of the same voxel in the atlas image. The resulting atlas was then used in conjunction with the JCs (multiplied by an appropriate scaling factor) to calculate volumes for each region in the brain and for the brains of all mice in the study. The regional volumetric values of the right and left sides of the brains were averaged. Since we used a genetically heterogeneous population of mice from 7 strains that significantly differed in their mean total brain volumes (A: 391 ± 2; B: 472 ± 3; AXB1: 417 ± 8; AXB24: 398 ± 5; AXB4: 384 ± 8; BXA14: 397 ± 8; BXA24: 461 ± 4 mm^3; $p < 0.0005$), the JC values used in this analysis were normalized for every mouse with respect to its overall brain volume. This approach allowed for examination of normalized regional brain volumes and comparison of anatomical differences across mice receiving tooth extraction or sham operation.

To test whether sMRI can detect significant differences between mice of different genetic background we utilized two strains, the BXA14 ($N = 7$ Extraction, 3 Sham) and BXA24 ($N = 12$ Extraction, 9 Sham) strains since they had the largest numbers of mice per group, they significantly differed in their total brain volume ($P < 0.0001$), and previous studies have shown they have contrasting tactile hypersensitivity following orofacial and lumbar nerve injuries (Seltzer et al., 2001; Zhang S. H. et al., 2006; Nissenbaum et al., 2010; Mashregi et al., 2011; Soleimannejad et al., 2012).

Statistical Analysis

Significance of the treatment effect in the regional brain volume analysis was carried out by analysis of variance (ANOVA). Resulting probabilities were adjusted for multiple comparisons with the False Discovery Rate (FDR) set at 1%. For the voxel-wise analysis, we performed a two-sample *t*-test to compare significant voxel-wise differences between tooth extraction and sham operation. The *p*-values were adjusted by FDR at 1, 5, and 10%. Thereafter, these voxels were annotated by their neuroanatomical region (Genovese et al., 2002). The t-statistic values of the voxel-wise analysis were then used for graphically displaying brain statistical maps of treatment effects in all mice (i.e., regardless of their genetic differences) and separately again when treatment effect was compared between mice of the BXA14 and BXA24 strains.

RESULTS

Anatomical Differences between Mice Receiving Tooth Extraction vs. Sham Operation

Regional Volumetric Analysis

Normalized volumetric sMRI data analysis of 160 brain regions revealed 34 brain regions that showed significant bilateral volumetric differences (FDR correction at 5 and 10%; none at 1%) between mice receiving tooth extraction and those receiving sham operation (**Table 1**). We found significantly decreased gray matter volumes in several forebrain regions, including the primary somatosensory (S1), primary motor (M1), and the cingulate cortices in mice receiving tooth extraction as compared with sham-operated mice. Decreased volume was also observed in components of the basal ganglia (striatum, globus pallidus, and nucleus accumbens). Also notably, several temporal limbic forebrain regions, including the amygdala, and subcortical sensory and motor nuclei showed significantly increased gray matter volumes following tooth extraction as compared with sham operation.

Voxel-Wise Analysis

Results of the voxel-wise comparison between mice receiving tooth extraction and those receiving sham operation are shown in **Figure 1**. Compared to sham operation, tooth extraction was associated with significantly decreased volume in many brain regions, including orofacial sensorimotor processing regions such as the S1, M1, and insular cortices, the basal ganglia (i.e., caudate, globus pallidus, and nucleus accumbens), paraventricular nucleus of the thalamus and trigeminal motor nucleus. Regions that showed significantly increased volume following tooth extraction included the entorhinal cortex, facial nerve and nucleus, cuneate nucleus, hypothalamus, inferior olivary complex, periaqueductal gray, pons, solitary tract nucleus, and trigeminal spinal tract nucleus. Notably, in no brain region were the observed effects of regional-based and voxel-wise analyses contradictory.

Anatomical Differences between Mice of Different Genetic Backgrounds

Voxel-Wise Analysis

When only mice of the BXA14 and BXA24 were included in the data analysis, we found that the normalized voxel-wise volumetric differences between mice receiving tooth extraction and those receiving sham operation (**Figure 2**) were similar but more significant than those obtained when all seven strains were included in the data analysis (**Figure 1**). In addition, voxel-wise comparison between the BXA14 mice and BXA24 mice (**Figure 3**) showed that irrespective of the dental manipulation, many normalized brain regions, including the periaqueductal gray and thalamus, were significantly larger ($FDR = 1\%$) in BXA24 mice than in BXA14 mice. Other brain regions such as

TABLE 1 | Regional volumes (mm^3) (Mean ± SEM) and % difference in the means of the normalized volumes between mice receiving tooth extraction and those receiving sham operation.

Brain region	Volume (mm^3) (Mean + SEM)		Effect of extraction vs. sham	% difference from sham (normalized)	*q*-values
	Extract	Sham			
FOREBRAIN CORTEX					
Lateral orbital cortex	2.86 ± 0.04	3.00 ± 0.05	Shrank	−2.86	0.083
Frontal association cortex	6.37 ± 0.11	6.71 ± 0.11	Shrank	−3.48	0.079
Primary motor cortex	6.50 ± 0.09	6.69 ± 0.09	Shrank	−2.12	0.076
Primary somatosensory cortex	4.58 ± 0.06	4.76 ± 0.06	Shrank	−2.22	0.057
Cingulate cortex (area 24a)	1.67 ± 0.02	1.74 ± 0.02	Shrank	−2.90	0.075
Cingulate cortex (area 25)	0.42 ± 0.01	0.45 ± 0.01	Shrank	−3.24	0.031
Cingulate cortex (area 32)	2.22 ± 0.04	2.34 ± 0.03	Shrank	−3.86	0.081
Medial entorhinal cortex	0.69 ± 0.01	0.68 ± 0.01	Expanded	2.91	0.037
Posteromedial cortical amygdalar area	1.18 ± 0.02	1.15 ± 0.02	Expanded	3.74	0.031
Amygdalopiriform transition area	23.00 ± 0.26	22.30 ± 0.27	Expanded	3.16	0.079
Posterolateral cortical amygdalar area	1.18 ± 0.02	1.15 ± 0.02	Expanded	2.24	0.086
Caudomedial entorhinal cortex	4.85 ± 0.09	4.77 ± 0.09	Expanded	3.20	0.030
Ventral intermediate entorhinal cortex	0.99 ± 0.02	0.98 ± 0.02	Expanded	3.03	0.065
CEREBELLUM					
Cerebellar lobule10 white matter	0.09 ± 0.00	0.08 ± 0.00	Expanded	7.08	0.031
Cerebellar lobule10 nodulus	1.50 ± 0.03	1.44 ± 0.03	Expanded	5.76	0.054
Cerebellar peduncle inferior	0.86 ± 0.01	0.84 ± 0.01	Expanded	3.75	0.054
Cerebellar peduncle (middle)	1.25 ± 0.02	1.23 ± 0.02	Expanded	3.22	0.085
FOREBRAIN SUBCORTEX					
Mammillary bodies	0.51 ± 0.01	0.49 ± 0.01	Expanded	5.82	0.031
Claustrum	0.30 ± 0.01	0.32 ± 0.01	Shrank	−5.32	0.020
Claustrum ventral part	0.51 ± 0.01	0.54 ± 0.01	Shrank	−2.48	0.044
Dorsal nucleus of the endopiriform	1.37 ± 0.02	1.43 ± 0.03	Shrank	−2.72	0.030
Striatum	19.94 ± 0.33	20.80 ± 0.43	Shrank	−2.35	0.076
Globus Pallidus	2.65 ± 0.05	2.75 ± 0.06	Shrank	−2.14	0.065
Nucleus accumbens	3.87 ± 0.06	4.03 ± 0.06	Shrank	−2.24	0.054
Fimbria	3.14 ± 0.06	3.28 ± 0.07	Shrank	−2.46	0.061
Bed nucleus of stria terminalis	1.12 ± 0.02	1.18 ± 0.03	Shrank	−3.18	0.036
TRACTS					
Mammilothalamic tract	0.24 ± 0.00	0.25 ± 0.00	Shrank	−2.18	0.077
Anterior commissure pars posterior	0.40 ± 0.01	0.42 ± 0.01	Shrank	−2.38	0.057
BRAINSTEM					
Periaqueductal gray	3.55 ± 0.07	3.67 ± 0.07	Shrank	−1.85	0.100
Pons	15.94 ± 0.28	15.87 ± 0.30	Expanded	2.08	0.061
Pontine nucleus	0.72 ± 0.01	0.69 ± 0.02	Expanded	5.65	0.061
Cuneate nucleus	0.25 ± 0.00	0.23 ± 0.00	Expanded	8.91	0.030
Superior olivary complex	0.79 ± 0.01	0.78 ± 0.01	Expanded	3.80	0.031
Medulla	26.25 ± 0.42	25.68 ± 0.42	Expanded	4.00	0.030

Negative values denote regions where volumes were smaller in mice receiving tooth extraction ("Shrank"). Positive values denote regions where volumes were larger in mice receiving tooth extraction ("Expanded"). q-values (<0.1) represent FDR-adjusted p-values.

the M1, S1, nucleus accumbens, arbor vita of the cerebellum, and corpus callosum, were significantly larger (FDR = 1%) in BXA14 than in BXA24 mice.

DISCUSSION

This is the first study to show that *post-mortem* sMRI is a sensitive method capable of detecting significant differences in the volume of brain regions between mice of different genetic background and between mice that had tooth extraction vs. sham operation. The study provides novel findings that tooth loss in a genetically heterogeneous population of mice leads to widespread bilateral gray matter changes. Specifically, we found that tooth extraction leads to: (1) reduced gray matter volume in several forebrain regions including the sensorimotor cortex, insula, cingulate cortex, and basal ganglia; (2) increased gray matter volume in several brainstem sensory and motor nuclei, and in the cerebellum; (3) increased gray matter

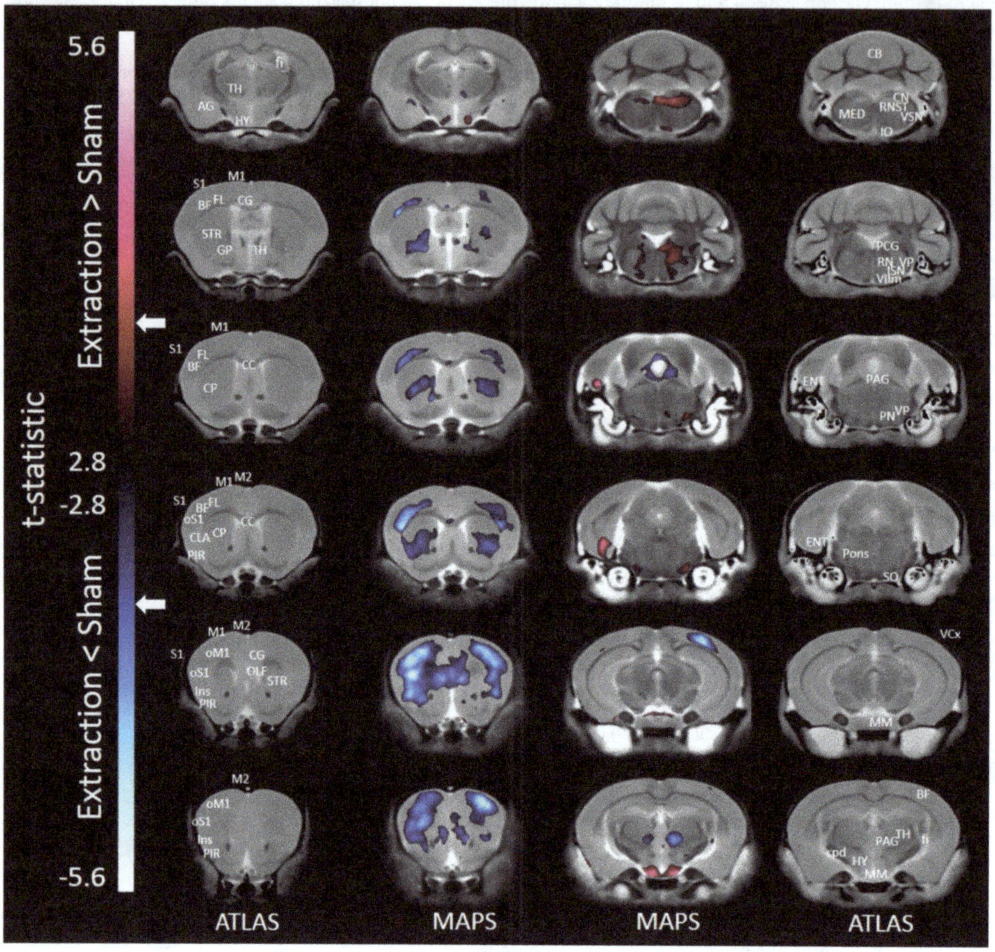

FIGURE 1 | Representative color-coded t-statistic maps (when all mouse strains were included) superimposed on high-resolution sMRI coronal slices of the mouse brain. Images of coronal slices in the 1st and 4th columns show anatomical annotations. The coronal slices in the 2nd and 3rd columns are presented in a rostrocaudal order from top-left to bottom-right. Maps show normalized voxel-wise volumetric differences between mice receiving tooth extraction and those receiving sham operation. Red indicate regions that have larger voxel volumes in mice receiving tooth extraction than in mice receiving sham operation, whereas those in blue indicate regions that have smaller voxel volumes in mice receiving tooth extraction. All t-statistics shown are significant at a 10% FDR. Peaks associated with t-statistic values < -3.53 or > 3.53 are significant at FDR = 5% ($t = 3.53$ and $t = -3.53$ are marked as white arrows on the color palettes). No voxel differences were significant at a 1% FDR. BF, barrel field; CC, corpus callosum; CB, cerebellum; CG, cingulate cortex; CLA, claustrum; CP, caudate putamen; cpd, cerebral peduncle; ENT, entorhinal cortex; fi, fimbria; FL, forelimb; GP, globus pallidus; HY, hypothalamus; Ins, insular cortex; IO, inferior olivary complex; ISN, inferior salivary nucleus; M1, primary motor cortex; M2, secondary motor cortex; MED, medulla; MM, mammillary nucleus; OLF, olfactory area; oM1, orofacial primary motor cortex; oS1, orofacial primary somatosensory cortex; PAG, periaqueductal gray; PCG, pontine central gray; PIR, piriform area; PN, pontine nuclei; RN, reticular nuclei; S1, primary somatosensory cortex; SO, superior olivary complex; ST, solitary tract nucleus; STR, striatum; TH, thalamus; VCx, visual cortex; VIIm, facial cranial nerve motor; VP, trigeminal principal nucleus; VSN, trigeminal spinal tract nucleus.

volume in several cognitive and limbic brain regions, including the anterior association cortex, nucleus accumbens, entorhinal cortex, mammillary bodies, and the amygdala. Together, these findings highlight the tremendous impact of tooth loss on brain structures across sensory, motor, and limbic systems.

Effects of Tooth Loss on Brain Anatomy

Tooth Loss Related Plasticity in Sensory and Motor Brain Regions

One of the main findings of this study was that tooth loss leads to gray matter decreases in the basal ganglia, and in the S1 and M1 cortices. The shrinkage of M1 and S1 is consistent with previous findings of decreased jaw and tongue motor representations and decreased excitability of orofacial M1 and S1 following molar tooth extraction in rodents (Avivi-Arber et al., 2015; Hayashi et al., 2015). Such changes may reflect the documented adaptive or maladaptative processes induced by the altered somatosensory inputs as a result of the missing teeth, injury to gingival, periodontal and pulpal nerves, and/or by compensatory sensorimotor functions caused by the loss of three major food-grinding dental elements (for review see Avivi-Arber et al., 2011; Sessle et al., 2013).

We also found that tooth extraction induced volumetric expansion in several brainstem regions involved in sensory and

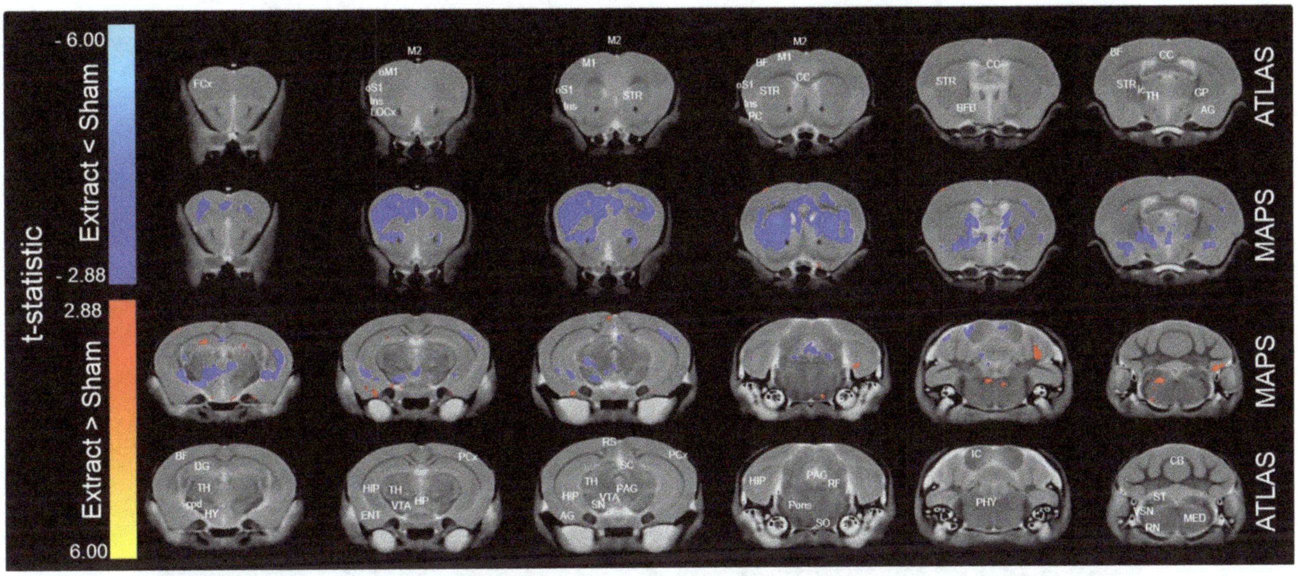

FIGURE 2 | Representative color-coded t-statistic maps (when only the BXA14 and BXA24 strains were included) superimposed on high-resolution sMRI coronal slices of the mouse brain. Images of coronal slices in the 1st and 4th rows show anatomical annotations. The coronal slices in the 2nd and 3rd rows are presented in a rostrocaudal order from top-left to bottom-right. Maps show normalized voxel-wise volumetric differences between mice receiving tooth extraction and those receiving sham operation. Red indicate regions that have larger voxel volumes in mice receiving tooth extraction than in mice receiving sham operation, whereas blue indicate regions that have smaller voxel volumes in mice receiving tooth extraction. All t-statistics shown are significant at a 10% FDR. White contour lines delineate regions where the statistical maps are significant at 5% FDR. No voxel differences were significant at a 1% FDR. AG, amygdalar cortex; BF, barrel field; BFB, basal forebrain; CC, corpus callosum; CB, cerebellum; cpd, cerebral peduncle; DG, dentate gyrus; ENT, entorhinal cortex; FCx, frontal cortex; GP, globus pallidus; HIP, hippocampus; HP, hypothalamic nucleus; HY, hypothalamus; ic, internal capsule; IC, inferior colliculus; Ins, insular cortex; LOCx, lateral orbital cortex; M1, primary motor cortex; M2, secondary motor cortex; MED, medulla; oM1, orofacial primary motor cortex; oS1, orofacial primary somatosensory cortex; PAG, periaqueductal gray; PCx, Parietal cortex; PC, Piriform cortex; PHY, perihypoglossal nuclei; RF, reticular formation; RN, reticular nucleus; RS, retrosplenial; SC, superior colliculus motor related; SN, substantia nigra; SO, superior olivary complex; ST, solitary tract nucleus; STR, striatum; TH, thalamus; VSN, trigeminal spinal nucleus; VTA, ventral tegmental area.

motor functions. These include the trigeminal motor nucleus, facial nucleus and nerve, the trigeminal sensory and solitary tract nuclei, pons, superior and inferior olivary complexes, and the cuneate nucleus. These novel findings, of changes in brainstem sensory and motor nuclei that are related to orofacial sensory and motor functions, are consistent with electrophysiological studies in rats. In these studies we and others have shown that acute or chronic dental pulpitis or trigeminal nerve damage induced functional neuroplasticity reflecting an increased glutamate-mediated excitability ("*central sensitization*") of nociceptive neurons within the brainstem trigeminal subnucleus caudalis that process orofacial nociceptive afferent inputs (for review see Sessle, 2011), and increased neuronal activity in the trigeminal motor nucleus (Sunakawa et al., 1999; Mostafeezur et al., 2014). Central sensitization following dental manipulations has also been documented in the rodent somatosensory thalamus (Park et al., 2006; Zhang S. et al., 2006; Kaneko et al., 2011). Central sensitization contributes to increased pain sensitivity (allodynia and hyperalgesia) and extraterritorial spread or referral of pain hypersensitivity that characterize many acute and chronic pain conditions (for review, see Sessle, 2011).

In addition, we showed here that tooth extraction was also associated with reduced gray matter volume in the frontal association cortex, an area that is mainly responsible for complex processes involving inputs to the cerebral cortex and the generation of behaviors including motor planning, working memory, and problem solving (Purves et al., 2012).

Compared to sham-operated mice, mice that underwent tooth extraction also had less gray matter volume in the basal ganglia, including the striatum, globus pallidus, and nucleus accumbens—regions related to motor processing and motivation. Specifically, nucleus accumbens is involved in reward processing and motor recovery after injury, and also shows abnormal response to noxious stimuli in subjects suffering from various chronic pain conditions (Pliakas et al., 2001; Perrotti et al., 2008; Baliki et al., 2010; Gustin et al., 2011; Desouza et al., 2013; Ikeda et al., 2015; Sawada et al., 2015; Elman and Borsook, 2016).

We are unaware of comparable MRI studies in humans following tooth loss, however, decreased gray matter volume in the premotor cortex has been associated with decreased masticatory performance (Lin et al., 2016). Functional brain imaging studies have revealed that dental stimulation, chewing, and tooth clenching are associated with activation of several nodes of the sensorimotor network, including the S1, M1, premotor and supplementary motor cortices, insula, cerebellum, striatum, and thalamus (Momose et al., 1997; Onozuka et al., 2002; Ettlin et al., 2004; Miyamoto et al., 2006; Luraschi et al.,

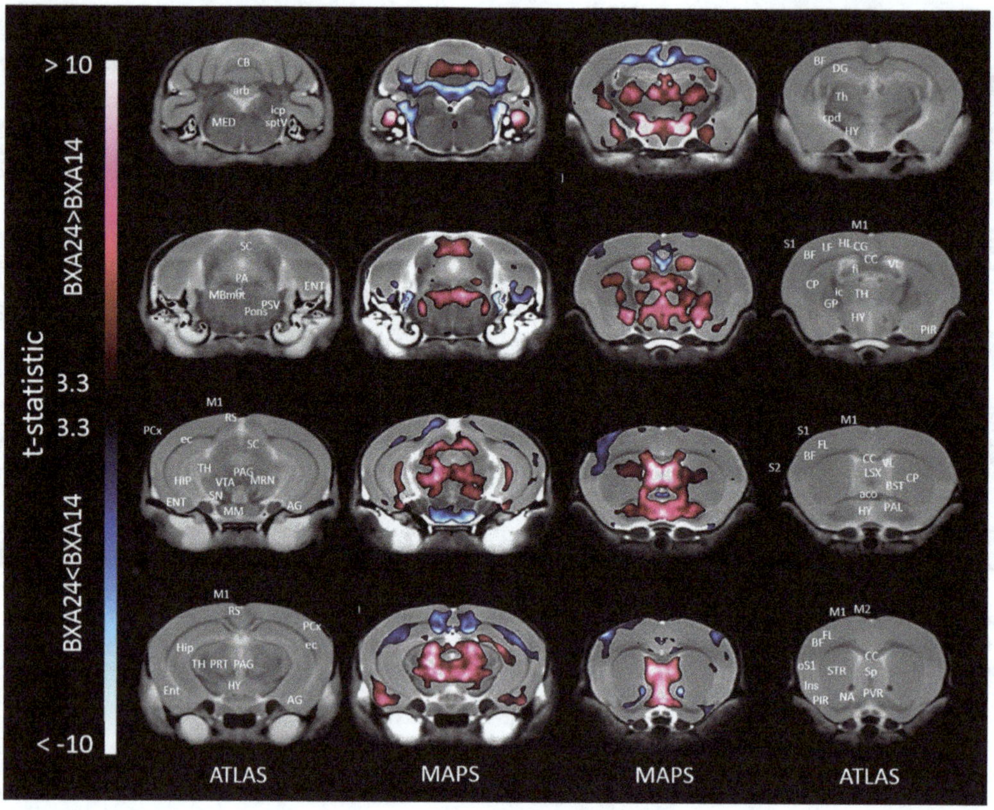

FIGURE 3 | Representative color-coded t-statistic maps superimposed on high-resolution sMRI coronal slices of the mouse brain. Images of coronal slices in the 1st and 4th columns show anatomical annotations. The coronal slices in the 2nd and 3rd columns are presented in a rostrocaudal order from bottom-right to top-left. Maps show normalized voxel-wise volumetric differences between BXA14 and BXA24 mice. Red indicate regions that have larger voxel volumes in BXA24 mice than in BXA14 mice, whereas those in blue indicate regions that have larger voxel volumes in BXA14 mice. All t-statistic values shown are significant at 1% FDR. Abbreviations: aco, anterior commissure; AG, amygdalar cortex; arb, arbor vitae; BF, barrel field; BST, bed nucleus of stria terminalis; CB, cerebellum; CC, corpus callosum; CG, cingulate cortex; CP, caudate putamen; cpd, cerebral peduncle; DG, dentate gyrus; ec, external capsule; ENT, entorhinal cortex; fi, fimbria; FL, forelimb; HIP, hippocampus; HL, hindlimb; HY, hypothalamus; ic, internal capsule; icp, inferior cerebellar peduncle; Ins, insular cortex; LSX, lateral septal complex; M1, primary motor cortex; M2, secondary motor cortex; MBmot, midbrain, motor related; MED, medulla; MM, mammillary nucleus; MRN, midbrain reticular nucleus; NA, nucleus accumbens; oS1, orofacial primary somatosensory cortex; PAG, periaqueductal gray; PAL, pallidum; PCx, posterior parietal association area; PIR, piriform area; PRT, pretectal region; PSV, principal sensory nucleus of the trigeminal; PVR, periventricular area; RS, retrosplenial; S1, primary somatosensory cortex; S2, secondary somatosensory cortex; SC, superior colliculus; SN, substantia nigra; Sp, septal nuclei; sptV, spinal tract of the trigeminal nerve; STR, striatum; TH, thalamus; VL, lateral ventricle; VTA, ventral tegmental area.

2013; Shoi et al., 2014; Jiang et al., 2015). Moreover, several of these studies have shown that the level of brain activity is related to the degree of biting force or dentitional state (i.e., whether it was fully dentate, partially- or completely edentate, or restored with dental implants). In addition, although tooth extraction is usually associated with a transient postoperative pain lasting up to 7 days, 0–3% of the patients undergoing tooth extraction develop chronic pain (Marbach and Raphael, 2000), and several fMRI studies have documented functional and structural changes in the brain of humans suffering from various chronic orofacial pain conditions. These studies identified structural abnormalities in brain regions such as the S1, M1, insular, and cingulate cortices (e.g., Nash et al., 2010; Gerstner et al., 2011; Gustin et al., 2011; Moayedi et al., 2011; Weissman-Fogel et al., 2011; Desouza et al., 2013; Youssef et al., 2014). Thus, the pattern of structural changes observed in the present study in mice, and those of other oral manipulations in humans, support the view that sMRI in mice can adequately detect quantitative brain volumetric changes following tooth loss, and that this method can serve as a research platform to better understand these changes so that treatments can be developed to maximize adaptation and minimize possible concomitant maladaptation following tooth loss.

Tooth Loss-Related Changes in Cognitive and Emotional Functions

Emerging evidence from human and animal studies have reported that tooth loss may be a contributing factor to cognitive and memory decline (for review see Klineberg et al., 2014; Palla, 2015; Cerutti-Kopplin et al., 2016). It is commonly known that tooth loss can induce intense emotional distress (Okoro et al., 2012; Wiener et al., 2015). In the present study, tooth loss was associated with volume loss in the frontal association cortex and nucleus accumbens. The frontal association cortex is involved in motor planning, working memory, and problem solving; whereas the nucleus accumbens has been implicated in the formation of emotional memories (e.g., pain, stress; Pliakas et al., 2001; Perrotti et al., 2008; Elman and Borsook, 2016). Volume loss in the frontal association cortex and nucleus accumbens in humans has been correlated with cognitive decline (de Jong et al., 2012). Moreover, the present study revealed that the mammillary bodies, which play a crucial role in memory consolidation (Vann and Aggleton, 2004), underwent significant expansion following tooth extraction. Tooth extraction was also associated with expansion of the amygdala and entorhinal cortex. These brain regions are part of the limbic system and were found to be enlarged in humans and animals subjected to fearful conditions (De Bellis et al., 2000; Lupien et al., 2009; van der Plas et al., 2010; Scholz et al., 2015b). Thus, the increased volume of these regions in the present study may be related to excessive fear or anxiety in response to the tooth loss.

Effects of Genetic Differences on Brain Anatomy

We report here significant volumetric differences between the BXA14 and BXA24 strains for which we had sufficient numbers of mice per group to determine a statistically significant genetic effect. The total brain volume of the BXA14 mice was strikingly smaller than that of BXA24. This is consistent with a previous histological report of significant differences in total brain size across all 25 strains of the AXB-BXA strain panel (including BXA14 and BXA24) (Cutler Strom, 2002). Since in the present study regional volumes were normalized by total brain volume, the differences between BXA14 vs. BXA24 reflect true strain-dependent volumetric plasticity following tooth extraction.

Using histological preparations to measure the size of the cerebral ventricles it was reported that there are significant differences across strains of the AXB-BXA panel (Zygourakis and Rosen, 2003). But the present study is the first to use sMRI to compare 160 different regions of known structural and functional importance in the whole brain of two of the strains of this panel. We have shown that the two strains significantly differ in the normalized voxel-wise volumes of many gray and white matter regions. For example, the M1 and S1 cortices, nucleus accumbens, arbor vita of the cerebellum and corpus callosum were significantly larger in BXA14 than in BXA24 mice whereas the periaqueductal gray and thalamus showed the opposite effect. Since the non-genetic, environmental parameters of this study were identical for all mice, the strain-dependent differences in brain regional volume indicate a difference in the genetic control of this trait. As these mice were derived from the A and B strains by recombinations, these parental strains must also differ in the genetic control of regional brain volumes. This feature can be used to study the genetic underpinning controlling this trait by capitalizing on the availability of the genetic map of all 25 strains of this panel (Sampson et al., 1998). Knowing the regional volumes of all 25 strains for intact mice and those receiving the sham-operation or tooth extraction will enable mapping the chromosomal regions that harbor the genes controlling the brain regional volumes of naïve female mice and those controlling the volumetric changes caused by tooth extraction (http://www.genenetwork.org/home.html). The present findings are the first step in this direction by demonstrating that sMRI is sensitive enough to quantify differences in regional brain volumes of strains in the AXB-BXA panel.

Possible Mechanisms Underlying Tooth Loss-Induced Volumetric Brain Changes

The mechanisms involved in changes in regional brain volume following intraoral injuries such as tooth extraction are not well known. Such volumetric alterations may reflect structural changes in glia, neurons, and blood vessels that result from changes in their number, function and/or volume (Zatorre et al., 2012), as well as volumetric changes caused by changes in the extracellular space. While there are many neurophysiological consequences of tooth loss, none of these can explain how they cause or relate to the different volumetric changes that we report here. The most obvious neurophysiological consequences of tooth loss are alterations in somatosensory (including nociceptive and proprioceptive) inputs from the lost teeth, injured gums and periodontal ligaments that are relayed via injured primary afferents, ascending tracts, and relay nuclei to multiple brain regions (Sessle, 2009; Avivi-Arber et al., 2011; Sessle et al., 2013). Somatosensory inputs from the tongue, jaw muscles, and temporomandibular joints may also be altered since tooth loss is associated with changes in masticatory patterns (Miehe et al., 1999; Klineberg and Jagger, 2004). Changes in the trigeminal brainstem sensory nuclei, thalamus, S1, M1 as well as in other higher order brain regions were documented by us previously (for review see Avivi-Arber et al., 2011; Sessle et al., 2013). For example, we have shown in rodents and humans that changes in somatosensory inputs or altered motor functions induced by intraoral manipulations, including tooth extraction, can result in short-term (days) and long-term (months) functional neuroplasticity in the orofacial S1 and M1 (Adachi et al., 2007; Avivi-Arber et al., 2010a, 2015; Awamleh et al., 2015; Pun et al., 2016). Tooth loss results in decreased motor representation of jaw and tongue muscles and decreased orofacial M1 excitability (Avivi-Arber et al., 2015). Moreover, acute dental stimulation, pulpectomy, or trigeminal nerve injury produces increased excitability of neurons within the ascending trigeminal somatosensory pathways including the trigeminal brainstem sensory nuclei, and decreased excitability in the orofacial sensorimotor cortex (e.g., Hu et al., 1986; Kwan et al., 1993; Adachi et al., 2007; Okada-Ogawa et al., 2009; Tsuboi et al., 2011; Chiang et al., 2012; Cao et al., 2013; Awamleh et al., 2015; Pun et al., 2016). We have also shown that these functional neuroplastic changes are dependent on the functional integrity of glial cells (Okada-Ogawa et al., 2009; Chiang et al., 2011, 2012; Tsuboi et al., 2011; Awamleh et al., 2015; Pun et al., 2016), and are associated with changes in the number and cytoarchitectural features of neurons and glia within the trigeminal brainstem sensory nuclei as well as the orofacial S1 and M1 (Okada-Ogawa et al., 2009; Tsuboi et al., 2011; Varathan et al., 2014; Avivi-Arber et al., 2015; Watase et al., 2016). However, as discussed above, none of these functional changes has ever been shown to causally drive the structural changes or *vice versa*. More research is needed to unravel the mechanisms underlying the sMRI plasticity observed in the current study and to link them to the documented neuronal and glial changes following intra-oral injuries.

CONCLUSIONS AND IMPLICATIONS FOR FUTURE STUDIES

The current study has demonstrated, for the first time, that high-resolution sMRI can be used for quantifying small volumetric brain differences between mice of different genetic background and between mice receiving tooth extraction vs. sham operation. The novel findings show that tooth loss is associated with widespread sMRI-defined structural changes in somatosensory, motor, cognitive, and limbic regions of the brain. The robust findings reported here were obtained from a genetically diverse population of mice of 7 different strains, thereby modeling the effect of tooth loss in heterogeneous cohorts of humans. The findings also show significant sMRI-defined structural differences between two strains (BXA14 and BXA24) of the AXB-BXA panel. Future studies using sMRI are warranted to phenotype brain structural plasticity in all 23 recombinant inbred strains of the AXB-BXA panel and their A and B parental strains, to map the murine genome for chromosomal regions harboring candidate genes controlling the volumetric brain changes induced by tooth loss, implementing the already documented high-resolution genetic map of this panel (Seltzer et al., 2001; Zhang S. H. et al., 2006; Zhang et al., 2014; Nissenbaum et al., 2010; Mashregi et al., 2011; Meloto et al., 2011; Soleimannejad et al., 2012; Seltzer, 2014). Additionally, the volumetric brain changes can be correlated with behavioral changes caused by tooth loss (e.g., altered cognitive behavior, orofacial mechanical sensitivity, patterns of mastication) as well as changes in gene expression and cellular, molecular, micro-functional, and micro-structural changes. Such studies can provide a powerful multidisciplinary approach to elucidate mechanisms underlying sMRI-defined macrostructural brain changes produced by tooth loss and other orofacial manipulations of clinical relevance in humans (Clarke et al., 2015). The findings of these studies have the potential to identify new targets for the prevention and treatment of maladaptive behaviors after tooth loss and other orofacial manipulations.

AUTHOR CONTRIBUTIONS

Conceived the study: LA, ZS, BS, JL, MM, and KD. Designed the experiments: LA, ZS, BS, MF, and JL. Performed the experiments: LA, MF, and JL. Analyzed the data: LA, ZS, BS, MF, and JL. Wrote the paper: LA, ZS, BS, MF, JL, MM, and KD.

ACKNOWLEDGMENTS

This research was supported by the Canadian Institutes of Health Research (to BS), NIH RO1 DE-018575 (to ZS), Canada Research Chair Program (tier I, to BS and ZS), and the Faculty of Dentistry Dental Research Institute Fund (to LA, BS, and ZS).

REFERENCES

Adachi, K., Lee, J.-C., Hu, J. W., Yao, D., and Sessle, B. J. (2007). Motor cortex neuroplasticity associated with lingual nerve injury in rats. *Somatosens. Mot. Res.* 24, 97–109. doi: 10.1080/08990220701470451

Arima, T., Yanagi, Y., Niddam, D. M., Ohata, N., Arendt-Nielsen, L., Minagi, S., et al. (2011). Corticomotor plasticity induced by tongue-task training in humans: a longitudinal fMRI study. *Exp. Brain Res.* 212, 199–212. doi: 10.1007/s00221-011-2719-7

Avivi-Arber, L., Friedel, M., Lerch, J., Hayashi, Y., Landzberg, G., Moayedi, M., et al. (2014). "Loss of teeth in genetically-mapped recombinant inbred mouse strains as a model to study the genetic control of orofacial sensorimotor functions and the associated functional and sMRI-defined plasticity of the orofacial sensorimotor cortex post-injury," in *Social Neuroscience Abstracts Annual Meeting* (Washington, DC).

Avivi-Arber, L., Lee, J. C., and Sessle, B. J. (2010a). Cortical orofacial motor representation: effect of diet consistency. *J. Dent. Res.* 89, 1142–1147. doi: 10.1177/0022034510373767

Avivi-Arber, L., Lee, J. C., and Sessle, B. J. (2010b). Effects of incisor extraction on jaw and tongue motor representations within face sensorimotor cortex of adult rats. *J. Comp. Neurol.* 518, 1030–1045. doi: 10.1002/cne.22261

Avivi-Arber, L., Lee, J. C., Sood, M., Lakschevitz, F., Fung, M., Barashi-Gozal, M., et al. (2015). Long-term neuroplasticity of the face primary motor cortex and adjacent somatosensory cortex induced by tooth loss can be reversed following dental implant replacement in rats. *J. Comp. Neurol.* 523, 2372–2389. doi: 10.1002/cne.23793

Avivi-Arber, L., Martin, R., Lee, J.-C., and Sessle, B. J. (2011). Face sensorimotor cortex and its neuroplasticity related to orofacial sensorimotor functions. *Arch. Oral Biol.* 56, 1440–1465. doi: 10.1016/j.archoralbio.2011.04.005

Awamleh, L., Pun, H., Lee, J. C., and Avivi-Arber, L. (2015). Decreased face primary motor cortex (face-m1) excitability induced by noxious stimulation of the rat molar tooth pulp is dependent on the functional integrity of face-m1 astrocytes. *Exp. Brain Res.* 233, 1261–1272. doi: 10.1007/s00221-015-4198-8

Baliki, M. N., Geha, P. Y., Fields, H. L., and Apkarian, A. V. (2010). Predicting value of pain and analgesia: nucleus accumbens response to noxious stimuli changes in the presence of chronic pain. *Neuron* 66, 149–160. doi: 10.1016/j.neuron.2010.03.002

Bennett, G. J., Chung, J. M., Honore, M., and Seltzer, Z. (2003). Models of neuropathic pain in the rat. *Curr. Protoc. Neurosci. Chapter* 9: Unit 9. 14. doi: 10.1002/0471142301.ns0914s22

Cahill, L. S., Laliberté, C. L., Ellegood, J., Spring, S., Gleave, J. A., Eede, M. C. et al. (2012). Preparation of fixed mouse brains for MRI. *Neuroimage* 60, 933–939. doi: 10.1016/j.neuroimage.2012.01.100

Cahill, L. S., Steadman, P. E., Jones, C. E., Laliberté, C. L., Dazai, J., Lerch, J. P., et al. (2015). MRI-detectable changes in mouse brain structure induced by voluntary exercise. *Neuroimage* 113, 175–183. doi: 10.1016/j.neuroimage.2015.03.036

Cao, Y., Wang, H., Chiang, C.-Y., Dostrovsky, J. O., and Sessle, B. J. (2013). Pregabalin suppresses nociceptive behavior and central sensitization in a rat trigeminal neuropathic pain model. *J. Pain* 14, 193–204. doi: 10.1016/j.jpain.2012.11.005

Carr, A. B., and Brown, D. T. (2015). *Mccracken's Removable Partial Prosthodontics*. St. Louis, MO: Elsevier - Health Sciences Division.

Cerutti-Kopplin, D., Feine, J., Padilha, D. M., De Souza, R. F., Ahmadi, M., Rompré, P., et al. (2016). Tooth loss increases the risk of diminished cognitive function: a systematic review and meta-analysis. *JDR Clin. Transl. Res.* 1, 10–19. doi: 10.1177/2380084416633102

Chen, H., Iinuma, M., Onozuka, M., and Kubo, K. Y. (2015). Chewing maintains hippocampus-dependent cognitive function. *Int. J. Med. Sci.* 12, 502–509. doi: 10.7150/ijms.11911

Chiang, C. Y., Dostrovsky, J. O., Iwata, K., and Sessle, B. J. (2011). Role of glia in orofacial pain. *Neuroscientist* 17, 303–320. doi: 10.1177/1073858410386801

Chiang, C. Y., Sessle, B. J., and Dostrovsky, J. O. (2012). Role of astrocytes in pain. *Neurochem. Res.* 37, 2419–2431. doi: 10.1007/s11064-012-0801-6

Clarke, H., Katz, J., Flor, H., Rietschel, M., Diehl, S. R., and Seltzer, Z. (2015). Genetics of chronic pain: a crucial step toward personal pain medicine. *Can. J. Anaesth.* 62, 294–303. doi: 10.1007/s12630-014-0287-6

Crocombe, L. A., Mejia, G. C., Koster, C. R., and Slade, G. D. (2009). Comparison of adult oral health in australia, the usa, germany and the uk. *Aust. Dent. J.* 54, 147–153. doi: 10.1111/j.1834-7819.2009.01108.x

Cutler Strom, R. (2002). *Genetic and Environmental Control of Brain Weight Variation.* Available online at: http://www.nervenet.org/papers/Strom99/Chapter2.html

De Bellis, M. D., Casey, B. J., Dahl, R. E., Birmaher, B., Williamson, D. E., Thomas, K. M., et al. (2000). A pilot study of amygdala volumes in pediatric generalized anxiety disorder. *Biol. Psychiatry* 48, 51–57. doi: 10.1016/S0006-3223(00)00835-0

de Jong, L. W., Wang, Y., White, L. R., Yu, B., van Buchem, M. A., and Launer, L. J. (2012). Ventral striatal volume is associated with cognitive decline in older people: a population based MR-study. *Neurobiol. Aging* 33, 424.e1-10 doi: 10.1016/j.neurobiolaging.2010.09.027

Desouza, D. D., Moayedi, M., Chen, D. Q., Davis, K. D., and Hodaie, M. (2013). Sensorimotor and pain modulation brain abnormalities in trigeminal neuralgia: a paroxysmal, sensory-triggered neuropathic pain. *PLoS ONE* 8:e66340. doi: 10.1371/journal.pone.0066340

Devor, M., Gilad, A., Arbilly, M., Nissenbaum, J., Yakir, B., Raber, P., et al. (2007). Sex-specific variability and a 'cage effect' independently mask a neuropathic pain quantitative trait locus detected in a whole genome scan. *Eur. J. Neurosci.* 26, 681–688. doi: 10.1111/j.1460-9568.2007.05704.x

Dorr, A. E., Lerch, J. P., Spring, S., Kabani, N., and Henkelman, R. M. (2008). High resolution three-dimensional brain atlas using an average magnetic resonance image of 40 adult c57bL/6J mice. *Neuroimage* 42, 60–69. doi: 10.1016/j.neuroimage.2008.03.037

Elman, I., and Borsook, D. (2016). Common brain mechanisms of chronic pain and addiction. *Neuron* 89, 11–36. doi: 10.1016/j.neuron.2015.11.027

Ettlin, D. A., Zhang, H., Lutz, K., Järmann, T., Meier, D., Gallo, L. M., et al. (2004). Cortical activation resulting from painless vibrotactile dental stimulation measured by functional magnetic resonance imaging (fMRI). *J. Dent. Res.* 83, 757–761. doi: 10.1177/154405910408301004

Feine, J. S., and Carlsson, G. E. (2003). *Implant Overdentures: The Standard of Care for Edentulous Patients.* Chicago, IL: Quintessence Publishing Company.

Genovese, C. R., Lazar, N. A., and Nichols, T. (2002). Thresholding of statistical maps in functional neuroimaging using the false discovery rate. *Neuroimage* 15, 870–878. doi: 10.1006/nimg.2001.1037

Gerstner, G., Ichesco, E., Quintero, A., and Schmidt-Wilcke, T. (2011). Changes in regional gray and white matter volume in patients with myofascial-type temporomandibular disorders: a voxel-based morphometry study. *J. Orofac. Pain* 25, 99–106.

Gustin, S. M., Peck, C. C., Wilcox, S. L., Nash, P. G., Murray, G. M., and Henderson, L. A. (2011). Different pain, different brain: thalamic anatomy in neuropathic and non-neuropathic chronic pain syndromes. *J. Neurosci.* 31, 5956–5964. doi: 10.1523/JNEUROSCI.5980-10.2011

Haraldson, T., Jemt, T., Stålblad, P. A., and Lekholm, U. (1988). Oral function in subjects with overdentures supported by osseointegrated implants. *Scan J. Dent. Res.* 96, 235–242. doi: 10.1111/j.1600-0722.1988.tb01550.x

Hayashi, Y., Lee, J.-C., Chocron, D., Cherkas, P., Sessle, B. J., and Avivi-Arber, L. (2015). "Neuroplasticity of face sensorimotor cortex induced by tooth extraction in c57bl/6 Mice," in *Social Neuroscience Abstracts Annual Meeting* (Chicago, IL).

Hu, J. W., Dostrovsky, J. O., Lenz, Y. E., Ball, G. J., and Sessle, B. J. (1986). Tooth pulp deafferentation is associated with functional alterations in the properties of neurons in the trigeminal spinal tract nucleus. *J. Neurophysiol.* 56, 1650–1668.

Ikeda, H., Adachi, K., Fujita, S., Tomiyama, K., Saigusa, T., Kobayashi, M., et al. (2015). Investigating complex basal ganglia circuitry in the regulation of motor behaviour, with particular focus on orofacial movement. *Behav. Pharmacol.* 26, 18–32. doi: 10.1097/FBP.0000000000000118

Jiang, H., Liu, H., Liu, G., Jin, Z., and Liu, X. (2010). The effects of chewing-side preference on human brain activity during tooth clenching: an fMRI study. *J. Oral Rehabil.* 37, 877–883. doi: 10.1111/j.1365-2842.2010.02115.x

Jiang, H., Liu, H., Liu, G., Jin, Z., Wang, L., Ma, J., et al. (2015). Analysis of brain activity involved in chewing-side preference during chewing: an fMRI study. *J. Oral Rehabil.* 42, 27–33. doi: 10.1111/joor.12224

Kaneko, M., Kaneko, T., Kaneko, R., Chokechanachaisakul, U., Kawamura, J., Sunakawa, M., et al. (2011). The role of N-methyl-D-aspartate receptor subunits in the rat thalamic mediodorsal nucleus during central sensitization. *Brain Res.* 1371, 16–22. doi: 10.1016/j.brainres.2010.11.054

Katz, J., and Seltzer, Z. (2009). Transition from acute to chronic postsurgical pain: risk factors and protective factors. *Expert Rev. Neurother.* 9, 723–744. doi: 10.1586/ern.09.20

Klineberg, I., and Jagger, R. (2004). *Occlusion and Clinical Practice - an Evidence Based Approach.* London: Elsevier.

Klineberg, I., Palla, S., and Trulsson, M. (2014). Contemporary relevance of occlusion and mastication. *Int. J. Prosthodont.* 27, 411–412. doi: 10.11607/ijp.2014.5.e

Kwan, C. L., Hu, J. W., and Sessle, B. J. (1993). Effects of tooth-pulp deafferentation on brain-stem neurons of the rat trigeminal subnucleus oralis. *Somatosens. Mot. Res.* 10, 115–131. doi: 10.3109/08990229309028828

Lerch, J. P., Sled, J. G., and Henkelman, R. M. (2011a). "MRI phenotyping of genetically altered mice," in *Magnetic Resonance Neuroimaging: Methods and Protocols*, eds M. Modo, and J. W. M. Bulte (New York, NY: Humana Press), 349–361.

Lerch, J. P., Yiu, A. P., Martinez-Canabal, A., Pekar, T., Bohbot, V. D., Frankland, P. W., et al. (2011b). Maze training in mice induces MRI-detectable brain shape changes specific to the type of learning. *Neuroimage* 54, 2086–2095. doi: 10.1016/j.neuroimage.2010.09.086

Lin, C.-S., Wu, S.-Y., Wu, C.-Y., and Ko, H.-W. (2016). Gray matter volume and resting-state functional connectivity of the motor cortex-cerebellum network reflect the individual variation in masticatory performance in healthy elderly people. *Front. Aging Neurosci.* 7:247. doi: 10.3389/fnagi.2015.00247

Lu, X., Skamene, E., and Richardson, P. M. (1994). Studies of axonal regeneration in c57bl/6j and a/j mice. *Brain Res.* 652, 174–176. doi: 10.1016/0006-8993(94)90335-2

Lupien, S. J., McEwen, B. S., Gunnar, M. R., and Heim, C. (2009). Effects of stress throughout the lifespan on the brain, behaviour and cognition. *Nat. Rev. Neurosci.* 10, 434–445. doi: 10.1038/nrn2639

Luraschi, J., Korgaonkar, M. S., Whittle, T., Schimmel, M., Müller, F., and Klineberg, I. (2013). Neuroplasticity in the adaptation to prosthodontic treatment. *J. Orofac. Pain* 27, 206–216. doi: 10.11607/jop.1097

MacFarlane, T. V. (2014). "Epidemiology of orofacial pain," in *Orofacial Pain: Recent Advances in Assessment, Management, and Understanding of Mechanisms*, ed B. J. Sessle (Washington, DC: IASP Press), 33–51.

Marbach, J. J., and Raphael, K. G. (2000). Phantom tooth pain: a new look at an old dilemma. *Pain Med.* 1, 68–77. doi: 10.1046/j.1526-4637.2000.00012.x

Marshall, J. D., Mu, J. L., Cheah, Y. C., Nesbitt, M. N., Frankel, W. N., and Paigen, B. (1992). The AXB and BXA set of recombinant inbred mouse strains. *Mamm. Genome* 3, 669–680. doi: 10.1007/BF00444361

Mashregi, M., Soleimannejad, E., Froimovitch, D., Biton, D., and Seltzer, Z. (2011). *Phenomics and QTL Mapping of Sensitivity to Noxious Heat in Naïve a/j, c57bl/6j and their 23 AXB-BXA Descendant Recombinant Mice Lines.* Montreal, QC: International Association for the Study of Pain.

Meloto, C. B., Serrano, P. O., Ribeiro-DaSilva, M. C., and Rizzatti-Barbosa, C. M. (2011). Genomics and the new perspectives for temporomandibular disorders. *Arch. Oral Biol.* 56, 1181–1191. doi: 10.1016/j.archoralbio.2011.03.012

Miehe, B., Fanghänel, J., Kubein-Meesenburg, D., Nägerl, H., and Schwestka-Polly, R. (1999). Masticatory musculature under altered occlusal relationships – a model study with experimental animals. *Ann. Anat.* 181, 37–40. doi: 10.1016/S0940-9602(99)80084-3

Mishra, B. K., Wu, T., Belfer, I., Hodgkinson, C. A., Cohen, L. G., Kiselycznyk, C., et al. (2007). Do motor control genes contribute to interindividual variability in decreased movement in patients with pain? *Mol. Pain* 3:20. doi: 10.1186/1744-8069-3-20

Missitzi, J., Gentner, R., Misitzi, A., Geladas, N., Politis, P., Klissouras, V., et al. (2013). Heritability of motor control and motor learning. *Physiol. Rep.* 1:e00188. doi: 10.1002/phy2.188

Miyamoto, J. J., Honda, M., Saito, D. N., Okada, T., Ono, T., Ohyama, K., et al. (2006). The representation of the human oral area in the somatosensory cortex: a functional MRI study. *Cereb. Cortex* 16, 669–675. doi: 10.1093/cercor/bhj012

Moayedi, M., Weissman-Fogel, I., Crawley, A. P., Goldberg, M. B., Freeman, B. V., Tenenbaum, H. C., et al. (2011). Contribution of chronic pain and neuroticism to abnormal forebrain gray matter in patients with temporomandibular disorder. *Neuroimage* 55, 277–286. doi: 10.1016/j.neuroimage.2010.12.013

Momose, T., Nishikawa, J., Watanabe, T., Sasaki, Y., Senda, M., Kubota, K., et al. (1997). Effect of mastication on regional cerebral blood flow in humans examined by positron-emission tomography with o-15-labelled water and magnetic resonance imaging. *Arch. Oral Biol.* 42, 57–61. doi: 10.1016/S0003-9969(96)00081-7

Mostafeezur, R. M., Shinoda, M., Unno, S., Zakir, H. M., Takatsuji, H., Takahashi, K., et al. (2014). Involvement of astroglial glutamate-glutamine shuttle in modulation of the jaw-opening reflex following infraorbital nerve injury. *Eur. J. Neurosci.* 39, 2050–2059. doi: 10.1111/ejn.12562

Nash, P. G., Macefield, V. G., Klineberg, I. J., Gustin, S. M., Murray, G. M., and Henderson, L. A. (2010). Changes in human primary motor cortex activity during acute cutaneous and muscle orofacial pain. *J. Orofac. Pain* 24, 379–390.

Nieman, B. J., Flenniken, A. M., Adamson, S. L., Henkelman, R. M., and Sled, J. G. (2006). Anatomical phenotyping in the brain and skull of a mutant mouse by magnetic resonance imaging and computed tomography. *Physiol. Genomics* 24, 154–162. doi: 10.1152/physiolgenomics.00217.2005

Nissenbaum, J., Devor, M., Seltzer, Z., Gebauer, M., Michaelis, M., Tal, M., et al. (2010). Susceptibility to chronic pain following nerve injury is genetically affected by CACNG2. *Genome Res.* 20, 1180–1190. doi: 10.1101/gr.104976.110

Ohkubo, C., Morokuma, M., Yoneyama, Y., Matsuda, R., and Lee, J. S. (2013). Interactions between occlusion and human brain function activities. *J. Oral Rehabil.* 40, 119–129. doi: 10.1111/j.1365-2842.2012.02316.x

Okada-Ogawa, A., Suzuki, I., Sessle, B. J., Chiang, C. Y., Salter, M. W., Dostrovsky, J. O., et al. (2009). Astroglia in medullary dorsal horn (trigeminal spinal subnucleus caudalis) are involved in trigeminal neuropathic pain mechanisms. *J. Neurosci.* 29, 11161–11171. doi: 10.1523/JNEUROSCI.3365-09.2009

Okoro, C. A., Strine, T. W., Eke, P. I., Dhingra, S. S., and Balluz, L. S. (2012). The association between depression and anxiety and use of oral health services and tooth loss. *Community Dent. Oral Epidemiol.* 40, 134–144. doi: 10.1111/j.1600-0528.2011.00637.x

Ono, Y., Yamamoto, T., Kubo, K. Y., and Onozuka, M. (2010). Occlusion and brain function: mastication as a prevention of cognitive dysfunction. *J. Oral Rehabil.* 37, 624–640. doi: 10.1111/j.1365-2842.2010.02079.x

Onozuka, M., Fujita, M., Watanabe, K., Hirano, Y., Niwa, M., Nishiyama, K., et al. (2002). Mapping brain region activity during chewing: a functional magnetic resonance imaging study. *J. Dent. Res.* 81, 743–746. doi: 10.1177/154405910208101104

Palla, S. (2015). Neurocognition and neuroplasticity: what does it all mean for clinical practice? *J. Oral Facial Pain Headache* 29, 113–114. doi: 10.11607/ofph.2015.2.e

Park, S. J., Zhang, S., Chiang, C. Y., Hu, J. W., Dostrovsky, J. O., and Sessle, B. J. (2006). Central sensitization induced in thalamic nociceptive neurons by tooth pulp stimulation is dependent on the functional integrity of trigeminal brainstem subnucleus caudalis but not subnucleus oralis. *Brain Res.* 1112, 134–145. doi: 10.1016/j.brainres.2006.06.115

Perrotti, L. I., Weaver, R. R., Robison, B., Renthal, W., Maze, I., Yazdani, S., et al. (2008). Distinct patterns of deltafosb induction in brain by drugs of abuse. *Synapse* 62, 358–369. doi: 10.1002/syn.20500

Pliakas, A. M., Carlson, R. R., Neve, R. L., Konradi, C., Nestler, E. J., and Carlezon, W. A. Jr. (2001). Altered responsiveness to cocaine and increased immobility in the forced swim test associated with elevated camp response element-binding protein expression in nucleus accumbens. *J. Neurosci.* 21, 7397–7403.

Prendergast, B. J., Onishi, K. G., and Zucker, I. (2014). Female mice liberated for inclusion in neuroscience and biomedical research. *Neurosci. Biobehav. Rev.* 40, 1–5. doi: 10.1016/j.neubiorev.2014.01.001

Pun, H., Awamleh, L., Lee, J. C., and Avivi-Arber, L. (2016). Decreased face primary motor cortex (face-m1) excitability induced by noxious stimulation of the rat molar tooth pulp is dependent on the functional integrity of medullary astrocytes. *Exp. Brain Res.* 234, 645–657. doi: 10.1007/s00221-015-4448-9

Purves, D., Augustine, G. J., and Fitzpatrick, D. (2012). "Chapter 26, the association cortices," in *Neuroscience 2nd Edn.*, eds D. Purves, G. J. Augustine, D. Fitzpatrick, L. C. Katz, A.-S. LaMantia, J. O. McNamara, and S. M. Williams (Sunderland, MA: Sinauer Associates), 587–606.

Sampson, S. B., Higgins, D. C., Elliot, R. W., Taylor, B. A., Lueders, K. K., Koza, R. A., et al. (1998). An edited linkage map for the AXB and BXA recombinant inbred mouse strains. *Mamm. Genome* 9, 688–694. doi: 10.1007/s003359900849

Sawada, M., Kato, K., Kunieda, T., Mikuni, N., Miyamoto, S., Onoe, H., et al. (2015). Function of the nucleus accumbens in motor control during recovery after spinal cord injury. *Science* 350, 98–101. doi: 10.1126/science.aab3825

Scholz, J., Allemang-Grand, R., Dazai, J., and Lerch, J. P. (2015a). Environmental enrichment is associated with rapid volumetric brain changes in adult mice. *Neuroimage* 109, 190–198. doi: 10.1016/j.neuroimage.2015.01.027

Scholz, J., Niibori, Y., Frankland, P. W., and Lerch, J. P. (2015b). Rotarod training in mice is associated with changes in brain structure observable with multimodal MRI. *Neuroimage* 107, 182–189. doi: 10.1016/j.neuroimage.2014.12.003

Seltzer, Z. (2014). Nothing in pain makes sense except in the light of genetics. *Pain* 155, 841–842. doi: 10.1016/j.pain.2014.02.001

Seltzer, Z., and Mogil, J. S. (2008). "Pain and genetics," in *Orofacial Pain and Related Conditions, 2nd Edn.*, eds B. J. Sessle, G. Lavigne, J. P. Lund, and R. Dubner (Hanover Park, IL: Quintessence Publishing Company), 69–75.

Seltzer, Z., Wu, T., Max, M. B., and Diehl, S. R. (2001). Mapping a gene for neuropathic pain-related behavior following peripheral neurectomy in the mouse. *Pain* 93, 101–106. doi: 10.1016/S0304-3959(01)00295-0

Seminowicz, D. A., Laferriere, A. L., Millecamps, M., Yu, J. S., Coderre, T. J., and Bushnell, M. C. (2009). MRI structural brain changes associated with sensory and emotional function in a rat model of long-term neuropathic pain. *Neuroimage* 47, 1007–1014. doi: 10.1016/j.neuroimage.2009.05.068

Sessle, B., Avivi-Arber, L., and Murray, G. (2013). "Motor control of masticatory muscles," in *Craniofacial Muscles*, eds L. K. McLoon and F. Andrade (New York, NY: Springer), 111–30.

Sessle, B. J. (2009). "Sensation from the face," in *Encyclopedia of Neuroscience*, Vol. 8, ed L. Squire (Oxford: Academic Press), 585–592.

Sessle, B. J. (2011). Peripheral and central mechanisms of orofacial inflammatory pain. *Int. Rev. Neurobiol.* 97, 179–206. doi: 10.1016/B978-0-12-385198-7.00007-2

Shoi, K., Fueki, K., Usui, N., Taira, M., and Wakabayashi, N. (2014). Influence of posterior dental arch length on brain activity during chewing in patients with mandibular distal extension removable partial dentures. *J. Oral Rehabil.* 41, 486–495. doi: 10.1111/joor.12169

Soleimannejad, E., Froimovitch, D., and Seltzer, Z. (2012). *QTL Mapping of Mechanical Sensitivity in Naïve a/j, c57bl/6j and their 23 AXB-BXA Recombinant Mice Lines.* Montreal, QC: International Congress of Human Genetics.

Steadman, P. E., Ellegood, J., Szulc, K. U., Turnbull, D. H., Joyner, A. L., Henkelman, R. M., et al. (2014). Genetic effects on cerebellar structure across mouse models of autism using a magnetic resonance imaging atlas. *Autism Res.* 7, 124–137. doi: 10.1002/aur.1344

Sunakawa, M., Chiang, C. Y., Sessle, B. J., and Hu, J. W. (1999). Jaw electromyographic activity induced by the application of algesic chemicals to the rat tooth pulp. *Pain* 80, 493–501. doi: 10.1016/S0304-3959(98)00241-3

Trulsson, M., van der Bilt, A., Carlsson, G. E., Gotfredsen, K., Larsson, P., Müller, F., et al. (2012). From brain to bridge: masticatory function and dental implants. *J. Oral Rehabil.* 39, 858–877. doi: 10.1111/j.1365-2842.2012.02340.x

Tsuboi, Y., Iwata, K., Dostrovsky, J. O., Chiang, C. Y., Sessle, B. J., and Hu, J. W. (2011). Modulation of astroglial glutamine synthetase activity affects nociceptive behaviour and central sensitization of medullary dorsal horn nociceptive neurons in a rat model of chronic pulpitis. *Eur. J. Neurosci.* 34, 292–302. doi: 10.1111/j.1460-9568.2011.07747.x

Ullmann, J. F, Watson, C., Janke, A. L., Kurniawan, N. D., and Reutens, D. C. (2013). A segmentation protocol and MRI atlas of the c57bl/6j mouse neocortex. *Neuroimage* 78, 196–203. doi: 10.1016/j.neuroimage.2013.04.008

van der Plas, E. A., Boes, A. D., Wemmie, J. A., Tranel, D., and Nopoulos, P. (2010). Amygdala volume correlates positively with fearfulness in normal healthy girls. *Soc. Cogn. Affect. Neurosci.* 5, 424–431. doi: 10.1093/scan/nsq009

Vann, S. D., and Aggleton, J. P. (2004). The mammillary bodies: two memory systems in one? *Nat. Rev. Neurosci.* 5, 35–44. doi: 10.1038/nrn1299

Varathan, V., Sood, M., Pun, H., Awamleh, L., Chocron, D., Bhatt, P., et al. (2014). "Neuroplasticity of orofacial sensorimotor cortex induced by dental manipulations: are glial cells involved?" in *Soc Neurosci Abst Annual Meeting* (Washington, DC).

Watase, T., Tang, D., Sessle, J. B., and Avivi-Arber, L. (2016). "Astroglial morphological changes induced by tooth extraction in mice," in *Soc Neurosci Abst Annual Meeting* (San Diego, CA).

Weissman-Fogel, I., Moayedi, M., Tenenbaum, H. C., Goldberg, M. B., Freeman, B. V., and Davis, K. D. (2011). Abnormal cortical activity in patients with temporomandibular disorder evoked by cognitive and emotional tasks. *Pain* 152, 384–396. doi: 10.1016/j.pain.2010.10.046

Wiener, R. C., Wiener, M. A., and McNeil, D. W. (2015). Comorbid depression/anxiety and teeth removed: behavioral risk factor surveillance system 2010. *Community Dent. Oral Epidemiol.* 43, 433–443. doi: 10.1111/cdoe.12168

Yan, C., Ye, L., Zhen, J., Ke, L., and Gang, L. (2008). Neuroplasticity of edentulous patients with implant-supported full dentures. *Eur. J. Oral Sci.* 116, 387–393. doi: 10.1111/j.1600-0722.2008.00557.x

Youssef, A. M., Gustin, S. M., Nash, P. G., Reeves, J. M., Petersen, E. T., Peck, C. C., et al. (2014). Differential brain activity in subjects with painful trigeminal neuropathy and painful temporomandibular disorder. *Pain* 155, 467–475. doi: 10.1016/j.pain.2013.11.008

Zarb, A. G., Hobkirk, J., Eckert, S. E., and Jacob, R. F. (2013). *Prosthodontic Treatment for Edentulous Patients: Complete Dentures and Implant-Supported Prostheses*. St. Louis, MO: Mosby.

Zatorre, R. J., Fields, R. D., and Johansen-Berg, H. (2012). Plasticity in gray and white: neuroimaging changes in brain structure during learning. *Nat. Neurosci.* 15, 528–536. doi: 10.1038/nn.3045

Zhang, S., Chiang, C. Y., Xie, Y. F., Park, S. J., Lu, Y., Hu, J. W., et al. (2006). Central sensitization in thalamic nociceptive neurons induced by mustard oil application to rat molar tooth pulp. *Neuroscience* 142, 833–842. doi: 10.1016/j.neuroscience.2006.06.063

Zhang, S. H., Deniz, B., Lu, Y., Sessle, B. J., Hu, J., and Seltzer, Z. (2006). "Neuropathic pain spread to ipsilateral and contralateral body regions after unilateral infraorbital neurectomy in mice is determined genetically," in *Social Neuroscience Abstracts Annual Meeting* (Atlanta, GA).

Zhang, S., Mogil, J. S., and Seltzer, Z. (2014). "Genetic risk factors for orofacial pain: insights from animal models," in *Orofacial Pain: Recent Advances in Assessment, Management, and Understanding of Mechanisms,* ed B. J. Sessle (Washington, DC: IASP Press), 373–392.

Zygourakis, C. C., and Rosen, G. D. (2003). Quantitative trait loci modulate ventricular size in the mouse brain. *J. Comp. Neurol.* 461, 362–369. doi: 10.1002/cne.10697

10

New Insights in Trigeminal Anatomy: A Double Orofacial Tract for Nociceptive Input

Dylan J. H. A. Henssen[1,2]**, *Erkan Kurt*[2], *Tamas Kozicz*[1], *Robert van Dongen*[3], *Ronald H. M. A. Bartels*[2] *and Anne-Marie van Cappellen van Walsum*[1]

[1] *Department of Anatomy, Donders Institute for Brain Cognition and Behavior, Radboud University Medical Center, Nijmegen, Netherlands,* [2] *Department of Neurosurgery, Radboud University Medical Center, Nijmegen, Netherlands,* [3] *Department of Anaesthesiology, Pain and Palliative Care, Radboud University Medical Center, Nijmegen, Netherlands*

Correspondence:
Dylan J. H. A. Henssen
dylan.henssen@radboudumc.nl

Orofacial pain in patients relies on the anatomical pathways that conduct nociceptive information, originating from the periphery towards the trigeminal sensory nucleus complex (TSNC) and finally, to the thalami and the somatosensorical cortical regions. The anatomy and function of the so-called trigeminothalamic tracts have been investigated before. In these animal-based studies from the previous century, the intracerebral pathways were mapped using different retro- and anterograde tracing methods. We review the literature on the trigeminothalamic tracts focusing on these animal tracer studies. Subsequently, we related the observations of these studies to clinical findings using fMRI trials. The intracerebral trigeminal pathways can be subdivided into three pathways: a ventral (contralateral) and dorsal (mainly ipsilateral) trigeminothalamic tract and the intranuclear pathway. Based on the reviewed evidence we hypothesize the co-existence of an ipsilateral nociceptive conduction tract to the cerebral cortex and we translate evidence from animal-based research to the human anatomy. Our hypothesis differs from the classical idea that orofacial pain arises only from nociceptive information via the contralateral, ventral trigeminothalamic pathway. Better understanding of the histology, anatomy and connectivity of the trigeminal fibers could contribute to the discovery of a more effective pain treatment in patients suffering from various orofacial pain syndromes.

Keywords: trigeminal nerve, trigeminothalamic tract, orofacial pain, trigeminal neuropathy, bilateral registration

INTRODUCTION

Facial pain can be caused by many factors. One of the most severe and highly incapacitating conditions in which pharmacological treatments have an insufficient effect, are called trigeminal neuropathies, clinically often known as trigeminal neuralgia (Tsubokawa et al., 1991, 1993; Nguyen et al., 2000; Raslan et al., 2011; Slotty et al., 2015; Kolodziej et al., 2016).

Abbreviations: ACC, Anterior cingulate cortex; BOLD, Blood oxygen level dependent; CS, Caudal subnucleus; DTI, Diffusion tensor imaging; DW-MRI, Diffusion weighted magnetic resonance imaging; fMRI, Functional magnetic resonance imaging; IS, Interpolar subnucleus; MeN, Mesencephalic nucleus; MoN, Motor nucleus; OS, Oral subnucleus; PAG, Periaquaductal gray; PO, Posterior nucleus; PSN, Principal sensory nucleus; RF, Reticular formation; SN, Spinal nucleus; ST, Spinal tract; TSNC, Trigeminal sensory nucleus complex; VPL, Ventral posterolateral nucleus; VPM, Ventral posteromedial nucleus; V1, Ophthalmic nerve; V2, Maxillary nerve; V3, Mandibular nerve.

Although trigeminal neuropathies were first described more than 300 years ago, little is known about the relationship with the trigeminal nerve itself and the origin of the pain (Burchiel, 2003; Jantsch et al., 2005). In order to gain insight in the pathophysiology of trigeminal neuropathy, the anatomical connections between the trigeminal nerve and the involved brain regions seem of great importance. In summary, it is generally believed that sensory fibers involved in the conduction of pain and temperature spread over the trigeminal sensory nucleus complex (TSNC) and then cross over to the contralateral thalamus and cerebral cortex (Greenspan and Winfield, 1992; Bushnell et al., 1999; Kanda et al., 2000; Nieuwenhuys et al., 2008). In 2010, however, Nash et al. (2010) reported a bilateral fMRI registration in humans after noxious orofacial stimulation. Twenty-eight human subjects were injected with hypertonic saline (0.3 ml) into the central belly of the right masseter muscle and into the overlaying skin. Using blood oxygen level dependent (BOLD) contrast, a 3T Scanner imaged a bilateral fMRI-activation of the thalamus, S1 and S2 cortices after noxious orofacial stimulation. As an explanation, the authors hypothesized an extra tract, originating from the trigeminal nuclei running towards both thalami. However, no anatomical details about topography, explanation or evidence can be found in the anatomical literature for this hypothesized extra tract. The aims of this review are: (1) to provide a detailed overview of existing knowledge of the anatomy and function of the trigeminal nerve, its nuclei and its intracerebral pathways in animals; (2) to present studies that use functional imaging in the discussion of cortical representation of pain; and (3) to gain new insights in trigeminal anatomy in humans by synthesizing animal-based studies and papers that discuss functional imaging in humans.

ANATOMY OF THE TRIGEMINAL NERVE AND THE TSNC

The extracerebral portion of the three divisions of the trigeminal nerve (V1: ophthalmic division, V2: maxillary division, V3: mandibular division) has been described extensively before by many authors (Lang, 1981; Usunoff et al., 1997; Sessle, 2000; Go et al., 2001; Williams et al., 2003; Schünke et al., 2006; Nieuwenhuys et al., 2008; Borges and Casselman, 2010; Sabancl et al., 2011; Bathla and Hegde, 2013; Joo et al., 2014; Marur et al., 2014). The three main divisions fuse at the trigeminal ganglion, which divides into motor and sensor rootlets. These rootlets enter the lateral pons and fibers course towards the four trigeminal nuclei: the (1) Principal Sensory Nucleus (PSN); (2) Mesencephalic Nucleus (MeN); (3) Spinal Nucleus (SN); and (4) Motor Nucleus (MoN; **Figure 1**). The PSN and the SN together are also called the trigeminal sensory nuclear complex (TSNC) and are held responsible for the conduction of pain and temperature information (Matsushita et al., 1982).

The trigeminal nuclei have been well described by many authors (Ramon y Cajal, 1909; Meessen and Olszewski, 1949; Olszewski, 1950; Astrom, 1953; Taber, 1961; Eisenmann et al., 1963). A histological example of all the trigeminal nuclei, except the SN, is presented in **Figure 2**. This histological blockface was obtained from the unpublished materials from Mollink et al. (2015) and with consent of the authors adapted and published here. The literature concerning the TSNC, is summarized below. The PSN or pontine nucleus of the trigeminal nerve is located dorsolaterally to the motor nucleus of the trigeminal nerve in the pons. Its afferent fibers contribute to the perception of discriminative sensations. The termination

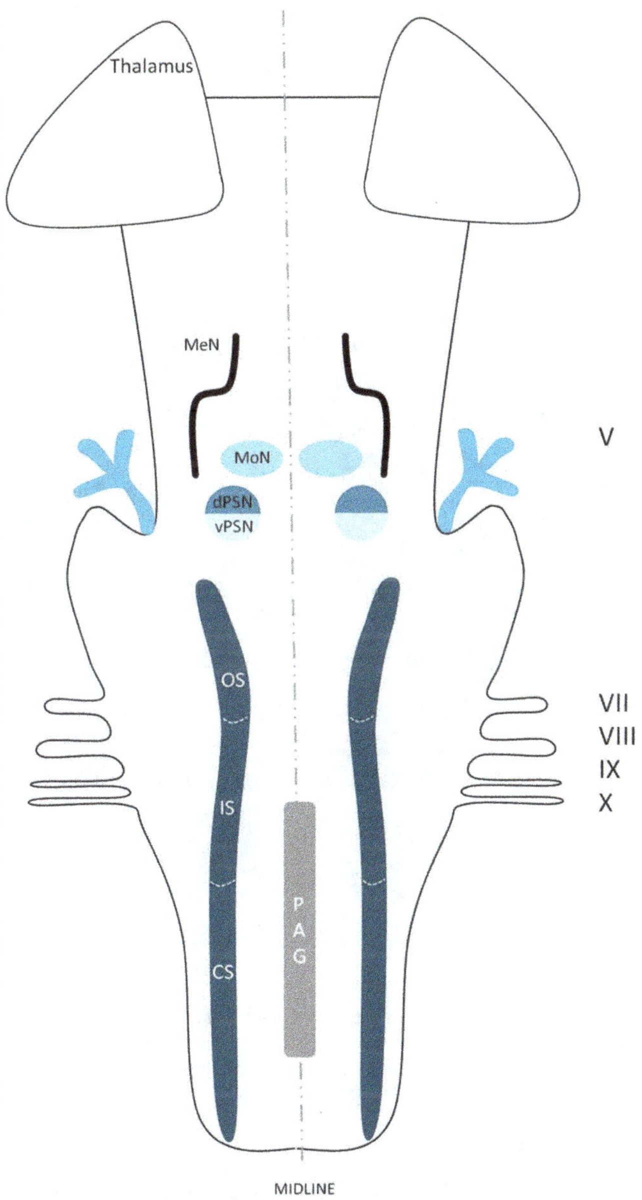

FIGURE 1 | Schematic overview of the trigeminal nuclei in the brainstem. MeN, Mesencephalic nucleus; MoN, Motor nucleus; dPSN, Dorsal part of the principal sensory nucleus; vPSN, Ventral part of the principal sensory nucleus; OS, Oral part of the spinal nucleus; IS, Interpolar part of the spinal nucleus; CS, Caudal part of the spinal nucleus; PAG, Periaquaductal gray; which receives afferents and courses more cranially as the intranuclear tract. V, Trigeminal nerve; VII, Facial nerve; VIII, Vestibulocochlear nerve; IX, Glossopharyngeal nerve; X, Vagus nerve.

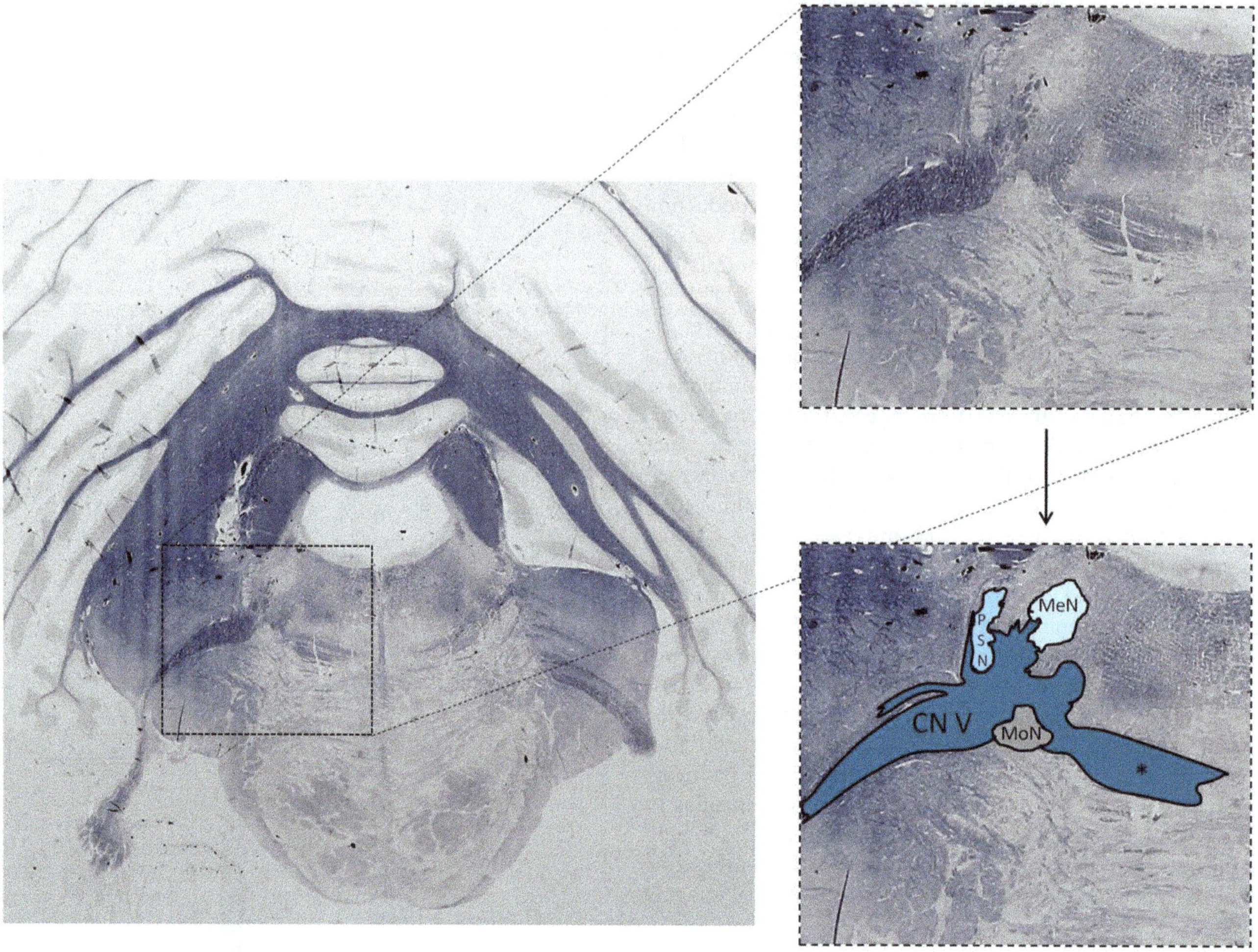

FIGURE 2 | Histological example of the anatomy of the trigeminal sensory nucleus complex (TSNC). Histological section stained for myelin with the modified Heidenhain-Woelcke stain at different levels of the cerebellum and the pons. The unstained areas are recognized as nuclei. CN V, Trigeminal nerve; MeN, Mesencephalic nucleus; PSN, Principal sensory nucleus of the trigeminal nerve; MoN, Motor nucleus of the trigeminal nerve. *Decussating fibers of the trigeminal nucleus. The spinal nucleus is not visible is this section. Unpublished data, published with consent of Mollink et al. (2015).

of these afferent fibers can be divided into a ventral and a dorsal projection site within the PSN. The PSN in the cat is a compact formation and consists of different shapes of neurons (round, stellar and triangular types; Gobel and Dubner, 1969). According to Kiknadze et al. (2001) however, the subdivision of the PSN into a ventral and dorsal part is arguable. Analysis of their data shows different-sized and different-shaped neurons throughout the entire nucleus, at equal frequencies. The SN is located medially to the descending spinal tract (ST) which is located in the dorsolateral region of the brainstem. The ST extends from the trigeminal entry zone (middle pons) to the third cervical spinal cord segment. The SN therefore is oriented in a longitudinal plane and can be subdivided into three subnuclei: the caudal (CS), interpolar (IS) and oral (OS) subnucleus. The CS extends from C3 to the obex and seems consistent with the dorsal horn of the cervical spinal cord. Due to this consistency, the subdivision into lamina according to Rexed (1952, 1954) can be used. Trigeminothalamic fibers are found in the layers I, V and VI of the CS and are thought to provide the anatomical and physiological substrate for pain and temperature perception in the facial region (Dubner et al., 1978). The IS on the other hand can be found in between the CS end of the obex and the CS part of the motor nucleus of the facial nerve. The medial and rostral borders have been described to be difficult to recognize under the light microscope (Capra and Dessem, 1992). The exact function remains unclear, but it is known that the IS enlarges when the vibrissae in rodents are well developed and therefore have a heavy central representation. The IS can be subdivided into different regions, receiving input from different terminal branches of the trigeminal nerve. The dorsolateral region receives input from the auriculotemporal nerve, whereas the ventrolateral region is the termination zone of the other ophthalmic and maxillary branches (Jacquin et al., 1983; Capra and Dessem, 1992). The OS or rostral subnucleus extends from the CS pole of the facial motor nucleus to the

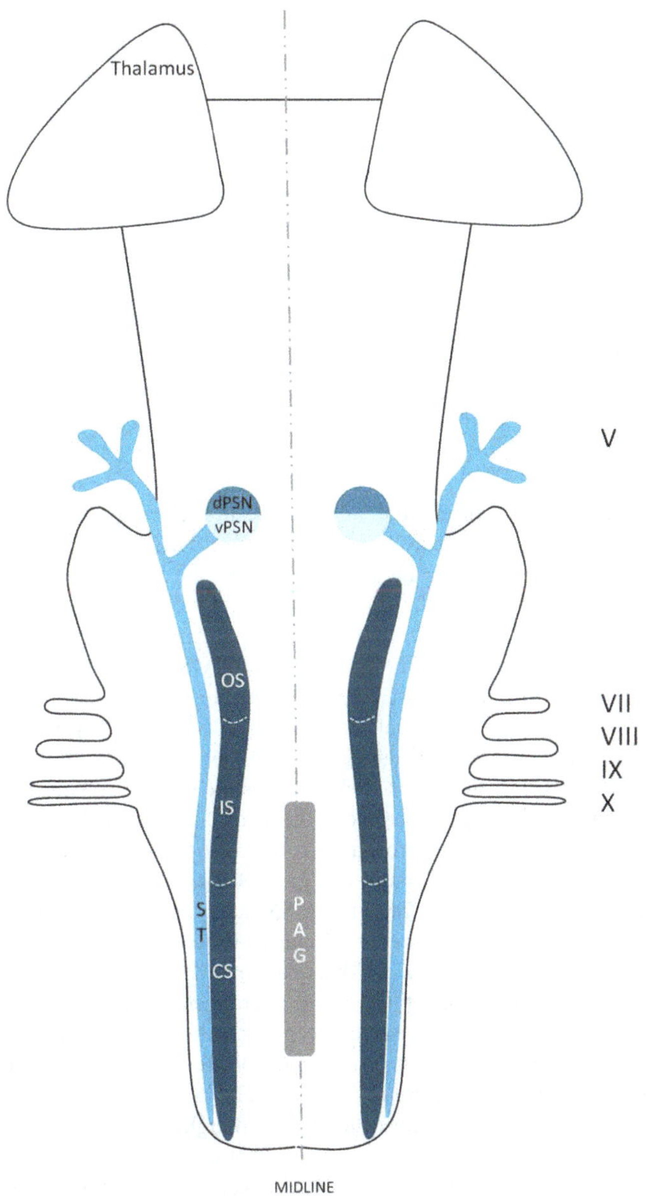

FIGURE 3 | Anatomy of the different trigeminal nuclei that are part of the TSNC. dPSN, Dorsal part of the principal sensory nucleus; vPSN, Ventral part of the principal sensory nucleus; OS, Oral part of the spinal nucleus; IS, Interpolar part of the spinal nucleus; CS, Caudal part of the spinal nucleus; ST, Spinal tract; PAG, Periaquaductal gray; which receives afferents and courses more cranially as the intranuclear tract. V, Trigeminal nerve; VII, Facial nerve; VIII, Vestibulocochlear nerve; IX, Glossopharyngeal nerve; X, Vagus nerve.

CS part of the motor nucleus of the trigeminal nerve (Crosby and Yoss, 1954). This subnucleus can be subdivided into a lateral and medial part. The medial subdivision receives afferents from intraoral structures, whereas the lateral part of the OS registers information from the dorsal structures of the face and the vibrissae (Eisenmann et al., 1963). **Figure 3** recapitulates the anatomy of the different trigeminal nuclei that are part of the TSNC.

INTRACEREBRAL ANATOMY OF FIBERS ORIGINATING FROM THE TSNC

Efferents from the PSN

Wallenberg (1905) dissected the brains of rabbits and observed uncrossed trigeminothalamic fibers, sprouting from the dorsal part of the PSN. After the example of Wallenberg (1905) others mentioned this ipsilateral circuit as well (Economo, 1911; Woodburne, 1936; Papez and Rundles, 1937; Walker, 1939; Papez, 1951; Carpenter, 1957) . Torvik (1957) studied the ascending pathways of the trigeminal nerve by means of a partial or complete transection of the rostral brains of 22 kittens and retrograde cellular alterations in the TSNC. It was concluded that from the PSN almost all fibers projected to one of both thalami and that these projections were both contralateral as ipsilateral. Smith (1975) carried out a partial unilateral stereotactic lesion of the PSN in cebus and rhesus monkeys and found a ventromedial decussation of fibers at the level of the pontine tegmentum and a dorsal collection of axons that form a smaller trigeminothalamic projection, originating from the dorsal one-third of the PSN. No neurons from the PSN appeared to project to the spinal cord (Matsushita et al., 1982). Matsushita et al. (1982) also used the retrograde horseradish peroxidase technique and injected it into the posterior ventral nucleus of the thalamus. A large number of neurons were observed in the ventral segment of the PSN and the IS of the SN on the contralateral side, whereas on the ipsilateral side, the dorsal aspect of the PSN was marked after injection. Rausell and Jones (1991) bilateral afferents to the VPM, originating from both the ipsilateral and the contralateral PSN using an anterograde tracing study in 3 cynomolgous monkeys (*Macaca fascicularis*). **Table 1** summarizes the mentioned tracing studies in animals. **Figure 4** depicts the trigeminothalamic tracts sprouting from the PSN.

Efferents from the SN

Ganchrow (1978) injected the CS of the SN with tritiated amino acids in the squirrel monkey and found that the efferents from the CS had a contralateral projection to the VPM. Also, bilateral connections were observed to the mediodorsal nucleus (MD), together with ipsilateral connections between the PSN and the CS of the SN. Burton et al. (1979) studied the projections from the CS of the spinal trigeminal complex with retrograde and anterograde axonal transport techniques in cats. Projections to the thalamus were both bilaterally to a dorsomedial region of the VPM as well as contralaterally to the main part of the VPM and PO (posterior nucleus) of the thalamus. Künzle (1998) a weak bilateral projection from the CS of the SN in the hedgehog tenrec (Echinops telfairi) after injection of trigeminal subdivisions with wheat germ agglutinin conjugated to horseradish peroxidase, biotinylated dextran amine and a solution of radioactive amino acids. There was little evidence for a trigeminal projection to the intralaminar nuclei but there was a distinct projection to the contralateral zona incerta of the thalamus. Furthermore, Ikeda et al. (1982) described intranuclear ascending fibers originating from the IS of the cat, after applying injections into the SN. The OS of the SN has been described

TABLE 1 | Tracing studies of the principal sensory nucleus (PSN).

Reference	Species	Tracing technique	Anatomical site of lesion/injection
Wallenberg (1905)	Rabbit	Marchi method after lesion	PSN
Economo (1911)	Macaque monkey	Degeneration	PSN
Woodburne (1936)	Series of vertebrates	Chroom silver preparation after sectioning	Section staining
Walker (1939)	Rhesus monkey	Marchi method	PSN
Papez (1951)	Series of quadrupeds	Weigert-Pal method	Section staining
Carpenter (1957)	Rhesus monkey	Marchi method after lesion	SCP/Mesencephalon
Torvik (1957)	Cat	Degeneration after lesion	PSN
Smith (1975)	Cebus monkey Rhesus monkey	Variety of Nauta silver impregnations	PSN
Matsushita et al. (1982)	Cat	Horseradish peroxidase	Posterior ventral nucleus of the thalamus
Rausell and Jones (1991)	Cynomolgus monkey	Horseradish peroxidase; Germ agglutin-conjugated horseradish peroxidase; Solution of 5% fast blue	Anterograde: CS Retrograde: S1-cortex, facial area

PSN, Principal sensory nucleus; SCP, Superior cerebellar peduncle.

to be consistent with the PSN. Efferents originating from the OS of the SN cross over to the contralateral VPM as a part of the trigeminal lemniscus (Nieuwenhuys et al., 2008). This would result in the trigeminothalamic tract sprouting from the SN as depicted in **Figure 5**. Furthermore, Panneton and Burton (1982) injected retrograde horseradish peroxidase into the rostral trigeminal region and showed that neurons in all laminae, however mainly III and IV of the medullary dorsal horn, project through an intranuclear pathway. Within layer III and IV orofacial fibers converge into their separate nuclei. Also, layer III and IV contain, next to orofacial fibers and trigeminal nuclei, many interneurons that can be responsible for the intranuclear pathway (Dubner et al., 1978). A third tract therefore can be described, the so-called intranuclear tract running towards or within the PAG from the IS and CS of the SN. This would result in the trigeminothalamic tract as depicted in **Figure 6**.

Table 2 provides an overview of the mentioned tracing studies.

FUNCTION OF THE DORSAL TRIGEMINOTHALAMIC TRACT

Although the trigeminothalamic connections and origins have extensively been described, little is known about the cells giving rise to these tracts. The dorsal trigeminothalamic tract in animals (cats and monkeys) consists of fibers originating from the dorsal PSN and the CS and OS of the SN (Burton and Craig, 1979; Matsushita et al., 1982; Nieuwenhuys et al., 2008). This is summarized in **Figure 7**. The dorsal PSN receives afferents originating from the oral cavity, hence it is associated with the intraoral sensitivity (Shigenaga et al., 1986). Takemura et al. (1993) by studying the afferent axons from the lower and upper teeth. They found that these fibers project to the PSN in monkeys. According to some authors, the PSN also receives mechanoreceptive afferents from the intraoral cavity (Zeigler and Witkovsky, 1968; Silver and Witkovsky, 1973; Kishida et al., 1985; Dubbeldam, 1998). In line with these studies, bird species that rely on tactile information while feeding, the complete PSN seems to be enlarged (Gutiérrez-Ibáñez et al., 2009). Shigenaga et al. (1986) showed that in cats, the branches supplying the anterior face, i.e., the frontal, infraorbital and mental nerves, also terminate in the ventral PSN. Furthermore, the alveolar (superior and inferior), buccal, lingual and pterygopalatine branches, responsible for the intraoral sensitivity, terminate not only in different areas of the PSN but also in the OS and IS of the SN. The IS of the SN also receives input from the anterior face region and the auriculotemporal, corneal, mylohyoid, and zygomatic afferent nerve fibers (Shigenaga et al., 1986). The projecting cells from the CS of the SN are held responsible for the transmission of pain and temperature from the orofacial region. However, dental pulp afferents projecting to the OS of the SN have also been described (Burton and Craig, 1979; Takemura et al., 1993). The afferents of the OS of the SN are described to convey noxious information after mechanical stimulation (Woda et al., 1977), but the OS has also been described as a CS extension of PSN (Eisenmann et al., 1963; Burton et al., 1979). Others described that the terminals from both the upper and lower pulpal afferents formed a connection between the PSN and the OS of the SN (Takemura et al., 1993). The IS and CS also receive afferents from the intra-oral cavity, though this projection is less dense compared to that of the PSN and the OS of the SN (Takemura et al., 1993). Therefore, the exact function of these separate subnuclei remains unclear. However, most assume that the ipsilateral, dorsal trigeminothalamic tract is responsible for proprioceptic sensorical information, it seems logical to assume that both the SN and the PSN receive pain, temperature and mechanoreceptive stimuli from the head and intraoral cavity.

FUNCTION OF THE CONTRALATERAL, VENTRAL TRIGEMINOTHALAMIC TRACT

The ventral trigeminothalamic tract, as depicted in **Figure 8**, consists of fibers originating from the ventral PSN, CS and IS of the SN. The fibers from this ventral tract decussate along the medial border of the medial lemniscus and are therefore also called the trigeminal lemniscus (Torvik, 1957; Smith, 1975; Matsushita et al., 1982; Nieuwenhuys et al., 2008). The ventral trigeminothalamic tract is held responsible for the conduction of vital information. The function of the various nuclei has been

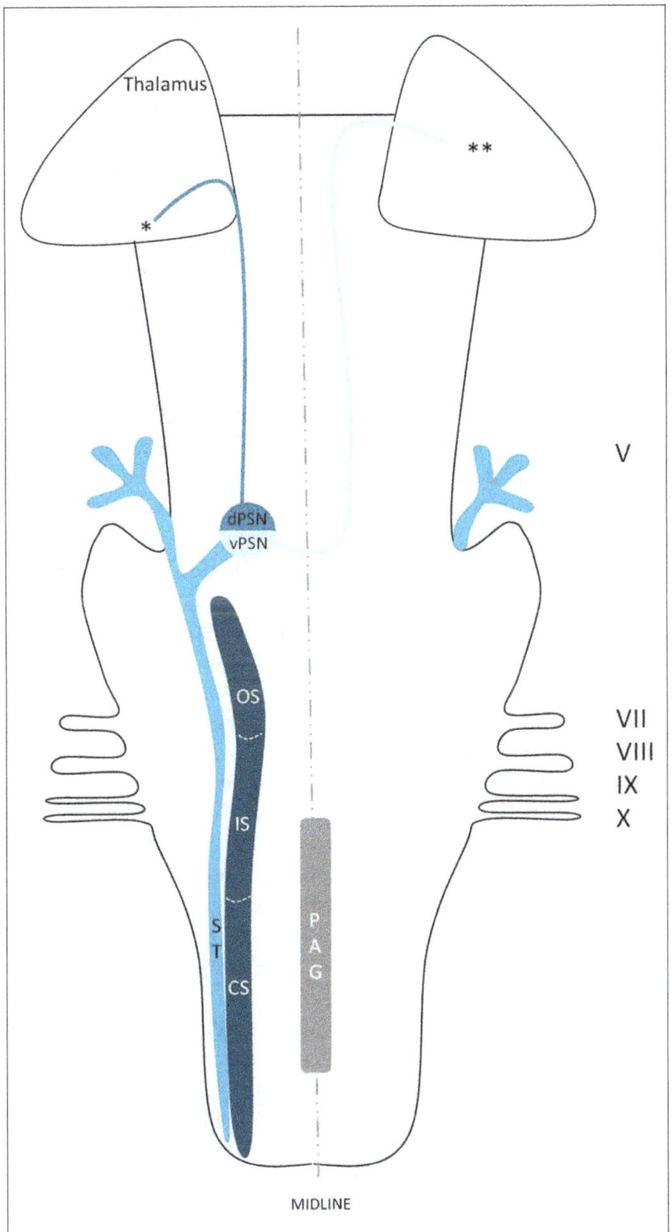

FIGURE 4 | Anatomy of the trigeminothalamic tracts sprouting from the principal sensory nucleus within the brainstem towards the diencephalon. dPSN, Dorsal part of the principal sensory nucleus; vPSN, Ventral part of the principal sensory nucleus; OS, Oral part of the spinal nucleus; IS, Interpolar part of the spinal nucleus; CS, Caudal part of the spinal nucleus; ST, Spinal tract; PAG, Periaquaductal gray; which receives afferents and courses more cranially as the intranuclear tract. V, Trigeminal nerve; VII, Facial nerve; VIII, Vestibulocochlear nerve; IX, Glossopharyngeal nerve; X, Vagus nerve. *Dorsal trigeminothalamic tract; **Ventral trigeminothalamic tract.

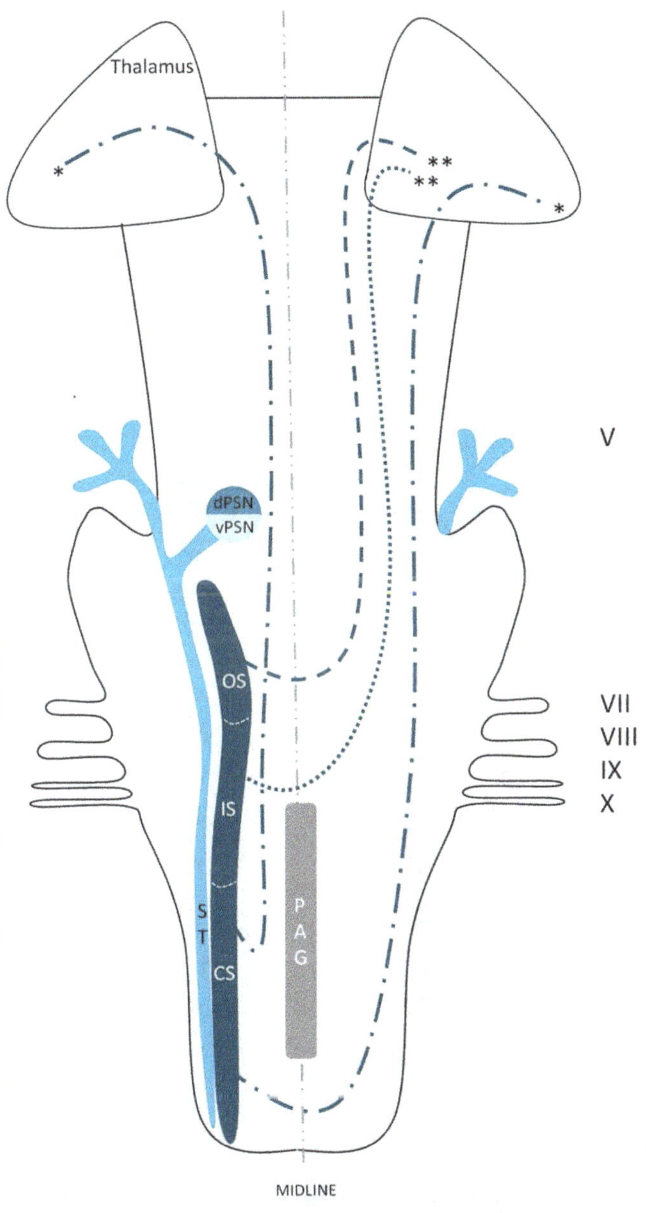

FIGURE 5 | Anatomy of the trigeminothalamic tracts sprouting from the spinal nucleus within the brainstem towards the diencephalon. dPSN, Dorsal part of the principal sensory nucleus; vPSN, Ventral part of the principal sensory nucleus; OS, Oral part of the spinal nucleus; IS, Interpolar part of the spinal nucleus; CS, Caudal part of the spinal nucleus; ST, Spinal tract; PAG, Periaquaductal gray; which receives afferents and courses more cranially as the intranuclear tract. V, Trigeminal nerve; VII, Facial nerve; VIII, Vestibulocochlear nerve; IX, Glossopharyngeal nerve; X, Vagus nerve. *Dorsal trigeminothalamic tract; **Ventral trigeminothalamic tract.

studied intensively before. The PSN is believed to be mainly involved in the conduction of tactile sensations and movement or position sense (Kruger, 1979). However, Kiknadze et al. (2001) showed that the same nucleus is also involved in the processing of orofacial and dental pain in cats. According to Shigenaga et al. (1986) the IS of the SN also receives input from the anterior orofacial region and several trigeminal peripheral branches. As we know from Sjögvist's tractotomy, the CS plays an important role in the transmission of vital information (Sjöqvist, 1938). These results would suggest that the ventral trigeminothalamic tract plays an important role in the contralateral registration of orofacial nociception, as suggested before by others (Sessle, 2000; Nieuwenhuys et al., 2008).

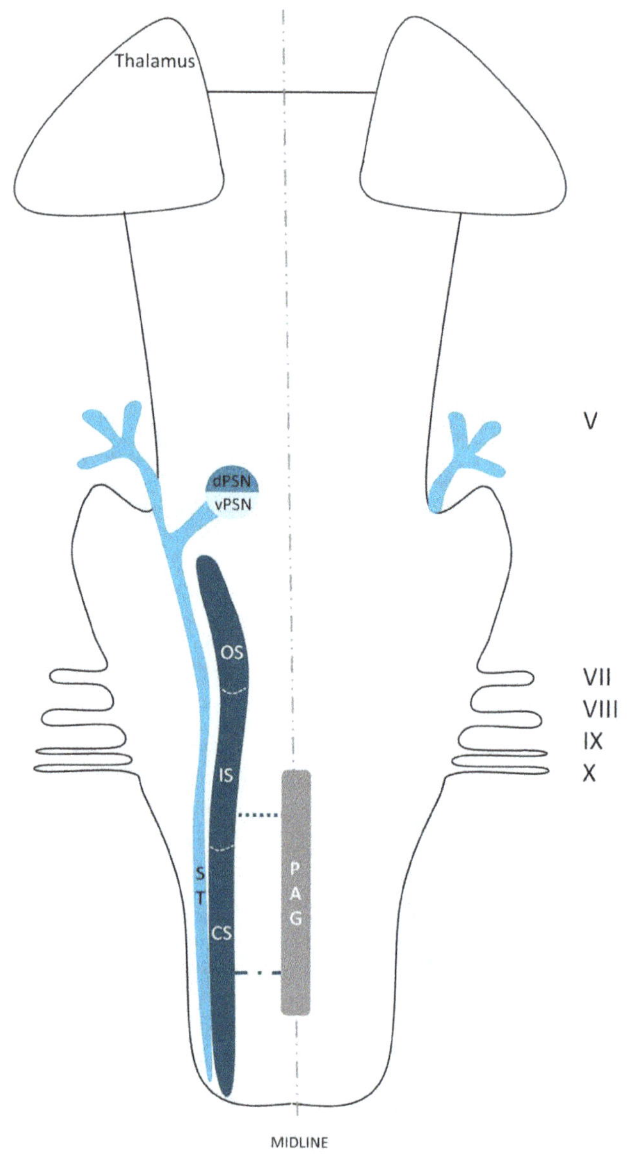

FIGURE 6 | Anatomy of the intranuclear tract within the brainstem. dPSN, Dorsal part of the principal sensory nucleus; vPSN, Ventral part of the principal sensory nucleus; OS, Oral part of the spinal nucleus, IS, Interpolar part of the spinal nucleus; CS, Caudal part of the spinal nucleus; ST, Spinal tract; PAG, Periaquaductal gray; which receives afferents and courses more cranially as the intranuclear tract. V, Trigeminal nerve; VII, Facial nerve; VIII, Vestibulocochlear nerve; IX, Glossopharyngeal nerve; X, Vagus nerve.

ACTIVATION OF BRAIN REGIONS IN RESPONSE TO OROFACIAL NOXIOUS STIMULATION

Pain, including that of orofacial origin, can be mediated by two systems. The medial system is composed of limbic structures and the anterior cingulate and insular cortices and is responsible for the emotional-affective and cognitive-behavioral dimensions of pain (Kulkarni et al., 2005; Wiech et al., 2006). The lateral pain network consists of the lateral spinothalamic tract, the VPL or VPM of the thalamus and the S1 cortex and processes the sensory-discriminative components of pain (Kenshalo et al., 1988; Bushnell and Duncan, 1989; Bushnell et al., 1999). The main components of the acute pain network are the prefrontal, M1, S2, anterior cingulate and insular cortices, the thalamus, supplementary motor areas, amygdala, PAG and basal ganglia (Apkarian et al., 2005). According to classical knowledge, it would be logical to assume that contralateral activation of the lateral system in response to unilateral noxious stimulation would occur. Surprisingly, according to Peyron et al. (2000) bilateral hemodynamic responses to acute noxious stimuli were observed in the thalamus and anterior cingulate, insular and SII cortices. An activation of S1, prefrontal and posterior parietal cortices, the striatum, cerebellum, PAG and supplementary motor areas was observed contralateral to the stimulus (Peyron et al., 2000). Bingel et al. (2004a,b) published a bilateral somatotopic cortical registration in event related fMRI after painful stimulation of the hand and foot. Touchless laser pain stimuli were applied to the dorsum of the hand and foot after which the neuronal response was measured using BOLD fMRI. In general, Bingel et al. (2004a,b) concluded that ipsilateral activity of S1 could be the result of an uncrossed ipsilateral tract or transcallosal excitatory pathways. Farrell et al. (2005) reviewed the literature on upper extremity noxious stimulation and showed a predominant contralateral activation of the anterior cingulate cortex (ACC), lentiform nucleus and the S1, S2 and M1 cortices, however the included reports discussed various activation patterns of cortical and subcortical structures. An ispilateral activation of the midbrain was also observed. The insular cortex, thalamus, cerebellum, premotor areas and inferior parietal lobule were regions that showed bilateral activation after noxious stimulation of the upper extremity.

Taking orofacial pain into account, in May et al. (1998) injected capsaicin in the foreheads of seven healthy volunteers. May et al. (1998) showed a bilateral activation of the cerebellum and the anterior insula and observed ipsilateral activation of the ACC and contralateral activation of the thalamus. DaSilva et al. (2002) showed an ipsilateral activation of the SN in patients that underwent noxious thermal stimulation of the skin of the trigeminal areas (V1, V2 and V3). Also, DaSilva et al. (2002) showed a contralateral activation of the thalamus and S1 cortex after stimulation. Brooks et al. (2005) showed a bilateral activation of the anterior insula, S2 and a contralateral activation of the posterior insula after noxious thermal stimulation of the face, hand or foot. When stimulating the face or hand, thalamic activity was also observed. Jantsch et al. (2005) discussed a bilateral fMRI activation of the S1 cortices after painful dental stimulation in eight healthy subjects. Interestingly, Jantsch et al. (2005) also mention a significant increase of BOLD-activation in the ipsilateral hemisphere after stimulation for which they do not give any explanation. Jantsch et al. (2005) that a complex cortical network must be responsible for a bilateral activation after orofacial stimulation. de Leeuw et al. (2006) observed brain activation with painful hot stimulation of the trigeminal nerve. In nine participants, the skin overlaying the left masseter muscle was triggered using thermal stimuli. Using fMRI, brain activity was registered. Bilateral activation was seen in the ACC, insula and thalamus. Ettlin et al. (2009) reported that bilateral non-nociceptive orofacial mechanical stimulation can provoke a bilateral activation of the insular cortex, whereas the S1-cortex was rarely activated. In the same year, Nash et al. (2009) investigated nociception in 30 humans (22 males, 19–52 years) using painful saline injections in the right masseter muscle. Both cutaneous and muscle nociceptive input activated the CS and OS subdivision of the SN. However, cutaneous nociceptive stimulation evoked a large response within the IS part of the SN, whereas muscle nociception was registered in the PSN. Weigelt et al. (2010) studied thirteen healthy volunteers that underwent stimulation of the dental pulp with a constant current tooth stimulator. After stimulation, they reported a bilateral activation of the S1, S2, the medial dorsal nuclei of the thalamus, insular cortices, ACC and precentral areas such as M1 as seen on fMRI. The information of the studies that discuss orofacial pain is presented in **Table 3**.

When investigated, the S2, insular and cingulate cortices seemed to be part of a bilateral projection system. Other structures, such as the thalamus, S1 cortex and the precentral gyrus, were also involved in the bilateral pain registration (Jantsch et al., 2005; de Leeuw et al., 2006; Staud et al., 2007; Cole et al., 2010; Weigelt et al., 2010). Nevertheless, Brügger et al. (2011) subdivided three lateralization patterns in the brain related to processing dental pain: (1) hemispheric lateralization irrespective of side of stimulation; (2) structures with predominant contralateral activation; and (3) structures showing hemispheric dominance and predominant contralateral activation. Pattern 1 shows that the right hemispheric effect is stronger to the cerebellar lobes and the parahippocampal area. The left hemispheric effect on the other hand is stronger to the putamen, pregenual, posterior and anterior cingulate cortices and supramarginal area. The second pattern shows five brain areas that are predominantly contralateral: the S1-cortex, thalamus, posterior insula, amygdala, and subcentral area. The subcentral area also shows lateralization to one hemisphere according to pattern 3. Also, they observe an activation of the contralateral amygdala in response to noxious dental stimulation.

DISCUSSION

We reviewed in animals that the somatosensory fibers of the fifth cranial nerve are distributed over the TSNC. From these nuclei, three tracts can be recognized. From the ventral part of the PSN, a large crossed tract, the trigeminal lemniscus or the ventral trigeminothalamic tract arises. This tract also receives efferents originating from the OS and IS of the SN. From the dorsal part of the PSN arises the dorsal trigeminothalamic tract, which also consists out of fibers from both the contra- and ipsilateral SN. Both tracts run to the thalamus, the VPL-region in specific. A third tract can be observed, originating from the distal two thirds of the SN. Fibers of this intranuclear tract course into the PAG (Wallenberg, 1905; Kohnstamm, 1910; Economo, 1911; Woodburne, 1936; Papez and Rundles, 1937; Walker, 1939; Papez, 1951; Torvik, 1957; Carpenter, 1957; Smith, 1975; Dubner et al., 1978; Ganchrow, 1978; Burton et al., 1979; Ikeda et al., 1982; Matsushita et al., 1982; Panneton and Burton, 1982; Rausell and Jones, 1991; Nieuwenhuys et al., 2008; Negredo et al., 2009; **Figure 9**). Although the mentioned ipsilateral tract has been described before, it has never been hypothesized to play a prominent role in the conduction of noxious stimulation. A full understanding of brain activation in response to nociceptive information is limited by the complexity of the multidimensional character of pain and the pain experience. Lateralization of the cortical areas involved in the medial pain system that seem predominantly active and are not influenced by the side of stimulation are the different parts of the cingulate gyrus (Brügger et al., 2011). This predominant activation could explain why fMRI studies show in some cases an ipsilateral activation. When the left cingulate gyrus gets activated after subjects are stimulated on the left side of the body, this may appear to be an ipsilateral activation pattern. Nevertheless, bilateral activation of the cingulate gyri has also been observed after unilateral noxious stimulation (Jantsch et al., 2005). The robust contralateral activation of the amygdala can only be speculated about. A high emotional value attributed to orofacial/dental pain could be one of the factors involved, but the emotional aspect of this kind of pain or noxious stimuli has never been investigated (Brügger et al., 2011). Even so, lateralization of the amygdala turns out to be inconsistent throughout human literature (Bingel et al., 2002; Bornhövd et al., 2002; Brügger et al., 2011). The subdivisions of the insular cortices showed a subdivision in activation. When bilateral activation was reported, this concerned mainly the anterior insular cortex (May et al., 1998; Jantsch et al., 2005). Contralateral activation was mainly seen in the posterior insular cortex (Brooks et al., 2005; Jantsch et al., 2005; Brügger et al., 2011). The posterior insular cortex is preferentially connected to other lateral structures, such as the S1 and S2 cortices (Wiech et al., 2014). The other structures of the lateral pain system are also predominantly contralateral according to Brooks's (2005) and Brüggers's (2011) studies but this is contradicted by various reports discussing a bilateral activation (de Leeuw et al., 2006; Nash et al., 2010; Weigelt et al., 2010). The activation of the ipsilateral S1 cortex is also held implausible, according to Brügger et al. (2011), but other reports do state a bilateral activation of S1 in response to noxious stimulation of the orofacial region (Bingel et al., 2004b; Jantsch et al., 2005; Nash et al., 2010; Weigelt et al., 2010; Brügger et al., 2011). The findings (Bingel et al., 2004b; Jantsch et al., 2005; Nash et al., 2010) could be in agreement with the results from animal-based studies about the intracerebral pathways. When we focus on facial pain, a double trigeminothalamic tract could be the answer to this clinical question, if both the ventral and dorsal trigeminothalamic tract are capable of nociceptive conduction. Another anatomical solution can be found in the transcallosal pathways. Nevertheless, this seems implausible bearing in mind the study of Stein et al. (1989) in which they investigated the pain perception of a split-brain patient after high intensity noxious stimulation was applied to the foot.

TABLE 2 | Tracing studies of the spinal nucleus (SN).

Reference	Species	Tracing technique	Anatomical site of lesion/injection
Ganchrow (1978)	Squirrel monkey	Degeneration after lesion; Injection with tritiated amino acids	CS
Burton and Craig (1979)	Cat and Cynomolgus monkey	Injection with horseradish peroxidase	Ventroposterior nucleus of the thalamus
Burton et al. (1979)	Cat	Injection with mixture of amino acids; Injection with horseradish peroxidase	Anterograde: CS Retrograde: ventroposterior nucleus of the thalamus
Ikeda et al. (1982)	Cat	Injection with horseradish peroxidase	IS
Panneton and Burton (1982)	Cat	Injection with horseradish peroxidase	Rostral trigeminal region
Künzle (1998)	Hedgehog tenre	Injection with a mixture of wheat germ agglutinin conjugated to horseradish peroxidase, biotinylated dextran amine and a solution of radioactive aminoacids	SN and PSN
Negredo et al. (2009)	Sprague-Dawley rat	Injection with dextran amine	Thalamus

CS, Caudal subnucleus; IS, Interpolar subnucleus; SN, Spinal nucleus; PSN, Principal sensory nucleus.

TABLE 3 | Synopsis of activated brain areas after noxious stimulation.

Reference	Site of stimulation	Medial dorsal thalamus	S1	S2	ACC	Insular cortical regions	Precentral gyrus
May et al. (1998)	Subcutaneous capsaicin injection into the forehead	Contralateral	N/A	N/A	Ipsilateral	Bilateral[B]	N/A
DaSilva et al. (2002)	Cutaneous thermal stimulation of right V1 region	Contralateral	Contralateral	N/A	N/A	N/A	N/A
	Cutaneous thermal stimulation of right V2 region	Contralateral	Contralateral	N/A	N/A	N/A	N/A
	Cutaneous thermal stimulation of right V3 region	Contralateral	Contralateral	N/A	N/A	N/A	N/A
Brooks et al. (2005)	Cutaneous thermal stimulation of the area below the right lower lip	Small activations[E]	N/A	Bilateral	N/A	Contralateral[D]	N/A
	Cutaneous thermal stimulation of the dorsum of the right hand	Small activations[E]	N/A	Bilateral	N/A	Contralateral[D]	N/A
	Cutaneous thermal stimulation of the dorsum of the right foot	N/A	N/A	Bilateral	N/A	Contralateral[D]	N/A
Jantsch et al. (2005)	Pneumatic mechanical stimulation of the middle phalanx	N/A	Contralateral[A]	Bilateral	Bilateral	Bilateral	Contra-lateral
	Constant electrical dental stimulation	N/A	Bilateral	Bilateral	Bilateral	Bilateral	Contra-lateral
de Leeuw et al. (2006)	Cutaneous thermal stimulation of the skin area overlying the left masseter muscle	Bilateral	Contra-lateral	N/A	Bilateral	Bilateral	Ipsilateral
Ettlin et al. (2009)	Electrical dental stimulation of one randomly selected canine with randomized intervals	N/A	N/A	N/A	Small activations[E]	Small activations[B,E]	Small activations[E]
Nash et al. (2010)	Subcutaneous hypertonic saline injection into the skin overlying the right masseter muscle and into the central belly of the right masseter muscle	Bilateral	Bilateral	Bilateral	N/A	N/A	N/A
Weigelt et al. (2010)	Constant electrical pulpal stimulation	Bilateral	Bilateral	Bilateral	Bilateral	Bilateral	Bilateral

N/A, not available from full text; [A]Hand-area on S1; [B]Anterior insular cortex; [C]Medial insular cortex; [D]Posterior insular cortex; [E]Author does not specify the results.

Limitations in the functional imaging of pain are: (1) anticipation of pain; (2) attentional modulation; and (3) emotional accounts of pain. The anticipation of pain is known to activate several brain regions, including the ACC, cerebellum, ventral premotor and ventromedial prefrontal cortex, the PAG and hippocampus (Hsieh et al., 1999; Ploghaus et al., 1999, 2001, 2003; Bantick et al., 2002). Brügger et al. (2011) study does indeed show that, when anticipation is ruled

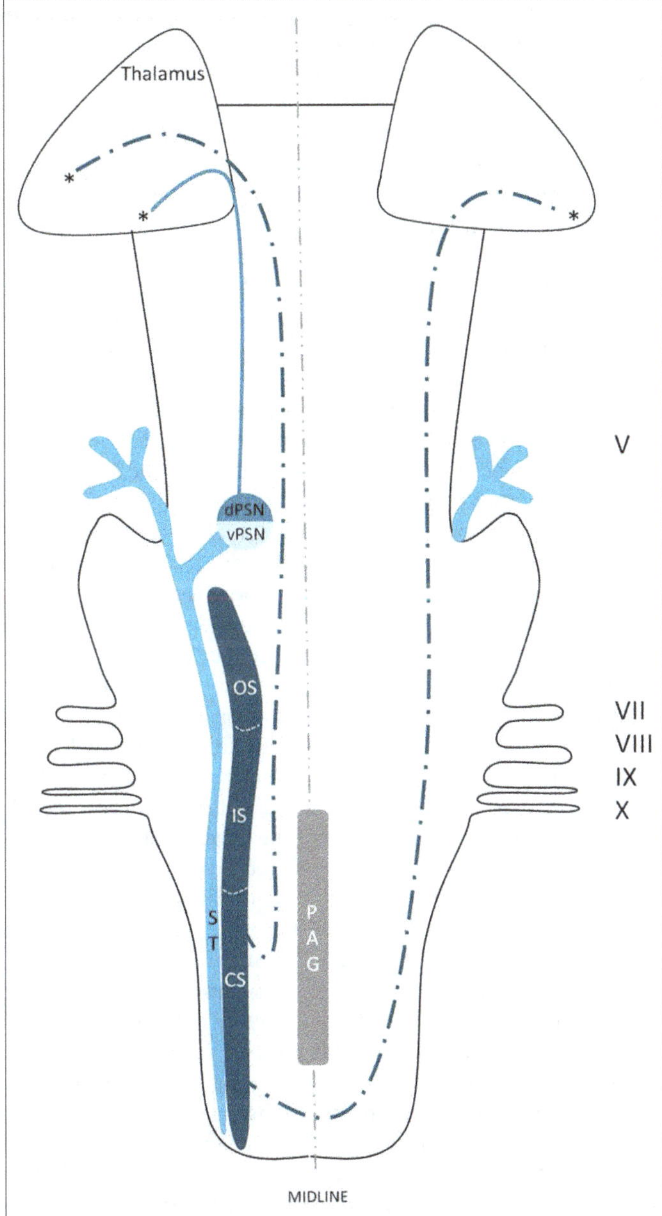

FIGURE 7 | Anatomy of the dorsal trigeminothalamic tract within the brainstem towards the diencephalon. dPSN, Dorsal part of the principal sensory nucleus; vPSN, Ventral part of the principal sensory nucleus; OS, Oral part of the spinal nucleus; IS, Interpolar part of the spinal nucleus; CS, Caudal part of the spinal nucleus; ST, Spinal tract; PAG, Periaquaductal gray; which receives afferents and courses more cranially as the intranuclear tract. V, Trigeminal nerve; VII, Facial nerve; VIII, Vestibulocochlear nerve; IX, Glossopharyngeal nerve; X, Vagus nerve. *Dorsal trigeminothalamic tract.

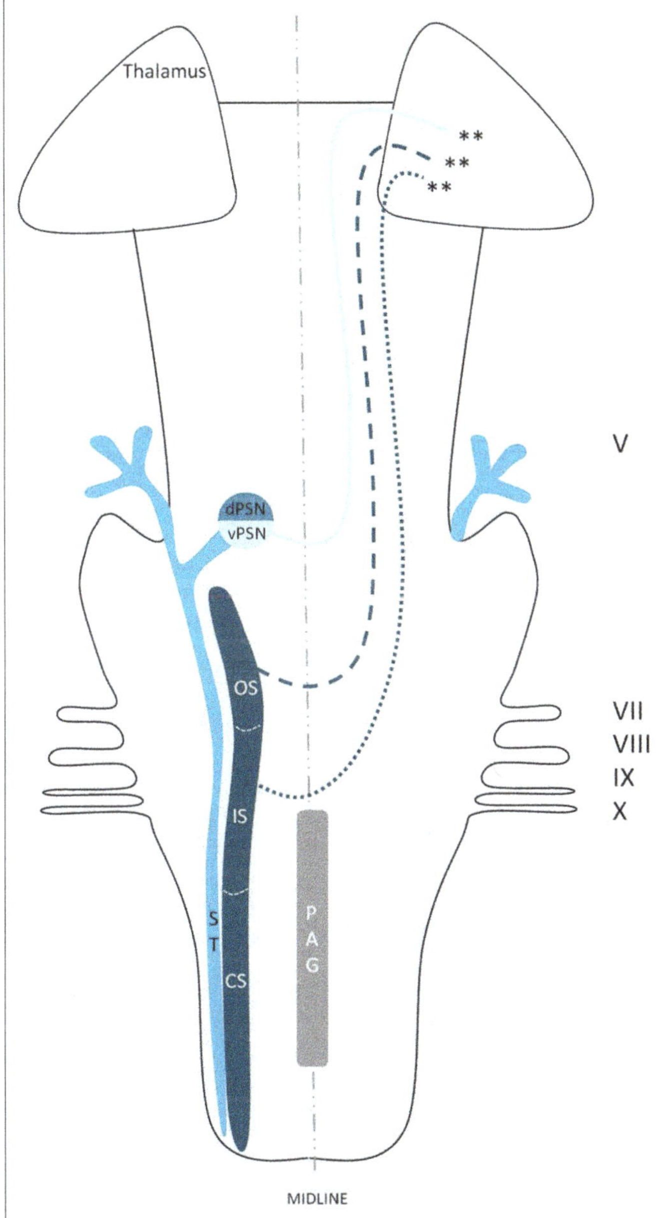

FIGURE 8 | Anatomy of the ventral trigeminothalamic tract within the brainstem towards the diencephalon. dPSN, Dorsal part of the principal sensory nucleus; vPSN, Ventral part of the principal sensory nucleus; OS, Oral part of the spinal nucleus; IS, Interpolar part of the spinal nucleus; CS, Caudal part of the spinal nucleus; ST, Spinal tract; PAG, Periaquaductal gray; which receives afferents and courses more cranially as the intranuclear tract. V, Trigeminal nerve; VII, Facial nerve; VIII, Vestibulocochlear nerve; IX, Glossopharyngeal nerve; X, Vagus nerve. **Ventral trigeminothalamic tract.

out, the bilateral activation decreases. This decrease in bilateral activity shows that anticipation of pain causes a bilateral network to be activated. Nevertheless, when anticipation is ruled out, there still seems to be a bilateral activation of cortical areas involved in the lateral pain system. This would suggest that both systems (pain and anticipation of pain) play a prominent role in registration of pain. Secondly, it is well known that pain related anxiety and fear are associated with difficulties in attention and result in an increased awareness of pain (Taylor et al., 2015). Chronic lower back pain patients have been shown to display activation of the insular cortex, supplementary motor area and pre-motor area, cerebellum, thalamus, pulvinar, posterior cingulate cortex, hippocampus, fusiform gyrus and angular gyrus after they saw a picture showing an aversive movement (Shimo et al., 2011). The emotional accounts have been studied extensively as well. When cued expectation of pain stimuli is

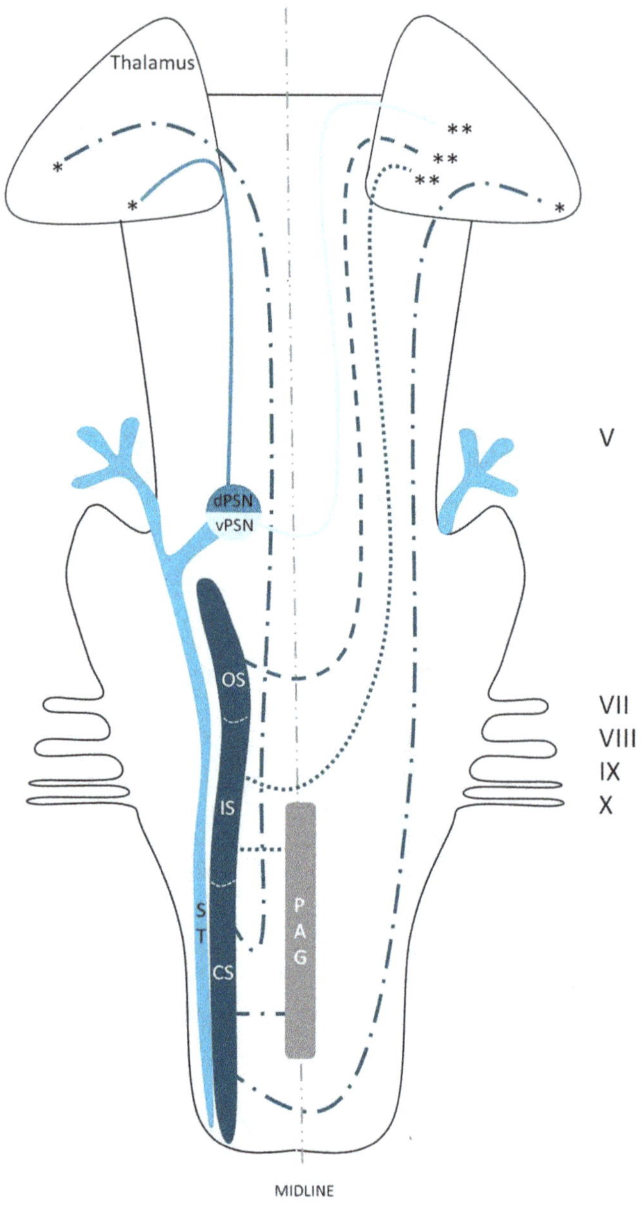

FIGURE 9 | Anatomy of the hypothesized bilateral orofacial pain registration system in humans. dPSN, Dorsal part of the principal sensory nucleus; vPSN, Ventral part of the principal sensory nucleus; OS, Oral part of the spinal nucleus; IS, Interpolar part of the spinal nucleus; CS, Caudal part of the spinal nucleus; ST, Spinal tract; PAG, Periaquaductal gray; which receives afferents and courses more cranially as the intranuclear tract. V, Trigeminal nerve; VII, Facial nerve; VIII, Vestibulocochlear nerve; IX, Glossopharyngeal nerve; X, Vagus nerve. *Dorsal trigeminothalamic tract; **Ventral trigeminothalamic tract.

studied, activation of various regions within the salience (insula and ACC), sensorimotor and attentional control (parietal and frontal) networks have been described (Yágüez et al., 2005; Carlsson et al., 2006; Seidel et al., 2015). Taking the mentioned regions into account, fMRI studies of the brain can be very useful and illustrative, but one must be careful when interpreting these results.

Lin (2014) states that a critical step in the future of fMRI investigations is to understand the chronic dental pain-related anatomy and cortical representations. The potential for investigating and understanding chronic orofacial pain is highlighted by their two major findings. First, the thalamus and S1 cortex were identified as two major sites of neuroplasticity and second, the increased connectivity between the thalamus and the insula. Although some other authors also state that the standard anatomy can change under the influence of chronic stimulation, such as pain (Wilcox et al., 2013, 2015), it seems logical to assume that orofacial pain is bilaterally registered in healthy humans as well, according to other investigations (Bingel et al., 2004b; Jantsch et al., 2005; de Leeuw et al., 2006; Staud et al., 2007; Cole et al., 2010; Nash et al., 2010; Weigelt et al., 2010). In order to gain more insight in the normal connectivity from the orofacial region and the related cortical areas, we subsequently make some proposals for future investigations. A post-mortem diffusion tensor imaging (DTI) study based on a diffusion weighted MRI (DW-MRI) scan could contribute to our insights in the trigeminal fibers, because this is currently the only capable method of mapping the detailed architecture of white matter fibers in human brain specimens (Jones et al., 2013). This technique could create a more profound insight in trigeminal anatomy, specifically concerning its intracerebral portion and is certain to contribute to clinical knowledge and decision making in the daily practice of trigeminal neuropathies. Nevertheless issues regarding high resolution MRI and reliable qualitative probabilistic tracking of the trigeminothalamic tracts may be important challenges to overcome (Jones et al., 2013). Beyond the challenges inherent in acquiring suitable DW-MRI data, there are currently many obstacles to overcome regarding the tractographic modeling of white matter tracts (O'Donnell and Pasternak, 2015). The use of post-mortem DTI could be a welcome supplement to the knowledge obtained by *in vivo* fMRI-studies, in which the activation of regions of the brain involved in the orofacial pain registration, have been mapped. There still remain outstanding questions that cannot be answered today. Is it possible that the trigeminothalamic tracts in humans are more comparable to those in animals? Is it possible that the several nuclei of the TSNC are indeed part of a conjoined complex which makes it difficult to separate several types of somatosensorical information and their conducting pathways? There is much left that we do not comprehend concerning orofacial pain, but knowledge of the involved trigeminothalamic and intranuclear pathways is believed to be of great importance in treating patients suffering from orofacial pain syndromes effectively .

CONCLUSION

The main aim of this review was to present new insights in trigeminal anatomy in humans, based on both animal-based papers and fMRI research studies. The classical point of view is that orofacial pain is conducted in a contralateral fashion. However by synthesizing animal-based literature and human functional imaging studies, we state that the exact neuroanatomy of orofacial pain is largely elusive, and we hypothesize the existence of a bilateral orofacial conduction system of nociceptive information in humans.

AUTHOR CONTRIBUTIONS

DJHAH undertook the action of collecting the literature and wrote the first draft of the article. After collecting multiple times the input from A-MvCvW, EK and RvD, he wrote the other versions. Together with EK, DJHAH created the **Figures 2–4**. **Figure 1** was created by A-MvCvW and DJHAH. RHMAB and TK reviewed the latest versions and gave valuable input from their point of expertise.

REFERENCES

Apkarian, A. V., Bushnell, M. C., Treede, R. D., and Zubieta, J. K. (2005). Human brain mechanisms of pain perception and regulation in health and disease. *Eur. J. Pain* 9, 463–484. doi: 10.1016/j.ejpain.2004.11.001

Astrom, K. E. (1953). On the central course of afferent fibers in the trigeminal, facial, glossopharyngeal and vagal nerves and their nuclei in the mouse. *Acta. Physiol. Scand.* 106, 209–320.

Bantick, S. J., Wise, R. G., Ploghaus, A., Clare, S., Smith, S. M., and Tracey, I. (2002). Imaging how attention modulates pain in humans using functional MRI. *Brain* 125, 310–319. doi: 10.1093/brain/awf022

Bathla, G., and Hegde, A. N. (2013). The trigeminal nerve: an illustrated review of its imaging anatomy and pathology. *Clin. Radiol.* 68, 203–213. doi: 10.1016/j.crad.2012.05.019

Bingel, U., Gläscher, J., Weiller, C., and Büchel, C. (2004a). Somatotopic representation of nociceptive information in the putamen: an event-related fMRI study. *Cereb. Cortex* 14, 1340–1345. doi: 10.1093/cercor/bhh094

Bingel, U., Lorenz, J., Glauche, V., Knab, R., Gläscher, J., Weiller, C., et al. (2004b). Somatotopic organization of human somatosensory cortices for pain: a single trial fMRI study. *Neuroimage* 23, 224–232. doi: 10.1016/j.neuroimage.2004.05.021

Bingel, U., Quante, M., Knab, R., Bromm, B., Weiller, C., and Büchel, C. (2002). Subcortical structures involved in pain processing: evidence from single-trial fMRI. *Pain* 99, 313–321. doi: 10.1016/s0304-3959(02)00157-4

Borges, A., and Casselman, J. (2010). Imaging the trigeminal nerve. *Eur. J. Radiol.* 74, 323–340. doi: 10.1016/j.ejrad.2010.02.006

Bornhövd, K., Quante, M., Glauche, V., Bromm, B., Weiller, C., and Büchel, C. (2002). Painful stimuli evoke different stimulus-response functions in the amygdala, prefrontal, insula and somatosensory cortex: a single-trial fMRI study. *Brain* 125, 1326–1336. doi: 10.1093/brain/awf137

Brooks, J. C., Zambreanu, L., Godinez, A., Craig, A. D., and Tracey, I. (2005). Somatotopic organisation of the human insula to painful heat studied with high resolution functional imaging. *Neuroimage* 27, 201–209. doi: 10.1016/j.neuroimage.2005.03.041

Brügger, M., Ettlin, D. A., Meier, M., Keller, T., Luechinger, R., Barlow, A., et al. (2011). Taking sides with pain–lateralization aspects related to cerebral processing of dental pain. *Front. Hum. Neurosci.* 5:12. doi: 10.3389/fnhum.2011.00012

Burchiel, K. J. (2003). A new classification for facial pain. *Neurosurgery* 53, 1164–1166; discussion 1166–1167. doi: 10.1227/01.neu.0000088806.11659.d8

Burton, H., and Craig, A. D. Jr. (1979). Distribution of trigeminothalamic projection cells in cat and monkey. *Brain Res.* 161, 515–521. doi: 10.1016/0006-8993(79)90680-2

Burton, H., Craig, A. D. Jr., Poulos, D. A., and Molt, J. T. (1979). Efferent projections from temperature sensitive recording loci within the marginal zone of the nucleus caudalis of the spinal trigeminal complex in the cat. *J. Comp. Neurol.* 183, 753–777. doi: 10.1002/cne.901830406

Bushnell, M. C., and Duncan, G. H. (1989). Sensory and affective aspects of pain perception: is medial thalamus restricted to emotional issues? *Exp. Brain Res.* 78, 415–418. doi: 10.1007/bf00228914

Bushnell, M. C., Duncan, G. H., Hofbauer, R. K., Ha, B., Chen, J. I., and Carrier, B. (1999). Pain perception: is there a role for primary somatosensory cortex? *Proc. Natl. Acad. Sci. U S A* 96, 7705–7709. doi: 10.1073/pnas.96.14.7705

Capra, N. F., and Dessem, D. (1992). Central connections of trigeminal primary afferent neurons: topographical and functional considerations. *Crit. Rev. Oral Biol. Med.* 4, 1–52.

Carlsson, K., Andersson, J., Petrovic, P., Petersson, K. M., Ohman, A., and Ingvar, M. (2006). Predictability modulates the affective and sensory-discriminative neural processing of pain. *Neuroimage* 32, 1804–1814. doi: 10.1016/j.neuroimage.2006.05.027

Carpenter, M. B. (1957). The dorsal trigeminal tract in the rhesus monkey. *J. Anat.* 91, 82–90.

Cole, L. J., Farrell, M. J., Gibson, S. J., and Egan, G. F. (2010). Age-related differences in pain sensitivity and regional brain activity evoked by noxious pressure. *Neurobiol. Aging* 31, 494–503. doi: 10.1016/j.neurobiolaging.2008.04.012

Crosby, E. C., and Yoss, R. E. (1954). The phylogenetic continuity of neural mechanisms of illustrated by the spinal tract of V and its nucleus. *Res. Publ. Assoc. Res. Nerv. Ment. Dis.* 33, 174–208.

DaSilva, A. F., Becerra, L., Makris, N., Strassman, A. M., Gonzalez, R. G., Geatrakis, N., et al. (2002). Somatotopic activation in the human trigeminal pain pathway. *J. Neurosci.* 22, 8183–8192.

de Leeuw, R., Davis, C. E., Albuquerque, R., Carlson, C. R., and Andersen, A. H. (2006). Brain activity during stimulation of the trigeminal nerve with noxious heat. *Oral Surg. Oral Med. Oral Pathol. Oral Radiol. Endod.* 102, 750–757. doi: 10.1016/j.tripleo.2005.12.018

Dubbeldam, J. L. (1998). The sensory trigeminal system in birds: input, organization and effects of peripheral damage. A review. *Arch. Physiol. Biochem.* 106, 338–345. doi: 10.1076/apab.106.5.338.4367

Dubner, R., Sessle, B. J., and Storey, A. T. (1978). *The Neurological Basis of Oral and Facial Function.* New York, NY: Plenum Press.

Economo, C. V. (1911). Über dissoziirte empfindungslähmung bei ponstumoren und über die zentralen bahnen des sensiblen trigeminus. *Jahr. f. Psychiat.* S2, 107–138.

Eisenmann, J., Landgren, S., and Novin, D. (1963). Functional organization in the main sensory trigeminal nucleus and in the rostral subdivision of the nucleus of the spinal trigeminal tract in the cat. *Acta Physiol. Scand. Suppl.* 214, 1–44.

Ettlin, D. A., Brügger, M., Keller, T., Luechinger, R., Jäncke, L., Palla, S., et al. (2009). Interindividual differences in the perception of dental stimulation and related brain activity. *Eur. J. Oral Sci.* 117, 27–33. doi: 10.1111/j.1600-0722.2008.00590.x

Farrell, M. J., Laird, A. R., and Egan, G. F. (2005). Brain activity associated with painfully hot stimuli applied to the upper limb: a meta-analysis. *Hum. Brain Mapp.* 25, 129–139. doi: 10.1002/hbm.20125

Ganchrow, D. (1978). Intratrigeminal and thalamic projections of nucleus caudalis in the squirrel monkey (Saimiri sciureus): a degeneration and autoradiographic study. *J. Comp. Neurol.* 178, 281–312. doi: 10.1002/cne.901780206

Go, J. L., Kim, P. E., and Zee, C. S. (2001). The trigeminal nerve. *Semin. Ultrasound CT MR* 22, 502–520. doi: 10.1016/S0887-2171(01)90004-6

Gobel, S., and Dubner, R. (1969). Fine structural studies of the main sensory trigeminal nucleus in the cat and rat. *J. Comp. Neurol.* 137, 459–493. doi: 10.1002/cne.901370405

Greenspan, J. D., and Winfield, J. A. (1992). Reversible pain and tactile deficits associated with a cerebral tumor compressing the posterior insula and parietal operculum. *Pain* 50, 29–39. doi: 10.1016/0304-3959(92)90109-o

Gutiérrez-Ibáñez, C., Iwaniuk, A. N., and Wylie, D. R. (2009). The independent evolution of the enlargement of the principal sensory nucleus of the trigeminal nerve in three different groups of birds. *Brain Behav. Evol.* 74, 280–294. doi: 10.1159/000270904

Hsieh, J. C., Stone-Elander, S., and Ingvar, M. (1999). Anticipatory coping of pain expressed in the human anterior cingulate cortex: a positron emission tomography study. *Neurosci. Lett.* 262, 61–64. doi: 10.1016/s0304-3940(99)00060-9

Ikeda, M., Matsushita, M., and Tanami, T. (1982). Termination and cells of origin of the ascending intra-nuclear fibers in the spinal trigeminal nucleus of the cat. A study with the horseradish peroxidase technique. *Neurosci. Lett.* 31, 215–220. doi: 10.1016/0304-3940(82)90022-2

Jacquin, M. F., Semba, K., Egger, M. D., and Rhoades, R. W. (1983). Organization of HRP-labeled trigeminal mandibular primary afferent neurons in the rat. *J. Comp. Neurol.* 215, 397–420. doi: 10.1002/cne.902150405

Jantsch, H. H. F., Kemppainen, P., Ringler, R., Handwerker, H. O., and Forster, C. (2005). Cortical representation of experimental tooth pain in humans. *Pain* 118, 390–399. doi: 10.1016/j.pain.2005.09.017

Jones, D. K., Knösche, T. R., and Turner, R. (2013). White matter integrity, fiber count and other fallacies: the do's and don'ts of diffusion MRI. *Neuroimage* 73, 239–254. doi: 10.1016/j.neuroimage.2012.06.081

Joo, W., Yoshioka, F., Funaki, T., Mizokami, K., and Rhoton, A. L. Jr. (2014). Microsurgical anatomy of the trigeminal nerve. *Clin. Anat.* 27, 61–88. doi: 10.1002/ca.22330

Kanda, M., Nagamine, T., Ikeda, A., Ohara, S., Kunieda, T., Fujiwara, N., et al. (2000). Primary somatosensory cortex is actively involved in pain processing in human. *Brain Res.* 853, 282–289. doi: 10.1016/s0006-8993(99)02274-x

Kenshalo, D. R. Jr., Chudler, E. H., Anton, F., and Dubner, R. (1988). SI nociceptive neurons participate in the encoding process by which monkeys perceive the intensity of noxious thermal stimulation. *Brain Res.* 454, 378–382. doi: 10.1016/0006-8993(88)90841-4

Kiknadze, G. I., Dzamoeva, E. I., and Lazriev, I. L. (2001). Ultrastructure of the main sensory nucleus of the trigeminal nerve of the cat in normal conditions and in conditions of threshold pain stimulation. *Neurosci. Behav. Physiol.* 31, 623–627. doi: 10.1023/A:1012377312817

Kishida, R., Dubbeldam, J. L., and Goris, R. C. (1985). Primary sensory ganglion cells projecting to the principal trigeminal nucleus in the mallard, Anas platyrhynchos. *J. Comp. Neurol.* 240, 171–179. doi: 10.1002/cne.902400207

Kohnstamm, O. (1910). Studien zur physiologischen anatomie des hirnstammes. Die tigrolytische methode nebst beispielen für ihre anwendung. *J. Psychol. u. Neurol.* 17, 33–57.

Kolodziej, M. A., Hellwig, D., Nimsky, C., and Benes, L. (2016). Treatment of central deafferentation and trigeminal neuropathic pain by motor cortex stimulation: report of a series of 20 patients. *J. Neurol. Surg. A Cent. Eur. Neurosurg.* 77, 52–58. doi: 10.1055/s-0035-1558419

Kruger, L. (1979). Functional subdivision of the brainstem sensory trigeminal nuclear complex. *Adv. Pain Res. Ther.* 3, 197–209.

Kulkarni, B., Bentley, D. E., Elliott, R., Youell, P., Watson, A., Derbyshire, S. W., et al. (2005). Attention to pain localization and unpleasantness discriminates the functions of the medial and lateral pain systems. *Eur. J. Neurosci.* 21, 3133–3142. doi: 10.1111/j.1460-9568.2005.04098.x

Künzle, H. (1998). Trigeminal projections to thalamus and subthalamus in the hedgehog tenrec. *Neuroscience* 86, 651–661. doi: 10.1016/s0306-4522(98)00056-6

Lang, J. (1981). Neuroanatomie der Nn. opticus, trigeminus, facialis, glossopharyngeus, vagus, accessorius und hypoglossus. *Arch. Oto-rhino-laryngology.* 231, 1–69. doi: 10.1007/bf00465556

Lin, C. S. (2014). Brain signature of chronic orofacial pain: a systematic review and meta-analysis on neuroimaging research of trigeminal neuropathic pain and temporomandibular joint disorders. *PLoS One* 9:e94300. doi: 10.1371/journal.pone.0094300

Marur, T., Tuna, Y., and Demirci, S. (2014). Facial anatomy. *Clin. Dermatol.* 32, 14–23. doi: 10.1016/j.clindermatol.2013.05.022

Matsushita, M., Ikeda, M., and Okado, N. (1982). The cells of origin of the trigeminothalamic, trigeminospinal and trigeminocerebellar projections in the cat. *Neuroscience* 7, 1439–1454. doi: 10.1016/0306-4522(82)90256-1

May, A., Kaube, H., Buchel, C., Eichten, C., Rijntjes, M., Juptner, M., et al. (1998). Experimental cranial pain elicited by capsaicin: a PET study. *Pain* 74, 61–66. doi: 10.1016/s0304-3959(97)00144-9

Meessen, H., and Olszewski, J. (1949). *A Cytoarchitectonic Atlas of the Rhombencephalon of the Rabbit.* Basel and New York: S. Karger.

Mollink, J., van Baarsen, K. M., Dederen, P. J., Foxley, S., Miller, K. L., Jbabdi, S., et al. (2015). Dentatorubrothalamic tract localization with postmortem MR diffusion tractography compared to histological 3D reconstruction. *Brain Struct Funct.* doi: 10.1007/s00429-015-1115-7 [Epub ahead of print].

Nash, P. G., Macefield, V. G., Klineberg, I. J., Gustin, S. M., Murray, G. M., and Henderson, L. A. (2010). Bilateral activation of the trigeminothalamic tract by acute orofacial cutaneous and muscle pain in humans. *Pain* 151, 384–393. doi: 10.1016/j.pain.2010.07.027

Nash, P. G., Macefield, V. G., Klineberg, I. J., Murray, G. M., and Henderson, L. A. (2009). Differential activation of the human trigeminal nuclear complex by noxious and non-noxious orofacial stimulation. *Hum. Brain Mapp.* 30, 3772–3782. doi: 10.1002/hbm.20805

Negredo, P., Martin, Y. B., Lagares, A., Castro, J., Villacorta, J. A., and Avendaño, C. (2009). Trigeminothalamic barrelette neurons: natural structural side asymmetries and sensory input-dependent plasticity in adult rats. *Neuroscience* 163, 1242–1254. doi: 10.1016/j.neuroscience.2009.07.065

Nguyen, J. P., Lefaucher, J. P., Le Guerinel, C., Eizenbaum, J. F., Nakano, N., Carpentier, A., et al. (2000). Motor cortex stimulation in the treatment of central and neuropathic pain. *Arch. Med. Res.* 31, 263–265. doi: 10.1016/S0188-4409(00)00078-3

Nieuwenhuys, R., Voogd, J., and Huijzen, C. V. (2008). *The Human Central Nervous System.* 4th Edn. New York, NY: Springer.

O'Donnell, L. J., and Pasternak, O. (2015). Does diffusion MRI tell us anything about the white matter? An overview of methods and pitfalls. *Schizophr. Res.* 161, 133–141. doi: 10.1016/j.schres.2014.09.007

Olszewski, J. (1950). On the anatomical and functional organization of the spinal trigeminal nucleus. *J. Comp. Neurol.* 92, 401–413. doi: 10.1002/cne.900920305

Panneton, W. M., and Burton, H. (1982). Origin of ascending intratrigeminal pathways in the cat. *Brain Res.* 236, 463–470. doi: 10.1016/0006-8993(82)90728-4

Papez, J. W. (1951). Dorsal trigemino-thalamic tract in the brain stem of quadrupeds. *Anat. Rec.* 109, 405.

Papez, J. W., and Rundles, W. (1937). The dorsal trigeminal tract and the centre median nucleus of Luys. *J. Nerv. Ment. Dis.* 85, 505–519. doi: 10.1097/00005053-193705000-00001

Peyron, R., Laurent, B., and García-Larrea, L. (2000). Functional imaging of brain responses to pain. A review and meta-analysis (2000). *Neurophysiol. Clin.* 30, 263–288. doi: 10.1016/s0987-7053(00)00227-6

Ploghaus, A., Becerra, L., Borras, C., and Borsook, D. (2003). Neural circuitry underlying pain modulation: expectation, hypnosis, placebo. *Trends Cogn. Sci.* 7, 197–200. doi: 10.1016/s1364-6613(03)00061-5

Ploghaus, A., Narain, C., Beckmann, C. F., Clare, S., Bantick, S., Wise, R., et al. (2001). Exacerbation of pain by anxiety is associated with activity in a hippocampal network. *J. Neurosci.* 21, 9896–9903.

Ploghaus, A., Tracey, I., Gati, J. S., Clare, S., Menon, R. S., Matthews, P. M., et al. (1999). Dissociating pain from its anticipation in the human brain. *Science* 284, 1979–1981. doi: 10.1126/science.284.5422.1979

Ramon y Cajal, S. (1909). *Histology of the Nervous System, Vol. 1.* Oxford, NY: Oxford University Press.

Raslan, A. M., Nasseri, M., Bahgat, D., Abdu, E., and Burchiel, K. J. (2011). Motor cortex stimulation for trigeminal neuropathic or deafferentation pain: an institutional case series experience. *Stereotact. Funct. Neurosurg.* 89, 83–88. doi: 10.1159/000323338

Rausell, E., and Jones, E. G. (1991). Chemically distinct compartments of the thalamic VPM nucleus in monkeys relay principal and spinal trigeminal pathways to different layers of the somatosensory cortex. *J. Neurosci.* 11, 226–237.

Rexed, B. (1952). The cytoarchitectonic organization of the spinal cord in the cat. *J. Comp. Neurol.* 96, 414–495. doi: 10.1002/cne.900960303

Rexed, B. (1954). A cytoarchitectonic atlas of the spinal cord in the cat. *J. Comp. Neurol.* 100, 297–379. doi: 10.1002/cne.901000205

Sabancl, P. A., Batay, F., Civelek, E., Al Mefty, O., Husain, M., Abdulrauf, S. I., et al. (2011). Meckel's cave. *World Neurosurg.* 76, 335–341; discussion 266–337. doi: 10.1016/j.wneu.2011.03.037

Schünke, M. S. E., Schumacher, U., Voll, M., and Wesker, K. (2006). *Prometheus LernAtlas der Anatomie-Kopf und Neuroanatomie.* Stuttgart: Georg Thieme Verlag.

Seidel, E. M., Pfabigan, D. M., Hahn, A., Sladky, R., Grahl, A., Paul, K., et al. (2015). Uncertainty during pain anticipation: the adaptive value of preparatory processes. *Hum. Brain Mapp.* 36, 744–755. doi: 10.1002/hbm.22661

Sessle, B. J. (2000). Acute and chronic craniofacial pain: brainstem mechanisms of nociceptive transmission and neuroplasticity and their clinical correlates. *Crit. Rev. Oral Biol. Med.* 11, 57–91. doi: 10.1177/10454411000110010401

Shigenaga, Y., Okamoto, T., Nishimori, T., Suemune, S., Nasution, I. D., Chen, I. C., et al. (1986). Oral and facial representation in the trigeminal principal and rostral spinal nuclei of the cat. *J. Comp. Neurol.* 244, 1–18. doi: 10.1002/cne.902440102

Shimo, K., Ueno, T., Younger, J., Nishihara, M., Inoue, S., Ikemoto, T., et al. (2011). Visualization of painful experiences believed to trigger the activation of affective and emotional brain regions in subjects with low back pain. *PLoS One* 6:e26681. doi: 10.1371/journal.pone.0026681

Silver, R., and Witkovsky, P. (1973). Functional characteristics of single units in the spinal trigeminal nucleus of the pigeon. *Brain Behav. Evol.* 8, 287–303. doi: 10.1159/000124359

Sjöqvist, O. (1938). Eine neue operationsmethode bei trigeminusneuralgie: durchschneidung des tractus spinalis trigemini. *Zentralbl. Neurochir.* 2, 274–281.

Slotty, P. J., Eisner, W., Honey, C. R., Wille, C., and Vesper, J. (2015). Long-term follow-up of motor cortex stimulation for neuropathic pain in 23 patients. *Stereotact. Funct. Neurosurg.* 93, 199–205. doi: 10.1159/000375177

Smith, R. L. (1975). Axonal projections and connections of the principal sensory trigeminal nucleus in the monkey. *J. Comp. Neurol.* 163, 347–375. doi: 10.1002/cne.901630307

Staud, R., Craggs, J. G., Robinson, M. E., Perlstein, W. M., and Price, D. D. (2007). Brain activity related to temporal summation of C-fiber evoked pain. *Pain* 129, 130–142. doi: 10.1016/j.pain.2006.10.010

Stein, B. E., Price, D. D., and Gazzaniga, M. S. (1989). Pain perception in a man with total corpus callosum transection. *Pain* 38, 51–56. doi: 10.1016/0304-3959(89)90072-9

Taber, E. (1961). The cytoarchitecture of the brain stem of the cat. I. Brain stem nuclei of cat. *J. Comp. Neurol.* 116, 27–69. doi: 10.1002/cne.901160104

Takemura, M., Nagase, Y., Yoshida, A., Yasuda, K., Kitamura, S., Shigenaga, Y., et al. (1993). The central projections of the monkey tooth pulp afferent neurons. *Somatosens. Mot. Res.* 10, 217–227. doi: 10.3109/08990229309028833

Taylor, A. M., Harris, A. D., Varnava, A., Phillips, R., Taylor, J. O., Hughes, O., et al. (2015). A functional magnetic resonance imaging study to investigate the utility of a picture imagination task in investigating neural responses in patients with chronic musculoskeletal pain to daily physical activity photographs. *PLoS One* 10:e0141133. doi: 10.1371/journal.pone.0141133

Torvik, A. (1957). The ascending fibers from the main trigeminal sensory nucleus. *Am. J. Anat.* 100, 1–15. doi: 10.1002/aja.1001000102

Tsubokawa, T., Katayama, Y., Yamamoto, T., Hirayama, T., and Koyama, S. (1991). Treatment of thalamic pain by chronic motor cortex stimulation. *Pacing Clin. Electrophysiol.* 14, 131–134. doi: 10.1111/j.1540-8159.1991.tb04058.x

Tsubokawa, T., Katayama, Y., Yamamoto, T., Hirayama, T., and Koyama, S. (1993). Chronic motor cortex stimulation in patients with thalamic pain. *J. Neurosurg.* 78, 393–401. doi: 10.3171/jns.1993.78.3.0393

Usunoff, K. G., Marani, E., and Schoen, J. H. R. (1997). *The Trigeminal System in Man.* Berlin, New York, NY: Springer.

Walker, A. E. (1939). The origin, course and termination of the secondary pathways of the trigeminal nerve in the primate. *J. Comp. Neurol.* 71, 59–89. doi: 10.1002/cne.900710105

Wallenberg, A. (1905). Sekundäre Bahnen aus den frontalen sensiblen Trigeminuskerne des Kaninchens. *Anat. Anz.* 26, 145–155.

Weigelt, A., Terekhin, P., Kemppainen, P., Dörfler, A., and Forster, C. (2010). The representation of experimental tooth pain from upper and lower jaws in the human trigeminal pathway. *Pain* 149, 529–538. doi: 10.1016/j.pain.2010.03.027

Wiech, K., Jbabdi, S., Lin, C. S., Andersson, J., and Tracey, I. (2014). Differential structural and resting state connectivity between insular subdivisions and other pain-related brain regions. *Pain* 155, 2047–2055. doi: 10.1016/j.pain.2014.07.009

Wiech, K., Kalisch, R., Weiskopf, N., Pleger, B., Stephan, K. E., and Dolan, R. J. (2006). Anterolateral prefrontal cortex mediates the analgesic effect of expected and perceived control over pain. *J. Neurosci.* 26, 11501–11509. doi: 10.1523/jneurosci.2568-06.2006

Wilcox, S. L., Gustin, S. M., Eykman, E. N., Fowler, G., Peck, C. C., Murray, G. M., et al. (2013). Trigeminal nerve anatomy in neuropathic and non-neuropathic orofacial pain patients. *J. Pain* 14, 865–872. doi: 10.1016/j.jpain.2013.02.014

Wilcox, S. L., Gustin, S. M., Macey, P. M., Peck, C. C., Murray, G. M., and Henderson, L. A. (2015). Anatomical changes at the level of the primary synapse in neuropathic pain: evidence from the spinal trigeminal nucleus. *J. Neurosci.* 35, 2508–2515. doi: 10.1523/JNEUROSCI.3756-14.2015

Williams, L. S., Schmalfuss, I. M., Sistrom, C. L., Inoue, T., Tanaka, R., Seoane, E. R., et al. (2003). MR imaging of the trigeminal ganglion, nerve and the perineural vascular plexus: normal appearance and variants with correlation to cadaver specimens. *AJNR Am. J. Neuroradiol.* 24, 1317–1323.

Woda, A., Azerad, J., and Albe-Fessard, D. (1977). Mapping of the trigeminal sensory complex of the cat. Characterization of its neurons by stimulations of peripheral field, dental pulp afferents and thalamic projections. *J. Physiol. (Paris)* 73, 367–378.

Woodburne, R. T. (1936). A phylogenetic consideration of the primary and secondary centers and connections of the trigeminal complex in a series of vertebrates. *J. Comp. Neurol.* 65, 403–501. doi: 10.1002/cne.900650113

Yágüez, L., Coen, S., Gregory, L. J., Amaro, E. Jr., Altman, C., Brammer, M. J., et al. (2005). Brain response to visceral aversive conditioning: a functional magnetic resonance imaging study. *Gastroenterology* 128, 1819–1829. doi: 10.1053/j.gastro.2005.02.068

Zeigler, H. P., and Witkovsky, P. (1968). The main sensory trigeminal nucleus in the pigeon: a single-unit analysis. *J. Comp. Neurol.* 134, 255–264. doi: 10.1002/cne.901340302

11

An *In vivo* Multi-Modal Structural Template for Neonatal Piglets using High Angular Resolution and Population-Based Whole-Brain Tractography

*Jidan Zhong[1], David Q. Chen[1,2], Matthew Walker[1,2], Adam Waspe[3], Thomas Looi[3], Karolina Piorkowska[3], James M. Drake[3,4] and Mojgan Hodaie[1,2,5]**

[1] Division of Brain, Imaging and Behaviour – Systems Neuroscience, Krembil Research Institute, University Health Network, Toronto, ON, Canada, [2] Institute of Medical Science, University of Toronto, Toronto, ON, Canada, [3] Centre for Image Guided Innovation and Therapeutic Intervention, The Hospital for Sick Children, Toronto, ON, Canada, [4] Division of Neurosurgery, The Hospital for Sick Children, Toronto, ON, Canada, [5] Division of Neurosurgery, Toronto Western Hospital – University of Toronto, Toronto, ON, Canada

***Correspondence:**
Mojgan Hodaie
mojgan.hodaie@uhn.ca

An increasing number of applications use the postnatal piglet model in neuroimaging studies, however, these are based primarily on T1 weighted image templates. There is a growing need for a multimodal structural brain template for a comprehensive depiction of the piglet brain, particularly given the growing applications of diffusion weighted imaging for characterizing tissue microstructures and white matter organization. In this study, we present the first multimodal piglet structural brain template which includes a T1 weighted image with tissue segmentation probability maps, diffusion weighted metric templates with multiple diffusivity maps, and population-based whole-brain fiber tracts for postnatal piglets. These maps provide information about the integrity of white matter that is not available in T1 images alone. The availability of this diffusion weighted metric template will contribute to the structural imaging analysis of the postnatal piglet brain, especially models that are designed for the study of white matter diseases. Furthermore, the population-based whole-brain fiber tracts permit researchers to visualize the white matter connections in the piglet brain across subjects, guiding the delineation of a specific white matter region for structural analysis where current diffusion data is lacking. Researchers are able to augment the tracts by merging tracts from their own data to the population-based fiber tracts and thus improve the confidence of the population-wise fiber distribution.

Keywords: neonatal piglet, template, multi-modal, diffusion imaging, population-based whole-brain fiber tracts

INTRODUCTION

The domestic piglet is a common animal model for translational research in pediatric neuroscience because of its neuroanatomical commonalities with the human brain (Lind et al., 2007; Sauleau et al., 2009; Mendl et al., 2010; Gieling et al., 2011), with respect to the morphological shape of the piglet brain including the gyral and sulcal pattern, and the rapid period of brain growth lasting from late prenatal to early postnatal (Dickerson and Dobbing, 1967; Thibault and Margulies, 1998). There is an additional advantage in that the piglet brain is of sufficient size to allow *in vivo* multimodal imaging and facilitates surgical procedures and electrode placement (Sauleau et al., 2009).

Previous imaging research based on imaging analysis of multiple piglets has required manual evaluation at the individual level due to lack of a common template (Conrad et al., 2012; Radlowski et al., 2014). Conrad et al. (2012) performed intensive manual segmentation of individual brain regions of interest (ROIs) over seven longitudinal scans of 15 piglets. Saikali et al. (2010) published a high-resolution surface-based three-dimensional (3D) digital template of a female pig (Sus scrofa domesticus), segmented into 178 cerebral structures. This template proved useful for localizing brain areas for the purposes of functional magnetic resonance imaging (MRI) studies or electrode implantation trials. However, the template was constructed based on a single brain of a 6-month old pig. This creates important limitations in its use since age results in a significant difference in the total brain volume (TBV) as well as the proportion of cortical volume over TBV in pigs (Conrad et al., 2012). In order to address this deficiency, two additional templates have been published recently, based on T1 images from neonatal piglets. Conrad et al. (2014) generated an *in vivo* 3D T1 template of the neonatal piglet (4-week old, Sus scrofa). Still, this template lacks adequate sulcal and gyral information because linear registration was performed to generate the template and non-linear deformation fields were only applied to compensate for template shape or morphology. Gan et al. (2014) generated a T1 template based on a group of neonatal piglets (38 days old, Suscrofa × Landrace × Large White F1). The Gan template shows improved gray matter/white matter (GM/WM) contrast, however, important anatomical areas such as the optic chiasm and bulbus olfactorius needed to be removed to allow for better positional accuracy, limiting the usability of this template. Importantly, both the Conrad and Gan templates provide very limited identification of specific WM tracts, since they are based on T1 images which provide a homogeneous WM appearance (Toga et al., 2006).

The limitations of the existing templates clarify the need for a multi-modal template for the neonatal pig that includes information on WM tracts. The most advantageous technique that permits information on WM tracts is diffusion weighted MR imaging (DWI). This technique non-invasively measures the diffusivity of water molecules and characterizes the integrity of white matter fibers within the tissue based on diffusion orientation information (Basser et al., 1994). By modeling the directional diffusion of water as an ellipsoid, or "tensor", quantitative information is provided, such as axial diffusivity (AD), radial diffusivity (RD; Song et al., 2003), mean diffusivity (MD; Cercignani et al., 2000) and fractional anisotropy (FA; Basser and Pierpaoli, 1996). With this technique, white matter has been shown to be implicated in children and adolescents in a wide range of disorders, including autism spectrum disorder (Mak-Fan et al., 2013; Conti et al., 2015), attention deficit hyperactivity disorder (ADHD; Lawrence et al., 2013) and Turner syndrome (Villalon-Reina et al., 2013). Other than quantitative measures, diffusion tractography derived from DWI is also a powerful measure to aid image interpretation through visualization of the orientation and 3D course of white matter tracts (Hiltunen et al., 2005). It helps clarify the architecture of tissues by integrating the estimates of voxel-based diffusion maximums (Feldman et al., 2010; Alexander et al., 2011). It also allows visualization of specific fiber connections and comparison across individuals (Witwer et al., 2002; Yeatman et al., 2009), definition of specific ROIs (Schlaier et al., 2015), as well as characterization of connectivity properties (e.g., fiber density and fiber count) between ROIs (Kim et al., 2011).

There is a clear paucity of literature exploring tractography in the piglet model. A few studies have applied diffusion imaging to detect brain WM alterations in piglets through comparison of FA values, as a consequence of low birth weight (Radlowski et al., 2014), perinatal choline deficiency (Mudd et al., 2015) and dietary treatment (Mudd et al., 2016). Winter et al. (2011) assessed the microstructural changes during pig brain development by measuring MD and FA values. However, none of the studies have reported tractography results. Furthermore, their relatively small number of direction of their diffusion-encoding gradient ($\leq$30) made it hard to resolve the crossing fibers (Tournier et al., 2011). High angular resolution diffusion imaging (HARDI) techniques allow reconstruction of more accurate models for the diffusion process to resolve multiple fiber routes in the same voxel, and thus provide a more accurate WM geometry in the brain (Alexander et al., 2002; Tuch et al., 2002). Thus, tractography that is based on HARDI in the piglet brain allows *in vivo* visualization of WM connections with more accurate presentation of crossing fibers, and can also guide specific ROI delineation and brain anatomy dissection for structural analysis.

Overall, a multi-modal template incorporating T1, DWI metrics and tractography would allow a comprehensive, multi-modal depiction of the piglet brain and serve as an important reference for piglet brain imaging studies. Our present study reports the creation of a multi-modal piglet brain template that includes T1, DWI metric map and population-based whole-brain fiber tracts. Each of the modalities provides an important component to the template. T1 images provide good contrast between GM and WM, and diffusion metrics characterize the integrity of white matter fibers. These metric maps also allow the possibility of advanced automated structural analysis to investigate the WM changes at the voxel-level. Furthermore, the population-based whole-brain fiber tracts can provide valuable information on WM connections across subjects, with fiber reliability and variability estimated through the inter-subject consistency of the fibers.

MATERIALS AND METHODS

Ethics Statement

These experiments were approved by the Animal Care Committee and Lab Animal Services at the Hospital for Sick Children. This study follows the Canadian Council on Animal Care (CCAC) standards.

Piglet *In vivo* Models

Eight male Yorkshire piglets of 22 ± 6 days old (body weight: 6.1 ± 1.2 kg) were used in this study. All piglets were housed in pairs in a temperature- and humidity-controlled environment with a 12-h light/dark cycle and fed with a commercial piglet milk replacer prior to MRI scanning. The piglets were euthanized by intravenous injection of pentobarbital sodium (120 mg/kg) upon the completion of all imaging procedures and while under general anesthesia.

Magnetic Resonance Imaging

The animals were pre-anesthetized with a Ketamine (10 mg/kg) solution intramuscularly, intubated and maintained under anesthesia with 2.5% isoflurane and 2 L of oxygen delivered via MRI-compatible ventilator during the MRI scanning. Heart rate and oxygen saturation were monitored and a circulating water blanket was used to maintain core body temperature of 37°C. The animals were placed prone and head first on the diagnostic table. In the Philips Achieva 3T MR scanner, a 32-channel receive-only head coil was placed around the head to provide MR imaging. A three-dimensional T1-weighted magnetization prepared gradient echo (MPRAGE) sequence was used. The sequence parameters were: repetition time (TR) = 8.15 ms, echo time (TE) = 3.72 ms, flip angle = 8°, matrix = 224 × 224, field of view (FOV) = 224 mm × 224 mm, slice thickness = 1.00 mm.

The diffusion-weighted images were collected with a spin-echo single-shot echo-planar imaging (EPI) sequence using sensitivity encoding (SENSE; TR = 5844.97 ms; TE = 105.90 ms; flip angle = 90°; matrix = 128 × 128, FOV = 205 mm × 205 mm; slice thickness/spacing = 1.60/1.60 mm; SENSE reduction factor = 2) with a b-value of 800 s/mm^2 along 128 directions. A baseline image with b = 0 s/mm^2 (b0 image) was acquired for both forward and reverse phase encoding directions.

Image Processing

T1 Template Generation

To minimize the manual work for the brain mask delineation, template generation was initiated with manual registration of the individual T1 images to the Conrad T1 template to provide a general individual brain mask using 3D Slicer (version 4.4)[1]. The mask was then manually corrected to remove possible remaining non-brain tissue (e.g., extra skull and cerebral spinal fluid (CSF) between the skull and brain). The T1 brain images were then collected to generate a population-averaged template using symmetric diffeomorphic registration (SyN) with Automated Normalization Tools (ANTs; Avants et al., 2011b). The template was then reoriented along a line connecting the centers of the anterior and posterior commissure (y-axis). The origin was set to be the anterior limit of the posterior commissure in the midsagittal plane, consistent with published pig templates (Felix et al., 1999; Watanabe et al., 2001; Saikali et al., 2010; Conrad et al., 2014; Gan et al., 2014). The FMRIB's Automated Segmentation Tool (FAST) of FSL (Analysis Group, FMRIB, Oxford, UK)[2] was applied to segment the individual brains into GM, WM, and CSF. The probability map for each segmentation was then transformed to the final template and averaged. To calculate the individual brain volume, the brain mask of the final T1 template was transformed back to individual space based on the transformation field generated during the template generation.

Landmark Variation

Distance variations between the individual subject and the template were calculated to validate the template. The anterior and posterior extents of the corpus callosum (CC), and the anterior extent of the posterior commissure were picked as the landmarks. These landmarks were transformed into the template space based on the registration and their spatial locations were compared to the template to compute the landmark variation. Mean (±standard deviation), minimum and maximum distances between individuals and the template in the landmarks were calculated in Matlab (version 2014b, MathWorks, Natick, MA, USA).

DWI Process

The DWI sequences were corrected for distortions induced by susceptibility-induced off-resonance field using "Topup" in FSL (Andersson et al., 2003). Following this, the images were aligned to their b0 images with an affine registration to correct for eddy-current and motion distortions using FLIRT in FSL (Jenkinson et al., 2002). Additionally, the gradient vectors were corrected with the appropriate rotational component of the motion correction to ensure that errors in the diffusion weighting that originate from these rotations could be minimized (Leemans and Jones, 2009). The data were resampled for a final voxel size of 1 mm × 1 mm × 1 mm. Diffusion tensors (DTs) were fitted at each voxel to calculate scalar maps: FA, AD, RD, and MD.

To perform whole-brain fiber tracking with the MRtrix software package (Brain Research Institute, Melbourne, VIC, Australia[3]), an intra-subject T1 to DWI space transformation was obtained through manual registration using FA as the feature using 3D Slicer. Individual brain masks were transformed from T1 space to DWI space to be the mask for whole brain tractography.

The response function for a single fiber population was estimated for those voxels with a FA > 0.3 using an iterative optimization method proposed by Tax et al. (2014). The response function was then used for constrained spherical deconvolution to accurately estimate the fiber orientation distribution (FOD; Tournier et al., 2007). Fibers were then generated with a deterministic tracking algorithm, referred as SD-Stream, that follows the orientation of the nearest FOD peak at each step (Tournier et al., 2012). The algorithm generated 10,000 fibers of minimum length 5 mm. Other tracking parameters included a step size of 0.1 mm, minimum radius of curvature of 1 mm and FOD cutoff of 0.2. All voxels in the white matter mask segmented in the previous mentioned step were used as seeds and the tracking procedure was stopped if a fiber reached a voxel outside the mask or if a stopping criterion was met (high

[1] https://www.slicer.org/

[2] http://fsl.fmrib.ox.ac.uk/fsl/fslwiki/

[3] http://www.brain.org.au/software/

fiber curvature or low FOD). To reduce the size of the data, we decreased the density of the points along the length of the streamline by half. Finally, all the scalar values (FA, AD, RD, and MD) were interpolated at each point of the fibers.

Based on the intra-subject registration between T1 and DWI and the inter-subject registration between T1 and the T1 template, all scalar maps were transformed into the template space and averaged to be the corresponding metric template. Using software developed in-house that non-linearly deforms fiber tracts based on the registration transformations, the individual whole-brain fiber tracts were transformed into the template space and merged as population-based whole-brain fiber tracts. The scalar information was also kept on the population fiber tracts.

Application: ROI-Specific Fiber Tracts

Specific ROI-based fiber tracts were extracted from the population-based whole-brain fiber tracts. The ROIs include genu and splenium of the CC, optic chiasm, fornix and middle cerebellar peduncle. 3D Slicer was used to extract the fibers passing through specific fibers.

Statistical Analysis

Mean (±standard deviation) body weight, age and brain size of the piglets used to generate the templates were calculated in Matlab (version 2014b, MathWorks, Natick, MA, USA).

RESULTS

Animal Modal Parameters

The average age of the eight piglets was 22 days (range: 17∼35 days old). The average brain size of the piglets was 65500 ± 3806 mm^3, and the template brain size was 67294 mm^3. For the six pigs used to generate the DWI related template, the average body weight, age, and brain size were 6.5 ± 1.2 kg, 23 ± 6 days old and 66434 ± 3927 mm^3. The body weight, age and brain size of the eight piglets used to generate T1 template are shown in **Table 1**.

TABLE 1 | Body weight, age and brain size information of the piglets used for T1 template and DWI template generation.

Pig index	Body weight (kg)	Age (days)	Brain size (mm^3)	Template generation
1	4.9	17	61606	T1
2	5.0	19	63787	T1
3	5.1	18	62279	T1, DWI
4	8.3	35	73946	T1, DWI
5	6.7	21	65359	T1, DWI
6	7.1	21	68884	T1, DWI
7	5.3	21	63573	T1, DWI
8	6.3	21	64563	T1, DWI
Avg for T1	6.1 ± 1.2	22 ± 6	65500 ± 3806	–
Avg for DWI	6.5 ± 1.2	23 ± 6	66434 ± 3927	–

Avg for T1- Average of the demographic information over the pigs used to generate the T1 template; Avg for DWI- Average of the demographic information over the pigs used to generate the diffusion related template.

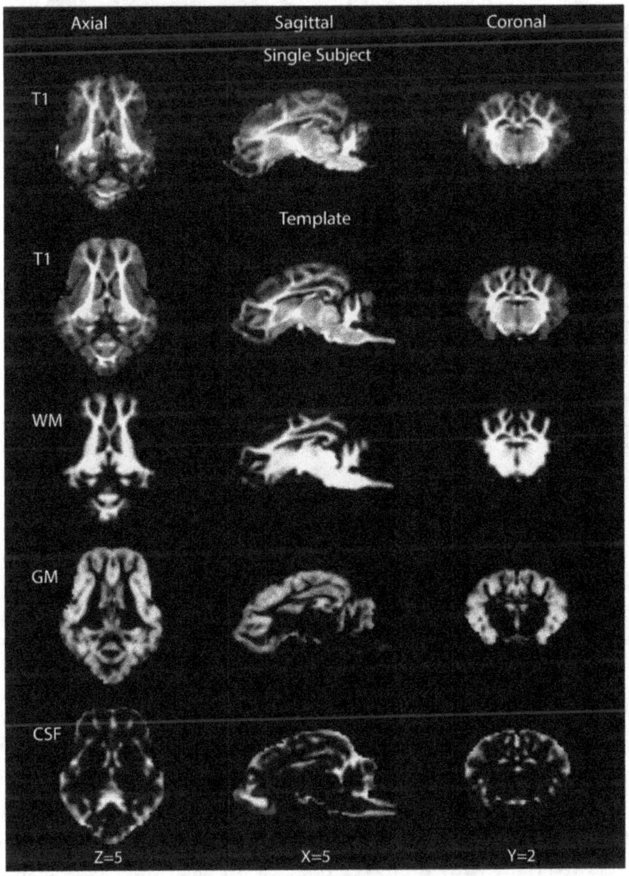

FIGURE 1 | Single subject T1 image (row 1) and template T1 image (row 2) are shown in the axial ($Z = 5$), sagittal ($X = 5$) and coronal ($Y = 2$) views. Rows 3∼5 show tissue probability maps for white matter (WM), gray matter (GM) and cerebrospinal fluid (CSF) in the template space.

T1 Template and Segmentation

The brain pattern is well preserved in the final T1 template brain compared to that of a single subject T1 image (**Figure 1**, row 1). The final T1 template brain is shown in **Figure 1** (row 2) in the axial, coronal and sagittal views. Qualitatively, the outline of brain structures and GM/WM contrast are clearer in the template than in the single subject. Based on the intensity differences, the T1 brain image could be segmented into GM, WM and CSF. **Figure 1**, rows 3–5 shows the probability maps of GM, WM and CSF in the template space.

T1 Template Validation

The maximum distance was 1.73 mm for one subject at the posterior CC, while the mean distances across subjects were smaller than 1 mm for all three landmarks. The differences between coordinates in selected landmarks are shown in **Table 2**.

DWI Template

DWI metric templates, including FA, AD, RD, and MD maps, were generated (**Figure 2**). **Figure 3** shows the population-based

TABLE 2 | The distance differences between individuals and the template in selected landmarks.

	Distance, mm (mean ± SD)	Max distance, mm	Min distance, mm
Anterior CC	0.85 ± 0.52	1.41	0
Posterior CC	0.72 ± 0.60	1.73	0
Anterior end of posterior commissure	0.50 ± 0.50	1.00	0

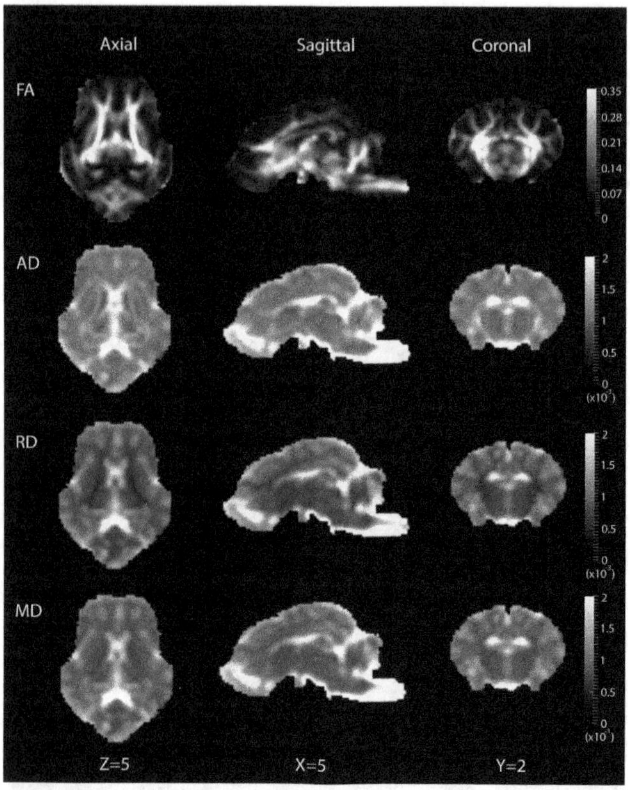

FIGURE 2 | Diffusion metric templates with FA, AD, RD and MD maps are shown in the axial (*Z* = 5), sagittal (*X* = 5) and coronal (*Y* = 2) views.

whole-brain fiber tracts transformed from individual space, with each color representing fibers from each individual. The top row shows the fibers from a single subject in the template space. In general, the whole brain fibers from different subjects were overlapped in the template space. **Figure 4** shows the merged tracts overlaid with the DWI metrics on each fiber. Consistent with the DWI metric maps, FA values on the fiber tracts were higher in the regions with highly aligned structures, such as the CC, fornix, and trigeminal nerve. On the contrary, AD, RD and MD values were higher in the regions with more fluid, such as olfactory bulbs, ventricles and cisterns.

ROI-Based Tracts

The ROI-specific tracts were extracted from the population-based whole-brain tracts, including tracts from the fornix, optic chiasm, middle cerebellar peduncle, genu and splenium of the CC (**Figure 5**). Column 1 and 3 represent fibers colored by the direction of the tensor and FA values, separately. Column 2 represents fibers colored by individual identities, showing that the tracts from restricted ROIs were consistently present across subjects. Specifically, the fornix could be visualized as the C-shaped fiber bundle from its body, approximately at the level of the anterior commissure, and reaching to the level of the crura. The crossing fibers of the optic chiasm were clearly visualized. The middle cerebellar peduncle fibers were visualized with projections deep into the cerebellum. Similarly, the genu of the CC projections to the bilateral dorsolateral prefrontal region were also seen, with fibers visualized distally and approaching the cortex. For the splenium, the majority of the tracts traveled along the external boundary of lateral ventricles, bilaterally to the temporal lobe (tapetum of the CC), while few tracts traveled to the visual cortex (forceps major).

This template images and tractography are available online[4], and can be visualized in 3D Slicer.

DISCUSSION

In this study, we present the first multi-modal piglet brain structural MR template. This template shares the same coordinate origin with existing piglet templates, thus allows for compatibility of the results based on different templates. The T1 template includes tissue segmentation probability maps, which allow for single image segmentation as *a priori* input. The DWI metric template, in the same space as the T1 template, includes FA, AD, RD, and MD maps. These maps make feasible the possibility for gathering a wealth of information on the integrity of WM that is otherwise not available in a T1 template. Over the tracts explored through specific ROIs, similarity of fiber arrangements between piglets and humans are found in the fornix, optic chiasm, the genu of the CC and middle cerebellar peduncles, while different shape is found in the splenium of the CC. The availability of population-based whole-brain fiber tracts allows visualization of the white matter connections at the group level, exploration of specific connections of interest, estimation of their reliability based on the inter-subject consistency, as well as guidance for specific ROI delineation. Additional data from new studies could also be added to this existing population-based fiber tracts to augment the tracts, and thus improve the confidence of the population-wise fiber distribution.

T1 Template

Compared to the existing two piglet T1 templates, this T1 template includes higher GM/WM contrast retaining more detailed information than the one from Conrad et al. (2014) and is more comprehensive, including both the optic chiasm and olfactory bulb, relative to the one generated by Gan et al. (2014).

A standard coordinate system is important for brain research, where reported brain locations could be easily compared across studies and imaging modalities. In order to maintain consistency

[4]http://www.hodaielab.com/resources.html

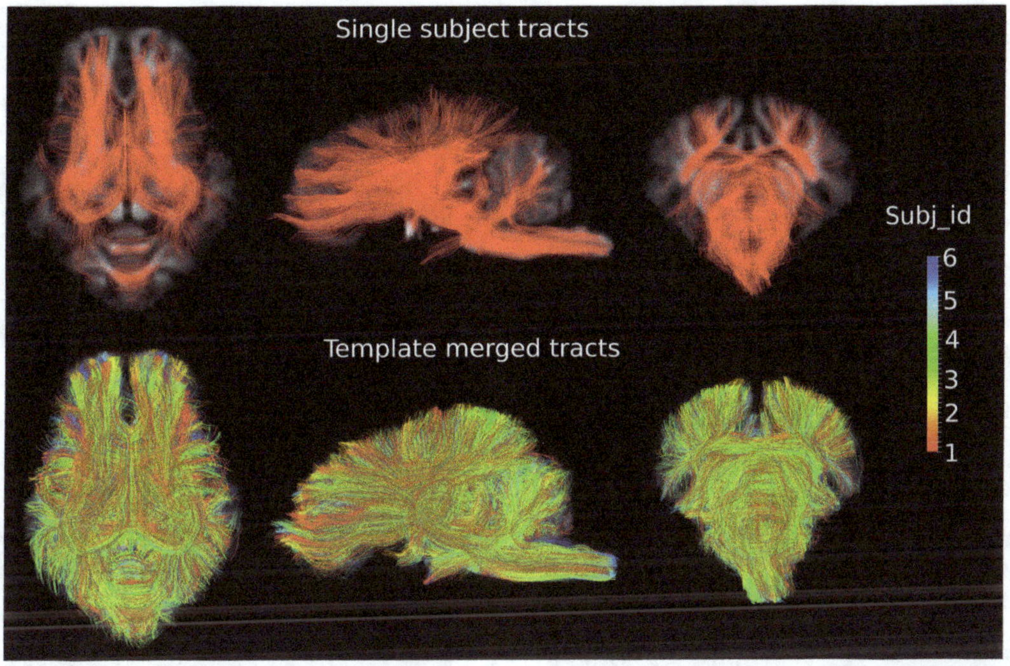

FIGURE 3 | Fiber tracts from a single subject and a group of subjects are shown in the axial ($Z = 3$), sagittal ($X = 0$) and coronal ($Y = -1$) views in the template space, with the template T1 image as the background. Different colors represent the fibers from different individuals.

with other templates (Felix et al., 1999; Watanabe et al., 2001; Saikali et al., 2010; Conrad et al., 2014; Gan et al., 2014), we set the same origin at the anterior limit of the posterior commissure in the midsagittal plane. This eases the comparison of results from studies with different templates. The validation results presented show only a small deviation (≤ 1 voxel) between the template and each individual brains. Probability maps of segmentation are also presented here to serve as *a priori* input to aid future single image segmentation.

DWI Template

Diffusion templates introduced for humans (Mori et al., 2008; Verhoeven et al., 2010; Wang et al., 2011), primates (Adluru et al., 2012; Zakszewski et al., 2014) and rats (Rumple et al., 2013), have played an important role in subsequent ROI-delineation and brain registration (Zhang et al., 2010; Turken and Dronkers, 2011; Vetreno et al., 2015). To date there has been no DWI metric template introduced for the piglet brain, which limits any significant level of information about WM anatomy. In this study, the DWI metric template was generated based on six piglets, providing voxel-wise diffusion information. The different scalar maps could be used as a template for brain normalization. Volumetric-based morphometry analysis of a DWI metric map can also be accomplished with this template.

In this study, with the conjunction uses of HARDI and the method proposed by Tournier et al. (2007) to determine the FOD, orientations that are separated by small angles could be resolved. The fiber tract model thus could represent crossing fibers reliably, e.g., the optic chiasm (**Figure 5**). The population-based whole-brain fiber tracts were generated through transformation of individual streamlines into the template space. These tracts thus represent homologous white matter connections between individual animals. The tracts connecting the same regions are highly overlapped across individuals, reflecting consistency of tracts across subjects (**Figures 3** and **5**), and suggesting that the inter-subject template registrations are within an acceptable range. On the contrary, tracts that show less overlaps may indicate higher structural variability across subjects or lower consistency from tracts generation. Merged tracts are different from tracts generated based on an average diffusion template (Verhoeven et al., 2010; Adluru et al., 2012; Zakszewski et al., 2014), where individual subject diffusion orientation information would have been lost. Furthermore, as the population-based tracts preserve individual tracts information, researchers are able to merge tracts from their own data to the population-based tracts. With the augmented fiber tracts from more subjects, the degree of consistency of the population-wise fiber distribution may be visualized and inspected more confidently.

Specific ROI analysis shows that fiber morphology is analogous in piglets to humans in the fornix (Chen et al., 2015; Kehoe et al., 2015), optic chiasm (Hofer et al., 2010), the genu of the CC (Verde et al., 2014) and middle cerebellar peduncles (Chanraud et al., 2009). However, the shape of the fibers passing through the splenium of the CC is different in piglets and humans. The majority of the splenium fibers project to the visual cortex (called forceps major) while other fibers were part of the tapetum that extended laterally into the temporal lobe in adult human brains (Hofer et al., 2010; Miller et al., 2011; Turken and Dronkers, 2011) as well as neonates (Gilmore et al., 2007; De Bruïne et al., 2011). However,

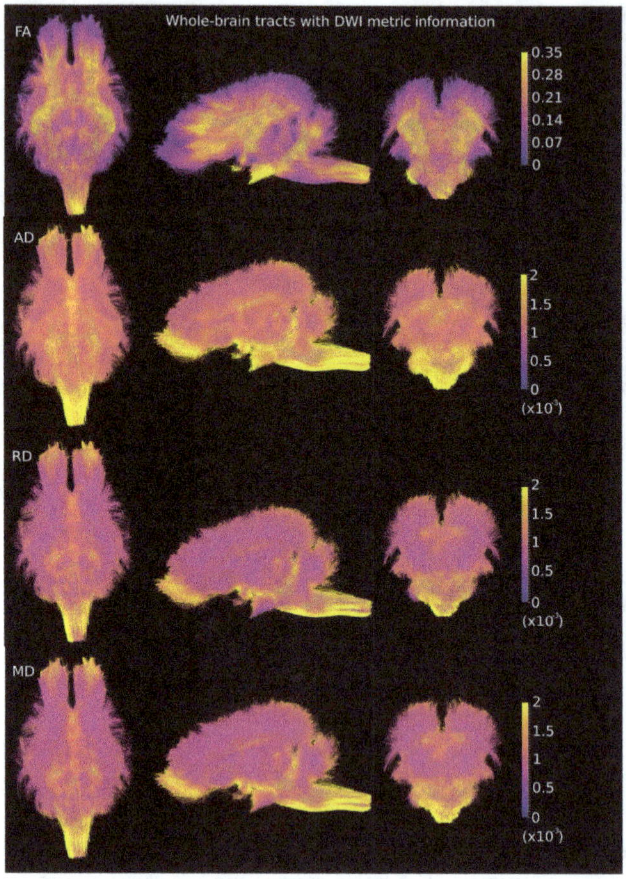

FIGURE 4 | Merged whole-brain fiber tracts overlaid with DWI metrics (with the same value scale as in Figure 2) in the axial, sagittal and coronal views. Brighter color represents higher values.

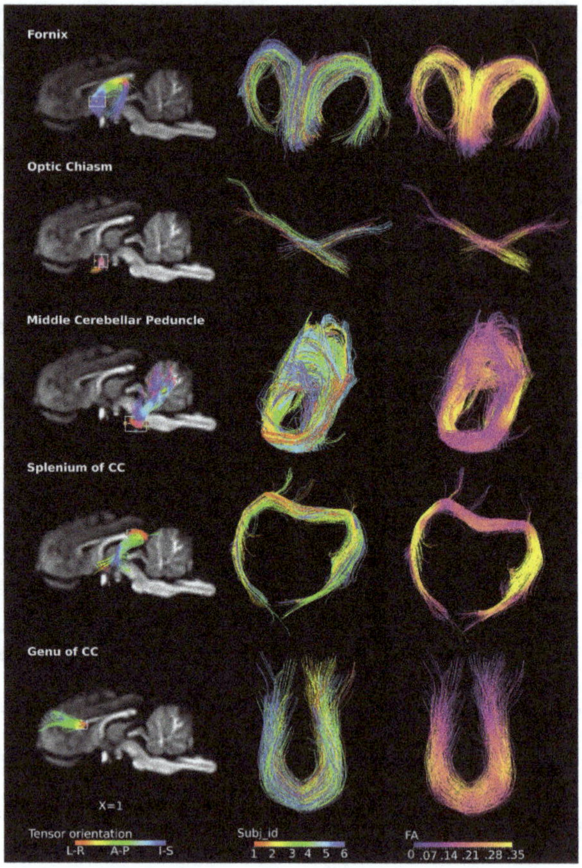

FIGURE 5 | ROI-specific fibers from fornix, optic chiasm, middle cerebellar peduncle, and splenium and genu of CC. Column 1 shows the location of the ROIs with a rectangular box, the overlaid fiber tracts are colored by the tensor orientation. Column 2 shows the extracted fibers, with each color representing fibers from each individual. Column 3 shows the extracted fibers colored by the FA values, with brighter color representing higher FA values.

in the piglets, the majority of these fibers form the tapetum, with only a small portion of the tracts projecting to the visual cortex (**Figure 5**). The discrepancy is expected as many brain structural differences exist between the two species (Sauleau et al., 2009). For example, the telencephalon of the pig brain is less curved than that of the human brain (Sauleau et al., 2009).

Subject Age and Size

The newborn human brain is approximately 36% the size of the adult human brain. With a fast growth speed, the TBV reaches ~72% of adult brain size at 1 year, and ~83% at 2 years (Knickmeyer et al., 2008). A similar developmental curve until the maximum is present in the pigs. It is suggested that the piglets reached its maximum brain growth rate at around week 4, when the TBV reached 50% of its maximum, and reached 95% of its maximum by 21–23 weeks of age (Conrad et al., 2012). The age of our piglets is between 17 and 35 days, with an average of 22 days old. The brain size of our piglets is similar to that of the piglets at around 2–5 weeks reported by Conrad et al. (2012). Thus, our template represents the brain with a total volume at around 50% of its maximum brain volume.

Limitations

The major limitation is that we have a small number of subjects to generate the population-averaged template. However, it has been previously reported that a template stabilizes at around 10 subjects for most human populations based on observations (Avants et al., 2011a). As one of the ungulates, piglets show less complicated convolutional pattern of the brain than humans (Turner, 1890; Welker, 1990; Roth and Dicke, 2005), this eight-subject-based template should therefore be a good representation of brain morphology and its variability of the normal population at this weight range. The mean squared difference comparison between 8-subject-based-template and 2-, 4-, 6-, 8-subject-based templates showed that the templates perceive small differences between the 6-subject-based and 8-subject-based templates (Supplementary Material, Table S1 and

Figure S1). Thus, although the sample size is small, the 6-subject-based DWI metric template can serve as a template for the normal piglets at this weight range. Furthermore, the fiber tracts were merged instead of averaged across subjects, extra number of subjects would not influence existing fiber locations or shape. Researchers can augment the tracts by merging tracts from their own data to the population-based tracts. To our knowledge, our atlas template study is the first study investigating the white matter connections of the piglet brain. The population-based fiber tracts presented here will facilitate ROI delineation study of the piglet brain.

AUTHOR CONTRIBUTIONS

All authors contributed to this work. The ideas of the manuscript were discussed with the whole project team. JZ, MW, AW, KP, and TL collected the data. JZ wrote the manuscript. DC, AW, KP, JD, MW, and MH commented on the manuscript and gave conceptual advice at the final stage.

ACKNOWLEDGMENT

We thank Marvin Estrada, Anson Lam in Lab Animal Services for their technical help with the animal care.

REFERENCES

Adluru, N., Zhang, H., Fox, A. S., Shelton, S. E., Ennis, C. M., Bartosic, A. M., et al. (2012). A diffusion tensor brain template for rhesus macaques. *Neuroimage* 59, 306–318. doi: 10.1016/j.neuroimage.2011.07.029

Alexander, A. L., Hurley, S. A., Samsonov, A. A., Adluru, N., Hosseinbor, A. P., Mossahebi, P., et al. (2011). Characterization of cerebral white matter properties using quantitative magnetic resonance imaging stains. *Brain Connect.* 1, 423–446. doi: 10.1089/brain.2011.0071

Alexander, D. C., Barker, G. J., and Arridge, S. R. (2002). Detection and modeling of non-gaussian apparent diffusion coefficient profiles in human brain data. *Magn. Reson. Med.* 48, 331–340. doi: 10.1002/mrm.10209

Andersson, J. L. R., Skare, S., and Ashburner, J. (2003). How to correct susceptibility distortions in spin-echo echo-planar images: application to diffusion tensor imaging. *Neuroimage* 20, 870–888. doi: 10.1016/S1053-8119(03)00336-7

Avants, B. B., Tustison, N., and Song, G. (2011a). *Advanced Normalization Tools (ANTS)*:1–35. Available at: https://sourceforge.net/projects/advants/files/Documentation/ants.pdf

Avants, B. B., Tustison, N. J., Song, G., Cook, P. A., Klein, A., and Gee, C. (2011b). A Reproducible evaluation of ANTs similarity metric performance in brain image registration. *Neuroimage* 54, 2033–2044. doi: 10.1016/j.neuroimage.2010.09.025

Basser, P. J., Mattiello, J., and LeBihan, D. (1994). MR diffusion tensor spectroscopy and imaging. *Biophys. J.* 66, 259–267. doi: 10.1016/S0006-3495(94)80775-1

Basser, P. J., and Pierpaoli, C. (1996). Microstructural and physiological features of tissues elucidated by quantitative-diffusion-tensor MRI. *J. Magn. Reson.* 111, 209–219. doi: 10.1006/jmrb.1996.0086

Cercignani, M., Iannucci, G., Rocca, M. A., Comi, G., Horsfield, M. A., and Filippi, M. (2000). Pathologic damage in MS assessed by diffusion-weighted and magnetization transfer MRI. *Neurology* 54, 1139–1144. doi: 10.1212/WNL.54.5.1139

Chanraud, S., Reynaud, M., Wessa, M., Penttilä, J., Kostogianni, N., Cachia, A., et al. (2009). Diffusion tensor tractography in mesencephalic bundles: relation to mental flexibility in detoxified alcohol-dependent subjects. *Neuropsychopharmacology* 34, 1223–1232. doi: 10.1038/npp.2008.101

Chen, D. Q., Strauss, I., Hayes, D. J., Davis, K. D., and Hodaie, M. (2015). Age-related changes in diffusion tensor imaging metrics of fornix subregions in healthy humans. *Stereotact. Funct. Neurosurg.* 93, 151–159. doi: 10.1159/000368442

Conrad, M. S., Dilger, R. N., and Johnson, R. W. (2012). Brain growth of the domestic pig (*Sus scrofa*) from 2 to 24 weeks of age: a longitudinal MRI study. *Dev. Neurosci.* 34, 291–298. doi: 10.1159/000339311

Conrad, M. S., Sutton, B. P., Dilger, R. N., and Johnson, R. W. (2014). An in vivo three-dimensional magnetic resonance imaging-based averaged brain collection of the neonatal piglet (*Sus scrofa*). *PLoS ONE* 9:e107650. doi: 10.1371/journal.pone.0107650

Conti, E., Calderoni, S., Gaglianese, A., Pannek, K., Mazzotti, S., Rose, S., et al. (2015). Lateralization of brain networks and clinical severity in toddlers with autism spectrum disorder: a hardi diffusion MRI study. *Autism Res.* 9, 382–392. doi: 10.1002/aur.1533

De Bruïne, F. T., Van Wezel-Meijler, G., Leijser, L. M., Van Den Berg-Huysmans, A. A., Van Steenis, A., Van Buchem, M. A., et al. (2011). Tractography of developing white matter of the internal capsule and corpus callosum in very preterm infants. *Eur. Radiol.* 21, 538–547. doi: 10.1007/s00330-010-1945-x

Dickerson, J. W. T., and Dobbing, J. (1967). Prenatal and postnatal growth and development of the central nervous system of the pig. *Proc. R. Soc. Lond. B Biol. Sci.* 166, 384–395. doi: 10.1098/rspb.1967.0002

Feldman, H. M., Yeatman, J. D., Lee, E. S., Barde, L. H. F., and Gaman-Bean, S. (2010). Diffusion tensor imaging: a review for pediatric researchers and clinicians. *J. Dev. Behav. Pediatr.* 31, 346–356. doi: 10.1097/DBP.0b013e3181dcaa8b

Felix, B., Léger, M. E., Albe-Fessard, D., Marcilloux, J. C., Rampin, O., Laplace, J. P., et al. (1999). Stereotaxic atlas of the pig brain. *Brain Res. Bull.* 49, 1–137. doi: 10.1016/S0361-9230(99)00012-X

Gan, H., Zhang, Q., Zhang, H., Chen, Y., Lin, J., Kang, T., et al. (2014). Development of new population-averaged standard templates for spatial normalization and segmentation of MR images for postnatal piglet brains. *Magn. Reson. Imaging* 32, 1396–1402. doi: 10.1016/j.mri.2014.08.036

Gieling, E. T., Nordquist, R. E., and van der Staay, F. J. (2011). Assessing learning and memory in pigs. *Anim. Cogn.* 14, 151–173. doi: 10.1007/s10071-010-0364-3

Gilmore, J. H., Lin, W., Corouge, I., Vetsa, Y. S. K., Smith, J. K., Kang, C., et al. (2007). Early postnatal development of corpus callosum and corticospinal white matter assessed with quantitative tractography. *Am. J. Neuroradiol.* 28, 1789–1795. doi: 10.3174/ajnr.A0751

Hiltunen, J., Suortti, T., Arvela, S., Seppä, M., Joensuu, R., and Hari, R. (2005). Diffusion tensor imaging and tractography of distal peripheral nerves at 3 T. *Clin. Neurophysiol.* 116, 2315–2323. doi: 10.1016/j.clinph.2005.05.014

Hofer, S., Karaus, A., and Frahm, J. (2010). Reconstruction and dissection of the entire human visual pathway using diffusion tensor MRI. *Front. Neuroanat.* 4:15. doi: 10.3389/fnana.2010.00015

Jenkinson, M., Bannister, P., Brady, M., and Smith, S. (2002). Improved optimization for the robust and accurate linear registration and motion correction of brain images. *Neuroimage* 17, 825–841. doi: 10.1006/nimg.2002.1132

Kehoe, E. G., Farrell, D., Metzler-Baddeley, C., Lawlor, B. A., Kenny, R. A., Lyons, D., et al. (2015). Fornix white matter is correlated with resting-state functional connectivity of the thalamus and hippocampus in healthy aging but not in mild cognitive impairment–a preliminary study. *Front. Aging Neurosci.* 7:10. doi: 10.3389/fnagi.2015.00010

Kim, D.-J., Skosnik, P. D., Cheng, H., Pruce, B. J., Brumbaugh, M. S., Vollmer, J. M., et al. (2011). Structural network topology revealed by white matter tractography in cannabis users: a graph theoretical analysis. *Brain Connect.* 1, 473–483. doi: 10.1089/brain.2011.0053

Knickmeyer, R. C., Gouttard, S., Kang, C., Evans, D., Wilber, K., Smith, J. K., et al. (2008). A structural MRI study of human brain development from birth to 2 years. *J. Neurosci.* 28, 12176–12182. doi: 10.1523/JNEUROSCI.3479-08.2008

Lawrence, K. E., Levitt, J. G., Loo, S. K., Ly, R., Yee, V., O'Neill, J., et al. (2013). White matter microstructure in subjects with attention-deficit/hyperactivity disorder and their siblings. *J. Am. Acad. Child Adolesc. Psychiatry* 52, 431–440.e4. doi: 10.1016/j.jaac.2013.01.010

Leemans, A., and Jones, D. K. (2009). The B-matrix must be rotated when correcting for subject motion in DTI data. *Magn. Reson. Med.* 61, 1336–1349. doi: 10.1002/mrm.21890

Lind, N. M., Moustgaard, A., Jelsing, J., Vajta, G., Cumming, P., and Hansen, A. K. (2007). The use of pigs in neuroscience: modeling brain disorders. *Neurosci. Biobehav. Rev.* 31, 728–751. doi: 10.1016/j.neubiorev.2007.02.003

Mak-Fan, K. M., Morris, D., Vidal, J., Anagnostou, E., Roberts, W., and Taylor, M. J. (2013). White matter and development in children with an autism spectrum disorder. *Autism* 17, 541–557. doi: 10.1177/1362361312442596

Mendl, M., Held, S., and Byrne, R. (2010). Pig cognition. *Curr. Biol.* 20, R796–R798. doi: 10.1016/j.cub.2010.07.018

Miller, K. L., Stagg, C. J., Douaud, G., Jbabdi, S., Smith, S. M., Behrens, T. E. J., et al. (2011). Diffusion imaging of whole, post-mortem human brains on a clinical MRI scanner. *Neuroimage* 57, 167–181. doi: 10.1016/j.neuroimage.2011.03.070

Mori, S., Oishi, K., Jiang, H., Jiang, L., Li, X., Akhter, K., et al. (2008). Stereotaxic white matter atlas based on diffusion tensor imaging in an ICBM template. *Neuroimage* 40, 570–582. doi: 10.1016/j.neuroimage.2007.12.035

Mudd, A. T., Alexander, L. S., Berding, K., Waworuntu, R. V., Berg, B. M., Donovan, S. M., et al. (2016). Dietary prebiotics, milk fat globule membrane, and lactoferrin affects structural neurodevelopment in the young piglet. *Front. Pediatr.* 4:4. doi: 10.3389/fped.2016.00004

Mudd, A. T., Getty, C., Sutton, B., and Dilger, R. (2015). Perinatal choline deficiency delays brain development and alters metabolite concentrations in the young pig. *Nutr. Neurosci.* doi: 10.1179/1476830515Y.0000000031 [Epub ahead of print].

Radlowski, E. C., Conrad, M. S., Lezmi, S., Dilger, R. N., Sutton, B., Larsen, R., et al. (2014). A neonatal piglet model for investigating brain and cognitive development in small for gestational age human infants. *PLoS ONE* 9:e91951. doi: 10.1371/journal.pone.0091951

Roth, G., and Dicke, U. (2005). Evolution of the brain and intelligence. *Trends Cogn. Sci.* 9, 250–257. doi: 10.1016/j.tics.2005.03.005

Rumple, A., McMurray, M., Johns, J., Lauder, J., Makam, P., Radcliffe, M., et al. (2013). 3-dimensional diffusion tensor imaging (DTI) atlas of the rat brain. *PLoS ONE* 8:e67334. doi: 10.1371/journal.pone.0067334

Saikali, S., Meurice, P., Sauleau, P., Eliat, P. A., Bellaud, P., Randuineau, G., et al. (2010). A three-dimensional digital segmented and deformable brain atlas of the domestic pig. *J. Neurosci. Methods* 192, 102–109. doi: 10.1016/j.jneumeth.2010.07.041

Sauleau, P., Lapouble, E., Val-Laillet, D., and Malbert, C.-H. (2009). The pig model in brain imaging and neurosurgery. *Animal* 3, 1138–1151. doi: 10.1017/S1751731109004649

Schlaier, J., Anthofer, J., Steib, K., Fellner, C., Rothenfusser, E., Brawanski, A., et al. (2015). Deep brain stimulation for essential tremor: targeting the dentato-rubro-thalamic tract? *Neuromodulation* 18, 105–112. doi: 10.1111/ner.12238

Song, S. K., Sun, S. W., Ju, W. K., Lin, S. J., Cross, A. H., and Neufeld, A. H. (2003). Diffusion tensor imaging detects and differentiates axon and myelin degeneration in mouse optic nerve after retinal ischemia. *Neuroimage* 20, 1714–1722. doi: 10.1016/j.neuroimage.2003.07.005

Tax, C. M., Jeurissen, B., Vos, S. B., Viergever, M. A., and Leemans, A. (2014). Recursive calibration of the fiber response function for spherical deconvolution of diffusion MRI data. *Neuroimage* 86, 67–80. doi: 10.1016/j.neuroimage.2013.07.067

Thibault, K. L., and Margulies, S. S. (1998). Age-dependent material properties of the porcine cerebrum: e ect on pediatric inertial head injury criteria. *J. Biomech.* 31, 1119–1126. doi: 10.1016/S0021-9290(98)00122-5

Toga, A. W., Thompson, P. M., Mori, S., Amunts, K., and Zilles, K. (2006). Towards multimodal atlases of the human brain. *Nat. Rev. Neurosci.* 7, 952–966. doi: 10.1038/nrn2012

Tournier, J., Mori, S., and Leemans, A. (2011). Diffusion tensor imaging and beyond. *Magn. Reson. Med.* 65, 1532–1556. doi: 10.1002/mrm.22924

Tournier, J. D., Calamante, F., and Connelly, A. (2007). Robust determination of the fibre orientation distribution in diffusion MRI: non-negativity constrained super-resolved spherical deconvolution. *Neuroimage* 35, 1459–1472. doi: 10.1016/j.neuroimage.2007.02.016

Tournier, J. D., Calamante, F., and Connelly, A. (2012). MRtrix: diffusion tractography in crossing fiber regions. *Int. J. Imaging Syst. Technol.* 22, 53–66. doi: 10.1002/ima.22005

Tuch, D. S., Reese, T. G., Wiegell, M. R., Makris, N., Belliveau, J. W., and Van Wedeen, J. (2002). High angular resolution diffusion imaging reveals intravoxel white matter fiber heterogeneity. *Magn. Reson. Med.* 48, 577–582. doi: 10.1002/mrm.10268

Turken, A. U., and Dronkers, N. F. (2011). The neural architecture of the language comprehension network: converging evidence from lesion and connectivity analyses. *Front. Syst. Neurosci.* 5:1. doi: 10.3389/fnsys.2011.00001

Turner, W. (1890). The convolutions of the brain: a study in comparative anatomy. *J. Anat. Physiol.* 25, 105–153.

Verde, A. R., Budin, F., Berger, J.-B., Gupta, A., Farzinfar, M., Kaiser, A., et al. (2014). UNC-Utah NA-MIC framework for DTI fiber tract analysis. *Front. Neuroinform.* 7:51. doi: 10.3389/fninf.2013.00051

Verhoeven, J. S., Sage, C. A., Leemans, A., Van Hecke, W., Callaert, D., Peeters, R., et al. (2010). Construction of a stereotaxic DTI atlas with full diffusion tensor information for studying white matter maturation from childhood to adolescence using tractography-based segmentations. *Hum. Brain Mapp.* 31, 470–486. doi: 10.1002/hbm.20880

Vetreno, R. P., Yaxley, R., Paniagua, B., and Crews, F. T. (2015). Diffusion tensor imaging reveals adolescent binge ethanol-induced brain structural integrity alterations in adult rats that correlate with behavioral dysfunction. *Addict. Biol.* 21, 939–953. doi: 10.1111/adb.12232

Villalon-Reina, J., Jahanshad, N., Beaton, E., Toga, A. W., Thompson, P. M., and Simon, T. J. (2013). White matter microstructural abnormalities in girls with chromosome 22q11.2 deletion syndrome, fragile X or turner syndrome as evidenced by diffusion tensor imaging. *Neuroimage* 81, 441–454. doi: 10.1016/j.neuroimage.2013.04.028

Wang, Y., Gupta, A., Liu, Z., Zhang, H., Escolar, M. L., Gilmore, J. H., et al. (2011). DTI registration in atlas based fiber analysis of infantile Krabbe disease. *Neuroimage* 55, 1577–1586. doi: 10.1016/j.neuroimage.2011.01.038

Watanabe, H., Andersen, F., Simonsen, C. Z., Evans, S. M., Gjedde, A., and Cumming, P. (2001). MR-based statistical atlas of the Göttingen minipig brain. *Neuroimage* 14, 1089–1096. doi: 10.1006/nimg.2001.0910

Welker, W. (1990). "Why does cerebral cortex fissure and fold? A review of determinants of gyri and sulci," in *Cerebral Cortex*, Vol. 8a, eds E. G. Jones and A. Peters (New York, NY: Plenum Press), 3–136.

Winter, J. D., Dorner, S., Lukovic, J., Fisher, J. A., St Lawrence, K. S., and Kassner, A. (2011). Noninvasive MRI measures of microstructural and cerebrovascular changes during normal swine brain development. *Pediatr. Res.* 69, 418–424. doi: 10.1203/PDR.0b013e3182110f7e

Witwer, B. P., Moftakhar, R., Hasan, K. M., Deshmukh, P., Haughton, V., Field, A., et al. (2002). Diffusion-tensor imaging of white matter tracts in patients with cerebral neoplasm. *J. Neurosurg.* 97, 568–575. doi: 10.3171/jns.2002.97.3.0568

Yeatman, J. D., Ben-Shachar, M., Bammer, R., and Feldman, H. M. (2009). Using diffusion tensor imaging and fiber tracking to characterize diffuse perinatal white matter injury: a case report. *J. Child Neurol.* 24, 795–800. doi: 10.1177/0883073808331080

Zakszewski, E., Adluru, N., Tromp, D. P. M., Kalin, N., and Alexander, A. L. (2014). A diffusion-tensor-based white matter atlas for rhesus macaques. *PLoS ONE* 9:e107398. doi: 10.1371/journal.pone.0107398

Zhang, Y., Zhang, J., Oishi, K., Faria, A. V., Jiang, H., Li, X., et al. (2010). Atlas-guided tract reconstruction for automated and comprehensive examination of the white matter anatomy. *Neuroimage* 52, 1289–1301. doi: 10.1016/j.neuroimage.2010.05.049

12

The Co-Evolution of Neuroimaging and Psychiatric Neurosurgery

*Timothy G. Dyster, Charles B. Mikell and Sameer A. Sheth**

Functional and Cognitive Neurophysiology Laboratory, Department of Neurological Surgery, Columbia University Medical Center, New York Presbyterian Hospital, New York, NY, USA

Correspondence:
Sameer A. Sheth
ss4451@cumc.columbia.edu

The role of neuroimaging in psychiatric neurosurgery has evolved significantly throughout the field's history. Psychiatric neurosurgery initially developed without the benefit of information provided by modern imaging modalities, and thus lesion targets were selected based on contemporary theories of frontal lobe dysfunction in psychiatric disease. However, by the end of the 20th century, the availability of structural and functional magnetic resonance imaging (fMRI) allowed for the development of mechanistic theories attempting to explain the anatamofunctional basis of these disorders, as well as the efficacy of stereotactic neuromodulatory treatments. Neuroimaging now plays a central and ever-expanding role in the neurosurgical management of psychiatric disorders, by influencing the determination of surgical candidates, allowing individualized surgical targeting and planning, and identifying network-level changes in the brain following surgery. In this review, we aim to describe the coevolution of psychiatric neurosurgery and neuroimaging, including ways in which neuroimaging has proved useful in elucidating the therapeutic mechanisms of neuromodulatory procedures. We focus on ablative over stimulation-based procedures given their historical precedence and the greater opportunity they afford for post-operative re-imaging, but also discuss important contributions from the deep brain stimulation (DBS) literature. We conclude with a discussion of how neuroimaging will transition the field of psychiatric neurosurgery into the era of precision medicine.

Keywords: neuroimaging, magnetic resonance imaging (MRI), psychiatric neurosurgery, cingulotomy, capsulotomy, obsessive-compulsive disorder (OCD), major depressive disorder (MDD)

PSYCHIATRIC SURGERY IN THE PRE-IMAGING ERA

Long before the advent of neuroimaging, psychiatric neurosurgery was born. At the time, knowledge about the human brain's functional anatomy was limited, and surgeons relied heavily on contemporary theory and scientific instinct to select neuroablative targets. In 1888, when Dr. Gottlieb Burckhardt removed the left frontotemporal cerebral cortex in six patients with psychiatric diagnoses, his surgical plan was based on results from animal studies and evidence of hypertrophic gyri in psychiatric patients (Burckhardt, 1891; Joanette et al., 1993). Burckhardt hypothesized that different regions of the cerebral cortex were responsible for different behavioral functions, and termed these localizations "psychic domains" (Burckhardt, 1891; Stone, 2001). He speculated aberrant activity in specific domains was responsible for psychiatric pathology, and that ablation of those regions would cure psychiatric disease. Burckhardt's operations, which lasted only a few hours and were performed with a sharp spoon (Burckhardt, 1891; Stone, 2001), were considered ethically dubious by his contemporaries (de Meuron, 1949; Joanette et al., 1993). Nonetheless, Burckhardt's work represented an effort to translate contemporary neuroscience into neurosurgical technique, and thus set the stage for further co-mingling of these nascent fields.

Half a century later, in the 1930s, Moniz developed the "prefrontal leucotomy," a procedure that involved coring small regions of the frontal lobes (Moniz, 1937). His surgical plan was inspired by emerging evidence of calmed behavior in animals after resection of the anterior frontal cortex, although performing a procedure based on this evidence was considered controversial (Munoz and Iniguez, 1949). The prefrontal leucotomy had highly inconsistent results, but Moniz (1937) reported improvement in some patients. In 1949, he was awarded the Nobel Prize for the leucotomy, although his body of work was also notable for pioneering cerebral angiography (Moniz, 1933). Freeman (1957), an American neurologist, learned from Moniz and promoted the modified "lobotomy" procedure in the United States. His infamous "icepick" lobotomies, formally the transorbital lobotomy (Freeman, 1949), fell out of favor and maligned the developing field due to overuse, unacceptable long-term morbidity, and Freeman's brazen self-promotion (Diefenbach et al., 1999).

In the following decades, psychiatric neurosurgery became safer and more precise with the introduction of stereotactic techniques. Developed in the early 1900s by Horsley and Clarke (1908) the stereotactic frame was first used to target specific locations in animal brains described by a Cartesian coordinate system. Spiegel et al. (1947) translated the technology to humans, and performed the first stereotactic human neurosurgical procedure. Using the "Horsley apparatus", Spiegel and Wycis were able to minimize injury to the cerebral cortex and white matter while performing a stereotactic medial thalamotomy to treat a behavioral disorder.

In addition to improved safety and precision, stereotactic neurosurgery offered increased reproducibility, and therefore an opportunity to evaluate a surgical target's efficacy when used across many patients. In 1962, Ballantine performed the first stereotactic bilateral cingulotomy (Ballantine et al., 1967, 1987), based on Fulton's (1951) proposal that the cingulate cortex should be considered as a surgical target. In the following 4 years, Ballantine et al. (1967) performed an additional 94 such procedures. The cingulotomy target used by Ballantine et al. (1967) was based on contemporary theory and on the work of Foltz and White (1962), who performed the procedure for intractable pain but had observed their best outcomes in patients with co-morbid anxiety or depression (Foltz and White, 1962; Ballantine et al., 1967). Similarly, in 1949, Talairach based his anterior capsulotomy target, the anterior limb of the internal capsule (ALIC), on the hypothesis that the internal capsule had connections with the "limbic system," a circuit proposed by Papez (1937) that included the cingulum bundle, hippocampus, thalamus, and hypothalamus and was believed to mediate emotional experience and expression (Papez, 1937; Talairach et al., 1949). Thus, by the mid-twentieth century, the field had made significant advances since its advent, but strong evidence to explain the mechanisms underlying neuroablative targets remained elusive.

PSYCHIATRIC NEUROSURGERY AND THE ADVENT OF NEUROIMAGING

The introduction of neuroimaging dramatically expanded the repertoire of techniques for explaining how neuroablation treated psychiatric disease. Neuroimaging made it possible to demonstrate where functional domains localized within the brain and to analyze structural differences between patients and healthy controls. Using these newly available methods, investigators could show that surgical targets selected decades earlier based on theory and trial-and-error were actually at sites that localized functions impaired in psychiatric disease or that exhibited structural correlates of a patient's functional pathology. To appreciate the neuroimaging data that shows why early ablative procedures such as the capsulotomy and cingulotomy are efficacious, one must first understand the functional and neurobiological models of the psychiatric disorders that the procedures are being used to treat.

Functional Models of Psychiatric Disorders

Within the last few decades, interest has grown in conceiving psychiatric disorders in a spectrum-based model, with emphasis on impairment in functional domains (Castle and Phillips, 2006). This model offers the advantage that a single functional domain may span multiple classic psychiatric diagnoses, and descriptions using several functional domains can help to subtype patients within a single diagnostic class (McElroy et al., 1994; Castle and Phillips, 2006). For example, the classic diagnostic criteria for obsessive-compulsive disorder (OCD) requires the presence of clinically significant obsessions (intrusive and unwanted thoughts), compulsions (ritualistic behavior or thoughts), or both (American Psychiatric Association, 2013). In a functional domain-based model, however, OCD might be conceived as dysfunction in such domains as cognitive control, attention, reward sensitivity, learning, memory, fear response, and mood stability (Hollander et al., 2012). Evidence for a possible deficit in memory confidence, or the ability to determine whether a recalled memory is true, also characterizes the disorder (MacDonald et al., 1997).

Similarly, the classic criteria for major depressive disorder (MDD) include anhedonia or depressed mood, with the addition of at least four more symptoms such as: change in sleep pattern, psychomotor status, or concentration; fatigue; feelings of worthlessness; or recurrent thoughts of death (American Psychiatric Association, 2013). In a functional domain-based model, MDD might be conceived as a dysfunction of cognitive control, learning, mood stability, and assigning value to self, actions, and objects (Austin et al., 1992; Veiel, 1997; American Psychiatric Association, 2013). OCD and MDD serve as prominent examples because they represent the majority of indications for psychiatric neurosurgical procedures, but many other examples exist, including schizophrenia (Mikell et al., 2016), autism (Sturm et al., 2012; Rutishauser et al., 2015; Sinha et al., 2015), post-traumatic stress disorder (Langevin et al., 2010, 2016), eating disorders (Halpern et al., 2008; Lipsman et al., 2013), and others.

Thus understanding the mechanism of stereotactic neuromodulatory procedures requires understanding the networks involved with these functional domains. This relationship between function and treatment is of course not limited to surgical procedures. Indeed, the National Institute of Mental Health (NIMH) has recently proposed a strategy for classifying all mental health disorders based on neurobiological measures as described above, termed the Research Domain Criteria (RDoC) project (Insel et al., 2010). The NIMH's strategic plan notes that the classification scheme for psychiatric disorders, the Diagnostic and Statistical Manual (DSM), is based on clinical observation of certain symptom clusters. While this scheme has been in use for decades, it does have important shortcomings, most notably that its diagnoses are not necessarily coherent pathophysiological entities, but rather heterogeneous collections of symptoms that at times describe a syndrome, rather than define a disease process (Clark et al., 1995; Cross-Disorder Group of the Psychiatric Genomics Consortium, 2013; Cuthbert, 2014). It is therefore often difficult to ascribe for these diagnostic entities a neurobiological substrate that can be systematically subjected to research, and consequently difficult for the research to be translated back into substrate-directed treatments.

The RDoC system, on the other hand, attempts to project observable symptoms and measurable variables onto a set of axes ("Domains", with sub-categories of "Constructs" and "Subconstructs") defined in terms of functional neurobiological systems. A phenomenological diagnosis such as "OCD" would thus be re-classified according to dysfunction of fundamental constituent aspects of behavior and circuitry. Some of the key aspects of dysfunction in OCD include performance monitoring, response inhibition, and goal selection, all of which are classified under the RDoC construct of Cognitive Control (which is contained within the larger domain of Cognitive Systems). OCD may also project onto domains of Negative Valence Systems (Sustained Threat construct) and Positive Valence Systems (Reward Learning construct). Similarly, the diagnosis "MDD" may involve dysfunction in domains of Positive Valence Systems (Approach Motivation), Negative Valence Systems (Loss), Cognitive Systems (Cognitive Control), Arousal, and perhaps others.

Another specifically mentioned motivation for creating the RDoC classification was to align the taxonomy of mental illness with neuroscience research (Insel et al., 2010; Cuthbert, 2014). Because the domains and constructs within them comprise defined fields of research, they may be studied using various "Units of Analysis," including behavioral, genetic, physiological, and especially relevant to this discussion, imaging studies. Thus the recognition that advanced neuroimaging has contributed to improvements in psychiatric neurosurgery runs parallel to, and in some ways represents a microcosm of, broader trends to align the diagnosis and treatment of mental health disorders with measurable biomarkers.

Contributions by the Pre-Frontal Cortex and Other Brain Regions to the Functional Domains Impaired in OCD and MDD

Through the use of neuroimaging, the functional domains impaired in psychiatric disease, including cognitive control, attention, reward sensitivity, memory, learning, fear response, and assignment of value, have been shown to involve specific regions of the brain relevant to psychiatric neurosurgery, including the cingulate cortex.

The cingulate cortex, especially the dorsal anterior cingulate cortex (dACC), has been linked to several functional domains relevant to OCD and MDD, including fear response, anxiety, reward response, and memory. In a neuroimaging meta-analysis, the dACC demonstrated increased activity in patients who underwent fear or anticipatory anxiety conditioning (Mechias et al., 2010), suggesting a role for the cingulate in fear response, anxiety, and threat appraisal, three of the functional domains impaired in OCD. Similarly, a meta-analysis of 171 functional magnetic resonance imaging (fMRI) studies revealed activation peaks in the dACC during tasks involving reward responses, memory, and negative outcomes, further underscoring the dACC's role in functional domains impaired in OCD and MDD (Beckmann et al., 2009). In a domain-based model of psychiatric disease, these results identify dACC as a key node in psychiatric pathology, and accordingly, as a possible therapeutic target.

Cognitive control, the cognitive process used to overcome interference or habitual responses, is another cognitive domain impaired in OCD and MDD, and has been linked to the cingulate cortex. Patients who are completing interference tasks demonstrate increased activity in the anterior cingulate cortex (ACC), dorsolateral prefrontal cortex (DLPFC), inferior frontal gyrus (IFG), and posterior parietal cortex (PPC; Nee et al., 2007). In addition to its role in cognitive control, anatomical, physiological, and functional data link the midcingulate cortex to negative affect and pain (Shackman et al., 2011). Anatomically, the cingulate cortex represents an intersection of fibers from the amygdala, thalamus, striatum, and other regions, and it has been proposed that its core function is to use input from these connected regions to determine an optimal course of action when the best course of action is uncertain (Shackman et al., 2011). Similarly, cognitive neuroscientists have proposed an overarching function for the dACC, termed "expected value of control" (Shenhav et al., 2013). In this model, the dACC determines whether to exert cognitive control by integrating three pieces of information: the predicted benefit of exerting cognitive control, the amount of control required to achieve the predicted benefit, and the expected cost in cognitive effort. Expected value of control provides another important link between the cingulate cortex and psychiatric pathology, as impaired ability to perform the cost-benefit calculation for cognitive control could cause some of the symptoms seen in

OCD and MDD. Unsurprisingly, cognitive control is considered a relevant RDoC construct for both pathologies.

Thus the cingulate cortex plays a clear role in domains impaired in psychiatric disease. However, evidence suggests other brain regions are also linked to relevant functional domains. The PFC has been implicated in cognitive control (Miller and Cohen, 2001), reward sensitivity (Ridderinkhof et al., 2004), memory and attention (Kane and Engle, 2002), fear (Mechias et al., 2010; Marek et al., 2013), memory confidence, (Chiang et al., 2014) and assignment of value (Murray et al., 2011). The thalamus has been implicated in memory and attention (de Bourbon-Teles et al., 2014), and has been shown to interact with the amygdala to produce the fear response (LeDoux et al., 1990; Ciocchi et al., 2010). The amygdala plays roles in fear (Davis, 1992), learning (Morris et al., 1998), and memory (Hamann et al., 1999). The hippocampus is crucial for memory formation (Tulving and Markowitsch, 1998), and the role of the nucleus accumbens in reward sensitivity is well-established (Ikemoto and Panksepp, 1999). In summary, while the list is ever expanding, the functions impaired in OCD and MDD localize to several specific areas of the brain, including the dACC, PFC, thalamus, amygdala, hippocampus, and nucleus accumbens.

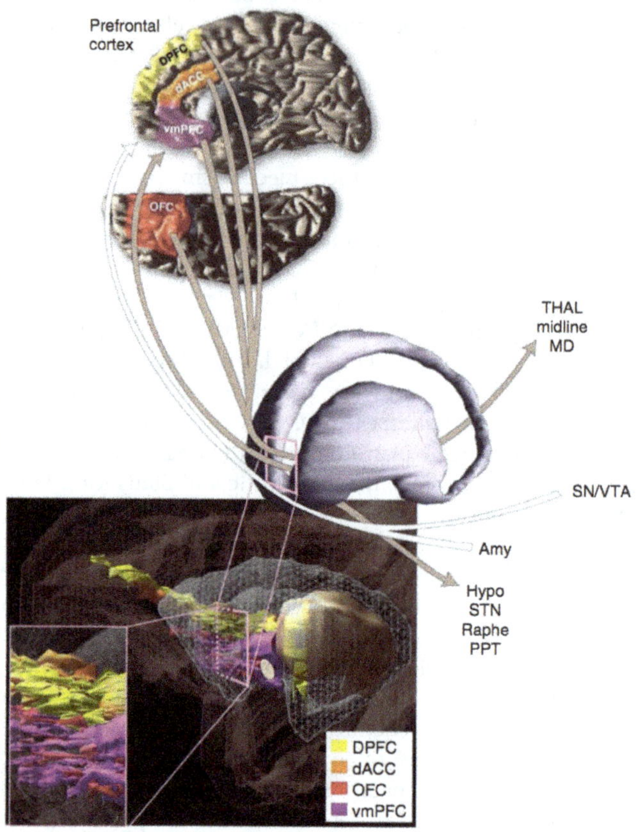

FIGURE 1 | A schematic representation of the network passing through the ventral portion of the anterior limb of the internal capsule (ALIC) that connects prefrontal cortex to several additional regions of the brain. Many of the depicted regions contribute to the proposed cortico-striato-thalamo-cortical (CSTC) loop that may underlie obsessive-compulsive disorder (OCD). Additional abbreviations used in the figure: DPFC, dorsolateral prefrontal cortex; dACC, dorsal anterior cingulate cortex; vmPFC, ventromedial prefrontal cortex; THAL, midline and mediodorsal (MD) nuclei of the thalamus; SN/VTA, substantia nigra and ventral tegmental area; Amy, amygdala; Hypo, hypothalamus; STN, subthalamic nucleus; Raphe, raphe nuclei; OFC, orbitofrontal cortex; PPT, pedunculopontine tegmental nucleus. Reprinted with permission from Greenberg et al. (2010b); Macmillan Publishers Ltd.

How Structural and Functional Imaging Inform Neurobiological Models of OCD and MDD

Obsessive-Compulsive Disorder

The current model of OCD's neurobiology was informed by a general neuroanatomical concept introduced in the late 20th century. In the 1980s, Alexander proposed that the cerebral cortex and subcortical structures might be organized into cortico-striato-thalamo-cortical (CSTC) loops (Alexander et al., 1986). Modell et al. (1989) extended this concept to psychiatric pathology, proposing that a CSTC loop involving the orbitofrontal cortex (OFC), basal ganglia, limbic striatum, and thalamus underlay OCD (**Figure 1**). In the model, the symptoms of OCD resulted from overactivity of the frontothalamic portion of the loop and failure of the limbic striatum to inhibit this activity (Modell et al., 1989). The caudate and cingulate were hypothesized to also play a central role in OCD pathogenesis (Modell et al., 1989; Insel, 1992). Thus the model made several critical predictions about patients with OCD: first, there should be overactivity in the frontal and thalamic structures; second, evidence for dysfunction in the limbic striatum should be present; third, structural changes, if present, should predominately exist in the OFC/PFC, cingulate, and caudate.

In the years after this model of OCD was proposed, new methods for imaging analysis that could test the critical predictions of the model were developed. Magnetic resonance diffusion tensor imaging (DTI), a technique that exploits the diffusion properties of water to determine fiber tract orientation (Basser et al., 1994), was combined with computational tractography methods to estimate neural fiber pathways in the white matter. Later modifications allowed the technique to evaluate gray matter structures, both for segmentation within the gray matter and to analyze the connectivity between different gray matter structures (Behrens et al., 2003).

These and other emerging imaging techniques provided *in vivo* evidence of structural abnormalities in patients with OCD. Neuroimaging studies indicated that patients with OCD had reduced PFC volume (Szeszko et al., 1999; Alonso et al., 2001; Choi et al., 2004; Kang et al., 2004; Pujol et al., 2004; Atmaca et al., 2006), reduced ACC volume (Szeszko et al., 2004), and changes in the size of the caudate nucleus (Scarone et al., 1992; Robinson et al., 1995). DTI studies suggested abnormalities in the white matter microstructure (Szeszko et al., 2005), left-lateralized asymmetry in cingulate connectivity, and left-lateralized asymmetry in connectivity between the thalamus and PFC (Chiu et al., 2011). Neuroimaging evidence also suggested structural changes in the amygdala (Szeszko et al., 1999; Kwon et al., 2003) and hippocampus (Kwon et al., 2003). These OCD-associated structural changes in the PFC, ACC, caudate, thalamus, amygdala, and hippocampus were consistent with the loop model of OCD and thus provided support for this proposed model.

In addition to evidence of structural change, emerging imaging techniques provided evidence of functional abnormalities in patients with OCD. Shortly after the development of fMRI, researchers evaluated neural activity in patients with OCD in response to stimuli that were known triggers for the patients' symptoms (Breiter et al., 1996). Compared to healthy controls, patients with OCD showed increased activation in lateral PFC, medial OFC, ACC, temporal and insular cortex, caudate, amygdala, and lenticulate nuclei when presented with the trigger stimulus. This pattern of functional change, which involved several frontal and limbic structures, corroborated existing structural evidence and further supported the loop model of OCD.

Major Depressive Disorder

The neurobiological mechanisms of normal mood and mood disturbances remain areas of active scientific investigation (Nestler et al., 2002). The proposed mechanisms for depression exist on multiple levels of analysis, and many are not mutually exclusive. Among the possibilities are dysfunction in the stress axis, altered glutamergic neurotransmission, reduced GABAergic transmission, abnormal circadian rhythms, and thyroxine abnormalities (Belmaker and Agam, 2008). In this review, we focus on how dysfunction in specific brain structures and circuits might underlie MDD, as this model of MDD has been strongly informed by neuroimaging.

Early neurobiological models of MDD were influenced by the CSTC loop model, similar to early models of OCD. Initially, data from PET scans implicated the cortico-basal ganglia circuits, OFC, mesencephalon, and basotemporal limbic regions in MDD (Mayberg, 1994). These data, combined with clinical observation, informed a three "compartment" model of MDD (Mayberg, 1997). In the three-compartment model, a dorsal compartment, comprising cortical and midline limbic structures (dACC, DLPFC, inferior parietal cortex, and striatum), and a ventral compartment, comprising paralimbic regions (hypothalamus, insula, subgenual cingulate, and brainstem), were regulated and kept in balance by a third region, the rostral cingulate. Disturbances in mood represented failure of the cingulate to coordinate the other compartments. This unbalanced activity caused the dorsal compartment to produce attentive-cognitive symptoms, and the ventral compartment to produce vegetative-somatic symptoms.

Advances in neuroimaging provided evidence that complicated the three-compartment model of MDD. Structural and functional MRI demonstrated changes in the cingulate cortex, PFC, amygdala, hippocampus, hypothalamus, and nucleus accumbens associated with MDD (Sheline et al., 1999; Nestler et al., 2002; Gutman et al., 2009; Mayberg, 2009; Murray et al., 2011; Patel et al., 2013). In 2009, an updated model

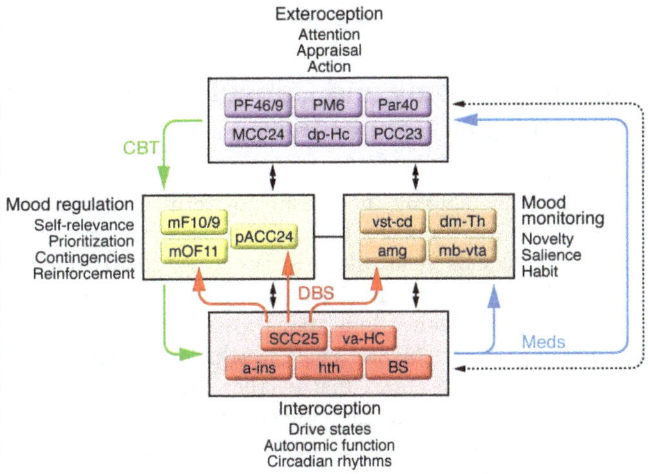

FIGURE 2 | A schematic representation of the network of connections between cortical, limbic, and paralimbic regions proposed to underlie major depressive disorder (MDD), and the four main functional compartments of the model, each of which represents a functional domain impaired in MDD and comprises a subset of brain regions that demonstrate robust anatomical connections to one another. Black arrows identify anatomical connections between compartments. Solid colored arrows identify connections that are proposed to mediate efficacy of a specific treatment: green indicates cognitive behavioral therapy; blue indicates pharmacotherapy; red indicates deep brain stimulation (DBS) at subcallosal cingulate. Additional abbreviations used in the figure: a-ins, anterior insula; amg, amygdala; dm-Th, dorsomedial thalamus; dp-Hc, dorsal-posterior hippocampus; mb-vta, midbrain-ventral tegmental area; mF10/9, medial frontal cortex BA10 and BA9; mOF11, medial orbital frontal cortex BA11; Par40, parietal cortex BA40; PF46/9, PFC BA46 and BA9; PM6, premotor cortex BA6; va-HC, ventral-anterior hippocampus; vst-cd, ventral striatum-caudate. Republished with permission of American Society for Clinical Investigation, from Mayberg (2009); permission conveyed through Copyright Clearance Center, Inc.

involving four regions was proposed (**Figure 2**; Mayberg, 2009). The four-region model included a more comprehensive set of brain regions; however, the "dorsal compartment" and "ventral compartment" from the prior model approximated the new model's "exteroceptive region" and "interoceptive region," respectively. The exteroceptive region controlled cognitive function (e.g., attention, appraisal, action), while the interoceptive region controlled visceral-motor function (e.g., drive states, autonomic function, circadian rhythms). The four-region model maintained that mood disturbances resulted from a lack of coordination between exteroceptive and interoceptive activity. Sustained loss of coordination produced major depressive episodes. Two regions in the model were new: a mood-monitoring region (comprising subcortical regions such as the dorsomedial thalamus, amygdala, and basal ganglia), and a mood regulation region (comprising regions of the medial frontal cortex including the rostral ACC). The mood-monitoring region processed both emotional and non-emotional stimuli, while the mood regulation region mediated cognitive control and overt control of emotional state. Thus in its final form, the model included the striatum, amygdala, dorsomedial thalamus, and cingulate cortex, among other regions (Mayberg, 2009), constituting a complex cortico-limbic-thalamic-striatal network.

The Cingulotomy and Capsulotomy: Target Anatomy and Connectivity

Cingulotomy

Currently, cingulotomy is mostly performed for severe, refractory OCD (Bourne et al., 2013; Sheth et al., 2013) and MDD (Shields et al., 2008; Steele et al., 2008), although chronic neuropathic pain (Viswanathan et al., 2013; Patel et al., 2015) and other indications also exist (Kanaka and Balasubramaniam, 1978; Baer et al., 1994). The cingulate cortex is a curved band of cortex that overlies the corpus callosum just off the midline, and the cingulotomy specifically targets a region approximately 15–20 mm posterior to the anterior-most point of the frontal horn of the lateral ventricles (Kim et al., 2003; Yang et al., 2014), placing it in the "anterior midcingulate," a region associated with cognitive control functions (Shackman et al., 2011; Cavanagh and Shackman, 2015).

The cingulotomy lesion also typically extends into the cingulum bundle, the white matter pathway immediately ventral to the cingulate cortex, and disrupts cingulate fibers projecting to other regions of the brain (Jellison et al., 2004; Steele et al., 2008). Therefore, to fully understand the cingulotomy's mechanism requires an understanding of the cingulate's connectivity. Anatomical tract-tracing in nonhuman primate demonstrates cingulate fibers running in distinct bundles to the striatum, corpus callosum, internal capsule, external capsule, OFC and DLPFC (Heilbronner and Haber, 2014). In healthy human subjects, DTI demonstrates cingulate fibers to PFC, amygdala, striatum, hypothalamus, and parietal cortex (Beckmann et al., 2009). The cingulate's rich network notably includes several regions with known structural and functional associations to MDD and OCD. Considering these connectivity data and the cingulate's proposed role in cognitive control, a plausible mechanism for the cingulotomy's efficacy emerges: the cingulotomy ablates neural regions and tracts that underlie OCD and MDD.

Capsulotomy

Capsulotomy (or anterior capsulotomy) has primarily been used to treat severe, refractory OCD (Rück et al., 2008; Kondziolka et al., 2011; Sheehan et al., 2013; Lopes et al., 2014) and MDD (Christmas et al., 2011; Hurwitz et al., 2012), although other indications also exist (Rück et al., 2003; Barbier et al., 2011). The general target for the procedure is in the ventral portion of the ALIC. Initially, capsulotomy lesions were made exclusively using radiofrequency thermal techniques (Talairach et al., 1949), but more recently stereotactic radiosurgery techniques have also been used (Rück et al., 2008; Kondziolka et al., 2011; Sheehan et al., 2013; Lopes et al., 2014). Early reports described a large target region between the anterior and middle third of the ALIC at the level of the foramen of Monro, 10 mm anterior to the anterior commissure, 8 mm superior to the intercommisural plane, and 17 mm from the midline (Kihlström et al., 1997), although similar targets have been reported using slightly different landmarks (Rück et al., 2008; D'Astous et al., 2013). The lesions made at the target were 15–20 mm long and 4–5 mm wide (Kihlström et al., 1997; Aouizerate et al., 2006; Rück et al., 2008; D'Astous et al., 2013). More recent reports describe a smaller target region, closer to the ventral portion of the ALIC, 7–10 mm anterior to the anterior commissure, near the level of the intercommisural plane (Kondziolka et al., 2011; Sheehan et al., 2013; Lopes et al., 2014). These lesions are spherical to slightly oblong, extend less dorsally, and are smaller overall, with a widest diameter of a few to several millimeters.

The internal capsule serves as a conduit for a large bundle of fibers that run to and from the cerebral cortex (Jellison et al., 2004). As with the cingulotomy, to fully understand capsulotomy's mechanism requires an understanding of the internal capsule's connectivity. The internal capsule can be subdivided into anterior and posterior limbs, and each limb has a distinct pattern of connectivity. The anterior limb, which is targeted by capsulotomy, lies between the head of the caudate and the lenticular nucleus (Jellison et al., 2004). Tractography reveals projections from the ALIC to cortex, pons and thalamus in the anterior-posterior plane, and projections from the posterior limb into corticospinal, corticobulbar, and corticopontine tracts, mostly in the superior-inferior plane (Jellison et al., 2004). Neuroimaging studies further suggest internal capsule fibers target the PFC, amygdala, hippocampus, nucleus accumbens, thalamus, and cingulate (Behrens et al., 2003; Haber et al., 2006; Gutman et al., 2009). Considering these data, a few important patterns emerge. First, the areas targeted by fibers from the ALIC and the cingulate cortex show significant overlap (Gutman et al., 2009). Further, evidence suggests the reciprocal connections running through ALIC to thalamus and OFC interface with caudate and brainstem, consistent with the CSTC loop model and suggesting the ALIC may be an important loop node (Modell et al., 1989). Finally, fibers projecting through the ALIC come from regions with known structural and functional associations to OCD and MDD, implying a conceivable mechanism, similar to the mechanism of the cingulotomy, for the capsulotomy: the procedure disrupts tracts between neural regions that underlie OCD and MDD.

In summary, a neurobiological mechanism for both cingulotomy and capsulotomy is supported by modern fMRI and structural MRI data. These neuroablative procedures target the regions and tracts that have been shown to functionally and structurally underlie OCD and MDD.

Relevant Examples from Deep Brain Stimulation

This review focuses on cingulotomy and capsulotomy over DBS due to neuroablative procedures' historical role in understanding functional anatomy, longer follow-up times, and ease of re-imaging; however, it is important to briefly discuss DBS as well, as DBS plays an increasingly important role in the treatment of psychiatric disease, including MDD and OCD. DBS targets for MDD have included ventral capsule/ventral striatum (VC/VS; Malone et al., 2009), nucleus accumbens (Bewernick et al., 2012), and subcallosal cingulate (Lozano et al., 2008, 2012; Holtzheimer et al., 2012), whereas targets for OCD have included VC/VS (Greenberg et al., 2006, 2010a; Goodman et al., 2010; Mian et al., 2010), ALIC (Abelson et al., 2005), nucleus accumbens (Denys et al., 2010; Huff et al., 2010), inferior thalamic peduncle (Jiménez-Ponce et al., 2009), and subthalamic nucleus (STN; Mallet et al., 2008; Chabardès et al., 2013).

The VC/VS is among the most well-studied DBS targets for the treatment of OCD (Greenberg et al., 2006, 2010a; Goodman et al., 2010; Mian et al., 2010; Dougherty et al., 2016). In 1999, four patients with severe OCD underwent bilateral electrode implantation rostral to the anterior commissure with extension into the VC/VS. The results with stimulation were modest but promising (Nuttin et al., 1999), and the target's efficacy continued to be evaluated in small controlled- and open-studies. In one open-label series, eight patients with severe or resistant OCD who underwent implantation were followed to three-years of follow up, and demonstrated an average improvement from severe to moderate, with four of the eight showing ≥35% improvement in Yale-Brown Obsessive Compulsive Scores (YBOCS) severity, and two additional patients showing 25–35% improvement in YBOCS severity (Greenberg et al., 2006). Over time, the VC/VS target was refined and moved to a more posterior location, where the anterior capsule, anterior commissure, and posterior ventral striatum intersected and CSTC circuit fibers were thought to be more densely packed (Greenberg et al., 2010a). With this posterior shift, response rates to the procedure improved (Greenberg et al., 2010a). In 2010, a randomized, blinded, staggered-onset study reported ≥35% improvement in YBOCS in four out of six patients, with no significant responses during the sham period. The evolution of the VC/VS target further underscores the important interplay between understanding the neurobiological substrate of psychiatric disease and selecting procedural targets. When a psychiatric process is better understood at the neurobiological level, hypothesis-driven target selection and refinement become possible, which, in turn, have the potential to meaningfully improve clinical outcomes and patient care.

THE FUTURE OF PSYCHIATRIC NEUROSURGERY AND NEUROIMAGING

Neuroimaging has helped describe a growing list of functions localized to the cingulate cortex, the internal capsule, and their networks. Perhaps unsurprisingly, this list includes many of the functional domains impaired in the psychiatric diseases treated by cingulotomy and capsulotomy. Moreover, neuroimaging has revealed new connections and confirmed known connections between the cingulate, internal capsule, and other regions of the brain. In many cases, the nodes of these networks are the same regions that demonstrate structural and functional changes in the setting of psychiatric pathology, providing additional rationale for the efficacy of cingulotomy and capsulotomy.

In the present day, nearly all fields of medicine are trending toward the use of biomarkers to practice more personalized, patient-specific, "precision medicine" (Mirnezami et al., 2012), and the approach to managing psychiatric illness is no exception to this trend (Costa e Silva, 2013). This transition offers neuroimaging a new role in the realm of psychiatric neurosurgery. Whereas in the past neuroimaging was used to retrospectively clarify procedural mechanisms, in the future, the same modalities will prospectively inform patient-specific clinical management.

Neuroimaging makes it possible to evaluate patient-specific regional volume and connectivity. Thus one way in which neuroimaging may inform patient-specific clinical management is via the discovery of biomarkers for predicting outcomes in psychiatric neurosurgery. For example, a recent retrospective study analyzed preoperative T1 and diffusion MRI sequences for 15 patients who underwent cingulotomy, of whom only eight had responded to the procedure (Banks et al., 2015). Using voxel based morphometry and probabilistic tractography to analyze the area immediately anterior to the lesion target, the investigators found patients with increased right-sided gray matter signal in ACC exhibited poorer clinical response, while patients with decreased gray matter signal in the same region exhibited improved clinical response. Improved clinical response was also correlated with increased right-sided connectivity between the lesion site and the caudate, putamen, thalamus, pallidum, and hippocampus. These results suggest interplay between individual neuroanatomical variation and clinical response to cingulotomy, and therefore that patient-specific neuroanatomical markers might be useful for predicting clinical outcome. While this analysis was restricted to cingulotomy, it is conceivable that similar findings may eventually be described in other neuroablative procedures.

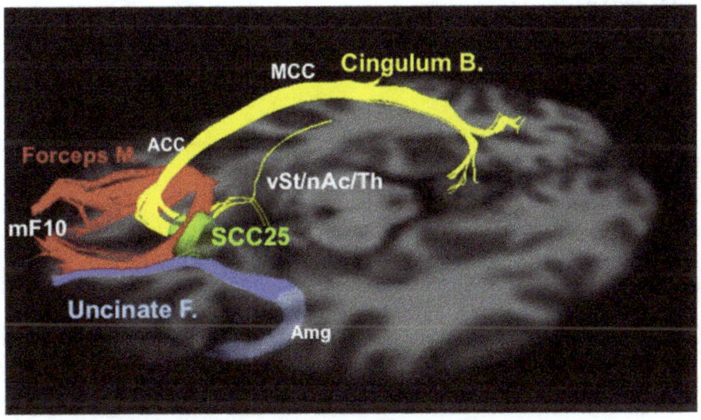

FIGURE 3 | Tractographic representation of a subcallosal cingulate fiber bundle optimal for DBS. Probabilistic tractography and similar techniques make it possible to evaluate patient-specific network connectivity when creating surgical plans. Using this information, physicians are able to select individualized stimulation targets at points where critical white matter tracts intersect. Red: forceps minor. Blue: uncinate fasciculus. Yellow: cingulate bundle. ACC, anterior cingulate cortex; Amg, amygdala; Cingulum B., cingulum bundle; Forceps M., forceps minor; MCC, middle cingulate cortex; mF10, medial frontal (Brodmann area 10); nAc, nucleus accumbens; SCC25, subcallosal cingulate cortex (Brodmann area 25); Th, thalamus; Uncinate F., uncinate fasciculus; vSt, ventral striatum. Reprinted from Riva-Posse et al. (2014); Copyright with permission from Elsevier; permission conveyed through Copyright Clearance Center, Inc.

Neuroimaging analysis techniques are also emerging as tools to refine surgical plans and select surgical targets. For example, neuroimaging and other data were used to select the "subgenual" or "subcallosal" cingulate (SCC), located near Brodmann area 25, as a DBS target for depression (Mayberg et al., 1999, 2005; Seminowicz et al., 2004; Mayberg, 2009). The early results from stimulation at SCC were promising, but highly variable, with reported 12-month response rates ranging from 29% to 62% in different series (Lozano et al., 2008, 2012; Hamani et al., 2009; Kennedy et al., 2011). Neuroimaging analysis revealed that the contact locations relative to neuroanatomical landmarks did not explain the differences in patient response (Hamani et al., 2009); however, tractographic analysis for a series of 16 patients who underwent DBS stimulation at SCC revealed that all responders shared bilateral pathways from their activation volumes to the medial frontal cortex, rostral and dorsal cingulate cortex, and subcortical nuclei; conversely, non-responders did not consistently show these connections (Riva-Posse et al., 2014). These results suggest tractography may be useful for optimizing electrode implantation on a patient-by-patient basis using patient-specific anatomical connectivity (**Figure 3**; Riva-Posse et al., 2014). Prospective trials are currently underway to further test these imaging-driven hypotheses for surgical targeting ([1]NCT00367003, NCT01984710). Similarly, tractography has helped identify the medial forebrain bundle as a node in a subcortical emotional system that may mediate elements of addiction and depression (Coenen et al., 2011). Based on these data, a trial is currently underway to evaluate a novel DBS for depression target, located lateral to the ventral tegmental area in the midbrain, where the superolateral medial forebrain bundle branch emerges from the main medial forebrain bundle ([1]NCT01095263).

[1]www.clinicaltrials.gov

In summary, the emerging literature surrounding neuroimaging biomarkers may forecast an era of "precision surgery," in which patient-specific neuroanatomy, elucidated by neuroimaging analysis, is used to refine surgical targets (Rück et al., 2008), patient selection (Banks et al., 2015), and electrode implantation (Riva-Posse et al., 2014). Undoubtedly, new and innovative uses of neuroimaging in psychiatric neurosurgery will continue to emerge.

CONCLUSION

The field of psychiatric neurosurgery has co-evolved with modern neuroimaging modalities. However, the relationship between psychiatric neurosurgery and neuroimaging has shifted dramatically since the field's advent. Whereas neuroimaging was once used to retrospectively clarify procedural mechanisms, in the future, the same modalities will directly inform clinical decision-making, and, perhaps, will usher in an era of "precision surgery" for psychiatric disease.

AUTHOR CONTRIBUTIONS

TGD, CBM, and SAS made substantial contributions to the conception and design of the work, drafted the work and revised it critically, gave final approval of the version to be published, and agree to be accountable for all aspects of the work in ensuring that questions related to the accuracy or integrity of any part of the work are appropriately investigated and resolved.

ACKNOWLEDGMENTS

This work was supported by the Dana Foundation. The authors would like to thank Dr. Yagna J. Pathak, and Dr. Elliot H. Smith, for their thoughtful suggestions during the drafting of this manuscript.

REFERENCES

Abelson, J. L., Curtis, G. C., Sagher, O., Albucher, R. C., Harrigan, M., Taylor, S. F., et al. (2005). Deep brain stimulation for refractory obsessive-compulsive disorder. *Biol. Psychiatry* 57, 510–516. doi: 10.1016/j.biopsych.2004.11.042

Alexander, G. E., DeLong, M. R., and Strick, P. L. (1986). Parallel organization of functionally segregated circuits linking basal ganglia and cortex. *Annu. Rev. Neurosci.* 9, 357–381. doi: 10.1146/annurev.neuro.9.1.357

Alonso, P., Pujol, J., Cardoner, N., Benlloch, L., Deus, J., Menchón, J. M., et al. (2001). Right prefrontal repetitive transcranial magnetic stimulation in obsessive-compulsive disorder: a double-blind, placebo-controlled study. *Am. J. Psychiatry* 158, 1143–1145. doi: 10.1176/appi.ajp.158.7.1143

American Psychiatric Association. (2013). *Diagnostic and Statistical Manual of Mental Disorders: DSM 5*. Washington, DC: American Psychiatric Association.

Aouizerate, B., Rotgé, J., Martin-Guehl, C., Cuny, E., Rougier, A., Guehl, D., et al. (2006). A systematic review of psychosurgical treatments for obsessive-compulsive disorder: does deep brain stimulation represent the future trend in psychosurgery? *Clin. Neuropsychiatry* 3, 391–403.

Atmaca, M., Yildirimb, H., Ozdemirb, H., Aydinb, A., Tezcana, E., and Ozlera, S. (2006). Volumetric MRI assessment of brain regions in patients with refractory obsessive-compulsive disorder. *Prog. Neuropsychopharmacol. Biol. Psychiatry* 30, 1051–1057. doi: 10.1016/j.pnpbp.2006.03.033

Austin, M. P., Ross, M., Murray, C., O'Carroll, R. E., Ebmeier, K. P., and Goodwin, G. M. (1992). Cognitive function in major depression. *J. Affect. Disord.* 25, 21–29. doi: 10.1016/0165-0327(92)90089-o

Baer, L., Rauch, S. L., Jenike, M. A., Cassem, N., Ballantine, H., Manzo, P., et al. (1994). Cingulotomy in a case of concomitant obsessive-compulsive disorder and tourette's syndrome. *Arch. Gen. Psychiatry* 51, 73–74. doi: 10.1001/archpsyc.1994.03950010073013

Ballantine, H. T., Bouckoms, A. J., Thomas, E. K., and Giriunas, I. E. (1987). Treatment of psychiatric illness by stereotactic cingulotomy. *Biol. Psychiatry* 22, 807–819. doi: 10.1016/0006-3223(87)90080-1

Ballantine, H. T. Jr., Cassidy, W. L., Flanagan, N. B., and Marino, R. Jr. (1967). Stereotaxic anterior cingulotomy for neuropsychiatric illness and intractable pain. *J. Neurosurg.* 26, 488–495. doi: 10.3171/jns.1967.26.5.0488

Banks, G. P., Mikell, C. B., Youngerman, B. E., Henriques, B., Kelly, K. M., Chan, A. K., et al. (2015). Neuroanatomical characteristics associated with response to dorsal anterior cingulotomy for obsessive-compulsive disorder. *JAMA Psychiatry* 72, 127–135. doi: 10.1001/jamapsychiatry.2014.2216

Barbier, J., Gabriëls, L., van Laere, K., and Nuttin, B. (2011). Successful anterior capsulotomy in comorbid anorexia nervosa and obsessive-compulsive disorder: case report. *Neurosurgery* 69, E745–E751; discussion E751. doi: 10.1227/NEU.0b013e31821964d2

Basser, P. J., Mattiello, J., and LeBihan, D. (1994). MR diffusion tensor spectroscopy and imaging. *Biophys. J.* 66, 259–267. doi: 10.1016/s0006-3495(94)80775-1

Beckmann, M., Johansen-Berg, H., and Rushworth, M. F. S. (2009). Connectivity-based parcellation of human cingulate cortex and its relation to functional specialization. *J. Neurosci.* 29, 1175–1190. doi: 10.1523/JNEUROSCI.3328-08.2009

Behrens, T. E. J., Johansen-Berg, H., Woolrich, M. W., Smith, S. M., Wheeler-Kingshott, C. A. M., Boulby, P. A., et al. (2003). Non-invasive mapping of connections between human thalamus and cortex using diffusion imaging. *Nat. Neurosci.* 6, 750–757. doi: 10.1038/nn1075

Belmaker, R. H., and Agam, G. (2008). Major depressive disorder. *N. Engl. J. Med.* 358, 55–68. doi: 10.1056/NEJMra073096

Bewernick, B. H., Kayser, S., Sturm, V., and Schlaepfer, T. E. (2012). Long-term effects of nucleus accumbens deep brain stimulation in treatment-resistant depression: evidence for sustained efficacy. *Neuropsychopharmacology* 37, 1975–1985. doi: 10.1038/npp.2012.44

Bourne, S. K., Sheth, S. A., Neal, J., Strong, C., Mian, M. K., Cosgrove, G. R., et al. (2013). Beneficial effect of subsequent lesion procedures after nonresponse to initial cingulotomy for severe, treatment-refractory obsessive-compulsive disorder. *Neurosurgery* 72, 196–202; discussion 202. doi: 10.1227/NEU.0b013e31827b9c7c

Breiter, H. C., Rauch, S. L., Kwong, K. K., Baker, J. R., Weisskoff, R. M., Kennedy, D. N., et al. (1996). Functional magnetic resonance imaging of symptom provocation in obsessive-compulsive disorder. *Arch. Gen. Psychiatry* 53, 595–606. doi: 10.1001/archpsyc.1996.01830070041008

Burckhardt, G. (1891). Ueber Rindenexcisionen, als Beitrag zur operativen Therapier der Psychosen. *Allg. Zeitschift fur Psychiatry* 47, 463–548.

Castle, D. J., and Phillips, K. A. (2006). Obsessive-compulsive spectrum of disorders: a defensible construct? *Aust. N Z J. Psychiatry* 40, 114–120. doi: 10.1080/j.1440-1614.2006.01757.x

Cavanagh, J. F., and Shackman, A. J. (2015). Frontal midline theta reflects anxiety and cognitive control: meta-analytic evidence. *J. Physiol. Paris* 109, 3–15. doi: 10.1016/j.jphysparis.2014.04.003

Chabardès, S., Polosan, M., Krack, P., Bastin, J., Krainik, A., David, O., et al. (2013). Deep brain stimulation for obsessive-compulsive disorder: subthalamic nucleus target. *World Neurosurg.* 80, S31.e1–e8. doi: 10.1016/j.wneu.2012.03.010

Chiang, T.-C., Lu, R.-B., Hsieh, S., Chang, Y.-H., and Yang, Y.-K. (2014). Stimulation in the dorsolateral prefrontal cortex changes subjective evaluation of percepts. *PLoS One* 9:e106943. doi: 10.1371/journal.pone.0106943

Chiu, C. H., Lo, Y. C., Tang, H. S., Liu, I. C., Chiang, W. Y., Yeh, F. C., et al. (2011). White matter abnormalities of fronto-striato-thalamic circuitry in obsessive-compulsive disorder: a study using diffusion spectrum imaging tractography. *Psychiatry Res.* 192, 176–182. doi: 10.1016/j.pscychresns.2010.09.009

Choi, J. S., Kang, D. H., Kim, J. J., Ha, T. H., Lee, J. M., Youn, T., et al. (2004). Left anterior subregion of orbitofrontal cortex volume reduction and impaired organizational strategies in obsessive-compulsive disorder. *J. Psychiatr. Res.* 38, 193–199. doi: 10.1016/j.jpsychires.2003.08.001

Christmas, D., Eljamel, M. S., Butler, S., Hazari, H., MacVicar, R., Steele, J. D., et al. (2011). Long term outcome of thermal anterior capsulotomy for chronic, treatment refractory depression. *J. Neurol. Neurosurg. Psychiatry* 82, 594–600. doi: 10.1136/jnnp.2010.217901

Ciocchi, S., Herry, C., Grenier, F., Wolff, S. B. E., Letzkus, J. J., Vlachos, I., et al. (2010). Encoding of conditioned fear in central amygdala inhibitory circuits. *Nature* 468, 277–282. doi: 10.1038/nature09559

Clark, L. A., Watson, D., and Reynolds, S. (1995). Diagnosis and classification of psychopathology: challenges to the current system and future directions. *Annu. Rev. Psychol.* 46, 121–153. doi: 10.1146/annurev.psych.46.1.121

Coenen, V. A., Schlaepfer, T. E., Maedler, B., and Panksepp, J. (2011). Cross-species affective functions of the medial forebrain bundle-Implications for the treatment of affective pain and depression in humans. *Neurosci. Biobehav. Rev.* 35, 1971–1981. doi: 10.1016/j.neubiorev.2010.12.009

Costa e Silva, J. A. (2013). Personalized medicine in psychiatry: new technologies and approaches. *Metabolism.* 62, S40–S44. doi: 10.1016/j.metabol.2012.08.017

Cross-Disorder Group of the Psychiatric Genomics Consortium. (2013). Identification of risk loci with shared effects on five major psychiatric disorders: a genome-wide analysis. *Lancet* 381, 1371–1379. doi: 10.1016/S0140-6736(12)62129-1

Cuthbert, B. N. (2014). Research domain criteria: toward future psychiatric nosology. *Asian J. Psychiatr.* 7, 4–5. doi: 10.1016/j.ajp.2013.12.007

D'Astous, M., Cottin, S., Roy, M., Picard, C., and Cantin, L. (2013). Bilateral stereotactic anterior capsulotomy for obsessive-compulsive disorder: long-term follow-up. *J. Neurol. Neurosurg. Psychiatry* 84, 1208–1213. doi: 10.1136/jnnp-2012-303826

Davis, M. (1992). The role of the amygdala in fear and anxiety. *Annu. Rev. Neurosci.* 15, 353–375. doi: 10.1146/annurev.ne.15.030192.002033

de Bourbon-Teles, J., Bentley, P., Koshino, S., Shah, K., Dutta, A., Malhotra, P., et al. (2014). Thalamic control of human attention driven by memory and learning. *Curr. Biol.* 24, 993–999. doi: 10.1016/j.cub.2014.03.024

de Meuron, P. (1949). *La Maison de Sante de Prefargier 1849–1949.* Neuchâtel: Attinger.

Denys, D., Mantione, M., Figee, M., van den Munckhof, P., Koerselman, F., Westenberg, H., et al. (2010). Deep brain stimulation of the nucleus accumbens for treatment-refractory obsessive-compulsive disorder. *Arch. Gen. Psychiatry* 67, 1061–1068. doi: 10.1001/archgenpsychiatry.2010.122

Diefenbach, G. J., Diefenbach, D., Baumeister, A., and West, M. (1999). Portrayal of lobotomy in the popular press: 1935–1960. *J. Hist. Neurosci.* 8, 60–69. doi: 10.1076/jhin.8.1.60.1766

Dougherty, D. D., Chou, T., Corse, A. K., Arulpragasam, A. R., Widge, A. S., Cusin, C., et al. (2016). Acute deep brain stimulation changes in regional cerebral blood flow in obsessive-compulsive disorder. *J. Neurosurg.* 19, 1–7. doi: 10.3171/2015.9.jns151387

Foltz, E. L., and White, L. E. Jr. (1962). Pain "relief" by frontal cingulumotomy. *J. Neurosurg.* 19, 89–100. doi: 10.3171/jns.1962.19.2.0089

Freeman, W. (1949). Transorbital lobotomy. *Am. J. Psychiatry* 105, 734–740. doi: 10.1176/ajp.105.10.734

Freeman, W. (1957). Frontal lobotomy 1936-1956: a follow-up study of 3000 patients from one to twenty years. *Am. J. Psychiatry* 113, 877–886. doi: 10.1176/ajp.113.10.877

Fulton, J. (1951). The physiological basis of psyhosurgery. *Proc. Am. Philos. Soc.* 95, 538–541.

Goodman, W. K., Foote, K. D., Greenberg, B. D., Ricciuti, N., Bauer, R., Ward, H., et al. (2010). Deep brain stimulation for intractable obsessive compulsive disorder: pilot study using a blinded, staggered-onset design. *Biol. Psychiatry* 67, 535–542. doi: 10.1016/j.biopsych.2009.11.028

Greenberg, B. D., Gabriels, L. A., Malone, D. A. Jr., Rezai, A. R., Friehs, G. M., Okun, M. S., et al. (2010a). Deep brain stimulation of the ventral internal capsule/ventral striatum for obsessive-compulsive disorder: worldwide experience. *Mol. Psychiatry* 15, 64–79. doi: 10.1038/mp.2008.55

Greenberg, B. D., Rauch, S. L., and Haber, S. N. (2010b). Invasive circuitry-based neurotherapeutics: stereotactic ablation and deep brain stimulation for OCD. *Neuropsychopharmacology* 35, 317–336. doi: 10.1038/npp.2009.128

Greenberg, B. D., Malone, D. A., Friehs, G. M., Rezai, A. R., Kubu, C. S., Malloy, P. F., et al. (2006). Three-year outcomes in deep brain stimulation for highly resistant obsessive-compulsive disorder. *Neuropsychopharmacology* 31, 2384–2393. doi: 10.1038/sj.npp.1301165

Gutman, D. A., Holtzheimer, P. E., Behrens, T. E. J., Johansen-Berg, H., and Mayberg, H. S. (2009). A tractography analysis of two deep brain stimulation white matter targets for depression. *Biol. Psychiatry* 65, 276–282. doi: 10.1016/j.biopsych.2008.09.021

Haber, S. N., Kim, K.-S., Mailly, P., and Calzavara, R. (2006). Reward-related cortical inputs define a large striatal region in primates that interface with associative cortical connections, providing a substrate for incentive-based learning. *J. Neurosci.* 26, 8368–8376. doi: 10.1523/jneurosci.0271-06.2006

Halpern, C. H., Wolf, J. A., Bale, T. L., Stunkard, A. J., Danish, S. F., Grossman, M., et al. (2008). Deep brain stimulation in the treatment of obesity. *J. Neurosurg.* 109, 625–634. doi: 10.3171/JNS/2008/109/10/0625

Hamani, C., Mayberg, H., Snyder, B., Giacobbe, P., Kennedy, S., and Lozano, A. M. (2009). Deep brain stimulation of the subcallosal cingulate gyrus for depression: anatomical location of active contacts in clinical responders and a suggested guideline for targeting. *J. Neurosurg.* 111, 1209–1215. doi: 10.3171/2008.10.jns08763

Hamann, S. B., Ely, T. D., Grafton, S. T., and Kilts, C. D. (1999). Amygdala activity related to enhanced memory for pleasant and aversive stimuli. *Nat. Neurosci.* 2, 289–293. doi: 10.1038/6404

Heilbronner, S. R., and Haber, S. N. (2014). Frontal cortical and subcortical projections provide a basis for segmenting the cingulum bundle: implications for neuroimaging and psychiatric disorders. *J. Neurosci.* 34, 10041–10054. doi: 10.1523/JNEUROSCI.5459-13.2014

Hollander, E., Poskar, S., and Gerard, A. (2012). "The obsessive-compulsive spectrum," in *Obsessive Compulsive Disorder: Current Science and Clinical Practice*, ed. J. Zohar (West Sussex, DE: John Wiley & Sons, Ltd.), 135–157.

Holtzheimer, P. E., Kelley, M. E., Gross, R. E., Filkowski, M. M., Garlow, S. J., Barrocas, A., et al. (2012). Subcallosal cingulate deep brain stimulation for treatment-resistant unipolar and bipolar depression. *Arch. Gen. Psychiatry* 69, 150–158. doi: 10.1001/archgenpsychiatry.2011.1456

Horsley, V., and Clarke, R. (1908). The structure and functions of the cerebellum examined by a new method. *Brain* 31, 45–124. doi: 10.1093/brain/31.1.45

Huff, W., Lenartz, D., Schormann, M., Lee, S., Kuhn, J., Koulousakis, A., et al. (2010). Unilateral deep brain stimulation of the nucleus accumbens in patients with treatment-resistant obsessive-compulsive disorder: outcomes after one year. *Clin. Neurol. Neurosurg* 112, 137–143. doi: 10.1016/j.clineuro.2009.11.006

Hurwitz, T. A., Honey, C. R., Allen, J., Gosselin, C., Hewko, R., Martzke, J., et al. (2012). Bilateral anterior capsulotomy for intractable depression. *J. Neuropsychiatry Clin. Neurosci.* 24, 176–182. doi: 10.1176/appi.neuropsych.11080189

Ikemoto, S., and Panksepp, J. (1999). The role of nucleus accumbens dopamine in motivated behavior. *Brain Res. Brain Res. Rev.* 31, 6–41. doi: 10.1016/s0165-0173(99)00023-5

Insel, T. R. (1992). Toward a neuroanatomy of obsessive-compulsive disorder. *Arch. Gen. Psychiatry* 49, 739–744. doi: 10.1001/archpsyc.1992.01820090067011

Insel, T., Cuthbert, B., Garvey, M., Heinssen, R., Pine, D. S., Quinn, K., et al. (2010). Research domain criteria (RDoC): toward a new classification framework for research on mental disorders. *Am. J. Psychiatry* 167, 748–751. doi: 10.1176/appi.ajp.2010.09091379

Jellison, B. J., Field, A. S., Medow, J., Lazar, M., Salamat, M. S., and Alexander, A. L. (2004). Diffusion tensor imaging of cerebral white matter: a pictorial review of physics, fiber tract anatomy and tumor imaging patterns. *AJNR Am. J. Neuroradiol.* 25, 356–369.

Jiménez-Ponce, F., Velasco-Campos, F., Castro-Farfán, G., Nicolini, H., Velasco, A. L., Salín-Pascual, R., et al. (2009). Preliminary study in patients with obsessive-compulsive disorder treated with electrical stimulation in the inferior thalamic peduncle. *Neurosurgery* 65, 203–209; discussion 209. doi: 10.1227/01.NEU.0000345938.39199.90

Joanette, Y., Stemmer, B., Assal, G., and Whitaker, H. (1993). From theory to practice: the unconventional contribution of gottlieb burckhardt to psychosurgery. *Brain Lang.* 45, 572–587. doi: 10.1006/brln.1993.1061

Kanaka, T., and Balasubramaniam, V. (1978). Stereotactic cingulumotomy for drug addiction. *Appl. Neurophysiol.* 41, 86–92. doi: 10.1159/000102404

Kane, M. J., and Engle, R. W. (2002). The role of prefrontal cortex in working-memory capacity, executive attention and general fluid intelligence: an individual-differences perspective. *Psychon. Bull. Rev.* 9, 637–671. doi: 10.3758/bf03196323

Kang, D.-H., Kim, J.-J., Choi, J.-S., Kim, Y. I., Kim, C.-W., Youn, T., et al. (2004). Volumetric investigation of the frontal-subcortical circuitry in patients with obsessive-compulsive disorder. *J. Neuropsychiatry Clin. Neurosci.* 16, 342–349. doi: 10.1176/appi.neuropsych.16.3.342

Kennedy, S. H., Giacobbe, P., Rizvi, S. J., Placenza, F. M., Nishikawa, Y., Mayberg, H. S., et al. (2011). Deep brain stimulation for treatment-resistant depression: follow-up after 3 to 6 years. *Am. J. Psychiatry* 168, 502–510. doi: 10.1176/appi.ajp.2010.10081187

Kihlström, L., Hindmarsh, T., Lax, I., Lippitz, B., Mindus, P., and Lindquist, C. (1997). Radiosurgical lesions in the normal human brain 17 years after gamma knife capsulotomy. *Neurosurgery* 41, 396–402; discussion 401–402. doi: 10.1097/00006123-199708000-00011

Kim, C.-H., Chang, J. W., Koo, M.-S., Kim, J. W., Suh, H. S., Park, I. H., et al. (2003). Anterior cingulotomy for refractory obsessive-compulsive disorder. *Acta Psychiatr. Scand.* 107, 283–290. doi: 10.1034/j.1600-0447.2003.00087.x

Kondziolka, D., Flickinger, J. C., and Hudak, R. (2011). Results following gamma knife radiosurgical anterior capsulotomies for obsessive compulsive disorder. *Neurosurgery* 68, 28–32; discussion 23–23. doi: 10.1227/NEU.0b013e3181fc5c8b

Kwon, J. S., Shin, Y.-W., Kim, C.-W., Kim, Y. I., Youn, T., Han, M. H., et al. (2003). Similarity and disparity of obsessive-compulsive disorder and schizophrenia in MR volumetric abnormalities of the hippocampus-amygdala complex. *J. Neurol. Neurosurg. Psychiatry* 74, 962–964. doi: 10.1136/jnnp.74.7.962

Langevin, J.-P., De Salles, A. A. F., Kosoyan, H. P., and Krahl, S. E. (2010). Deep brain stimulation of the amygdala alleviates post-traumatic stress disorder symptoms in a rat model. *J. Psychiatr. Res.* 44, 1241–1245. doi: 10.1016/j.jpsychires.2010.04.022

Langevin, J.-P., Koek, R. J., Schwartz, H. N., Chen, J. W. Y., Sultzer, D. L., Mandelkern, M. A., et al. (2016). Deep brain stimulation of the basolateral amygdala for treatment-refractory posttraumatic stress disorder. *Biol. Psychiatry* 79, e82–e84. doi: 10.1016/j.biopsych.2015.09.003

LeDoux, J. E., Cicchetti, P., Xagoraris, A., and Romanski, L. M. (1990). The lateral amygdaloid nucleus: sensory interface of the amygdala in fear conditioning. *J. Neurosci.* 10, 1062–1069.

Lipsman, N., Woodside, D. B., Giacobbe, P., Hamani, C., Carter, J. C., Norwood, S. J., et al. (2013). Subcallosal cingulate deep brain stimulation for treatment-refractory anorexia nervosa: a phase 1 pilot trial. *Lancet* 381, 1361–1370. doi: 10.1016/S0140-6736(12)62188-6

Lopes, A. C., Greenberg, B. D., Canteras, M. M., Batistuzzo, M. C., Hoexter, M. Q., Gentil, A. F., et al. (2014). Gamma ventral capsulotomy for obsessive-compulsive disorder: a randomized clinical trial. *JAMA Psychiatry* 71, 1066–1076. doi: 10.1001/jamapsychiatry.2014.1193

Lozano, A. M., Giacobbe, P., Hamani, C., Rizvi, S. J., Kennedy, S. H., Kolivakis, T. T., et al. (2012). A multicenter pilot study of subcallosal cingulate area deep brain stimulation for treatment-resistant depression. *J. Neurosurg.* 116, 315–322. doi: 10.3171/2011.10.JNS102122

Lozano, A. M., Mayberg, H. S., Giacobbe, P., Hamani, C., Craddock, R. C., and Kennedy, S. H. (2008). Subcallosal cingulate gyrus deep brain stimulation for treatment-resistant depression. *Biol. Psychiatry* 64, 461–467. doi: 10.1016/j.biopsych.2008.05.034

MacDonald, P. A., Antony, M. M., MacLeod, C. M., and Richter, M. A. (1997). Memory and confidence in memory judgements among individuals with obsessive compulsive disorder and non-clinical controls. *Behav. Res. Ther.* 35, 497–505. doi: 10.1016/s0005-7967(97)00013-2

Mallet, L., Polosan, M., Jaafari, N., Baup, N., Welter, M. L., Fontaine, D., et al. (2008). Subthalamic nucleus stimulation in severe obsessive-compulsive disorder. *N. Engl. J. Med.* 16, 2121–2134. doi: 10.1056/NEJMoa0708514

Malone, D. A., Dougherty, D. D., Rezai, A. R., Carpenter, L. L., Friehs, G. M., Eskandar, E. N., et al. (2009). Deep brain stimulation of the ventral capsule/ventral striatum for treatment-resistant depression. *Biol. Psychiatry* 65, 267–275. doi: 10.1016/j.biopsych.2008.08.029

Marek, R., Strobel, C., Bredy, T. W., and Sah, P. (2013). The amygdala and medial prefrontal cortex: partners in the fear circuit. *J. Physiol.* 591, 2381–2391. doi: 10.1113/jphysiol.2012.248575

Mayberg, H. S. (1994). Frontal lobe dysfunction in secondary depression. *J. Neuropsychiatry Clin. Neurosci.* 6, 428–442. doi: 10.1176/jnp.6.4.428

Mayberg, H. S. (1997). Limbic-cortical dysregulation: a proposed model of depression. *J. Neuropsychiatry Clin. Neurosci.* 9, 471–481. doi: 10.1176/jnp.9.3.471

Mayberg, H. S. (2009). Targeted electrode-based modulation of neural circuits for depression. *J. Clin. Invest.* 119, 717–725. doi: 10.1172/JCI38454

Mayberg, H. S., Liotti, M., Brannan, S. K., McGinnis, S., Mahurin, R. K., Jerabek, P. A., et al. (1999). Reciprocal limbic-cortical function and negative mood: converging PET findings in depression and normal sadness. *Am. J. Psychiatry* 156, 675–682.

Mayberg, H. S., Lozano, A. M., Voon, V., McNeely, H. E., Seminowicz, D., Hamani, C., et al. (2005). Deep brain stimulation for treatment-resistant depression. *Neuron* 45, 651–660. doi: 10.1016/j.neuron.2005.02.014

McElroy, S. L., Phillips, K. A., and Keck, P. E. Jr. (1994). Obsessive compulsive spectrum disorder. *J. Clin. Psychiatry* 55, 33–51; discussion 52–53. doi: 10.1007/springerreference_44589

Mechias, M. L., Etkin, A., and Kalisch, R. (2010). A meta-analysis of instructed fear studies: implications for conscious appraisal of threat. *Neuroimage* 49, 1760–1768. doi: 10.1016/j.neuroimage.2009.09.040

Mian, M. K., Campos, M., Sheth, S. A., and Eskandar, E. N. (2010). Deep brain stimulation for obsessive-compulsive disorder: past, present and future. *Neurosurg. Focus* 29:E10. doi: 10.3171/2010.4.FOCUS10107

Mikell, C. B., Sinha, S., and Sheth, S. A. (2016). Neurosurgery for schizophrenia: an update on pathophysiology and a novel therapeutic target. *J. Neurosurg.* 124, 917–928. doi: 10.3171/2015.4.JNS15120

Miller, E. K., and Cohen, J. D. (2001). An integrative theory of prefrontal cortex function. *Annu. Rev. Neurosci.* 24, 167–202. doi: 10.1146/annurev.neuro.24.1.167

Mirnezami, R., Nicholson, J., and Darzi, A. (2012). Preparing for precision medicine. *N. Engl. J. Med.* 366, 489–491. doi: 10.1056/NEJMp1114866

Modell, J. G., Mountz, J. M., Curtis, G. C., and Greden, J. F. (1989). Neurophysiologic dysfunction in basal ganglia/limbic striatal and thalamocortical circuits as a pathogenetic mechanism of obsessive-compulsive disorder. *J. Neuropsychiatry Clin. Neurosci.* 1, 27–36. doi: 10.1176/jnp.1.1.27

Moniz, E. (1933). Cerebral angiography: its application in clinical practice and physiology. *Lancet* 222, 1144–1147. doi: 10.1016/s0140-6736(00)89520-3

Moniz, E. (1937). Prefrontal leucotomy in the treatment of mental disorders. *Am. J. Psychiatry* 93, 1379–1385. doi: 10.1176/ajp.93.6.1379

Morris, J. S., Ohman, A., and Dolan, R. J. (1998). Conscious and unconscious emotional learning in the human amygdala. *Nature* 393, 467–470. doi: 10.1038/30976

Munoz, G. J., and Iniguez, A. R. (1949). "Mechanism of action of prefrontal leucotomy," in 1st Int. Conf. Psychosurgery (Lisboa), 51–62.

Murray, E. A., Wise, S. P., and Drevets, W. C. (2011). Localization of dysfunction in major depressive disorder: prefrontal cortex and amygdala. *Biol. Psychiatry* 69, e43–e54. doi: 10.1016/j.biopsych.2010.09.041

Nee, D. E., Wager, T. D., and Jonides, J. (2007). Interference resolution: insights from a meta-analysis of neuroimaging tasks. *Cogn. Affect. Behav. Neurosci.* 7, 1–17. doi: 10.3758/cabn.7.1.1

Nestler, E. J., Barrot, M., DiLeone, R. J., Eisch, A. J., Gold, S. J., and Monteggia, L. M. (2002). Neurobiology of depression. *Neuron* 34, 13–25. doi: 10.1016/S0896-6273(02)00653-0

Nuttin, B., Cosyns, P., Demeulemeester, H., Gybels, J., and Meyerson, B. (1999). Electrical stimulation in anterior limbs of internal capsules in patients with obsessive-compulsive disorder. *Lancet* 354:1526. doi: 10.1016/S0140-6736(99)02376-4

Papez, J. W. (1937). A proposed mechanism of emotion. *Arch. Neurol. Psychiatry* 38, 725–743. doi: 10.1001/archneurpsyc.1937.02260220069003

Patel, N. V., Agarwal, N., Mammis, A., and Danish, S. F. (2015). Frameless stereotactic magnetic resonance imaging-guided laser interstitial thermal therapy to perform bilateral anterior cingulotomy for intractable pain: feasibility, technical aspects and initial experience in 3 patients. *Neurosurgery* 2, 17–25. doi: 10.1227/NEU.0000000000000581

Patel, S. R., Aronson, J. P., Sheth, S. A., and Eskandar, E. N. (2013). Lesion procedures in psychiatric neurosurgery. *World Neurosurg.* 80, S31.e9–e16. doi: 10.1016/j.wneu.2012.11.038

Pujol, J., Soriano-Mas, C., Alonso, P., Cardoner, N., Menchón, J. M., Deus, J., et al. (2004). Mapping structural brain alterations in obsessive-compulsive disorder. *Arch. Gen. Psychiatry* 61, 720–730. doi: 10.1001/archpsyc.61.7.720

Ridderinkhof, K. R., van den Wildenberg, W. P. M., Segalowitz, S. J., and Carter, C. S. (2004). Neurocognitive mechanisms of cognitive control: the role of prefrontal cortex in action selection, response inhibition, performance monitoring and reward-based learning. *Brain Cogn.* 56, 129–140. doi: 10.1016/j.bandc.2004.09.016

Riva-Posse, P., Choi, K. S., Holtzheimer, P. E., McIntyre, C. C., Gross, R. E., Chaturvedi, A., et al. (2014). Defining critical white matter pathways mediating successful subcallosal cingulate deep brain stimulation for treatment-resistant depression. *Biol. Psychiatry* 76, 963–969. doi: 10.1016/j.biopsych.2014.03.029

Robinson, D., Wu, H., Munne, R. A., Ashtari, M., Alvir, J. M. J., Lerner, G., et al. (1995). Reduced caudate nucleus volume in obsessive compulsive disorder. *Arch. Gen. Psychiatry* 52, 393–398. doi: 10.1001/archpsyc.1995.03950170067009

Rück, C., Andréewitch, S., Flyckt, K., Edman, G., Nyman, H., Meyerson, B. A., et al. (2003). Capsulotomy for refractory anxiety disorders: long-term follow-up of 26 patients. *Am. J. Psychiatry* 160, 513–521. doi: 10.1176/appi.ajp.160.3.513

Rück, C., Karisson, A., Steele, D., Edman, G., Meyerson, B. A., Ericson, K., et al. (2008). Capsulotomy for obsessive-compulsive disorder: long-term follow-up of 25 patients. *Arch. Gen. Psychiatry* 65, 914–922. doi: 10.1001/archpsyc.65.8.914

Rutishauser, U., Mamelak, A. N., and Adolphs, R. (2015). The primate amygdala in social perception—insights from electrophysiological recordings and stimulation. *Trends Neurosci.* 38, 295–306. doi: 10.1016/j.tins.2015.03.001

Scarone, S., Colombo, C., Livian, S., Abbruzzese, M., Ronchi, P., Locatelli, M., et al. (1992). Increased right caudate nucleus size in obsessive-compulsive disorder: detection with magnetic resonance imaging. *Psychiatry Res.* 45, 115–121. doi: 10.1016/0925-4927(92)90005-o

Seminowicz, D., Mayberg, H. S., McIntosh, A., Goldapple, K., Kennedy, S., Segal, Z., et al. (2004). Limbic-frontal circuitry in major depression: a path modeling metanalysis. *Neuroimage* 22, 409–418. doi: 10.1016/j.neuroimage.2004.01.015

Shackman, A. J., Salomons, T. V., Slagter, H. A., Fox, A. S., Winter, J. J., and Davidson, R. J. (2011). The integration of negative affect, pain and cognitive control in the cingulate cortex. *Nat. Rev. Neurosci.* 12, 154–167. doi: 10.1038/nrn2994

Sheehan, J. P., Patterson, G., Schlesinger, D., and Xu, Z. (2013). γ knife surgery anterior capsulotomy for severe and refractory obsessive-compulsive disorder. *J. Neurosurg.* 119, 1112–1118. doi: 10.3171/2013.5.JNS13201

Sheline, Y. I., Sanghavi, M., Mintun, M. A., and Gado, M. H. (1999). Depression duration but not age predicts hippocampal volume loss in medically healthy women with recurrent major depression. *J. Neurosci.* 19, 5034–5043.

Shenhav, A., Botvinick, M., and Cohen, J. (2013). The expected value of control: an integrative theory of anterior cingulate cortex function. *Neuron* 79, 217–240. doi: 10.1016/j.neuron.2013.07.007

Sheth, S. A., Neal, J., Tangherlini, F., Mian, M. K., Gentil, A., Cosgrove, G. R., et al. (2013). Limbic system surgery for treatment-refractory obsessive-compulsive disorder: a prospective long-term follow-up of 64 patients. *J. Neurosurg.* 118, 491–497. doi: 10.3171/2012.11.JNS12389

Shields, D. C., Asaad, W., Eskandar, E. N., Jain, F. A., Cosgrove, G. R., Flaherty, A. W., et al. (2008). Prospective assessment of stereotactic ablative surgery for intractable major depression. *Biol. Psychiatry* 64, 449–454. doi: 10.1016/j.biopsych.2008.04.009

Sinha, S., McGovern, R. A., and Sheth, S. A. (2015). Deep brain stimulation for severe autism: from pathophysiology to procedure. *Neurosurg. Focus* 38:E3. doi: 10.3171/2015.3.FOCUS1548

Spiegel, E., Wycis, H., Marks, M., and Lee, A. (1947). Stereotaxic appartus for operations on the human brain. *Science* 80, 349–350. doi: 10.1126/science.106.2754.349

Steele, J. D., Christmas, D., Eljamel, M. S., and Matthews, K. (2008). Anterior cingulotomy for major depression: clinical outcome and relationship to lesion characteristics. *Biol. Psychiatry* 63, 670–677. doi: 10.1016/j.biopsych.2007.07.019

Stone, J. L. (2001). Dr. Gottlieb Burckhardt–the pioneer of psychosurgery. *J. Hist. Neurosci.* 10, 79–92. doi: 10.1076/jhin.10.1.79.5634

Sturm, V., Fricke, O., Bührle, C. P., Lenartz, D., Maarouf, M., Treuer, H., et al. (2012). DBS in the basolateral amygdala improves symptoms of autism and related self-injurious behavior: a case report and hypothesis on the pathogenesis of the disorder. *Front. Hum. Neurosci.* 6:341. doi: 10.3389/fnhum.2012.00341

Szeszko, P. R., Ardekani, B. A., Ashtari, M., Malhotra, A. K., Robinson, D. G., Bilder, R. M., et al. (2005). White matter abnormalities in obsessive-compulsive disorder: a diffusion tensor imaging study. *Arch. Gen. Psychiatry* 62, 782–790. doi: 10.1001/archpsyc.62.7.782

Szeszko, P. R., Robinson, D., Alvir, J. M., Bilder, R. M., Lencz, T., Ashtari, M., et al. (1999). Orbital frontal and amygdala volume reductions in obsessive-compulsive disorder. *Arch. Gen. Psychiatry* 56, 913–919. doi: 10.1001/archpsyc.56.10.913

Szeszko, P. R., Szeszko, P. R., MacMillan, S., MacMillan, S., McMeniman, M., McMeniman, M., et al. (2004). Brain structural abnormalities in psychotropic drug-naive pediatric patients with obsessive-compulsive disorder. *Am. J. Psychiatry* 161, 1049–1056. doi: 10.1176/appi.ajp.161.6.1049

Talairach, J., Hecaen, H., and David, M. (1949). Lobotomie préfrontale limitée par électrocoagulation des fibres thalamo-frontales à leur émergence du bras antérieur de la capsule interne. *Rev. Neurol.* 83:59.

Tulving, E., and Markowitsch, H. J. (1998). Episodic and declarative memory: role of the hippocampus. *Hippocampus* 8, 198–204. doi: 10.1002/(sici)1098-1063(1998)8:3<198::aid-hipo2>3.3.co;2-j

Veiel, H. O. (1997). A preliminary profile of neuropsychological deficits associated with major depression. *J. Clin. Exp. Neuropsychol.* 19, 587–603. doi: 10.1080/01688639708403745

Viswanathan, A., Harsh, V., Pereira, E. A. C., and Aziz, T. Z. (2013). Cingulotomy for medically refractory cancer pain. *Neurosurg. Focus* 35:E1. doi: 10.3171/2013.6.FOCUS13236

Yang, J. C., Ginat, D. T., Dougherty, D. D., Makris, N., and Eskandar, E. N. (2014). Lesion analysis for cingulotomy and limbic leucotomy: comparison and correlation with clinical outcomes. *J. Neurosurg.* 120, 152–163. doi: 10.3171/2013.9.JNS13839

13

Diffusion Tractography in Deep Brain Stimulation Surgery

Evan Calabrese *

Center for In Vivo Microscopy, Department of Radiology, Duke University Medical Center, Durham, NC, USA

***Correspondence:**
Evan Calabrese
edc15@duke.edu

Deep brain stimulation (DBS) is believed to exert its therapeutic effects through modulation of brain circuitry, yet conventional preoperative planning does not allow direct targeting or visualization of white matter pathways. Diffusion MRI tractography (DT) is virtually the only non-invasive method of visualizing structural connectivity in the brain, leading many to suggest its use to guide DBS targeting. DT-guided DBS not only has the potential to allow direct white matter targeting for established applications [e.g., Parkinson's disease (PD), essential tremor (ET), dystonia], but may also aid in the discovery of new therapeutic targets for a variety of other neurologic and psychiatric diseases. Despite these exciting opportunities, DT lacks standardization and rigorous anatomic validation, raising significant concern for the use of such data in stereotactic brain surgery. This review covers the technical details, proposed methods, and initial clinical data for the use of DT in DBS surgery. Rather than focusing on specific disease applications, this review focuses on methods that can be applied to virtually any DBS target.

Keywords: diffusion tractography, deep brain stimulation, neuroanatomy, magnetic resonance imaging, tractography, diffusion tensor imaging

INTRODUCTION AND BACKGROUND

Deep brain stimulation (DBS) has become an established therapy for medically refractory movement disorders including Parkinson's disease (PD), essential tremor (ET), and dystonia. DBS is also currently under investigation for use in a variety of other neurologic and psychiatric conditions including depression, chronic pain, and obsessive compulsive disorder.

Diffusion MRI tractography (DT) refers to 3D models of white matter pathways generated from diffusion weighted MRI data, most commonly diffusion tensor imaging (DTI). Here, the term DT is used to refer to all forms of tractography derived from diffusion MRI data including but not limited to DTI (Mori et al., 1999), Q-ball (Tuch, 2004; Descoteaux et al., 2007), constrained spherical deconvolution (CSD; Tournier et al., 2008), BEDPOSTX (Behrens et al., 2007), and diffusion spectrum imaging (DSI; Wedeen et al., 2005). DT is currently the only non-invasive method for modeling structural brain connectivity in humans.

This review covers recent work on integrating DT into DBS surgical planning. Several facets of this complex topic have been previously reviewed (Henderson, 2012; Torres et al., 2014). The current review differs from previous work in that it focuses on DT methods in DBS surgery, and associated technical concerns, rather than on their use for the treatment specific diseases. In addition, it incorporates new research that was published in the approximately 2 years since the most recent review was written. Nonetheless, previous reviews are valuable counterparts to this work, particularly for researchers with interest in a specific disease.

As the use of DBS increases both in scope and in patient numbers, there is a need to evaluate and improve each step of the surgical process. Several groups have suggested and even implemented a variety of DT-based DBS targeting techniques (Coenen et al., 2011a; Hunsche et al., 2013; Schlaepfer et al., 2013). The rationale for incorporating DT into DBS planning is based on two prominent, though not rigorously proven theories in DBS research. First, that DBS functions, at least in part, by modulation of neural circuitry, and second, that direct targeting of the circuitry on which DBS is believed to exert its effects will improve patient outcomes (Coenen et al., 2012).

Unlike its predecessor, ablative brain lesioning, DBS theoretically leaves brain connections intact. Due to the similar efficacy of DBS and brain lesioning for movement disorders, it was initially thought that DBS functioned by creating a "functional lesion" via continuous depolarization lock of local neurons (Benabid et al., 2002). While appealing as a heuristic, the functional lesion theory fails to explain several aspects of DBS including, for example, the fact that lesions of the globus pallidus externus produce Parkinsonism, while DBS of the same region can reverse Parkinsonian symptoms (Vitek et al., 2004). High-frequency stimulation does appear to inhibit local neurons, but there is also evidence that it simultaneously produces downstream excitatory activity (Hashimoto et al., 2003; McIntyre et al., 2004a). In fact, evidence from a variety of different sources including functional MRI, optogenetics, and DT connectivity analysis suggests that DBS may exert effects in sites distant from, but structurally connected to, stimulation sites (McIntyre et al., 2004b; Gradinaru et al., 2009; Schweder et al., 2010). Exactly how DBS exerts therapeutic effects through neurocircuitry is less clear but several theories exist. For example, substantial evidence suggests that ET is caused by aberrant neural activity in the dentatorubrothalamic tract (DRT; Coenen et al., 2014), a pathway connecting the dentate nucleus of the cerebellum to the contralateral red nucleus, ventral intermediate thalamus, and motor cortex (**Figure 1A**). It has therefore been suggested that DBS for ET functions through normalization of, or indirect inhibition of, pathological activity (Chiken and Nambu, 2015). It is also possible that DBS causes global brain changes that extend beyond the area of stimulation and immediate downstream connections (Montgomery and Gale, 2008). For example, experiments on DBS of the subgenual cingulum for depression have demonstrated both modulation of neural activity and changes in gene expression at various distant cortical sites, many of which are not directly connected to the stimulation region (Lujan et al., 2013; Riva-Posse et al., 2014). The exact mechanisms of DBS remain largely unknown and are more thoroughly discussed elsewhere (Benabid et al., 2002; Montgomery and Gale, 2008). However, it is clear that white matter connections play a role in DBS, and exploring this role will be an important area for future research.

Interestingly, while surgical treatment for movement disorders has evolved from ablation to DBS-mediated neuromodulation, stereotactic targeting methods have not followed suit. Conventional DBS preoperative planning uses essentially the same stereotactic targeting methods as ablative procedures. While conventional stereotactic targeting methods have served functional neurosurgeons for decades, they have two major drawbacks that limit their use for DBS targeting. First, stereotactic coordinates are often derived from histology-based human brain atlases, which are 2D and prone to spatial distortions from fixing, sectioning, and staining of tissue slices. Second, available targets consist largely of brain nuclei, and direct targeting or visualization of white matter pathways is typically not possible. If indeed DBS exerts its therapeutic effects through direct modulation of neural circuitry, it stands to reason that DBS targeting should be focused on neural circuits. There are many potential benefits of direct targeting of neurocircuitry for DBS. First, it may improve targeting accuracy, allowing fewer passes, fewer ineffective surgeries, and perhaps even obviate the need for intraoperative contact stimulation testing. Second, it may expand DBS therapy to new diseases by allowing targeting of structures that are not visible using conventional methods. Finally, it may aid in our understanding of the mechanisms of DBS by revealing the exact pathways affected by stimulation.

To date, DT remains the only non-invasive method for visualizing human brain connections. DT suffers from both fundamental and practical limitations that limit its use for modeling brain connections. Unlike many invasive modalities, DT is incapable of determining the direction of information flow, nor can it distinguish single- and multi-neuron connections. DT may also have difficulty resolving complex intra-voxel fiber crossings or non-dominant fiber populations due to limitations in scan time, hardware, or processing methods. Despite its many limitations, DT has been successfully used to model human neuronal connections for over two decades, including several pathways that are putative DBS targets (Sedrak et al., 2008).

This review contains two main discussion sections. The first addresses technical considerations for designing DT-based studies in DBS patients. This section includes discussion of the details of diffusion data acquisition, preprocessing, and DT generation. The second is a review of recent studies on integrating DT into DBS surgery. This is not meant to be an exhaustive analysis of DT-based DBS studies, but rather a broad overview of common methods and their applications. A majority of these studies can be divided into three broad groups based on the primary methodology. In this review, we will refer to these broad methodologies as: Tract stimulation modeling (TSM); Tract proximity analysis (TPA); and Direct tract targeting (DTT). **Figures 1B–D** show graphic representations of these three research techniques. Each method has a different goal, and each will be discussed separately. Throughout this review, implantable quadripolar brain stimulator leads will be referred to as "electrodes", while the individual stimulation elements will be referred to as "contacts". DT based models of white matter pathways will be referred to as "tracts". **Table 1** provides a list of abbreviations used throughout the manuscript.

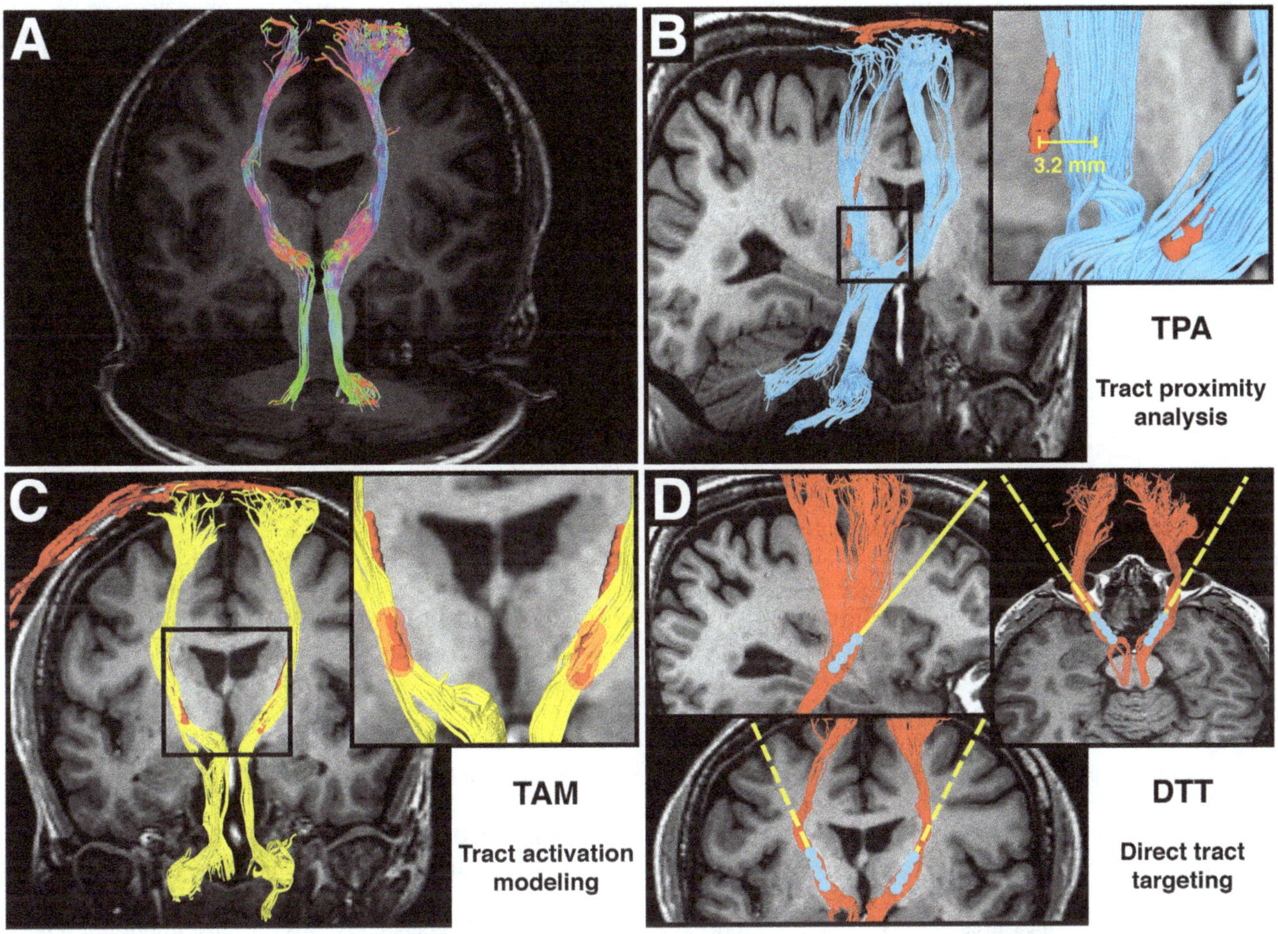

FIGURE 1 | Adapted from Calabrese et al. (2015b) Figure 6, with permission. (A) Directionally colored diffusion MRI tractography (DT) of the dentatorubrothalamic tract (DRT), which connects the dentate nucleus of the cerebellum, red nucleus, ventral intermediate thalamus, and motor cortex. Note the absence of a midline crossing in the midbrain, which is a limitation of the diffusion tensor imaging (DTI) technique. **(B)** Tract proximity analysis (TPA). Distances between the DRT (blue) and the deep brain stimulation (DBS) electrode (red) are compared with treatment outcomes. **(C)** Tract activation modeling. Fiber tracts (yellow) are generated from a region of interest surrounding the DBS contacts (red). **(D)** Direct tract targeting (DTT). The DT model of the DRT (red) is used for preoperative DBS electrode targeting.

TECHNICAL CONSIDERATIONS

DT generation can be divided into three separate steps: data acquisition, data processing, and tracking. Each of these steps has several variables that must be considered in order to ensure accurate DT. Many of the most common and important variables are discussed here.

Data Acquisition

Data acquisition involves the collection of diffusion weighted MRI data from subjects. For DT studies, the most important acquisition parameters include image resolution, diffusion weighting factor (*b*-value), and the number and distribution of diffusion measurements. Image resolution is important for DT because some fiber configurations, such as intra-voxel curving, can only be resolved by increasing spatial resolution (Calabrese et al., 2014). Image resolution also affects the accuracy of tract volume estimates, which is essential for DT-based DBS targeting (Lebel et al., 2011). In clinical MRI, resolution is typically limited by signal-to-noise ratio (SNR), and it is uncommon to achieve voxel sizes smaller than 2 mm isotropic at 3T. Many studies report spatial resolutions of 1 mm or less in plane, but typically have much larger (e.g., 3 mm) slice thickness. The use of anisotropic voxels should be discouraged for DT studies as it complicates accurate determination of fiber angles and fiber crossings due to partial volume effects (Mukherjee et al., 2008). SNR, and therefore resolution, can be improved by averaging or repeating scans, but a doubling of total scan time only increases SNR by a factor of $\sqrt{2}$ or approximately 1.4. Other important yet infrequently mentioned parameters that contribute to effective image resolution are sense factor, and incomplete *k*-space acquisition strategies like partial Fourier acquisition or zerofilling in *k*-space (Paschal and Morris, 2004). In general, it is best to use the highest isotropic resolution achievable without compromising SNR, and within a scan time compatible with clinical constraints

TABLE 1 | List of abbreviations used in this review.

Abbreviation	Definition
CSD	Constrained spherical deconvolution
DBS	Deep brain stimulation
DRT	Dentatorubrothalamic tract
DSI	Diffusion spectrum imaging
DT	Diffusion tractography
DTI	Diffusion tensor imaging
DTT	Direct tract targeting
ET	Essential tremor
HARDI	High angular resolution diffusion imaging
MRI	Magnetic resonance imaging
PD	Parkinson's disease
SNR	Signal-to-noise ratio
TPA	Tract proximity analysis
TSM	Tract stimulation modeling

(Jones and Cercignani, 2010). Increased resolution is unlikely to reduce accuracy, but it may not always be beneficial. For example, McNab et al. (2009) showed good correspondence between standard 2 mm isotropic preoperative DT and 0.73 mm isotropic postmortem DT in a patient who received DBS of the subgenual cingulum. In DBS studies, image resolutions as high as 1.6 mm isotropic have been used (Sudhyadhom et al., 2012).

In addition to spatial resolution, diffusion MRI requires consideration of intravoxel *diffusion* resolution. All DT techniques, in essence, use measurements of the 3D diffusion function in each voxel (often referred to as the diffusion propagator) to determine underlying fiber orientation. By convention, MRI measures diffusion in a spherical coordinate system known as *q*-space, which has a Fourier transform relationship with the diffusion propagator. All points in *q*-space can be defined by two angles (the diffusion measurement direction) and a radius (the diffusion weighting factor, or *b*-value). Increasing the number of diffusion measurement directions increases the angular resolution of the fiber reconstruction, which can allow multiple fibers to be reconstructed from a single voxel with appropriate processing. In general, higher *b*-values yield a larger signal difference between restricted and unrestricted diffusion at the cost of lower SNR. This increased signal difference affects the ability to accurately detect certain fiber populations (Frank, 2001; Basser, 2002). Both the number and the arrangement of *q*-space measurements required for accurate fiber reconstruction depends heavily on the constraints and assumptions of the DT technique being used.

The simplest case, DTI, assumes that there is a single fiber population, and that the diffusion propagator is a tensor. As such, it requires only six unique diffusion measurement directions and a *b*-value sufficient to distinguish the primary diffusion direction from the two perpendicular diffusion directions (usually $b \geq 800$ s/mm^2). In practice, using only six diffusion measurements is problematic because the reconstruction algorithm is highly sensitive to error with minimal inputs (Lebel et al., 2011). Increasing the number of diffusion measurement directions improves the accuracy of DTI fiber orientation estimations, but diminishing returns are reached at around 30 unique directions (Jones, 2004). Similarly, for DTI low *b*-values can introduce error, but there is little benefit to increasing *b*-value above $b = 1500$ s/mm^2 (Dyrby et al., 2011). In contrast, multi-fiber methods such as spherical harmonic Q-ball (Descoteaux et al., 2007), have far fewer model assumptions, and therefore require more diffusion measurement angles and higher *b*-values. Typical values are 30–120 directions and *b*-values in the 2000–5000 s/mm^2 range. Diminishing returns are reached at around 90 directions and $b = 4000$ s/mm^2 (Tournier et al., 2013). DSI, a DT reconstruction method that is often described as "model free", requires hundreds of diffusion measurement angles and *b*-values in the 10,000–50,000 s/mm^2 range because it attempts to directly calculate the underlying diffusion propagator in each voxel using the Fourier transform relationship (Wedeen et al., 2008). *b*-values in this range are often difficult or impossible to achieve on certain scanners because of hardware and/or SNR limitations. Even if appropriate hardware is available, lengthy diffusion sampling schemes may be impractical or cost-prohibitive in DBS patients. In general, diffusion sampling scheme should be chosen based on the data processing method, and should be as complete as possible given scan time limitations. In the existing DBS literature, 12–60 diffusion directions have been used, typically at $b = 1000$ s/mm^2 (Johansen-Berg et al., 2008; Klein et al., 2012; Sudhyadhom et al., 2012; Anthofer et al., 2014).

Data Processing

There are many different DT data processing methods available, each with different requirements, assumptions, limitations and benefits. Perhaps the most important processing difference for DBS studies is single-fiber (e.g., DTI) vs. multi-fiber reconstruction (e.g., Q-ball; Tuch, 2004). Multi-fiber methods may be preferable since many putative tract targets for DBS are located in structurally complex brain regions. Further, it has been shown that at clinical image resolution, 60–90% of white matter voxels contain crossing fibers (Jeurissen et al., 2012). Another important processing difference is direct fiber estimation methods (e.g., BEDPOSTX, CSD) vs. orientation distribution function-based methods (e.g., Q-ball, DSI). Orientation distribution function based methods attempt to reconstruct the diffusion propagator in each voxel, and then infer fiber orientation from the peaks of this function. In contrast, direct fiber estimation methods attempt to recover fiber orientation directly from diffusion MRI data. Direct methods may be less prone to error, and more flexible in terms of sampling requirements, but often have dramatically increased computational requirements (Behrens et al., 2007; Tournier et al., 2008, 2013).

DTI is by far the most common DT method used in DBS studies (Torres et al., 2014). This technique has the advantage of being readily available on most commercial scanners, as well as having a relatively quick acquisition, and a simple reconstruction. The major drawbacks of this method are the assumptions of the model and the fact that it only accounts for a single fiber population per voxel, which is insufficient for a majority of voxels in the human brain (Jeurissen et al., 2012). The strengths and weaknesses of other fiber reconstruction methods like Q-ball, CSD, and DSI are less clear, and depend heavily on the diffusion measurement scheme and the particular fiber tract of interest (Calabrese et al., 2014). These advanced DT methods are almost certainly more anatomically accurate than DTI, but their sampling requirements may be prohibitive in DBS patients, and it is not known if the added anatomic accuracy actually improves DBS surgical planning or electrode targeting. It is also important to note that many tractography data processing methods are neither designed for nor approved for use in surgical planning. Nonetheless, as DBS targets become more complex and nuanced, it stands to reason that advanced DT processing methods may play an important role in accurately visualizing the underlying anatomy. For instance, there are several examples of DBS studies that utilize BEDPOSTX fiber reconstruction for complex anatomic targets (Johansen-Berg et al., 2008; Klein et al., 2012; Clelland et al., 2014; Choi et al., 2015).

Tracking

Even with the exact same data and processing method, differences in tracking algorithms can dramatically affect the size, shape, and extent of resultant tracts, which has obvious implications for DT-based DBS targeting (Fillard et al., 2011). Most of the differences in tracking algorithms can be distilled to deterministic vs. probabilistic tracking, and the choice of tracking thresholds. Deterministic DT algorithms use only the calculated fiber orientations, while probabilistic algorithms randomly draw from a probability distribution of fiber orientations based on estimated error. Deterministic algorithms thus generate the same set of tracts every time, while probabilistic methods yield a random set of probability distributed tracts. This random, iterative process makes probabilistic methods much more computationally expensive and time consuming. The data formats for probabilistic and deterministic DT are also quite different, and often require different analysis methods. Deterministic data are typically stored as a set of 3D streamlines, while probabilistic data usually takes the form of an image, where intensity values reflect strength or probability of connection between a given voxel and a seed region. Probabilistic DT data can be easily adjusted using thresholding, which adds an additional layer of complexity. For example, contact between a DBS electrode and deterministic fiber tract is all or none, while contact with a probabilistic tract can be expressed in terms of contact strength or probability (Pouratian et al., 2011). In addition, probabilistic methods can be more sensitive than deterministic methods for non-dominant fiber pathways, but are also likely to have more false positives (Behrens et al., 2007). The choice of deterministic vs. probabilistic DT depends on the application, but for complex pathways probabilistic methods may be preferable (Behrens et al., 2007; Kwon et al., 2011). Although deterministic tractography is significantly more common for DBS applications, there are a number of published studies that use probabilistic methods (Johansen-Berg et al., 2008; Pouratian et al., 2011; Sudhyadhom et al., 2012; Riva-Posse et al., 2014).

The choice of DTI tracking thresholds (e.g., angle threshold, fractional anisotropy threshold) also depends on the application, and should generally be tailored to the specific tract of interest. For example, DT of cortical areas, or regions with many crossing fibers requires a very low fractional anisotropy threshold, and tracts with high curvature obviously require larger angle thresholds.

There are several other important differences between different tracking algorithms, particularly with regard to how tracts are propagated. The most basic tracking algorithms follow the calculated fiber orientation exactly when moving from voxel to voxel, while others integrate fiber direction over several adjacent voxels (Mori et al., 1999; Lazar et al., 2003). These differences affect anatomic accuracy and propagation of error, and can yield wildly different tracts even when performed on the same dataset (Lazar and Alexander, 2003; Fillard et al., 2011).

The choice of what to track is also important, particularly for DBS applications. If a pathway is known *a priori*, it may be possible to develop a standard set of seed and waypoint regions to allow reliable tracking (Coenen et al., 2011c, 2012; Anthofer et al., 2015). If the goal is to investigate the pathways being affected by given DBS electrode, a seed region can be generated around the implantation site using co-registered pre- and post-operative imaging. Such seed regions can range from simple cubes (Barkhoudarian et al., 2010) to elaborate electric field models based on stimulation parameters and the electrical properties of surrounding tissue (Butson et al., 2006, 2007). While electric field modeling adds considerable complexity to a study, it might also provide a more accurate estimation of the fiber populations that are modulated by DBS electrodes.

Another major issue with tracking is the lack of full-featured software suite for tracking and surgical planning in the surgical context. Many of the techniques described here, including probabilistic tractography and electric field modeling, are not commonly available in surgical planning software packages. In the absence of clinically tested or approved software, these techniques remain primarily research tools.

Anatomic Accuracy

Recently, several groups have shown that DT has relatively poor anatomic accuracy, particularly in areas of neuronal complexity (Thomas et al., 2014; Calabrese et al., 2015a). DT has both practical and fundamental limitations that decrease its anatomic accuracy. From a practical standpoint, diffusion MRI data derived from human subjects is never ideal due to factors like scan time considerations, hardware limitations, patient motion, cardiac pulsation, and bulk flow. Each of these factors has the potential to affect the anatomic accuracy of DT by introducing error into DT processing algorithms. Even in the absence of practical concerns, there are fundamental limitations to the DT method (Thomas et al., 2014). First, DT is based on the assumption that the diffusion of water in the brain follows axonal pathways, which may not always be correct. Second, DT is constrained by the assumptions of the reconstruction and tracking models. For example, many reconstruction algorithms assume that water diffusion in the brain is Gaussian in nature, and there is often an implicit or explicit limit in the number of fiber populations that can be reconstructed from a single voxel. Even so-called "model free" fiber reconstruction methods are still subject to the assumptions of tracking algorithms including tract initiation and termination criteria, and step length (Wedeen et al., 2008). Fortunately, for DBS targeting applications, the absolute accuracy of DT is not important as long as it is accurate enough to guide effective electrode placement. This question, "is DT accurate enough for effective DBS targeting?" is one of the fundamental motivations for the studies reviewed in the next section.

DT-BASED DBS METHODS

A number of different studies have been conducted with the goal of incorporating DT into DBS surgery. **Table 2** is a list of the DT/DBS studies discussed in this section. This is a representative rather than comprehensive list. Studies are organized into three broad categories based on methodology rather than the specific disease or DBS target.

Tract Stimulation Modeling

TSM (**Figure 1B**) refers to the practice of seeding DT from the region surrounding previously implanted DBS electrodes. The goal of TSM is to identify the population of brain connections that are likely to be modulated by a given DBS contact. This technique can be used to confirm that efficacious contacts are near or within a tract of interest. For example, Coenen et al. (2011b) performed TSM in a patient who received DBS for PD, and found that DT of the most efficacious contact yielded the expected DRT. The DRT was also identified by TSM of efficacious contacts in a patient with SCA1 dystonia by Copeland et al. (2014). Using similar methods, Kovanlikaya et al. (2014) found that TSM of efficacious contacts in a patient who received DBS for chronic pain demonstrated connections to the somatosensory cortex. TSM can also be used to identify pathways that lead to undesired side effects. Barkhoudarian et al. (2010) used TSM to demonstrate why stimulation of specific contacts at high voltages caused motor side effects in three patients who received DBS for movement disorders.

Another major use of TSM is to elucidate the activation patterns of successful vs. unsuccessful DBS for investigational applications. This exploratory (rather than confirmatory) use of TSM has been most widely used for depression, where the mechanism of DBS therapy is poorly understood. Johansen-Berg et al. (2008) generated a DT atlas of the subgenual cingulum from 17 healthy controls and then analyzed TSM of electrodes projected onto the atlas from nine patients who received DBS in the anterior cingulate cortex for refractory depression. They identified unique TSM patterns of efficacious contacts extending into frontal, limbic, and visceromotor regions. These results were built upon by Lujan et al. (2013) and Riva-Posse et al. (2014) in one and 17 patient(s) respectively. In both cases, TSM was compared between efficacious and non-efficacious contacts using simulated electric field models based on stimulation parameters. Both studies clearly showed different connectivity patterns of efficacious vs. non-efficacious contacts. Lujan et al. (2011) also performed a similar study in seven patients with refractory depression who received DBS of the ventral anterior internal capsule and ventral striatum. Once again, they found unique TSM patterns in responders and non-responders. Choi et al. (2015) performed intraoperative behavioral analysis on nine patients implanted for treatment-resistant depression, and found that contacts associated with acute positive mood changes were connected to the bilateral ventromedial frontal cortex and cingulate cortex. These TSM results lead the authors to suggest this specific connectivity pattern as a biomarker for effective DBS contact positioning.

Studies with similar methodologies have been conducted in patients who received DBS for cluster headache (Clelland et al., 2014), PD (Klein et al., 2012), primary dystonia (Rozanski et al., 2014), and chronic pain (Owen et al., 2007, 2008). In each case, authors analyzed TSM of efficacious vs. non-efficacious contacts in an effort to understand the neural networks that, when stimulated, lead to effective DBS therapy. These studies improve our understanding of the neurophysiologic underpinnings of brain diseases, and may eventually lead to more accurate and efficacious DBS targeting for the treatment of those diseases.

Tract Proximity Analysis

TPA (**Figure 1C**) refers to retrospective analysis of the location of DBS contacts with respect to a specific tract of interest. This method can be used to answer the question of whether the proximity of a contact to a specific tract correlates with treatment efficacy, as well as for retrospective analysis of electrode targeting accuracy. TPA has been most commonly used in the study of DBS for movement disorders where putative tracts of interest (e.g., the DRT) are well described in the literature. Pouratian et al. (2011) performed TPA on a total of 10 DBS tremor patients and found that efficacious contacts were most likely to be associated with thalamic projections to the premotor cortex. Subsequent TPA studies have largely focused on the DRT as a putative target for the therapeutic effects of DBS in tremor patients. Sweet et al. (2014) found a non-significant trend in improved tremor control with increased contact proximity to the DRT in a study of 14 patients who received DBS for tremor-dominant PD. Similarly, Coenen et al. (2014) found a non-significant trend towards improved efficacy with increased proximity of the DRT to simulated contact electrical fields in 11 ET patients. Anthofer et al. (2014) also found that efficacious contacts were frequently near or within the DRT in a study of 10 ET patients, however no statistical analysis was performed. Finally, Calabrese et al. (2015b) were able to show a weak, but statistically significant correlation between treatment efficacy and contact proximity to the DRT, however, they used a high-resolution postmortem fiber atlas to generate the DRT model.

TPA has also been used to investigate DBS-related adverse effects in tremor patients including motor, sensory, and psychiatric side effects. Motor side effects have been studied both by Calabrese et al. (2015b), who showed no significant correlation between side effects and contact proximity to the

TABLE 2 | List of articles on DT/DBS discussed in this review.

Reference	Title	Patients	Disease
Anthofer et al. (2015)	DTI-based deterministic fiber tracking of the medial forebrain bundle	10	ET
Anthofer et al. (2014)	The variability of atlas-based targets in relation to surrounding major fiber tracts in thalamic deep brain stimulation	11	Depression
Barkhoudarian et al. (2010)	A role of diffusion tensor imaging in movement disorder surgery	3	PD, ET, Dystonia
Bhatia et al. (2012)	Diffusion tensor imaging to Aid subgenual cingulum target selection for deep brain stimulation in depression	59	Depression
Butson et al. (2006)	Predicting the effects of deep brain stimulation with diffusion tensor based electric field models	1	PD
Butson et al. (2007)	Patient-specific analysis of the volume of tissue activated during deep brain stimulation	1	PD
Calabrese et al. (2015a,b)	Postmortem diffusion MRI of the human brainstem and thalamus for deep brain stimulator electrode localization	1	ET
Choi et al. (2015)	Mapping the "Depression switch" during intraoperative testing of subcallosal cingulate deep brain stimulation	9	Depression
Clelland et al. (2014)	Common cerebral networks associated with distinct deep brain stimulation targets for cluster headache	7	Cluster headace
Coenen et al. (2009)	Medial forebrain bundle stimulation as a pathophysiological mechanism for hypomania in subthalamic nucleus deep brain stimulation for Parkinson's disease	6	PD
Coenen et al. (2011a)	A role of diffusion tensor imaging fiber tracking in deep brain stimulation surgery: DBS of the dentato-rubro-thalamic tract (drt) for the treatment of therapy-refractory tremor	1	Dystonia
Coenen et al. (2011b)	Individual fiber anatomy of the subthalamic region revealed with DTI A concept to identify the DBS target for tremor suppression	1	PD
Coenen et al. (2012)	Diffusion tensor imaging and neuromodulation: DTI as key technology for deep brain stimulation	N/A	N/A
Coenen et al. (2014)	Modulation of the cerebello-thalamo-cortical network in thalamic deep brain stimulation for tremor	11	PD, ET, Dystonia
Copeland et al. (2014)	Deep brain stimulation of the internal globus pallidus for generalized dystonia associated with spinocerebellar ataxia type 1: a case report	1	Dystonia
Henderson (2012)	"Connectomic surgery": diffusion tensor imaging (DTI) tractography as a targeting modality for surgical modulation of neural networks	N/A	N/A
Hunsche et al. (2013)	Tractography-guided stimulation of somatosensory fibers for thalamic pain relief	4	Chronic pain
Johansen-Berg et al. (2008)	Anatomical connectivity of the subgenual cingulate region targeted with deep brain stimulation for treatment-resistant depression	9	Depression
Klein et al. (2012)	The tremor network targeted by successful VIM deep brain stimulation in humans	12	PD
Kovanlikaya et al. (2014)	Treatment of chronic pain: diffusion tensor imaging identification of the ventroposterolateral nucleus confirmed with successful deep brain stimulation	1	Chronic pain
Lujan et al. (2011)	Axonal pathways linked to therapeutic and nontherapeutic outcomes during psychiatric deep brain stimulation	7	Depression
Lujan et al. (2013)	Tractography-activation models applied to subcallosal cingulate deep brain stimulation	1	Depression
McIntyre et al. (2004a,b)	Uncovering the mechanism(s) of action of deep brain stimulation: activation, inhibition, or both	N/A	N/A
McNab et al. (2009)	Reduced limbic connections may contraindicate subgenual cingulate deep brain stimulation for intractable depression	1	Depression
Owen et al. (2007)	Preoperative DTI and probabilistic tractography in an amputee with deep brain stimulation for lower limb stump pain	1	Chronic pain
Owen et al. (2008)	Pre-operative DTI and probabilisitic tractography in four patients with deep brain stimulation for chronic pain	4	Chronic pain
Pouratian et al. (2011)	Multi-institutional evaluation of deep brain stimulation targeting using probabilistic connectivity-based thalamic segmentation	10	ET
Riva-Posse et al. (2014)	Defining critical white matter pathways mediating successful subcallosal cingulate deep brain stimulation for treatment-resistant depression	16	Depression
Rozanski et al. (2014)	Connectivity patterns of pallidal DBS electrodes in focal dystonia: a diffusion tensor tractography study	8	Dystonia
Said et al. (2014)	Correlation of diffusion tensor tractography and intraoperative macrostimulation during deep brain stimulation for Parkinson disease	17	PD
Schlaepfer et al. (2013)	Rapid effects of deep brain stimulation for treatment-resistant major depression	7	Depression
Schweder et al. (2010)	Chronic pedunculopontine nucleus stimulation restores functional connectivity	1	PD
Sedrak et al. (2008)	The role of modern imaging modalities on deep brain stimulation targeting for mental illness	15	PD, ET, Dystonia
Sudhyadhom et al. (2012)	Delineation of motor and somatosensory thalamic subregions utilizing probabilistic diffusion tractography and electrophysiology	5	ET
Sweet et al. (2014)	Fiber tractography of the axonal pathways linking the basal ganglia and cerebellum in Parkinson disease: implications for targeting in deep brain stimulation	14	PD
Torres et al. (2014)	Integrating diffusion tensor imaging-based tractography into deep brain stimulation surgery: a review of the literature	N/A	N/A

DRT, and by Said et al. (2014) who show a non-significant trend towards greater contact voltage tolerability thresholds with increasing distance from the corticospinal tracts. Sensory side effects have also been studied, including work by Sajonz et al. (2015) who showed that contact proximity to the medial lemniscus was significantly correlated with hypogeusia and ageusia. Additionally, Coenen et al. (2009) suggested that stimulation of the median forebrain bundle was responsible for hypomania symptoms in a patient who received DBS for PD.

TPA studies serve as an important first step towards prospective targeting of DT-derived tracts with DBS electrodes. TPA has the benefit of allowing a specific tract hypothesis to be tested, however, unlike TSM, it requires *a priori* identification of a pathway of interest, which may not always be feasible. Once a tract of interest is identified for a given disease, TPA can be used to retrospectively test whether or not electrode proximity to that tract results in improved treatment efficacy. This in turn can provide initial evidence towards DT-based targeting of the tract of interest.

Direct Tract Targeting

DTT (**Figure 1D**) refers to prospective targeting of DT-derived tracts with DBS electrodes. DTT requires not only *a priori* knowledge of a tract of interest, but also requires sufficient supporting evidence to justify targeting that tract in humans. Few putative tract targets meet these criteria, and as a result DTT studies are rare, and generally limited to cases where conventional methods are infeasible or ineffective. For example, Coenen et al. (2011a) describes successful DTT of the DRT in a patient with myoclonus dystonia. Conventional targeting, which employs intraoperative efficacy testing, was not possible because the patient's head-dominant symptoms were obscured by the DBS stereotaxic head frame. Successful symptomatic control was achieved, and simulated electric fields from efficacious contacts were shown to overlap the DRT but not other adjacent tracts such as the corticospinal tracts. Schlaepfer et al. (2013) used DTT of the medial forebrain bundle to successfully treat six of seven patients with refractory depression, with the rationale that this tract cannot be reliably identified using conventional MRI images. Indeed, previous work by Bhatia et al. (2012) showed that DT based coordinates of the subgenual cingulum—a related DBS target for depression—differed significantly from coordinates derived from conventional T2-weighted MRI. Hunsche et al. (2013) used a hybrid DTT approach to target the posterior limb of the internal capsule in four patients with thalamic pain syndrome. The stereotaxic target was based on conventional targeting methods, but the electrode implantation trajectory was adjusted to provide at least 20 mm of overlap with DT of the spinothalamic tract. This approach lead to a 40% or greater pain relief in three of four patients.

In many ways, DTT is the ultimate goal of studies seeking to integrate DT into DBS planning. It is appealing because it allows targeting of structures that may not be visible using conventional methods, and it incorporates a mechanistic view of DBS as a neuromodulatory therapy. Unfortunately, to date there have been no controlled clinical trials comparing DTT to conventional targeting methods. Without such studies, it is impossible to say for certain whether DTT can improve DBS patient outcomes.

CONCLUSIONS

While DT-based DBS targeting is still in its infancy, considerable progress has been made in incorporating DT into DBS surgery. These advances represent an exciting opportunity for both the DT and DBS communities. For DT researchers, DBS could become the second major clinical use for DT, the first being preoperative mapping of eloquent white matter pathways for brain tumor resection (Witwer et al., 2002; Nimsky et al., 2005). For the DBS community, DT provides a novel method for targeting structures that are not visible with conventional imaging methods, and may eventually help to elucidate the mechanisms underlying DBS therapy.

Interestingly, the three types of studies discussed here provide a reasonable workflow for DT-based investigation of novel DBS applications. For investigational DBS, TSM can be used to identify putative tracts of interest, which can in turn be validated using TPA, and then accurately targeted using DTT. This workflow is perhaps best exemplified by DBS of frontal lobe white matter pathways for refractory depression, where all three types of studies have been successfully performed (Coenen et al., 2012; Schlaepfer et al., 2013; Riva-Posse et al., 2014; Anthofer et al., 2015). If the issues facing DT-based DBS targeting are addressed, this workflow may become a valuable method for DT-based DBS target discovery, validation, and effective implementation.

Two major issues currently limit the potential of DT-based DBS targeting. First is the need for validation and standardization of DT, and second is the lack of randomized controlled trials. DT validation in humans is hindered by the inability to use "gold standard" methods like neuronal tracer studies. For this reason, animal studies, particularly those in non-human primates, are an important source of validation for DT (Schmahmann et al., 2007; Calabrese et al., 2014). However, no method is without limitations, and comparisons between DT and other neuronal mapping techniques are problematic because the data are fundamentally different (Thomas et al., 2014). Further, any information gleaned from animals will have to be extrapolated to humans, which reduces its utility for DBS planning. Interestingly, the integration of DT into DBS planning may itself provide important validation for DT. For example, comparisons of DT results with intraoperative microelectrode recording during DBS implantation has been used to validate DT-based segmentation of the thalamus (Sudhyadhom et al., 2012). The pathway towards standardization of DT is less clear, particularly since optimal methods are largely undefined. Knowledge of previous studies, like those discussed here, should help investigators make informed decisions on reasonable DT methods for their particular application.

Given these uncertainties it is no surprise that randomized controlled trials of DT-guided DBS have not been attempted to date. However, as with any emerging medical therapy, such trials will be essential for widespread adoption. The major challenge to the community will be in selecting the proper DBS application, DT methods, and the appropriate patient population for comparing DT-guided DBS to conventional methods.

AUTHOR CONTRIBUTIONS

EC performed the literature review and wrote the manuscript.

ACKNOWLEDGMENTS

The author would like to thank the following people for support and guidance: G. Allan Johnson, Shivanand P. Lad, Patrick Hickey, Beth Parente, Sally Zimney and Tawynna Gordon. The author acknowledges the National Institutes of Health and the National Institute of Biomedical Imaging and Bioengineering Grant number: P41 EB015897.

REFERENCES

Anthofer, J., Steib, K., Fellner, C., Lange, M., Brawanski, A., and Schlaier, J. (2014). The variability of atlas-based targets in relation to surrounding major fibre tracts in thalamic deep brain stimulation. *Acta Neurochir. (Wien)* 156, 1497–1504. doi: 10.1007/s00701-014-2103-z

Anthofer, J. M., Steib, K., Fellner, C., Lange, M., Brawanski, A., and Schlaier, J. (2015). DTI-based deterministic fibre tracking of the medial forebrain bundle. *Acta Neurochir. (Wien)* 157, 469–477. doi: 10.1007/s00701-014-2335-y

Barkhoudarian, G., Klochkov, T., Sedrak, M., Frew, A., Gorgulho, A., Behnke, E., et al. (2010). A role of diffusion tensor imaging in movement disorder surgery. *Acta Neurochir. (Wien)* 152, 2089–2095. doi: 10.1007/s00701-010-0742-2

Basser, P. J. (2002). Relationships between diffusion tensor and q-space MRI. *Magn. Reson. Med.* 47, 392–397. doi: 10.1002/mrm.10052

Behrens, T. E. J., Berg, H. J., Jbabdi, S., Rushworth, M. F. S., and Woolrich, M. W. (2007). Probabilistic diffusion tractography with multiple fibre orientations: what can we gain? *Neuroimage* 34, 144–155. doi: 10.1016/j.neuroimage.2006.09.018

Benabid, A. L., Benazzous, A., and Pollak, P. (2002). Mechanisms of deep brain stimulation. *Mov. Disord.* 17, S73–S74. doi: 10.1002/mds.10145

Bhatia, K. D., Henderson, L., Ramsey-Stewart, G., and May, J. (2012). Diffusion tensor imaging to aid subgenual cingulum target selection for deep brain stimulation in depression. *Stereotact. Funct. Neurosurg.* 90, 225–232. doi: 10.1159/000338083

Butson, C. R., Cooper, S. E., Henderson, J. M., and McIntyre, C. C. (2006). Predicting the effects of deep brain stimulation with diffusion tensor based electric field models. *Med. Image Comput. Comput. Assist. Interv.* 9, 429–437. doi: 10.1007/11866763_53

Butson, C. R., Cooper, S. E., Henderson, J. M., and McIntyre, C. C. (2007). Patient-specific analysis of the volume of tissue activated during deep brain stimulation. *Neuroimage* 34, 661–670. doi: 10.1016/j.neuroimage.2006.09.034

Calabrese, E., Badea, A., Coe, C. L., Lubach, G. R., Styner, M. A., and Johnson, G. A. (2014). Investigating the tradeoffs between spatial resolution and diffusion sampling for brain mapping with diffusion tractography: time well spent? *Hum. Brain Mapp.* 35, 5667–5685. doi: 10.1002/hbm.22578

Calabrese, E., Badea, A., Cofer, G., Qi, Y., and Johnson, G. A. (2015a). A diffusion MRI tractography connectome of the mouse brain and comparison with neuronal tracer data. *Cereb. Cortex* 25, 4628–4637. doi: 10.1093/cercor/bhv121

Calabrese, E., Hickey, P., Hulette, C., Zhang, J., Parente, B., Lad, S. P., et al. (2015b). Postmortem diffusion MRI of the human brainstem and thalamus for deep brain stimulator electrode localization. *Hum. Brain Mapp.* 36, 3167–3178. doi: 10.1002/hbm.22836

Chiken, S., and Nambu, A. (2015). Mechanism of deep brain stimulation: inhibition, excitation, or disruption? *Neuroscientist* doi: 10.1177/1073858415581986 [Epub ahead of print].

Choi, K. S., Riva-Posse, P., Gross, R. E., and Mayberg, H. S. (2015). Mapping the "depression switch" during intraoperative testing of subcallosal cingulate deep brain stimulation. *JAMA Neurol.* 72, 1252–1260. doi: 10.1001/jamaneurol.2015.2564

Clelland, C. D., Zheng, Z., Kim, W., Bari, A., and Pouratian, N. (2014). Common cerebral networks associated with distinct deep brain stimulation targets for cluster headache. *Cephalalgia* 34, 224–230. doi: 10.1177/0333102413509431

Coenen, V. A., Allert, N., and Mädler, B. (2011a). A role of diffusion tensor imaging fiber tracking in deep brain stimulation surgery: DBS of the dentato-rubro-thalamic tract (drt) for the treatment of therapy-refractory tremor. *Acta Neurochir. (Wien)* 153, 1579–1585. doi: 10.1007/s00701-011-1036-z

Coenen, V. A., Mädler, B., Schiffbauer, H., Urbach, H., and Allert, N. (2011b). Individual fiber anatomy of the subthalamic region revealed with diffusion tensor imaging: a concept to identify the deep brain stimulation target for tremor suppression. *Neurosurgery* 68, 1069–1076. doi: 10.1227/NEU.0b013e31820a1a20

Coenen, V. A., Schlaepfer, T. E., Maedler, B., and Panksepp, J. (2011c). Cross-species affective functions of the medial forebrain bundle-implications for the treatment of affective pain and depression in humans. *Neurosci. Biobehav. Rev.* 35, 1971–1981. doi: 10.1016/j.neubiorev.2010.12.009

Coenen, V. A., Allert, N., Paus, S., Kronenbürger, M., Urbach, H., and Mädler, B. (2014). Modulation of the cerebello-thalamo-cortical network in thalamic deep brain stimulation for tremor: a diffusion tensor imaging study. *Neurosurgery* 75, 657–670. doi: 10.1227/NEU.0000000000000540

Coenen, V. A., Honey, C. R., Hurwitz, T., Rahman, A. A., McMaster, J., Bürgel, U., et al. (2009). Medial forebrain bundle stimulation as a pathophysiological mechanism for hypomania in subthalamic nucleus deep brain stimulation for Parkinson's disease. *Neurosurgery* 64, 1106–1115. doi: 10.1227/01.NEU.0000345631.54446.06

Coenen, V. A., Panksepp, J., Hurwitz, T. A., Urbach, H., and Mädler, B. (2012). Human medial forebrain bundle (MFB) and anterior thalamic radiation (ATR): imaging of two major subcortical pathways and the dynamic balance of opposite affects in understanding depression. *J. Neuropsychiatry Clin. Neurosci.* 24, 223–236. doi: 10.1176/appi.neuropsych.11080180

Copeland, B. J., Fenoy, A., Ellmore, T. M., Liang, Q., Ephron, V., and Schiess, M. (2014). Deep brain stimulation of the internal globus pallidus for generalized dystonia associated with spinocerebellar ataxia type 1: a case report. *Neuromodulation* 17, 389–392. doi: 10.1111/ner.12081

Descoteaux, M., Angelino, E., Fitzgibbons, S., and Deriche, R. (2007). Regularized, fast and robust analytical Q-ball imaging. *Magn. Reson. Med.* 58, 497–510. doi: 10.1002/mrm.21277

Dyrby, T. B., Baaré, W. F. C., Alexander, D. C., Jelsing, J., Garde, E., and Søgaard, L. V. (2011). An *ex vivo* imaging pipeline for producing high-quality and high-resolution diffusion-weighted imaging datasets. *Hum. Brain Mapp.* 32, 544–563. doi: 10.1002/hbm.21043

Fillard, P., Descoteaux, M., Goh, A., Gouttard, S., Jeurissen, B., Malcolm, J., et al. (2011). Quantitative evaluation of 10 tractography algorithms on a realistic diffusion MR phantom. *Neuroimage* 56, 220–234. doi: 10.1016/j.neuroimage.2011.01.032

Frank, L. R. (2001). Anisotropy in high angular resolution diffusion-weighted MRI. *Magn. Reson. Med.* 45, 935–939. doi: 10.1002/mrm.1125

Gradinaru, V., Mogri, M., Thompson, K. R., Henderson, J. M., and Deisseroth, K. (2009). Optical deconstruction of parkinsonian neural circuitry. *Science* 324, 354–359. doi: 10.1126/science.1167093

Hashimoto, T., Elder, C. M., Okun, M. S., Patrick, S. K., and Vitek, J. L. (2003). Stimulation of the subthalamic nucleus changes the firing pattern of pallidal neurons. *J. Neurosci.* 23, 1916–1923.

Henderson, J. M. (2012). "Connectomic surgery": diffusion tensor imaging (DTI) tractography as a targeting modality for surgical modulation of neural networks. *Front. Integr. Neurosci.* 6:15. doi: 10.3389/fnint.2012.00015

Hunsche, S., Sauner, D., Runge, M. J. R., Lenartz, D., El Majdoub, F., Treuer, H., et al. (2013). Tractography-guided stimulation of somatosensory fibers for thalamic pain relief. *Stereotact. Funct. Neurosurg.* 91, 328–334. doi: 10.1159/000350024

Jeurissen, B., Leemans, A., Tournier, J.-D., Jones, D. K., and Sijbers, J. (2012). Investigating the prevalence of complex fiber configurations in white matter tissue with diffusion magnetic resonance imaging. *Hum. Brain Mapp.* 34, 2747–2766. doi: 10.1002/hbm.22099

Johansen-Berg, H., Gutman, D. A., Behrens, T. E. J., Matthews, P. M., Rushworth, M. F. S., Katz, E., et al. (2008). Anatomical connectivity of the subgenual cingulate region targeted with deep brain stimulation for treatment-resistant depression. *Cereb. Cortex* 18, 1374–1383. doi: 10.1093/cercor/bhm167

Jones, D. K. (2004). The effect of gradient sampling schemes on measures derived from diffusion tensor MRI: a monte carlo study. *Magn. Reson. Med.* 51, 807–815. doi: 10.1002/mrm.20033

Jones, D. K., and Cercignani, M. (2010). Twenty-five pitfalls in the analysis of diffusion MRI data. *NMR Biomed.* 23, 803–820. doi: 10.1002/nbm.1543

Klein, J. C., Barbe, M. T., Seifried, C., Baudrexel, S., Runge, M., Maarouf, M., et al. (2012). The tremor network targeted by successful VIM deep brain stimulation in humans. *Neurology* 78, 787–795. doi: 10.1212/WNL.0b013e318249f702

Kovanlikaya, I., Heier, L., and Kaplitt, M. (2014). Treatment of chronic pain: diffusion tensor imaging identification of the ventroposterolateral nucleus confirmed with successful deep brain stimulation. *Stereotact. Funct. Neurosurg.* 92, 365–371. doi: 10.1159/000366002

Kwon, H. G., Hong, J. H., Hong, C. P., Lee, D. H., Ahn, S. H., and Jang, S. H. (2011). Dentatorubrothalamic tract in human brain: diffusion tensor tractography study. *Neuroradiology* 53, 787–791. doi: 10.1007/s00234-011-0878-7

Lazar, M., and Alexander, A. L. (2003). An error analysis of white matter tractography methods: synthetic diffusion tensor field simulations. *Neuroimage* 20, 1140–1153. doi: 10.1016/s1053-8119(03)00277-5

Lazar, M., Weinstein, D. M., Tsuruda, J. S., Hasan, K. M., Arfanakis, K., Meyerand, M. E., et al. (2003). White matter tractography using diffusion tensor deflection. *Hum. Brain Mapp.* 18, 306–321. doi: 10.1002/hbm.10102

Lebel, C., Benner, T., and Beaulieu, C. (2011). Six is enough? Comparison of diffusion parameters measured using six or more diffusion-encoding gradient directions with deterministic tractography. *Magn. Reson. Med.* 68, 474–483. doi: 10.1002/mrm.23254

Lujan, J. L., Chaturvedi, A., Choi, K. S., Holtzheimer, P. E., Gross, R. E., Mayberg, H. S., et al. (2013). Tractography-activation models applied to subcallosal cingulate deep brain stimulation. *Brain Stimul.* 6, 737–739. doi: 10.1016/j.brs.2013.03.008

Lujan, J. L., Chaturvedi, A., Malone, D. A., Rezai, A. R., Machado, A. G., and McIntyre, C. C. (2011). Axonal pathways linked to therapeutic and nontherapeutic outcomes during psychiatric deep brain stimulation. *Hum. Brain Mapp.* 33, 958–968. doi: 10.1002/hbm.21262

McIntyre, C. C., Grill, W. M., Sherman, D. L., and Thakor, N. V. (2004a). Cellular effects of deep brain stimulation: model-based analysis of activation and inhibition. *J. Neurophysiol.* 91, 1457–1469. doi: 10.1152/jn.00989.2003

McIntyre, C. C., Savasta, M., Kerkerian-Le Goff, L., and Vitek, J. L. (2004b). Uncovering the mechanism(s) of action of deep brain stimulation: activation, inhibition, or both. *Clin. Neurophysiol.* 115, 1239–1248. doi: 10.1016/j.clinph.2003.12.024

McNab, J. A., Voets, N. L., Jenkinson, N., Squier, W., Miller, K. L., Goodwin, G. M., et al. (2009). Reduced limbic connections may contraindicate subgenual cingulate deep brain stimulation for intractable depression. *J. Neurosurg.* 111, 780–784. doi: 10.3171/2009.2.JNS081299

Montgomery, E. B., Jr., and Gale, J. T. (2008). Mechanisms of action of deep brain stimulation (DBS). *Neurosci. Biobehav. Rev.* 32, 388–407. doi: 10.1016/j.neubiorev.2007.06.003

Mori, S., Crain, B. J., Chacko, V. P., and van Zijl, P. C. M. (1999). Three-dimensional tracking of axonal projections in the brain by magnetic resonance imaging. *Ann. Neurol.* 45, 265–269. doi: 10.1002/1531-8249(199902)45:2<265::aid-ana21>3.0.co;2-3

Mukherjee, P., Chung, S. W., Berman, J. I., Hess, C. P., and Henry, R. G. (2008). Diffusion tensor MR imaging and fiber tractography: technical considerations. *AJMR Am. J. Neuroradiol.* 29, 843–852. doi: 10.3174/ajnr.A1052

Nimsky, C., Ganslandt, O., Hastreiter, P., Wang, R., Benner, T., Sorensen, A. G., et al. (2005). Preoperative and intraoperative diffusion tensor imaging-based fiber tracking in glioma surgery. *Neurosurgery* 56, 130–137; discussion 138. doi: 10.1227/01.NEU.0000144842.18771.30

Owen, S. L. F., Heath, J., Kringelbach, M., Green, A. L., Pereira, E. A. C., Jenkinson, N., et al. (2008). Pre-operative DTI and probabilisitic tractography in four patients with deep brain stimulation for chronic pain. *J. Clin. Neurosci.* 15, 801–805. doi: 10.1016/j.jocn.2007.06.010

Owen, S. L. F., Heath, J., Kringelbach, M. L., Stein, J. F., and Aziz, T. Z. (2007). Preoperative DTI and probabilistic tractography in an amputee with deep brain stimulation for lower limb stump pain. *Br. J. Neurosurg.* 21, 485–490. doi: 10.1080/02688690701558358

Paschal, C. B., and Morris, H. D. (2004). *K*-space in the clinic. *J. Magn. Reson. Imaging* 19, 145–159. doi: 10.1002/jmri.10451

Pouratian, N., Zheng, Z., Bari, A. A., Behnke, E., Elias, W. J., and Desalles, A. A. F. (2011). Multi-institutional evaluation of deep brain stimulation targeting using probabilistic connectivity-based thalamic segmentation. *J. Neurosurg.* 115, 995–1004. doi: 10.3171/2011.7.JNS11250

Riva-Posse, P., Choi, K. S., Holtzheimer, P. E., McIntyre, C. C., Gross, R. E., Chaturvedi, A., et al. (2014). Defining critical white matter pathways mediating successful subcallosal cingulate deep brain stimulation for treatment-resistant depression. *Biol. Psychiatry* 76, 963–969. doi: 10.1016/j.biopsych.2014.03.029

Rozanski, V. E., Vollmar, C., Cunha, J. P., Tafula, S. M. N., Ahmadi, S.-A., Patzig, M., et al. (2014). Connectivity patterns of pallidal dbs electrodes in focal dystonia: a diffusion tensor tractography study. *Neuroimage* 84, 435–442. doi: 10.1016/j.neuroimage.2013.09.009

Said, N., Elias, W. J., Raghavan, P., Cupino, A., Tustison, N., Frysinger, R., et al. (2014). Correlation of diffusion tensor tractography and intraoperative macrostimulation during deep brain stimulation for Parkinson disease. *J. Neurosurg.* 121, 929–935. doi: 10.3171/2014.6.JNS131673

Sajonz, B. E. A., Mädler, B., Herberhold, S., Paus, S., Allert, N., and Coenen, V. A. (2015). Stimulation induced hypogeusia in thalamic deep brain stimulation for tremor: an underestimated yet common side effect. *J. Neurol. Neurosurg. Psychiatry* doi: 10.1136/jnnp-2015-310368 [Epub ahead of print].

Schlaepfer, T. E., Bewernick, B. H., Kayser, S., Mädler, B., and Coenen, V. A. (2013). Rapid effects of deep brain stimulation for treatment-resistant major depression. *Biol. Psychiatry* 73, 1204–1212. doi: 10.1016/j.biopsych.2013.01.034

Schmahmann, J. D., Pandya, D. N., Wang, R., Dai, G., D'Arceuil, H. E., de Crespigny, A. J., et al. (2007). Association fibre pathways of the brain: parallel observations from diffusion spectrum imaging and autoradiography. *Brain* 130, 630–653. doi: 10.1093/brain/awl359

Schweder, P. M., Joint, C., Hansen, P. C., Green, A. L., Quaghebeur, G., and Aziz, T. Z. (2010). Chronic pedunculopontine nucleus stimulation restores functional connectivity. *Neuroreport* 21, 1065–1068. doi: 10.1097/WNR.0b013e32833ce607

Sedrak, M., Gorgulho, A., De Salles, A. F., Frew, A., Behnke, E., Ishida, W., et al. (2008). The role of modern imaging modalities on deep brain stimulation targeting for mental illness. *Acta. neurochirurgica.* 101, 3–7.

Sudhyadhom, A., McGregor, K., Okun, M. S., Foote, K. D., Trinastic, J., Crosson, B., et al. (2012). Delineation of motor and somatosensory thalamic subregions utilizing probabilistic diffusion tractography and electrophysiology. *J. Magn. Reson. Imaging* 37, 600–609. doi: 10.1002/jmri.23861

Sweet, J. A., Walter, B. L., Gunalan, K., Chaturvedi, A., McIntyre, C. C., and Miller, J. P. (2014). Fiber tractography of the axonal pathways linking the basal ganglia and cerebellum in Parkinson disease: implications for targeting in deep brain stimulation. *J. Neurosurg.* 120, 988–996. doi: 10.3171/2013.12.JNS131537

Thomas, C., Ye, F. Q., Irfanoglu, M. O., Modi, P., Saleem, K. S., Leopold, D. A., et al. (2014). Anatomical accuracy of brain connections derived from diffusion MRI tractography is inherently limited. *Proc. Natl. Acad. Sci. U S A* 111, 16574–16579. doi: 10.1073/pnas.1405672111

Torres, C. V., Manzanares, R., and Sola, R. G. (2014). Integrating diffusion tensor imaging-based tractography into deep brain stimulation surgery: a review of the literature. *Stereotact. Funct. Neurosurg.* 92, 282–290. doi: 10.1159/000362937

Tournier, J.-D., Calamante, F., and Connelly, A. (2013). Determination of the appropriate bvalue and number of gradient directions for high-angular-resolution diffusion-weighted imaging. *NMR Biomed.* 26, 1775–1786. doi: 10.1002/nbm.3017

Tournier, J.-D., Yeh, C.-H., Calamante, F., Cho, K.-H., Connelly, A., and Lin, C.-P. (2008). Resolving crossing fibres using constrained spherical deconvolution: validation using diffusion-weighted imaging phantom data. *Neuroimage* 42, 617–625. doi: 10.1016/j.neuroimage.2008.05.002

Tuch, D. S. (2004). Q-ball imaging. *Magn. Reson. Med.* 52, 1358–1372. doi: 10.1002/mrm.20279

Vitek, J. L., Hashimoto, T., Peoples, J., DeLong, M. R., and Bakay, R. A. E. (2004). Acute stimulation in the external segment of the globus pallidus improves parkinsonian motor signs. *Mov. Disord.* 19, 907–915. doi: 10.1002/mds.20137

Wedeen, V. J., Hagmann, P., Tseng, W.-Y. I., Reese, T. G., and Weisskoff, R. M. (2005). Mapping complex tissue architecture with diffusion spectrum magnetic resonance imaging. *Magn. Reson. Med.* 54, 1377–1386. doi: 10.1002/mrm.20642

Wedeen, V. J., Wang, R. P., Schmahmann, J. D., Benner, T., Tseng, W. Y. I., Dai, G., et al. (2008). Diffusion spectrum magnetic resonance imaging (DSI) tractography of crossing fibers. *Neuroimage* 41, 1267–1277. doi: 10.1016/j.neuroimage.2008.03.036

Witwer, B. P., Moftakhar, R., Hasan, K. M., Deshmukh, P., Haughton, V., Field, A., et al. (2002). Diffusion-tensor imaging of white matter tracts in patients with cerebral neoplasm. *J. Neurosurg.* 97, 568–575. doi: 10.3171/jns.2002.97.3.0568

14

Subcomponents and Connectivity of the Inferior Fronto-Occipital Fasciculus Revealed by Diffusion Spectrum Imaging Fiber Tracking

Yupeng Wu [1], Dandan Sun [2], Yong Wang [1] and Yibao Wang [1]*

[1] *Department of Neurosurgery, The First Affiliated Hospital of China Medical University, Shenyang, China,* [2] *Department of Cardiovascular Ultrasound, The First Affiliated Hospital of China Medical University, Shenyang, China*

Correspondence:
Yibao Wang
cmuwyb@hotmail.com

The definitive structure and functional role of the inferior fronto-occipital fasciculus (IFOF) are still controversial. In this study, we aimed to investigate the connectivity, asymmetry, and segmentation patterns of this bundle. High angular diffusion spectrum imaging (DSI) analysis was performed on 10 healthy adults and a 90-subject DSI template (NTU-90 Atlas). In addition, a new tractography approach based on the anatomic subregions and two regions of interest (ROI) was evaluated for the fiber reconstructions. More widespread anterior-posterior connections than previous "standard" definition of the IFOF were found. This distinct pathway demonstrated a greater inter-subjects connective variability with a maximum of 40% overlap in its central part. The statistical results revealed no asymmetry between the left and right hemispheres and no significant differences existed in distributions of the IFOF according to sex. In addition, five subcomponents within the IFOF were identified according to the frontal areas of originations. As the subcomponents passed through the anterior floor of the external capsule, the fibers radiated to the posterior terminations. The most common connection patterns of the subcomponents were as follows: IFOF-I, from frontal polar cortex to occipital pole, inferior occipital lobe, middle occipital lobe, superior occipital lobe, and pericalcarine; IFOF-II, from orbito-frontal cortex to occipital pole, inferior occipital lobe, middle occipital lobe, superior occipital lobe, and pericalcarine; IFOF-III, from inferior frontal gyrus to inferior occipital lobe, middle occipital lobe, superior occipital lobe, occipital pole, and pericalcarine; IFOF-IV, from middle frontal gyrus to occipital pole, and inferior occipital lobe; IFOF-V, from superior frontal gyrus to occipital pole, inferior occipital lobe, and middle occipital lobe. Our work demonstrates the feasibility of high resolution diffusion tensor tractography with sufficient sensitivity to elucidate more anatomical details of the IFOF. And we provides a new framework for subdividing the IFOF for better understanding its functional role in the human brain.

Keywords: inferior fronto-occipital fasciculus, diffusion spectrum imaging, asymmetry, language, tractography

INTRODUCTION

The inferior fronto-occipital fasciculus (IFOF) is one of the first major association fiber systems to be recognized and depicted in the human brain (Schmahmann and Pandya, 2007). As a long associative bundle, the IFOF passes through in the depth of temporal lobe and insula, connecting occipital cortex, temporo-basal areas, and superior parietal lobe to the frontal lobe (Martino et al., 2010). Also, there are some natural crossings of the IFOF with other tracts, including the superior longitudinal fasciculus (SLF), arcuate fascicle (AF), inferior longitudinal fasciculus (ILF), and middle longitudinal fascicle (MdLF). Several studies suggested that the IFOF possibly played an important role in reading, attention, and visual processing (Catani and Thiebaut de Schotten, 2008).

Traditionally, modern autoradiography in monkeys are considered as the "gold standard" for guiding human white matter connective patterns, however, it has been demonstrated that there is not existence of a human equivalent of the IFOF in the monkey brain (Schmahmann et al., 2007; Forkel et al., 2014). As for this, post-mortem dissection and diffusion tensor imaging (DTI) technique have been widely adopted to explore the anatomical structures of the IFOF. In 2013, Sarubbo et al. investigated the frontal terminations of the IFOF on 10 hemispheres using fiber dissection technique, and proposed that this fiber bundle could be segmented into different subcomponents for future functional analysis (Sarubbo et al., 2013). Two possible layers of the IFOF were identified by Sarubbo et al. according to the fiber frontal terminations. The first layer was superficial and antero-superiorly directed, associating with the inferior frontal gyrus. The second one was deeper and composed of three discrete fan-shaped portions: Anterior, middle, and posterior. The anterior component was connected with the orbito-frontal cortex and frontal pole. The middle component was directed to the lateral orbito-frontal cortex and middle frontal gyrus. The posterior one terminated in the dorso-lateral prefrontal cortex and middle frontal gyrus (Sarubbo et al., 2013). Coincident results were found by De Benedictis et al. (2012). However, neither of them mentioned the connections of the subcomponents to the posterior terminations. In another post-mortem dissection study, Martino et al. firstly reported new cortical terminations (i.e., postero-basal temporal portions and superior parietal lobe) except as the occipital cortex. And they suggested that there were two different subcomponents in the IFOF. One was a dorsal and superficial subpart that connected the superior parietal lobe and the posterior part of the superior and middle occipital cortex with the frontal lobe. The other was a ventral and deep subpart that connected the posterior part of the inferior occipital cortex and the posterior temporo-basal portions with the frontal lobe. But, they failed to identify their cortical terminations within the frontal lobe (Martino et al., 2010). The controversial results between studies might be attributed to the limitations of fiber dissection methods. First, this technique depends on the quality of the specimens, especially difficult to be performed in brains of elderly subjects with lacunar infarcts (Martino et al., 2011). Second, the dissection is limited to be applied in different crossing fiber termination regions.

As an alternative method, DTI technique provides a unique opportunity to study white matter architecture *in vivo* as 3D space. For the last decades, it has strongly contributed to our knowledge about fiber pathways in the human brain (Catani et al., 2002). Still, the detailed anatomical definition of the IFOF exists some controversies within reported DTI studies. For instance, some researchers described that the IFOF connected the fronto-marginal gyrus and lateral orbito-frontal gyrus with the lingual gyrus, inferior occipital gyrus, and inferior part of the middle occipital gyrus (Lawes et al., 2008). Whereas, others considered that the posterior terminations of the IFOF was at the level of the middle and posterior temporal lobe (Fernandez-Miranda et al., 2008a). Recently, Thiebaut de Schotten et al. reported that it probably had a contribution from the medial parietal lobe (Thiebaut de Schotten et al., 2012). We speculate that the technique DTI limitations may impede accurate depiction of the IFOF, such as the inability to map fiber ends of the white matter before contacting the cortical mantle, failure to solve complicated fiber crossings and to follow bundles within fiber tracts, and excessive false fiber continuity generating pseudotracts (Fernandez Miranda, 2013). In order to resolve the complex fiber crossings and partial-volume effect that typically affect DTI tractography data, tractography algorithms based on diffusion spectrum imaging (DSI) reconstructed by generalized q-sampling imaging (GQI) as a high-angular-resolution diffusion imaging (HARDI) method have been developed (Wedeen et al., 2005; Yeh et al., 2010). This approach leverages high directional sampling of diffusion imaging space to get better resolution of underlying white matter geometry for tractography. Our previous studies have provided accurate replication of complex known neuroanatomical features where DTI failed (Wang et al., 2013; Fernandez-Miranda et al., 2014; Leng et al., 2016; Wu et al., 2016).

In this study, we aimed to investigate the connectivity, asymmetry and segmentation of the left and right IFOF in a subject-specific approach (10 subjects) and a template approach (NTU-90 Atlas) using HARDI tractography. In addition, we evaluated a new tractography approach for the fiber tracking of IFOF based on the anatomic subregions and two regions of interest (ROI). We complemented this analysis compared with recent post-mortem dissection and functional neuroimaging studies of the IFOF to confirm the underlying neuroanatomy. Our study provides a more accurate and detailed description of the connectional architecture of the subcomponents within the IFOF, allowing a comprehensive morphological basis for further functional studies in the human brain.

MATERIALS AND METHODS

Participants

Ten volunteers (3 males, 7 females; all right handed; age range: 23–40 years) were included in the present study. No history of neurological and psychiatric disorders was present in study sample. All participants gave informed written consent prior to testing. The procedures used here were approved by the institutional review board, including the ethics committee at China Medical University.

Except as subject-specific analysis, we also conducted fiber tracking on a publicly available DSI template of 90 subjects (NTU-90 atlas). It includes 45 males and 45 female subjects. The age of the 90 subjects ranges from 18 to 60 years, and the mean ages of the male and female subjects are 32.58 and 33.58 years. The spatial resolution of the template is 2 mm (Yeh and Tseng, 2011). The NTU-90 template is freely downloadable at http://dsi-studio.labsolver.org.

Image Acquisition and Reconstruction

All studies were performed on a 3-T Tim Trio System (Siemens) with a 32-channel head coil to acquire DSI data. A head stabilizer was used to prevented head motion. This involved a 43-min, 257-direction scan using a twice-refocused spin-echo echo-planar imaging sequence and multiple q-values [echo time (TE) = 157 ms, repetition time (TR) = 9.916 ms, field of view (FoV) = 231 × 231 mm, voxel size = 2.4 × 2.4 × 2.4 mm, b max = 7000 s/mm^2] (Wedeen et al., 2005). We also included the high-resolution anatomical imaging to be as the anatomical comparisons, employing a 9-min T1-weighted axial magnetization prepared rapid gradient echo (MPRAGE) sequence (TE = 2.63 ms, TR = 2110 ms, flip angle = 8°, 176 slices, voxel size = 0.5 × 0.5 × 1.0 mm^3, FoV = 256 × 256 mm^2). DSI data was reconstructed with a generalized Q-sampling imaging (GQI) approach (Yeh et al., 2010). The orientation distribution functions (ODFs) were reconstructed to 362 discrete sampling directions and a mean diffusion distance of 1.2 mm.

Fiber Tracking and Analysis

The DSI Studio software was used for the fiber-tracking performing a multiple fiber version of the streamline tracking algorithm. The DSI Studio software is an open-source diffusion MRI analysis tool, which is freely downloadable at http://dsi-studio.labsolver.org. The fiber tracts were generated by whole brain seeding, and the tracts passing the ROI were implemented. In voxels with multiple fiber orientations, fiber tracking was initiated separately for each orientation, and fiber progression continued with a step size of 1.0 mm, minimum fiber length of 20 mm, and turning angle threshold of 60°. If multiple fiber orientations existed in the current progression location, the fiber orientation that was nearest to the incoming direction and formed a turning angle smaller than 60° was selected to determine the next moving direction (Fernandez-Miranda et al., 2014). To smooth each track, the next moving directional estimate of each voxel was weighted by 20% of the previous incoming direction and 80% of the nearest fiber orientation. This progression was repeated until the quantitative anisotropy (QA) of the fiber orientation dropped below a preset threshold (0.03–0.06 depending on the subject) or there was no fiber selected within the 60° angular range in the progression (Yeh et al., 2013). Once tracked, all streamlines were saved in the TrackVis file format.

For reconstruction of the IFOF, we assumed that the IFOF fibers only originated from the frontal lobe. The bilaterally frontal lobe cortical ROIs were all employed acting as the seeding regions, including the superior frontal gyrus, middle frontal gyrus, inferior frontal gyrus (i.e., pars opercularis, pars triangularis, and pars orbitalis), frontomarginal gyrus, transverse fronto-polar gyrus, and orbito-frontal cortex(i.e., lateral and medial orbito-frontal cortex). Two ROI masks were drawn to select only the fibers that passed from the frontal lobe to the posterior region. One was around the ventral part of the external capsule on the coronal QA color map, the other was on the coronal plane at the level of the central sulcus (**Figure 1**). In addition, for analyzing the spatial relationship of the IFOF with adjacent association tracts, we performed fiber reconstruction of the inferior longitudinal fascicles (ILF), optic radiation (OR), uncinate fasciculus (UF) and middle longitudinal fascicle (MdLF). For the ILF, two different ROIs were used: One along the anterior temporal region and another

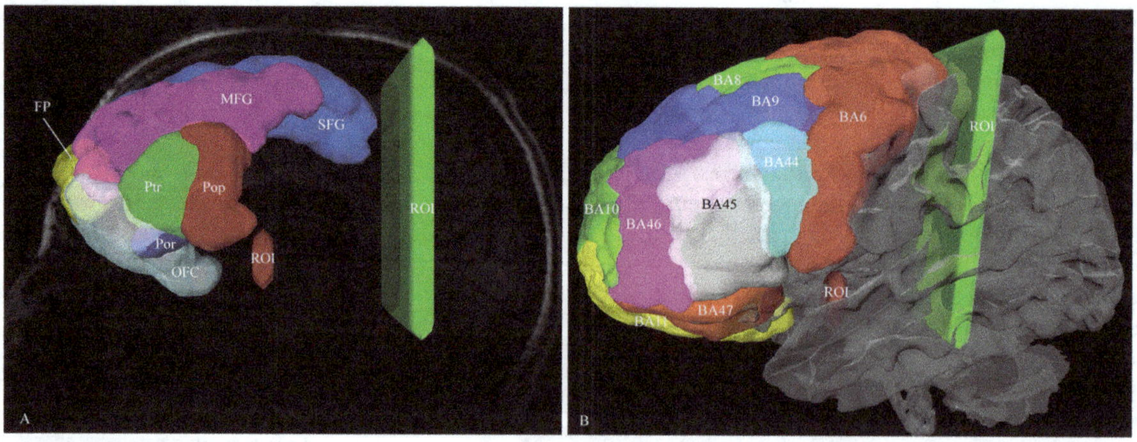

FIGURE 1 | *In vivo* fiber tractography of the IFOF. (A) Frontal lobe labels were used as the seeding regions for the reconstruction of the IFOF, including the superior frontal gyrus (SFG, blue), middle frontal gyrus (MFG, pink), inferior frontal gyrus [i.e., pars opercularis (Pop, red), pars triangularis (Ptr, green), and pars orbitalis (Por, blue)], frontal polar (FP, yellow) and orbito-frontal cortex (OFC, cyan). Two ROI masks were drawn to select only the fibers that passed from the frontal lobe to the posterior region. One was around the ventral part of the external capsule on the coronal quantitative anisotropy color map, the other was on the coronal plane at the level of the central sulcus. **(B)** Brodmann areas (BA) overlaid on the white matter surface. ROI, region of interest.

at the occipital region (Fernandez-Miranda et al., 2008a). For the OR, two different ROIs were applied: One at the thalamus region and another at the occipital region (Kamali et al., 2014). For the UF, the superior temporal gyrus, middle temporal gyrus, and temporal pole were performed as the seed regions (Leng et al., 2016). For the MdLF, the superior temporal gyrus was served as the seed region. The ROI mask was used on the coronal plane along the precentral region (Wang et al., 2013).

Cytoarchitectonic and Anatomic Segmentation

Brodmann areas and anatomical segmentation were both used to perform the cortical parcellation. DSI Studio uses linear transformation to register Talairach atlas on subject's diffusion space. The Talairach coordinate system provides anatomical and functional information (Nowinski, 2005). For comparison, FreeSurfer (http://surfer.nmr.mgh.harvard.edu) was used to segment cortical gyral ROIs based on previous brain atlases using each participant's T_1-weighted magnetization prepared rapid axial gradient echo (MPRAGE) image (Desikan et al., 2006). For the template, ICBM-152 T_1 template image was performed in FreeSurfer (Fonov et al., 2011).

Statistical Analysis

Statistical analyses were carried out using SPSS 16.0 (SPSS, Chicago, IL). For quantifying and comparing the right and left IFOF as well as the contribution of each seeding region, we calculated the volume of streamlines based on counting the number of voxels occupied by the fiber trajectories (streamlines). Continuous variables were presented as mean $\pm$ standard deviation. *T*-test was used to determine variances between the tract volume of left hemispheres and that of right hemispheres. All originating and terminating distributions of the five subcomponents between males and females were evaluated by chi-square ($\chi 2$) test. $P \leq 0.05$ was considered to be statistically significant.

RESULTS

The Trajectory of the IFOF in "Subject-Specific" Tractography Approach

In this study, the fiber tractography study consistently noted a large bundle of fibers projecting from the frontal seed regions toward the posterior terminations in all 20 hemispheres (**Figure 2**). Importantly, this distinct pathway demonstrated a greater inter-subjects connective variability with a maximum of 40% overlap in its central part. This group of fibers mainly originated from the orbito-frontal cortex (lateral and medial orbito-frontal cortex), frontal polar cortex (i.e., fronto-marginal gyrus and transverse fronto-polar gyrus), superior frontal gyrus and inferior frontal gyrus (i.e., pars opercularis, pars triangularis, pars orbitalis), some fibers also came from the middle frontal gyrus (12 out of 20 hemispheres). As the fibers leaved the originations, they narrowed as a compact fascicle at the level of the external/extreme capsules. Then, the fibers continued posteriorly through the temporal lobe. Subsequently, they fanned out before radiating to the terminations. In the sagittal view, it can be clearly noticed that the IFOF was a long-ranged and bowtie-shaped pathway at the inferior base of the cerebrum. The posterior terminations of the IFOF mainly included the pericalcarine (cuneus and lingual gyrus), fusiform gyrus, occipital pole, inferior occipital lobe, middle occipital lobe, and superior occipital lobe. Some fibers also terminated in the superior parietal lobe (10 out of 20 hemispheres), angular gyrus (10 out of 20 hemispheres) and postcentral gyrus (5 out of 20 hemispheres), and with a minor connection probably in the inferior temporal gyrus (1 out of 20 hemispheres) and middle temporal gyrus (1 out of 20 hemispheres) (**Table 1**).

Segmentation and Brain Connectivity of the IFOF

In order to find common patterns of connectivity within the IFOF, we investigated the structural interconnectivity between frontal lobe and posterior regions. Anatomical comparisons between the anterior and posterior cortex regions in the human brain, the frontal lobe is more easily recognizable for the fiber tracking. As for this, five different cortical areas of originations of the IFOF fibers in the frontal region were identified: Frontal polar cortex (i.e., fronto-marginal gyrus and transverse fronto-polar gyrus), orbito-frontal cortex (i.e., lateral and medial orbito-frontal cortex), inferior frontal gyrus (i.e., pars opercularis, pars triangularis and pars orbitalis), middle frontal gyrus, and superior frontal gyrus. Based on the frontal anatomic landmarks, five potential subcomponents of the IFOF connecting the different cortical and subcortical regions were visualized. IFOF-I originated from the frontal polar cortex, via the external/extreme capsules, then connected with the inferior occipital lobe [19/20, (19 out of 20 hemispheres)], the occipital pole (19/20), the middle occipital lobe (15/20), the pericalcarine (14/20), the superior occipital lobe (11/20), the superior parietal lobe (8/20), the fusiform gyrus (8/20), the postcentral gygus (1/20), and the precuneus (1/20). IFOF-II originated from the orbito-frontal cortex, via the external/extreme capsules, then connected with the occipital pole (19/20), the inferior occipital gyrus (18/20), the pericalcarine (18/20), the middle occipital lobe (15/20), the superior occipital lobe (12/20), the fusiform gyrus (9/20), the superior parietal lobe (8/20), the angular gyrus (4/20), and the precuneus (1/20). IFOF-III originated from the inferior frontal gyrus, via the external/extreme capsules, then connected with the inferior occipital gyrus (19/20), the middle occipital lobe (18/20), the occipital pole (18/20), the superior occipital lobe (13/20), the pericalcarine (12/20), the angular gyrus (9/20), the superior parietal lobe (8/20), the fusiform gyrus (6 /20), the postcentral gygus (5/20), the inferior temporal gyrus (1/20), and the middle temporal gyrus (1/20). IFOF-IV originated from the middle frontal gyrus, via the external/extreme capsules, then connected with the occipital pole (12/20), the inferior occipital gyrus (10/20), the middle occipital lobe (9/20), the pericalcarine (9/20), the superior occipital lobe (4/20), the angular gyrus (2/20), the superior parietal lobe (2/20), the postcentral gygus (1/20), and the fusiform gyrus (1/20). Finally, IFOF-V originated from the

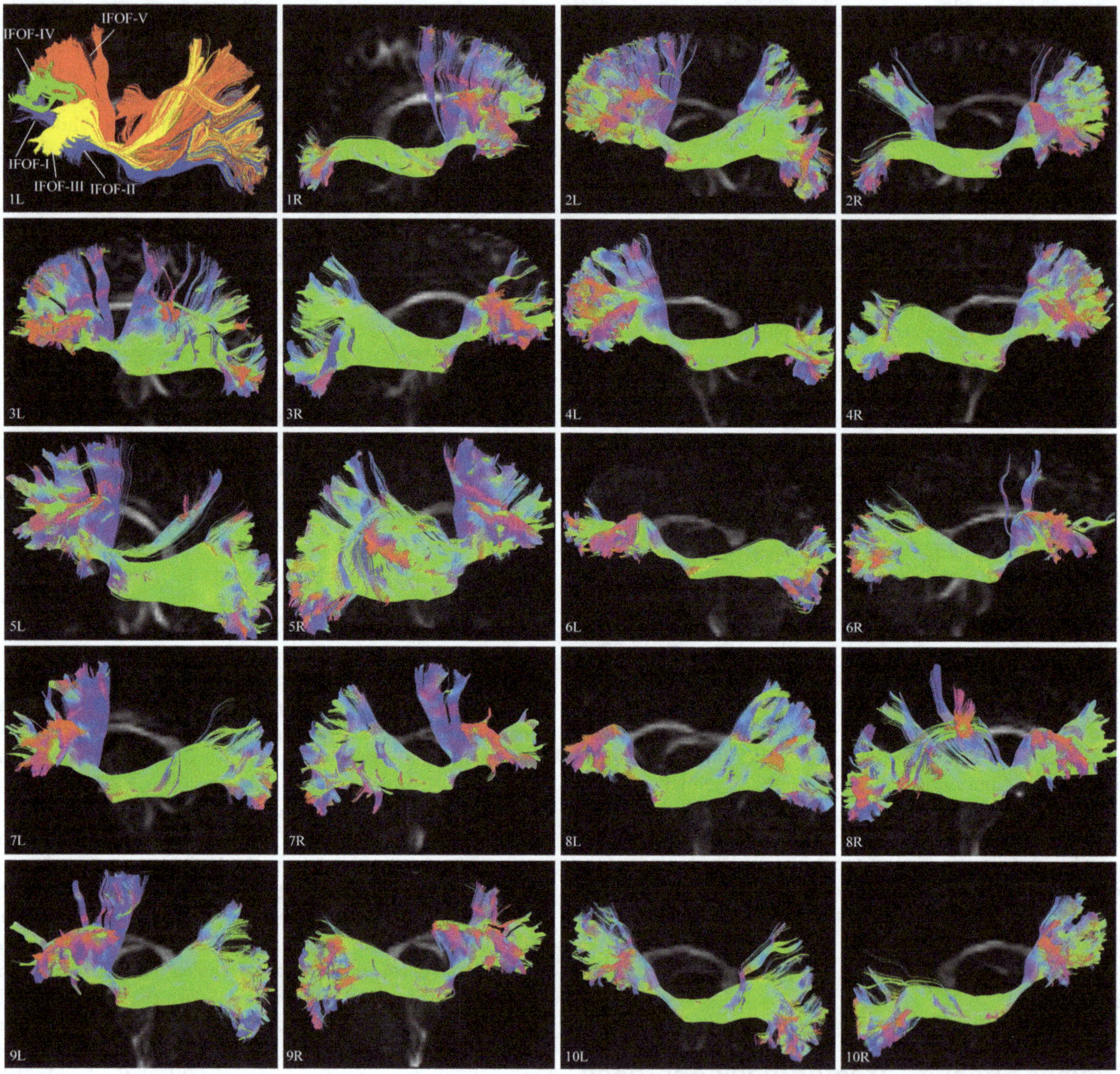

FIGURE 2 | DSI tractography studies of the IFOF in 20 hemispheres of 10 subjects on sagittal view. Order: Subject 1, 2, 3, 4, 5, 6, 7, 8, 9, 10. The IFOF was noted as a long-ranged and bowtie-shaped pathway at the inferior base of the cerebrum in all 20 hemispheres. As the fibers leaved the originations, they narrowed as a compact fascicle at the level of the external/extreme capsules, then fanned out to the terminations. Greater inter-subjects connective variabilities were demonstrated with a maximum of 40% overlap in the central part. L, left; R, right.

superior frontal gyrus, via the external/extreme capsules, then connected with the occipital pole (16/20), the inferior occipital gyrus (12/20), the middle occipital lobe (10/20), the superior occipital lobe (8/20), the pericalcarine (8/20), the superior parietal lobe (6/20), the fusiform gyrus (4/20), the angular gyrus (3/20), the postcentral gygus (2/20), and the inferior temporal gyrus (1/20) (**Table 1**).

As the subcomponents passed through the anterior floor of the external capsule, the fibers were mixed together and radiated to the posterior terminations (**Figure 4**). In fact, it was impossible for us to differentiate the subcomponents if we portrayed the fiber course from the posterior connections. Even so, two characteristic connections in the subcomponents were found. First, the IFOF-I was largely located on the bottom to the others, while the IFOF-V was slightly more superior than the others, despite their overlaps. Second, the fibers terminating in the angular gyrus was mainly come from the IFOF-III (**Figure 4A**).

TABLE 1 | Cortical connections of the five segments of the IFOF.

No	Side	IFOF-I connection		IFOF-II connection		IFOF-III connection		IFOF-IV connection		IFOF-V connection	
		Anterior	Posterior	Anterior	Posterior	Anterior	Posterior	Anterior	Posterior	Anterior	Posterior
1	L	FP	IOL,MOL,SOL,SPL,Opo	OFC	IOL,MOL,SOL,Opo, SPL,Pca,FG	Pop,Ptr,Por	PG,IOL,MOL,SOL,Opo, AG,SPL	MFG	PG,IOL,MOL,SOL, Opo,AG,SPL	SFG	PG,IOL,MOL,SOL,Opo, AG,SPL
	R	FP	IOL,Opo	OFC	IOL,MOL,Opo,Pca,FG	Pop,Ptr,Por	IOL,MOL,Opo	–		SFG	IOL,MOL,Opo
2	L	FP	IOL,SOL,SPL,Opo,Pre, Pca	OFC	IOL,SOL,SPL,Opo,Pre, Pca	Pop,Ptr,Por	AG,IOL,MOL,Opo	MFG	AG,IOL,MOL,Opo, Pca	SFG	AG,IOL,MOL,SPL,Opo, Pca
	R	FP	IOL,Opo,SPL	OFC	IOL,Opo,SPL	Ptr,Por	IOL,Opo,Pca	MFG	IOL,Opo	SFG	IOL,Opo,SPL,Pca
3	L	FP	IOL,MOL,SOL,Opo,Pca	OFC	IOL,MOL,SOL,Opo,Pca	Ptr,Por	PG,AG,IOL,MOL,SOL, Opo,FG	MFG	IOL,MOL,Opo,Pca, FG	SFG	IOL,MOL,Opo,Pca,FG
	R	FP	IOL,MOL,SOL,Opo, SPL,Pca,FG	OFC	IOL,MOL,SOL,Opo,Pca, FG	Ptr,Por	AG,IOL,MOL,SOL,Opo, SPL,Pca,FG	MFG	IOL,Opo,Pca,FG	SFG	IOL,Opo
4	L	FP	IOL,MOL,Opo,FG	OFC	IOL,MOL,Opo,Pca	Pop,Ptr,Por	IOL,MOL,SOL,Opo,Pca	MFG	IOL,MOL,SOL,Opo, Pca	SFG	IOL,MOL,SOL,Opo,Pca
	R	FP	IOL,MOL,SOL,Opo,Pca, FG	OFC	IOL,MOL,SOL,Opo,Pca, FG	Ptr,Por	IOL,MOL,SOL,Opo,Pca	MFG	MOL,SOL,Opo,Pca	SFG	MOL,SOL,Opo,Pca
5	L	FP	IOL,Opo,Pca,FG	OFC	IOL,MOL,SOL,SPL, Opo,Pca,FG	Pop,Ptr,Por	PG,IOL,MOL,SOL,SPL, Opo,Pca,FG	MFG	IOL,MOL,SPL,Opo, Pca	SFG	PG,IOL,MOL,SOL,Opo, AG,SPL,Pca
	R	FP	PG,IOL,MOL,SOL,Opo, SPL,Pca	OFC	AG,IOL,MOL,SOL,Opo, SPL,Pca	Ptr,Por	PG,AG,IOL,MOL,SOL, Opo,SPL,Pca	–		SFG	SOL,SPL
6	L	FP	IOL,MOL,Opo,Pca	OFC	IOL,MOL,Opo,Pca	Ptr,Por	IOL,MOL,Opo	–		–	
	R	FP	IOL,MOL,Opo,Pca,FG	OFC	Opo,Pca,FG	Pop,Ptr,Por	IOL,MOL,Opo,Pca,FG	–		SFG	Opo,MOL
7	L	FP	IOL,MOL,SOL,SPL, Opo,Pca	OFC	IOL,MOL,Opo,Pca	Pop,Ptr,Por	IOL,MOL,Opo,Pca	MFG	IOL,MOL,Opo,Pca	SFG	IOL,MOL,Opo,Pca
	R	FP	IOL,MOL,SOL,Opo,Pca, FG	OFC	IOL,MOL,SOL,Opo,Pca	Ptr,Por	AG,IOL,MOL,SOL,SPL, Pca,ITG	MFG	IOL,MOL,Opo,Pca	SFG	SOL,ITG
8	L	FP	AG,IOL,MOL,SOL,SPL	OFC	AG,IOL,MOL,SOL,SPL	Ptr,Por	AG,IOL,MOL,SOL,SPL	–		–	
	R	FP	IOL,Opo,Pca,FG	OFC	IOL,Opo,FG,Pca	Pop,Ptr,Por	PG,MTG,IOL,MOL,SOL, SPL,Opo.FG	–		SFG	IOL,Opo,FG
9	L	FP	MOL,SPL,Opo	OFC	AG,SOL,SPL,Opo,Pca	Pop,Ptr,Por	AG,SOL,SPL,Opo,Pca	–		SFG	SOL,SPL,Opo
	R	FP	IOL,MOL,SOL,,Opo,Pca	OFC	AG,IOL,MOL,SOL,SPL, Opo,Pca	Pop,Ptr,Por	AG,IOL,MOL,SOL,Opo, Pca	–		SFG	Opo
10	L	FP	IOL,MOL,SOL,Opo,Pca	OFC	IOL,MOL,SOL,Opo,FG, Pca	Ptr,Por	IOL,MOL,SOL,Opo	MFG	IOL,MOL,SOL,Opo, FG	SFG	IOL,MOL,SOL,FG,Opo
	R	FP	IOL,MOL,Opo,FG,Pca	OFC	IOL,MOL,Opo,FG,Pca	Pop,Ptr,Por	IOL,MOL,Opo,FG,Pca	MFG	Opo,Pca	SFG	IOL,Opo,FG,Pca
NTU-90	L	FP	IOL,LG	OFC	IOL,MOL,LG	Ptr,Por	PG,IOL,MOL,SOL,SPL, LG	MFG	IOL,MOL,SOL,SPL	SFG	PG,IOL,MOL,SOL,SPL, FG,Supa
	R	FP	LG	OFC	IOL,LG	Pop,Ptr,Por	AG,STG,MTG,IOL,MOL, SOL,SPL,LG	MFG	IOL,MOL,SOL,SPL	SFG	AG,STG,MTG,PG,IOL, MOL,SOL,SPL,FG

SFG, superior frontal gyrus; MFG, middle frontal gyrus; Pop, pars opercularis; Ptr, pars triangularis; Por, pars orbitalis; FP, frontal polar cortex; OFC, orbito-frontal cortex; STG, superior temporal gyrus; MTG, middle temporal gyrus; ITG, inferior temporal gyrus; FG, fusiform gyrus; LG, lingual gygus; PG, postcentral gygus; IOL, inferior occipital gyrus; AG, angular gyrus; SOL, superior occipital lobe; MOL, middle occipital lobe; SPL, superior parietal lobe; Supra, supramarginal gyrus; Opo, occipital pole; Pca, pericalcarine; Pre, precuneus; L, left hemisphere; R, right hemisphere.

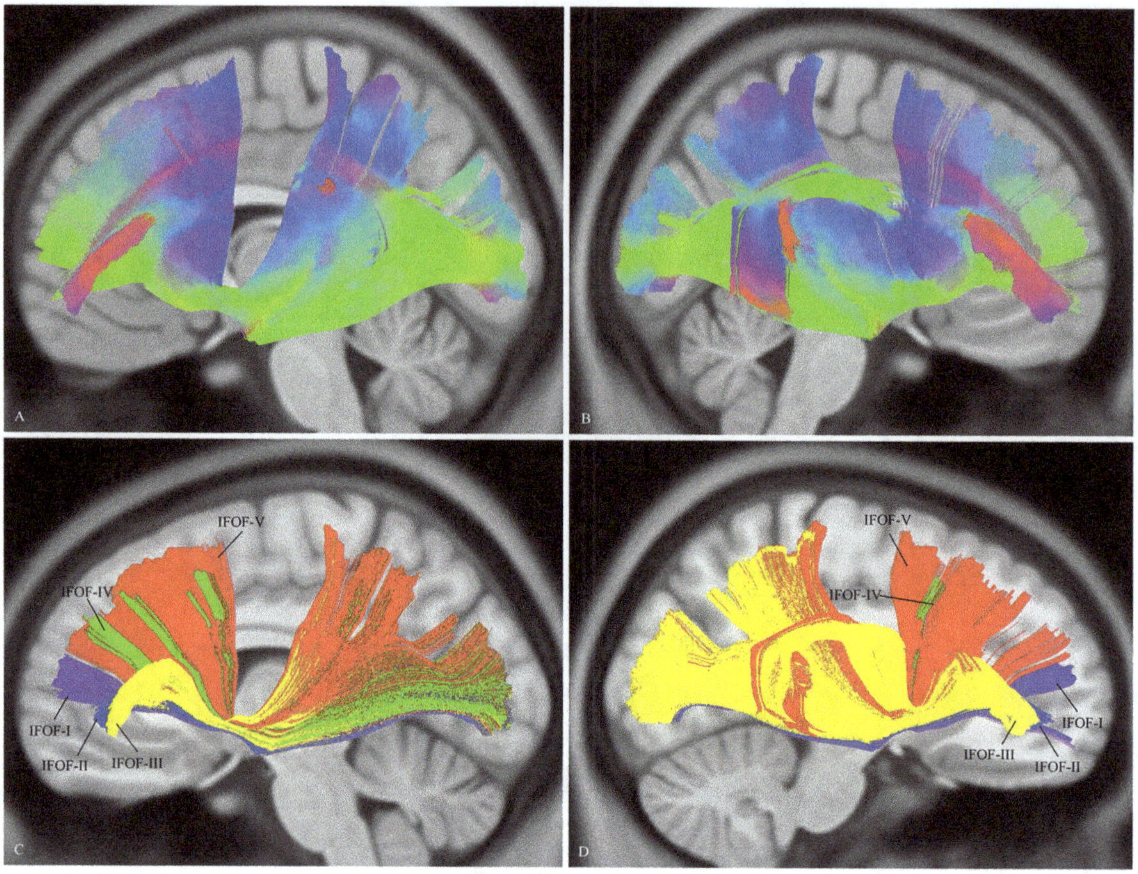

FIGURE 3 | *In vivo* fiber tractography of the IFOF on the DSI template. (A,B) The NTU-90 showed an extended pattern compared with the subject-specific results. **(C,D)** A consistent pattern of five segmentations was confirmed within both hemispheres of the template. L, left; R, right.

"Template" Tractography Approach

The DSI template (NTU-90) showed an extended pattern compared with the subject-specific results, similarly to the analysis of the subject 1L and the subject 5R. Moreover, a consistent pattern of five segmentations was confirmed within both hemispheres of the NTU-90 template (**Figure 3**). Briefly, IFOF-I connected the frontal polar cortex with the inferior occipital gyrus and the lingual gygus. IFOF-II connected the orbito-frontal cortex with the inferior occipital gyrus, the middle occipital lobe, and the lingual gygus. IFOF-III connected the inferior frontal gyrus with the inferior occipital gyrus, the middle occipital lobe, the superior occipital lobe (13/20), the pericalcarine, the angular gyrus, the superior parietal lobe, the superior temporal gyrus, the middle temporal gyrus, and the lingual gygus. IFOF-IV connected the middle frontal gyrus with the inferior occipital gyrus, the middle occipital lobe, the superior occipital lobe, and the superior parietal lobe. IFOF-V connected the superior frontal gyrus with the postcentral gygus, the inferior occipital lobe, the middle occipital lobe, the superior occipital lobe, the superior parietal lobe, the fusiform gyrus, the supramarginal gyrus, the angular gyrus, the superior temporal gyrus, and the postcentral gygus (**Table 1**).

The Spatial Relationship of the IFOF with Adjacent Association Tracts

In order to visualize the spatial relationship of the IFOF with adjacent association tracts, the ILF, OR, MdLF, and UF were reconstructed (**Figure 5**).

At the roof of the temporal horn, the fibers of the IFOF are located medially to the ILF and superficially to the OR (Martino et al., 2010). The MdLF interconnects the superior temporal gyrus with the superior parietal lobe and parieto-occipital region, immediately superficial to the fibers of the IFOF (Wang et al., 2013). Based on the different orientation of the fibers of these three fascicles, they were clearly separated. The UF is a hook-shaped short-range tract connecting the frontal and temporal lobes (Leng et al., 2016). In previous DTI studies, the IFOF was often confused with the UF, as they are near each other in the region of the insula (Kier et al., 2004). According to our results, at the level of the external/extreme capsule, the IFOF narrows just above and medial to the UF.

Quantitative Study of the IFOF

The data of ILOF volume in 10 subjects were presented in **Table 2**. The relative volume of the IFOF in relation to the whole brain white matter volume was 18.5% (15.3–24.5%). The

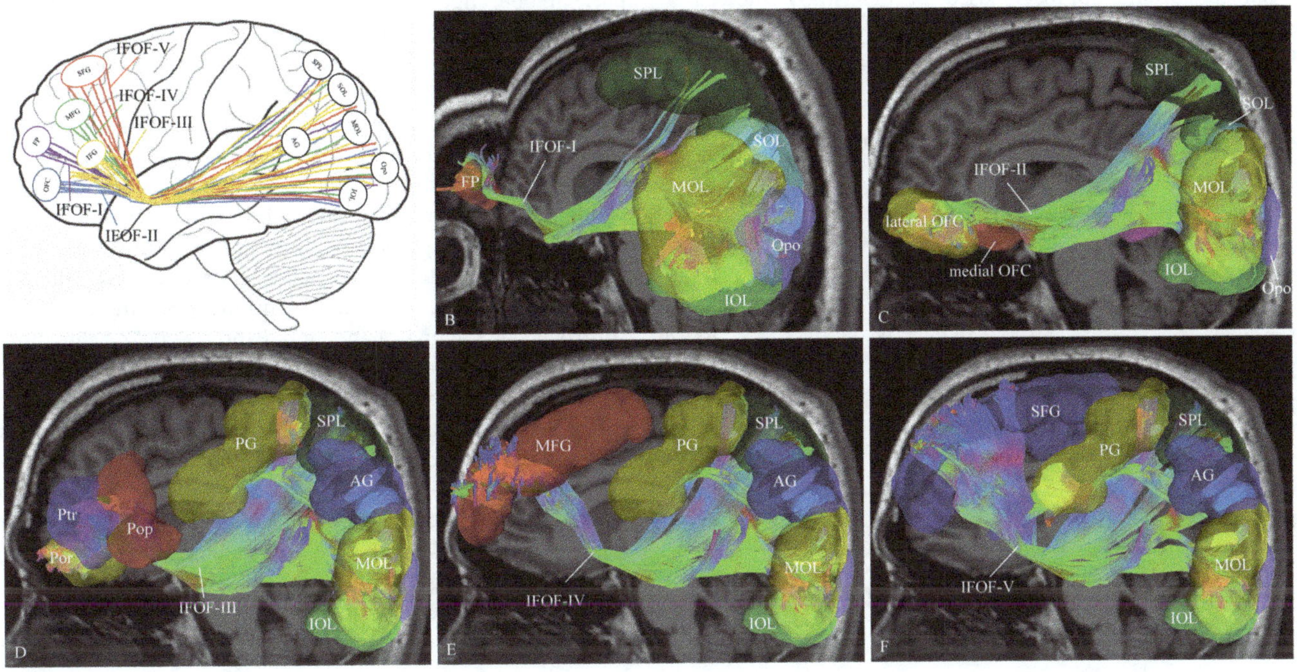

FIGURE 4 | The cortical endpoints of the IFOF and its five subcomponents (subject 1, left hemisphere). (A) A diagram of the five subcomponents. **(B)** IFOF-I originated from the frontal pole cortex to the inferior occipital lobe, the occipital pole, the middle occipital lobe, the superior occipital lobe, and the superior parietal lobe. **(C)** IFOF-II originated from the orbito-frontal cortex to the occipital pole, the inferior occipital gyrus, the pericalcarine, the middle occipital lobe, the superior occipital lobe and the fusiform gyrus, and the superior parietal lobe. **(D)** IFOF-III originated from the inferior frontal gyrus (i.e., pars opercularis, pars triangularis, and pars orbitalis) to the inferior occipital gyrus, the middle occipital lobe, the occipital pole, the superior occipital lobe, the angular gyrus, the superior parietal lobe, and the postcentral gygus. **(E)** IFOF-IV originated from the middle frontal gyrus to the occipital pole, the inferior occipital gyrus, the middle occipital lobe, the superior occipital lobe, the angular gyrus, the superior parietal lobe, and the postcentral gygus. **(F)** IFOF-V originated from the superior frontal gyrus to the occipital pole, the inferior occipital gyrus, the middle occipital lobe, the superior occipital lobe, the superior parietal lobe, the angular gyrus, and the postcentral gygus. FP, frontal pole; OFC, orbito-frontal cortex; Pop, pars opercularis; Ptr, pars triangularis; Por, pars orbitalis; MFG, middle frontal gyrus; SFG, superior frontal gyrus; AG, angular gyrus; SPL, superior parietal lobule; PG, postcentral gygus; SOL, superior occipital lobe; MOL, middle occipital lobe; IOL, inferior occipital lobe; FG, fusiform gyrus; Opo, occipital pole.

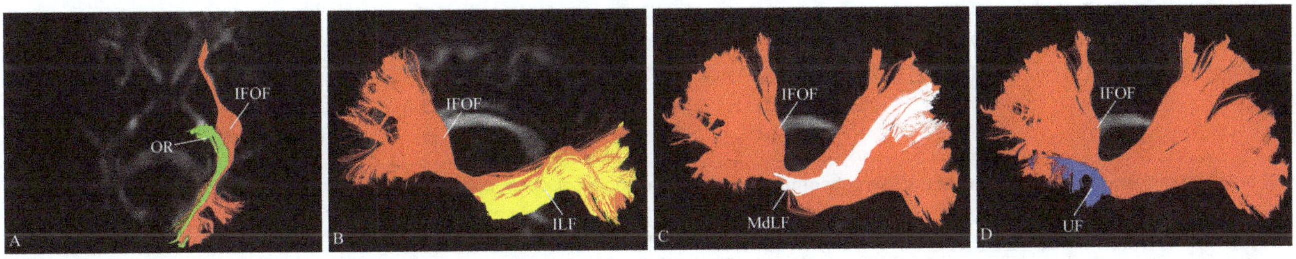

FIGURE 5 | Spatial relationship of the IFOF with adjacent association tracts. (A) Axial slice showed the IFOF located superficially to the OR. **(B)** Sagittal view showed the IFOF located medially to the ILF. **(C)** Sagittal view showed the MdLF was immediately superficial to the fibers of the IFOF. **(D)** Sagittal view showed the IFOF was just above and medial to the UF at the level of the external/extreme capsule. OR, optic radiation; ILF, inferior longitudinal fascicles; MdLF, middle longitudinal fascicle; UF, uncinate fasciculus.

statistical results revealed no significant difference in the total volume of the IFOF between the left and right hemispheres (62.79 ± 19.77 ml vs. 54.43 ± 8.96 ml, $P = 0.205$). All originating and terminating distributions of the five subcomponents between males and females were listed in **Tables 3-1, 3-2**. There were no significant differences existed in distributions of the IFOF according to the sex, no matter in originating or terminating distributions ($P > 0.05$).

DISCUSSION

In the present study, we investigated the trajectory, anatomical connectivity, and descriptive analysis of the IFOF in 10 subjects and a template of 90 subjects using high-angular-resolution fiber tractography. As for previous DTI reports, DSI approach demonstrated more higher resolution, and thus revealed a more complete connectivity pattern of the IFOF. Meanwhile, the subject-specific approach used in our study showed a greater inter-subjects variability, especially on the connection with the middle frontal gyrus, superior frontal gyrus, superior parietal lobe, angular gyrus, and postcentral gyrus. Furthermore, we also investigated whether there were discernible structural subdivisions in the IFOF based on white matter cortico-cortical connections. Five potentially different subcomponents were found within the IFOF, which could be achieved across 10 subjects and the template group.

TABLE 2 | Volume studies of the IFOF in 10 individual subjects.

Volume(ml)	L	R
1(male)	63.88	42.08
2(female)	84.75	66.67
3(female)	103.68	49.04
4(male)	64.89	63.32
5(female)	70.13	69.69
6(female)	40.72	49.58
7(male)	43.02	51.25
8(female)	44.91	52.61
9(female)	58.64	51.11
10(female)	53.26	48.90

The IFOF relative volume in relation to the whole brain white matter volume was 18.5% (15.3–24.5%). No significant difference in the total volume of the IFOF between the left and right hemispheres (62.79 ± 19.77 ml vs. 54.43 ± 8.96 ml, P = 0.205). L, left hemisphere; R, right hemisphere.

Descriptions of the IFOF have a long history. In the last century, Curran described the IFOF for the first time as one of the major long-range association tracts integrating anatomically distant brain cortex. Over several decades, its anatomical existence has been frequently mentioned, but the results were controversial (Schmahmann and Pandya, 2007; Schmahmann et al., 2007). Recent advances in DTI technique, allowing "*in vivo*" dissection of the white matter, demonstrated the existence of IFOF in the human brain (Catani et al., 2002). However, tractography based on DTI failed to solve the problem of "kissing" and crossing fibers or to determine with accuracy the origin and termination of white matter tracts. It would produce false tracts and artifacts (Wedeen et al., 2008). We assumed that the long-range connection and the natural crossing of the IFOF with other tracts were the main roots of the biases in previous DTI results. In our study, we not only employed

TABLE 3-1 | The originating distributions of the five subcomponents between males and females.

Variable	Total	FMG	MFG	MG	OFC	Pop	Por	Ptr	SFG	TFPG	P
IFOF-L (M/F)	23/47	2/4	3/4	0/3	3/7	3/3	3/7	3/7	3/5	3/7	0.946
IFOF-R (M/F)	20/48	1/4	2/3	1/3	3/7	1/3	3/7	3/7	3/7	3/7	1.000
IFOF-I-L (M/F)	5/14	2/4	0/0	0/3	0/0	0/0	0/0	0/0	0/0	3/7	0.524
IFOF-I-R (M/F)	5/14	1/4	0/0	1/3	0/0	0/0	0/0	0/0	0/0	3/7	0.916
IFOF-II-L (M/F)	3/7	0/0	0/0	0/0	3/7	0/0	0/0	0/0	0/0	0/0	–
IFOF-II-R (M/F)	3/7	0/0	0/0	0/0	3/7	0/0	0/0	0/0	0/0	0/0	–
IFOF-III-L (M/F)	9/17	0/0	0/0	0/0	0/0	3/3	3/7	3/7	0/0	0/0	0.665
IFOF-III-R (M/F)	7/17	0/0	0/0	0/0	0/0	1/3	3/7	3/7	0/0	0/0	0.980
IFOF-IV-L (M/F)	3/4	0/0	3/4	0/0	0/0	0/0	0/0	0/0	0/0	0/0	–
IFOF-IV-R (M/F)	2/3	0/0	2/3	0/0	0/0	0/0	0/0	0/0	0/0	0/0	–
IFOF-V-L (M/F)	3/5	0/0	0/0	0/0	0/0	0/0	0/0	0/0	3/5	0/0	–
IFOF-V-R (M/F)	3/7	0/0	0/0	0/0	0/0	0/0	0/0	0/0	3/7	0/0	–

TABLE 3-2 | The terminating distributions of the five subcomponents between males and females.

Variable	Total	IOL	MOL	SOL	Opo	Pca	SPL	AG	FG	PG	Pre	ITG	MTG	P
IFOF-L (M/F)	79/153	15/26	14/24	9/19	15/27	11/19	6/14	3/10	2/9	3/3	1/2	0/0	0/0	0.956
IFOF-R (M/F)	62/140	11/26	12/16	9/11	12/30	10/22	1/11	1/5	4/15	0/3	0/0	2/0	0/1	0.152
IFOF-I-L (M/F)	16/32	3/6	2/5	2/4	3/6	2/5	2/3	0/1	1/1	0/0	1/1	0/0	0/0	0.996
IFOF-I-R (M/F)	14/36	3/7	2/5	2/3	3/7	2/6	0/3	-	2/4	0/1	0/0	0/0	0/0	0.956
IFOF-II-L (M/F)	15/38	3/6	3/5	1/6	3/6	3/6	1/4	0/2	1/2	0/0	0/1	0/0	0/0	0.950
IFOF-II-R (M/F)	16/35	3/6	3/4	2/3	3/7	3/6	0/3	0/2	2/4	0/0	0/0	0/0	0/0	0.891
IFOF-III-L (M/F)	16/36	3/6	3/6	2/5	3/6	2/2	1/3	1/4	0/2	1/2	0/0	0/0	0/0	0.980
IFOF-III-R (M/F)	15/43	3/7	3/6	2/4	2/7	2/6	1/3	1/3	0/4	0/2	0/0	1/0	0/1	0.832
IFOF-IV-L (M/F)	16/20	3/4	3/4	2/1	3/4	2/3	1/1	1/1	0/2	1/0	0/0	0/0	0/0	0.894
IFOF-IV-R (M/F)	8/8	1/2	2/0	1/0	2/3	2/2	0/0	0/0	0/1	0/0	0/0	0/0	0/0	0.475
IFOF-V-L (M/F)	16/27	3/4	3/4	2/3	3/5	2/3	1/3	1/2	0/2	1/1	0/0	0/0	0/0	0.986
IFOF-V-R (M/F)	9/18	1/4	2/1	2/1	2/6	1/2	0/2	0/0	0/2	0/0	0/0	1/0	0/0	0.364

Sexual originating and terminating distributions of the five subcomponents. There were no significant differences existed in distributions of the IFOF according to the sex, no matter in originating or terminating distributions (P> 0.05). M, male; F, female.

an advanced DSI scan involving a dense sampling of angular space for underlying water diffusion, but also reconstructed the tractography by GQI engaging a high-angular-resolution-based approach. They enabled us to acquire a significantly improved resolution to trace the fibers from one cortical region to another cortical or subcortical regions through complex crossings areas (Wedeen et al., 2008; Fernandez-Miranda, 2013). It provided detailed cortical site of the origin or termination of the IFOF without need for approximation (Wang et al., 2013; Fernandez-Miranda et al., 2014).

Previously, one ROI was widely used for the definition of the origin or termination of IFOF (Fernandez-Miranda et al., 2008a,b; Caverzasi et al., 2014). The manual ROI drawing was usually placed around the ventral part of the external capsule, which was somewhat subjective, and thus the fibers of IFOF could not avoid being influenced by the adjacent crossing tracts such as the UF and corona radiata. In our study, we reconstructed the IFOF based on the cortical ROIs defining by the Automated Anatomical Labeling. The anatomic subregions were automatically generated in light of individuality which were viewed as ideal for generating tracts (Desikan et al., 2006). Two ROI masks were used to select the fibers that only originated from the frontal lobe to the posterior regions. In our experience, the data acquired by this method were more accurate and more intuitive than that obtained by other methods (Wang et al., 2013; Fernandez-Miranda et al., 2014; Leng et al., 2016; Wu et al., 2016).

As the "gold standard", post-mortem dissections have been widely employed to validate fiber tractography findings of the human white matter connective patterns. Over the past decades, although numerous microdissection studies have provided some basic anatomical information of the IFOF, a detailed analysis of the complex composition of this fiber bundle has not been reported. Only recently have two studies systematically investigated the anterior or the posterior cortical terminations of IFOF using post-mortem microdissection technique (Martino et al., 2010; Sarubbo et al., 2013). Now *in vivo*, we have not only reconstructed the results of these two studies in 10 healthy subjects and the template of 90 subjects, but also compared the connective difference among the subjects.

According to the anatomical dissection results, Martino et al. focused on the posterior terminations of IFOF, and firstly identified the posterior terminations both within and outside of the occipital lobes (Martino et al., 2010). However, they failed to identify the cortical terminations of IFOF within the frontal lobe. And they did not further confirm the results in the living human brain. Our results of *in vivo* tractography were consistent with their anatomical findings, well making up for the blanks. Moreover, we also found that there were some other terminations toward the angular gyrus, postcentral gyrus, and lingual gyrus. Indeed, the existence of the above cortex connections have been mentioned in some functional researches previously, which may be related to semantic processing (Hoeren et al., 2013; Moritz-Gasser et al., 2013; Willmes et al., 2014). This time, our results firstly provided importantly visible evidence to support the actual existence of these connections.

Recently, Sarubbo et al. has analyzed the frontal anatomical distribution of the IFOF by the post-mortem method, and attempted to confirm their findings using DTI (Sarubbo et al., 2013). They reported some new cortical terminations (i.e., middle frontal gyrus and superior frontal gyrus) in addition to the inferior frontal gyrus and orbito-frontal cortex. However, the study by Sarubbo et al. only involved the frontal connections, and not revealed the posterior components of the IFOF. Also, they performed DTI fiber tracking on just one left hemisphere. In accord with the anatomical findings of Sarubbo et al. our study identified more extended frontal connections beyond the previous "standard" IFOF. However, our results showed that there was a greater inter-subjects variability on the connections with the middle frontal gyrus and superior frontal gyrus, especially the fibers from the middle frontal gyrus, that we named as the IFOF-IV. This bundle of fibers was identified in 12 out of 20 hemispheres. And further investigation revealed that the above fiber tract was just a minor connectivity from the middle frontal gyrus to the posterior terminations in 8 out of 12 hemispheres. Similar results were obtained in the DSI template. Interesting, the inter-subjects variability was also revealed on the dorsal parieto occipital connections among our 10 subjects. Indeed, this inter-subjects variability has been mentioned previously. For example, Martino et al. identified the superior parietal lobe connection of the IFOF in 9 out of the 14 hemispheres, while the posterior and basal temporal connections were showed in 8 out of the 14 hemispheres (Martino et al., 2010). From the above, we assumed that the individual variation might be the main root of previous controversies about the detailed anatomical definition of the IFOF.

To better understand the functional role of the white matter pathway, recent studies have revealed that the SLF and the AF are constituted by different subcomponents (Makris et al., 2005). In the same way, based on our tractography results, we proposed that the IFOF was not a single pathway, but rather was composed of distinct subcomponents of white matter at different levels. And thus we trend to define the IFOF as a "multi-function" bundle. Previously, Sarubbo et al. pointed out that there were two subdivisions within the IFOF (Sarubbo et al., 2013). Given that distinct characteristics of the frontal cortical areas might be ascribed to different functional roles, we suggested that the IFOF could be further segmented into five subcomponents.

IFOF-I

The polar part of the frontal lobe (i.e., fronto-marginal gyrus and transverse fronto-polar gyrus, connected with the IFOF-I) is often designated as a single brain region, approximately corresponds to Brodmann's area (BA) 10 in the human brain. It is associated with many aspects of complex cognitive functions, such as social cognition, attention, multitasking, and episodic memory (Ramnani and Owen, 2004; Liu et al., 2013; Moayedi et al., 2015). These significant functions are primarily supported by white matter connectivity associating with the BA10 including the IFOF. Indeed, comparative morphological studies between human and non-human primate brains have showed that the human BA10 is proportionately much larger in absolute size. However, it is not disproportionately enlarged as comparisons with brain size (Semendeferi and Damasio, 2000). In addition, comparative analyses of the spatial organization of human BA10 cellular columns with BA10 in great apes, some significant differences have been identified between them, including cortical neuron organization. It means that the human BA10 contains more columnar interconnectivity (Semendeferi et al., 2011). In a recent study, Moayedi et al. used DTI to assess tractographic based dissections of the BA10 in 35 healthy subjects. They speculated that the white matter connections with the BA 10 (we named it as the IFOF-I) may play an important role in recent human cognitively special functions, which remained to be confirmed in further functional studies (Moayedi et al., 2015).

IFOF-II

Obsessive compulsive disorder (OCD) is a chronically debilitating psychiatric disease, associating with considerable anxiety and socio-occupational dysfunction (Horwath and Weissman, 2000). Functional neuroimaging studies have shown that the cognitive abnormalities in OCD patients, such as insufficient cognitive-behavioral flexibility, executive function deficits and alteration in decision-making, are associated with white matter structures connecting with the frontal lobes (Saxena et al., 2001; Lawrence et al., 2009). A recent study by Garibotto and colleagues evaluated the patterns of directionality and organization of the major fiber bundles in 15 OCD patients. The significant changes were revealed in the anatomical connectivity of the orbito-frontal cortex of the frontal lobe with the parietal and occipital cortices along the IFOF-II (Garibotto et al., 2010).

IFOF-III

For a long time, the Broca–Wernicke model of language implementation was widely adopt by generations of neuroscientists to solve language processing issues. The dorsal association via the SLF is the structural realization of these fiber connections (Poeppel and Hickok, 2004). Today, more studies have rediscovered a novel ventral stream connecting occipital, parietal, and posterior temporal regions to the Broca's areas as an independent second fiber connection of language network (Brauer et al., 2011, 2013). The fibers run through the extreme/external capsule confirming with our description on the IFOF-III. However, the distinctive roles of the dorsal and the ventral pathways playing in the language are still a matter of debate. Comparing with adults, more activities was found via the ventral fiber system for the language in children (Brauer et al., 2011). Recent studies on the neural connectivity of semantic memory has shown that a distributed left-lateralized association is consisted of the inferior frontal gyrus, the posterior lateral temporal region, the anterior temporal cortex, and the temporo-parietal junction (Nugiel et al., 2016). Therefore, Duffau et al. supported that the IFOF is the main structural pathway for semantic processing of the language (Duffau et al., 2013, 2014).

IFOF-IV and IFOF-V

The superior frontal gyrus and the middle frontal gyrus components of the IFOF, as identified in our findings, are not always shown as parts of the IFOF in previous researches (Lawes et al., 2008; Voineskos et al., 2010; Vandermosten et al., 2012). Our frontal connection findings are in line with *ex vivo* fiber dissection results that can prove our data is not artificial (Sarubbo et al., 2013). This major discrepancy is probably based on different fiber-tracking resolution of our study. According to the fiber connections, Sarubbo et al. assumed that the IFOF-IV and the IFOF-V might take part in the semantic processing of language, visual conceptualization, and recognition, however, further clinical analysis are needed to confirm their hypothesis (Sarubbo et al., 2013).

There were several limitations in our study. First, only 10 subjects were traced using the subject-specific approach, which was still relatively inadequate. More subjects are required to provide a more detailed understanding of IFOF pathway variability in the human brain, and even to investigate the IFOF variability according to different gender and age. Second, our study only explored structural connectivity of IFOF, and further anatomical and functional investigations are needed to confirm our proposal related to subcomponents.

CONCLUSIONS

The present study demonstrated the feasibility of high resolution diffusion tensor tractography with sufficient sensitivity to elucidate more anatomical details of the IFOF in the human brain. Our results were the first *in vivo* to present a more extended frontal and posterior connections beyond the previous 'standard' IFOF. In addition, according to our findings, we provided a novel framework for subdividing the IFOF, based both on its connectivity and function roles.

AUTHOR CONTRIBUTIONS

Conceived and designed the experiments: YiW and YuW. Performed the experiments: YuW, YiW, and YoW. Data interpretation and picture preparation: YuW and DS. Contributed reagents/materials/analyses tools: YiW. Wrote the paper and revised the manuscript: YuW, DS, and YiW.

ACKNOWLEDGMENTS

This study was supported by grants from the National Natural Science Foundation of China (No.31540077 to YiW).

REFERENCES

Brauer, J., Anwander, A., and Friederici, A. D. (2011). Neuroanatomical prerequisites for language functions in the maturing brain. *Cereb. Cortex* 21, 459–466. doi: 10.1093/cercor/bhq108

Brauer, J., Anwander, A., Perani, D., and Friederici, A. D. (2013). Dorsal and ventral pathways in language development. *Brain Lang.* 127, 289–295. doi: 10.1016/j.bandl.2013.03.001

Catani, M., Howard, R. J., Pajevic, S., and Jones, D. K. (2002). Virtual *in vivo* interactive dissection of white matter fasciculi in the human brain. *Neuroimage* 17, 77–94. doi: 10.1006/nimg.2002.1136

Catani, M., and Thiebaut de Schotten, M. (2008). A diffusion tensor imaging tractography atlas for virtual *in vivo* dissections. *Cortex* 44, 1105–1132. doi: 10.1016/j.cortex.2008.05.004

Caverzasi, E., Papinutto, N., Amirbekian, B., Berger, M. S., and Henry, R. G. (2014). Q-ball of inferior fronto-occipital fasciculus and beyond. *PLoS ONE* 9:e100274. doi: 10.1371/journal.pone.0100274

De Benedictis, A., Sarubbo, S., and Duffau, H. (2012). Subcortical surgical anatomy of the lateral frontal region: human white matter dissection and correlations with functional insights provided by intraoperative direct brain stimulation: laboratory investigation. *J. Neurosurg.* 117, 1053–1069. doi: 10.3171/2012.7.JNS12628

Desikan, R. S., Segonne, F., Fischl, B., Quinn, B. T., Dickerson, B. C., Blacker, D., et al. (2006). An automated labeling system for subdividing the human cerebral cortex on MRI scans into gyral based regions of interest. *Neuroimage* 31, 968–980. doi: 10.1016/j.neuroimage.2006.01.021

Duffau, H., Herbet, G., and Moritz-Gasser, S. (2013). Toward a pluri-component, multimodal, and dynamic organization of the ventral semantic stream in humans: lessons from stimulation mapping in awake patients. *Front. Syst. Neurosci.* 7:44. doi: 10.3389/fnsys.2013.00044

Duffau, H., Moritz-Gasser, S., and Mandonnet, E. (2014). A re-examination of neural basis of language processing: proposal of a dynamic hodotopical model from data provided by brain stimulation mapping during picture naming. *Brain Lang.* 131, 1–10. doi: 10.1016/j.bandl.2013.05.011

Fernandez-Miranda, J. C. (2013). Editorial: beyond diffusion tensor imaging. *J. Neurosurg.* 118, 1363–1365. discussion: 1365–1366. doi: 10.3171/2012.10.JNS121800

Fernandez-Miranda, J. C., Rhoton, A. L. Jr., Alvarez-Linera, J., Kakizawa, Y., Choi, C., and de Oliveira, E. P. (2008a). Three-dimensional microsurgical and tractographic anatomy of the white matter of the human brain. *Neurosurgery* 62(6 Suppl. 3), 989–1026. discussion: 1026–1028. doi: 10.1227/01.neu.0000333767.05328.49

Fernandez-Miranda, J. C., Rhoton, A. L. Jr., Kakizawa, Y., Choi, C., and Alvarez-Linera, J. (2008b). The claustrum and its projection system in the human brain: a microsurgical and tractographic anatomical study. *J. Neurosurg.* 108, 764–774. doi: 10.3171/JNS/2008/108/4/0764

Fernandez-Miranda, J. C., Wang, Y., Pathak, S., Stefaneau, L., Verstynen, T., and Yeh, F. C. (2014). Asymmetry, connectivity, and segmentation of the arcuate fascicle in the human brain. *Brain Struct. Funct.* 11, 341–352. doi: 10.1007/s00429-014-0751-7

Fonov, V., Evans, A. C., Botteron, K., Almli, C. R., McKinstry, R. C., Collins, D. L., et al. (2011). Unbiased average age-appropriate atlases for pediatric studies. *Neuroimage* 54, 313–327. doi: 10.1016/j.neuroimage.2010.07.033

Forkel, S. J., Thiebaut de Schotten, M., Kawadler, J. M., Dell'Acqua, F., Danek, A., and Catani, M. (2014). The anatomy of fronto-occipital connections from early blunt dissections to contemporary tractography. *Cortex* 56, 73–84. doi: 10.1016/j.cortex.2012.09.005

Garibotto, V., Scifo, P., Gorini, A., Alonso, C. R., Brambati, S., Bellodi, L., et al. (2010). Disorganization of anatomical connectivity in obsessive compulsive disorder: a multi-parameter diffusion tensor imaging study in a subpopulation of patients. *Neurobiol. Dis.* 37, 468–476. doi: 10.1016/j.nbd.2009.11.003

Hoeren, M., Kaller, C. P., Glauche, V., Vry, M. S., Rijntjes, M., Hamzei, F., et al. (2013). Action semantics and movement characteristics engage distinct processing streams during the observation of tool use. *Exp. Brain Res.* 229, 243–260. doi: 10.1007/s00221-013-3610-5

Horwath, E., and Weissman, M. M. (2000). The epidemiology and cross-national presentation of obsessive-compulsive disorder. *Psychiatr. Clin. North Am.* 23, 493–507.

Kamali, A., Hasan, K. M., Adapa, P., Razmandi, A., Keser, Z., Lincoln, J., et al. (2014). Distinguishing and quantification of the human visual pathways using high-spatial-resolution diffusion tensor tractography. *Magn. Reson. Imaging* 32, 796–803. doi: 10.1016/j.mri.2014.04.002

Kier, E. L., Staib, L. H., Davis, L. M., and Bronen, R. A. (2004). Anatomic dissection tractography: a new method for precise MR localization of white matter tracts. *AJNR Am. J. Neuroradiol.* 25, 670–676.

Lawes, I. N., Barrick, T. R., Murugam, V., Spierings, N., Evans, D. R., Song, M., et al. (2008). Atlas-based segmentation of white matter tracts of the human brain using diffusion tensor tractography and comparison with classical dissection. *Neuroimage* 39, 62–79. doi: 10.1016/j.neuroimage.2007.06.041

Lawrence, N. S., Jollant, F., O'Daly, O., Zelaya, F., and Phillips, M. L. (2009). Distinct roles of prefrontal cortical subregions in the Iowa Gambling Task. *Cereb. Cortex* 19, 1134–1143. doi: 10.1093/cercor/bhn154

Leng, B., Han, S., Bao, Y., Zhang, H., Wang, Y., Wu, Y., et al. (2016). The uncinate fasciculus as observed using diffusion spectrum imaging in the human brain. *Neuroradiology* 58, 595–606. doi: 10.1007/s00234-016-1650-9

Liu, H., Qin, W., Li, W., Fan, L., Wang, J., Jiang, T., et al. (2013). Connectivity-based parcellation of the human frontal pole with diffusion tensor imaging. *J. Neurosci.* 33, 6782–6790. doi: 10.1523/JNEUROSCI.4882-12.2013

Makris, N., Kennedy, D. N., McInerney, S., Sorensen, A. G., Wang, R., Caviness, V. S. Jr., et al. (2005). Segmentation of subcomponents within the superior longitudinal fascicle in humans: a quantitative, *in vivo*, DT-MRI study. *Cereb. Cortex* 15, 854–869. doi: 10.1093/cercor/bhh186

Martino, J., Brogna, C., Robles, S. G., Vergani, F., and Duffau, H. (2010). Anatomic dissection of the inferior fronto-occipital fasciculus revisited in the lights of brain stimulation data. *Cortex* 46, 691–699. doi: 10.1016/j.cortex.2009.07.015

Martino, J., De Witt Hamer, P. C., Vergani, F., Brogna, C., de Lucas, E. M., Vazquez-Barquero, A., et al. (2011). Cortex-sparing fiber dissection: an improved method for the study of white matter anatomy in the human brain. *J. Anat.* 219, 531–541. doi: 10.1111/j.1469-7580.2011.01414.x

Moayedi, M., Salomons, T. V., Dunlop, K. A., Downar, J., and Davis, K. D. (2015). Connectivity-based parcellation of the human frontal polar cortex. *Brain Struct. Funct.* 220, 2603–2616. doi: 10.1007/s00429-014-0809-6

Moritz-Gasser, S., Herbet, G., and Duffau, H. (2013). Mapping the connectivity underlying multimodal (verbal and non-verbal) semantic processing: a brain electrostimulation study. *Neuropsychologia* 51, 1814–1822. doi: 10.1016/j.neuropsychologia.2013.06.007

Nowinski, W. L. (2005). The cerefy brain atlases: continuous enhancement of the electronic talairach-tournoux brain atlas. *Neuroinformatics* 3, 293–300. doi: 10.1385/NI:3:4:293

Nugiel, T., Alm, K. H., and Olson, I. R. (2016). Individual differences in white matter microstructure predict semantic control. *Cogn. Affect. Behav. Neurosci.* doi: 10.3758/s13415-016-0448-x. [Epub ahead of print].

Poeppel, D., and Hickok, G. (2004). Towards a new functional anatomy of language. *Cognition* 92, 1–12. doi: 10.1016/j.cognition.2003.11.001

Ramnani, N., and Owen, A. M. (2004). Anterior prefrontal cortex: insights into function from anatomy and neuroimaging. *Nat. Rev. Neurosci.* 5, 184–194. doi: 10.1038/nrn1343

Sarubbo, S., De Benedictis, A., Maldonado, I. L., Basso, G., and Duffau, H. (2013). Frontal terminations for the inferior fronto-occipital fascicle: anatomical dissection, DTI study and functional considerations on a multi-component bundle. *Brain Struct. Funct.* 218, 21–37. doi: 10.1007/s00429-011-0372-3

Saxena, S., Bota, R. G., and Brody, A. L. (2001). Brain-behavior relationships in obsessive-compulsive disorder. *Semin. Clin. Neuropsychiatry* 6, 82–101.

Schmahmann, J. D., and Pandya, D. N. (2007). The complex history of the fronto-occipital fasciculus. *J. Hist. Neurosci.* 16, 362–377. doi: 10.1080/09647040600620468

Schmahmann, J. D., Pandya, D. N., Wang, R., Dai, G., D'Arceuil, H. E., de Crespigny, A. J., et al. (2007). Association fibre pathways of the brain: parallel observations from diffusion spectrum imaging and autoradiography. *Brain* 130(Pt 3), 630–653. doi: 10.1093/brain/awl359

Semendeferi, K., and Damasio, H. (2000). The brain and its main anatomical subdivisions in living hominoids using magnetic resonance imaging. *J. Hum. Evol.* 38, 317–332. doi: 10.1006/jhev.1999.0381

Semendeferi, K., Teffer, K., Buxhoeveden, D. P., Park, M. S., Bludau, S., Amunts, K., et al. (2011). Spatial organization of neurons in the frontal pole sets humans apart from great apes. *Cereb. Cortex* 21, 1485–1497. doi: 10.1093/cercor/bhq191

Thiebaut de Schotten, M., Dell'Acqua, F., Valabregue, R., and Catani, M. (2012). Monkey to human comparative anatomy of the frontal lobe association tracts. *Cortex* 48, 82–96. doi: 10.1016/j.cortex.2011.10.001

Vandermosten, M., Boets, B., Poelmans, H., Sunaert, S., Wouters, J., and Ghesquiere, P. (2012). A tractography study in dyslexia: neuroanatomic correlates of orthographic, phonological and speech processing. *Brain* 135(Pt 3), 935–948. doi: 10.1093/brain/awr363

Voineskos, A. N., Lobaugh, N. J., Bouix, S., Rajji, T. K., Miranda, D., Kennedy, J. L., et al. (2010). Diffusion tensor tractography findings in schizophrenia across the adult lifespan. *Brain* 133(Pt 5), 1494–1504. doi: 10.1093/brain/awq040

Wang, Y., Fernandez-Miranda, J. C., Verstynen, T., Pathak, S., Schneider, W., and Yeh, F. C. (2013). Rethinking the role of the middle longitudinal fascicle in language and auditory pathways. *Cereb. Cortex* 23, 2347–2356. doi: 10.1093/cercor/bhs225

Wedeen, V. J., Hagmann, P., Tseng, W. Y., Reese, T. G., and Weisskoff, R. M. (2005). Mapping complex tissue architecture with diffusion spectrum magnetic resonance imaging. *Magn. Reson. Med.* 54, 1377–1386. doi: 10.1002/mrm.20642

Wedeen, V. J., Wang, R. P., Schmahmann, J. D., Benner, T., Tseng, W. Y., Dai, G., et al. (2008). Diffusion spectrum magnetic resonance imaging (DSI) tractography of crossing fibers. *Neuroimage* 41, 1267–1277. doi: 10.1016/j.neuroimage.2008.03.036

Willmes, K., Moeller, K., and Klein, E. (2014). Where numbers meet words: a common ventral network for semantic classification. *Scand. J. Psychol.* 55, 202–211. doi: 10.1111/sjop.12098

Wu, Y., Sun, D., Wang, Y., Wang, Y., and Wang, Y. (2016). Tracing short connections of the temporo-parieto-occipital region in the human brain using diffusion spectrum imaging and fiber dissection. *Brain Res.* 1646, 152–159. doi: 10.1016/j.brainres.2016.05.046

Yeh, F. C., and Tseng, W. Y. (2011). NTU-90: a high angular resolution brain atlas constructed by q-space diffeomorphic reconstruction. *Neuroimage* 58, 91–99. doi: 10.1016/j.neuroimage.2011.06.021

Yeh, F. C., Verstynen, T. D., Wang, Y., Fernandez-Miranda, J. C., and Tseng, W. Y. (2013). Deterministic diffusion fiber tracking improved by quantitative anisotropy. *PLoS ONE* 8:e80713. doi: 10.1371/journal.pone.0080713

Yeh, F. C., Wedeen, V. J., and Tseng, W. Y. (2010). Generalized q-sampling imaging. *IEEE Trans. Med. Imaging* 29, 1626–1635. doi: 10.1109/TMI.2010.2045126

15

Computational Modeling and Neuroimaging Techniques for Targeting during Deep Brain Stimulation

Jennifer A. Sweet, Jonathan Pace, Fady Girgis and Jonathan P. Miller*

Department of Neurosurgery, University Hospitals Case Medical Center, Case Western Reserve University, Cleveland, OH, USA

Correspondence:
Jonathan P. Miller
jonathan.miller@UHHospitals.org

Accurate surgical localization of the varied targets for deep brain stimulation (DBS) is a process undergoing constant evolution, with increasingly sophisticated techniques to allow for highly precise targeting. However, despite the fastidious placement of electrodes into specific structures within the brain, there is increasing evidence to suggest that the clinical effects of DBS are likely due to the activation of widespread neuronal networks directly and indirectly influenced by the stimulation of a given target. Selective activation of these complex and inter-connected pathways may further improve the outcomes of currently treated diseases by targeting specific fiber tracts responsible for a particular symptom in a patient-specific manner. Moreover, the delivery of such focused stimulation may aid in the discovery of new targets for electrical stimulation to treat additional neurological, psychiatric, and even cognitive disorders. As such, advancements in surgical targeting, computational modeling, engineering designs, and neuroimaging techniques play a critical role in this process. This article reviews the progress of these applications, discussing the importance of target localization for DBS, and the role of computational modeling and novel neuroimaging in improving our understanding of the pathophysiology of diseases, and thus paving the way for improved selective target localization using DBS.

Keywords: deep brain stimulation, computational modeling, neuroimaging, tractography, targeting

INTRODUCTION

Deep brain stimulation (DBS) has been used to treat neurological disorders for several decades, but we still have little understanding of the mechanism by which it reverses pathological brain activity. This is in part due to the inherent difficulty in visualizing aberrant neural networks, thus challenging our ability to modulate such pathways via electrical stimulation. However, innovative developments in stereotaxy, computational modeling, engineering, and neuroimaging techniques have made it possible to identify complex connections of circuitry within the brain, improving our understanding of the pathophysiology of various diseases and facilitating our ability to influence these aberrant processes to produce therapeutic results. With continued advancements in engineering and neuroimaging, which enhance our targeting and delivery of stimulation, patients currently treated with DBS may experience improved, patient-specific outcomes, and those with other neurologic and psychiatric disorders may soon become candidates for surgical intervention using DBS.

MECHANISM OF ACTION OF DBS

DBS involves the surgical implantation of electrodes into deep structures of the brain to modulate brain circuitry in an effort to restore normal physiological function. DBS has been used effectively for the treatment of movement disorders, including Parkinson's disease (PD), Essential tremor (ET), and dystonia, as well as for psychiatric disorders such as obsessive compulsive disorder (OCD). It is currently under investigation for the treatment of additional psychiatric disorders, cognitive dysfunction, epilepsy, and other potentially neurologically-mediated diseases. However, our lack of understanding of the exact mechanism of action of DBS remains a limiting factor in our ability to successfully treat such disease entities.

Given that the clinical effects of DBS produce outcomes comparable to those seen with lesioning techniques, the postulated mechanism of action of DBS was initially thought to be due to widespread neuronal inhibition (Kern and Kumar, 2007; Johnson et al., 2008). Such inhibitory effects were thought to occur from a depolarization blockade or a jamming of neural networks (Grafton et al., 2006; Kern and Kumar, 2007; Hamel et al., 2003). Interestingly, despite various studies demonstrating decreased activity of the targeted cells with high-frequency DBS, the output from these cells is not necessarily lessened (Johnson et al., 2008). In fact, studies in which the activity of cells receiving input from a stimulated target were recorded suggest that the stimulated cells may release more neurotransmitters with electrical stimulation (Hashimoto et al., 2003). Despite such seemingly contradictory evidence, it is now appreciated that the delivery of stimulation is vastly more complex, resulting in the activation of some elements and the inhibition of others, each of which results in a multitude of downstream effects (Lozano et al., 2002; Kringelbach et al., 2007; Kahan et al., 2012).

In addition, DBS may exert its influence via the correction of aberrant neuronal activity. For example, in the setting of DBS for the treatment of PD, the loss of dopamine, which is known to be largely responsible for the pathophysiology of the disease, results in changes in the underlying activity of cells within the basal ganglia (Galvan et al., 2015). Analyses of the electrical activity of neurons using local field potentials, electroencephalography, and electrocorticography have demonstrated alterations of inter-spike intervals, specific firing patterns, and oscillatory activities of neuronal cells in PD (Galvan et al., 2015). It is now believed that DBS acts to disrupt the abnormal activity of these cell populations, for instance, interfering with pathologically synchronous cell groups, thus further contributing to the clinical efficacy of stimulation (Lozano et al., 2002; Kahan et al., 2012).

Finally, our notion of the target of stimulation has also changed over time. While it was once assumed that DBS affected only the regional gray matter structures in which the electrodes were placed, it is currently recognized that the effects of the electrical current are more far-reaching, modulating nearby white matter tracts as well as local and distant cortical and subcortical structures (Miocinovic et al., 2006; Kahan et al., 2012; Sweet et al., 2014b). Again looking at the model of DBS for PD, investigations have demonstrated similar motor outcomes with stimulation of either the globus pallidus interna (GPi) or the subthalamic nucleus (STN; Burchiel et al., 1999; Follett et al., 2010). Neuroimaging studies performed on patients following DBS of the STN demonstrate that the therapeutic contact is frequently positioned at the dorsolateral border of the STN and overlaps with white matter tracts from the zona incerta and fields of Forel H2, which carry fibers from the GPi (Miocinovic et al., 2006; Hamel et al., 2003). Thus, stimulation of adjacent white matter tracts, potentially affecting larger neuronal networks, may in part explain the similar effects of DBS with STN and GPi stimulation.

This concept of the activation of diffuse fiber pathways has been demonstrated in numerous imaging studies, in which widespread alterations in blood flow, glucose metabolism, and blood oxygenation level dependence (BOLD) across the brain as a result of DBS are shown, again suggesting its likely influence on the connectivity of networks (Mayberg, 1997; Grafton et al., 2006; Laxton et al., 2010; Kahan et al., 2012; Figee et al., 2013; Van Hartevelt et al., 2015). In addition, computational models replicating the effects of DBS on cell body firing patterns and subsequent downstream axonal activation reveal that stimulation of the STN influences the firing of cells within the GPi, thus altering the output of pallidothalamic projection fibers, which in turn affect thalamic processing. Once again, this reinforces the idea that DBS modulates complex neuronal systems (McIntyre et al., 2004; Rubin and Terman, 2004; Miocinovic et al., 2006; Maks et al., 2009; Hahn and McIntyre, 2010).

However, despite our incomplete understanding of the mechanism of action of DBS, there is substantial evidence to show its clinical efficacy for the treatment of movement disorders. In 1998, Limousin et al. (1998) assessed 24 patients with advanced motor symptoms of PD, who underwent bilateral STN DBS for 1 year. The patients had a 60% improvement in their motor scores of dopaminergic medications, and their daily activities also significantly improved. Moreover, the mean dose of medication was reduced by half and there was no change in their cognitive outcomes. Other studies have demonstrated similar results (Burchiel et al., 1999; Volkmann et al., 2001; Walter and Vitek, 2004), and a long-term study of 42 PD patients with STN DBS assessed for 5 years showed sustained efficacy (Krack et al., 2003). In a randomized controlled trial in 2006, Deuschl et al. (2006) found a 25% improvement in quality of life and 41% improvement in motor symptoms in patients with PD, which was superior to the best medical management. Similarly, in a randomized open-label trial, DBS of the STN plus medical treatment had better outcomes medical treatment alone for PD (Williams et al., 2010).

These impressive outcomes are not unique to the treatment of PD, as such improvements in motor symptoms have also been shown in patients with ET and dystonia. In another randomized controlled trial, patients with severe tremor due to PD and ET were implanted with electrodes into the ventrointermediate (VIM) nucleus of the thalamus. The authors found almost complete cessation in tremor in 90% of patients (Schuurman et al., 2000). Moreover, in a follow-up study of the ET patients, up to 7 years after DBS, a significant reduction in tremor score was maintained (Blomstedt et al., 2007; Kocabicak et al., 2015). Similarly, prospective randomized controlled trials assessing GPi DBS for primary dystonias also reveal significant benefits in motor symptoms and quality of life measures (Vidailhet et al., 2005; Kupsch et al., 2006; Panov et al., 2013), with sustained and even improved effects many years following surgical intervention (Vidailhet et al., 2007; Volkmann et al., 2012; Panov et al., 2013).

While there are fewer long-term studies investigating the effects of DBS for psychiatric disorders, the results are still promising. Several small studies evaluating DBS of the anterior limb of the internal capsule have been done for the treatment of OCD, based on data from capsulotomy lesions, demonstrating notable efficacy in treatment-refractory patients (Nuttin et al., 1999, 2003; Greenberg et al., 2006). Other targets have also been studied for OCD including the nucleus accumbens and the STN (Sturm et al., 2003; Mallet et al., 2008; Huff et al., 2010; Hamani et al., 2014; Kocabicak et al., 2015). Additionally, DBS for the treatment of psychiatric disorders, such as major depression (MD), have also been assessed. Targets for these various trials include the subgenual cingulate cortex, the nucleus accumbens, and the anterior limb of the internal capsule (Mayberg et al., 2005; Lozano et al., 2008; Malone et al., 2009; Kennedy et al., 2011; Bewernick et al., 2012; Holtzheimer et al., 2012). The fact that each of these studies, targeting different structures within the brain, resulted in comparable outcomes, again suggests that a complex and inter-related network is influenced by electrode stimulation.

However, while the smaller studies yielded encouraging findings, these results could not be replicated in larger, multi-center trials (Dougherty et al., 2015). This may in part be due to the heterogeneous patient population, high rates of concomitant psychiatric comorbidities among patients, or an overall still poor understanding of the involved neural circuitry (Coenen et al., 2011b). Moreover, given the vulnerability of patients with psychiatric disease and the inconsistent outcomes shown with surgical interventions, ethical considerations must be taken into account prior to proceeding to surgery for such disease states. The potentially devastating consequences of poor clinical judgment is evidenced by historical events that transpired during the psychosurgery era. Led largely by Walter Freeman in the 1940s and 1950s, the rampant and unregulated practice of the frontal lobotomy, adapted from the frontal leucotomy procedure that was initially described in Europe by Egas Moniz, was performed indiscriminately in patients of all ages with diverse symptomatology across the United States. These surgeries resulted in unacceptably high complication rates with minimal evidence to support their efficacy (Robinson et al., 2013). This underscores the importance of careful patient selection and the need for stringent pre-surgical criteria.

Therefore, although the exact mechanism of DBS remains unclear, our understanding of the complex interplay of systems involved continues to grow. In addition, there is a great deal of evidence demonstrating the benefits of DBS in appropriately selected patients. However, if we are to further optimize observable outcomes by delivering patient-specific stimulation or treating novel neurological and psychiatric diseases in a successful and consistent manner, then utilization of sophisticated and innovative targeting, engineering, and imaging techniques is required. Advancements in computational modeling and neuroimaging that can better demonstrate neuronal activity within the context of widespread connection networks has largely contributed to our progress thus far. Such strategies and technologies are discussed in the duration of this review.

Surgical Targeting

History of Surgical Targeting

As noted in the preceding section, the mechanism by which DBS exerts its clinical effects is incompletely understood. However, we do know that both the therapeutic benefits as well as many of the adverse symptoms resulting from DBS depend largely on the location of the electrode contacts within the brain. Thus surgical targeting is an essential factor contributing to the success of a DBS procedure.

Stereotaxis is the process by which deep regions of the brain may be surgically targeted via a minimally invasive approach using a three-dimensional coordinate system for spatial localization in reference to a targeting image (Schiefer et al., 2011). The role of stereotaxy for the treatment of neurological disorders dates to the 1940s when frame-based localization was used to aid in the precise targeting of intracranial structures (Leksell, 1949). The necessity for such precise and accurate localization is easily understood when considering the size and location of commonly targeted structures. For instance, the STN measures approximately 6 mm by 4 mm by 5 mm in size and is obliquely oriented in all three planes (Aboshch et al., 2010; Sweet et al., 2014a). In addition, the STN has been postulated to be somatotopically organized in a tripartite manner with respect to functional territories, such that the desired location of the DBS electrode is in the dorsolateral aspect of the nucleus, believed to correspond to the motor region of the STN (**Figure 1**; Joel and Weiner, 1997; Lambert et al., 2012; Tewari et al., 2016).

Historically, surgical targeting was done via a ventriculogram, to visualize the location of the anterior and posterior commissures which were used as reference points, and a standard stereotactic atlas, allowing for the determination of the desired target relative to its distance from these points (Walter and Vitek, 2004). The advent of computed tomography (CT) and magnetic resonance imaging (MRI), later replaced the use of the ventriculogram for indirect targeting. Yet, due to the potential error intrinsic to the process of indirect targeting, the practice of intraoperative microelectrode recording was developed. Microelectrode recording uses electrophysiology and somatosensory mapping to further confirm the precise location of the electrode within the brain (Walter and Vitek, 2004).

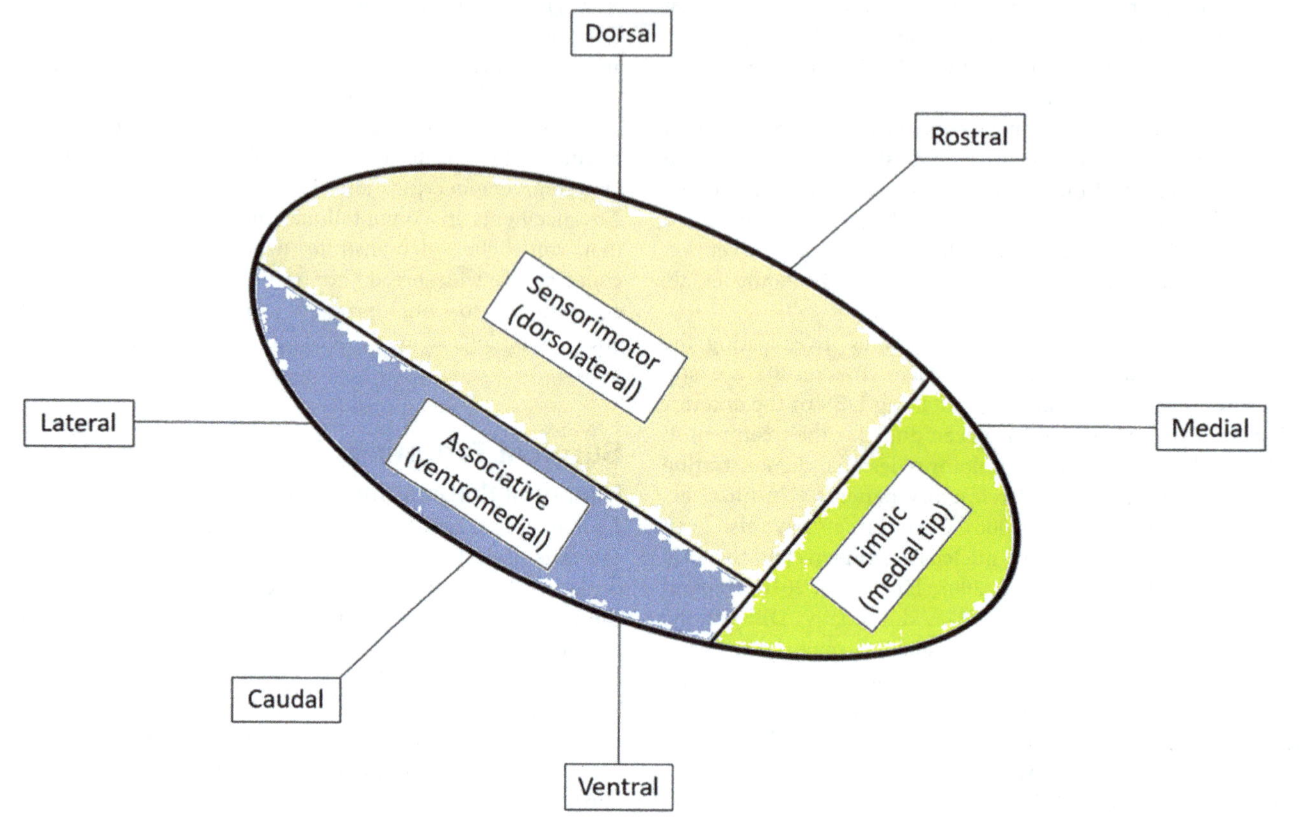

FIGURE 1 | Functional organization of subthalamic nucleus (STN) with cortical inputs into specific regions of the STN. Adapted from Tewari et al. (2016).

Further improvements in MRI technology and software targeting platforms has led to the practice of "direct" targeting, either alone or in combination with indirect targeting, to facilitate DBS electrode placement. This involves directly visualizing the target, such as the STN, using high-resolution MR images, rather than relying solely on the position of the target relative to the anterior and posterior commissures. Additional developments in neuroimaging, computational modeling, novel stimulation parameters, and improved electrode designs, are all drastically changing the way in which surgical targeting is performed. These developments aim to improve patient outcomes and aid in the understanding of both DBS and the pathophysiology of diseases.

High-Resolution MRI and Software Targeting Platforms

Improvements in neuroimaging modalities have revolutionized the process of DBS lead implantation. Advancements in MRI technology and the utilization of 3 tesla (T) MRI scanners rather than 1.5T MRI machines have made it possible to visualize deep structures of the brain to allow direct targeting of the structure with less reliance on indirect targeting based on standard landmarks (Rezai et al., 2006; Cho et al., 2010). Such visualization is even more impressive with 7-T MR systems, even allowing for detection of the VIM for ET (Aboshch et al., 2010; Cho et al., 2010).

In 2007, Guo et al. (2007) looked at six methods of targeting, including a T2-weighted MRI-based approach, a brain atlas, T1 and T2 maps, an electrophysiological database, a collection of final surgical targets from previous patients, and the combination of all of these functional and anatomical data. These were compared against the "gold standard," expert localization with intraoperative electrophysiologic confirmation. The displacement between the planned targets and the actual surgical targets compared to the gold standard ranged from 1.7 to 3 mm, with the technique combining anatomical and functional data being the most accurate (Guo et al., 2007). Additional advances enabling MRI-guided stereotaxy using a clinical workstation has been shown in animal models to be accurate to within 0.3–0.5 mm (Bjarkam et al., 2009).

Integration of imaging techniques with computer software platforms can further facilitate identification of brain structures and aid in targeting. Many such systems allow for the fusion of multiple imaging sequences while also superimposing standard brain atlases (D'haese et al., 2005; Castro et al., 2006; Duay et al., 2008). In addition, fusing different neuroimaging methodologies such as CT and MRI have also been found to ameliorate target localization (Chen et al., 2011).

Such targeting platforms have also been integrated into both frame-based and frameless stereotaxy systems. Traditionally, the placement of stereotactic head frames followed by a volumetric head CT prior to DBS surgery has been used for determination of stereotactic coordinates within the frame space, and this has been shown to be a highly accurate method of stereotaxy (Acar et al., 2007; Balachandran et al., 2009). Yet, frame placement can be uncomfortable for the patient, and requires repeated imaging once the frame is placed prior to surgery, therefore potentially adding to the length of surgery. As such, novel technologies have been developed in an effort to alleviate these concerns, allowing for the accurate targeting of deep structures without a frame. "Frameless" skull-mounted stereotactic platforms have been evaluated and found to have comparable accuracy with frame-based systems, although the use of these systems require operating through a narrow working field that can make neurophysiological recordings, if performed, more challenging (Fukaya et al., 2010).

Computational Modeling Techniques

Whole-Brain Activity Models

Computational modeling techniques have also contributed both to our understanding of and our progress in DBS. These techniques include a number of complex engineering technologies that allow us to better understand the pathophysiology of diseases treated with DBS, and the resultant effects of stimulation on the system as a whole. In particular, much work has been done looking at whole-brain network activity resulting from electrical stimulation. As previously mentioned, it is unclear as to how high-frequency DBS exerts its effects on surrounding structures. Thus, mathematical algorithms and computational models have been devised to help answer this question.

In 2004, Rubin and Terman (2004) created a computational network model to demonstrate how DBS of the STN results in the disruption of downstream pathological thalamic rhythms in PD. They did this by first creating mathematical equations and algorithms representative of the individual cell properties of each neuronal population with respect to the channels and molecular transporters comprising the cell membranes, the membrane capacitance, current flux across membranes, and additional factors in order to accurately model each cell type and its surrounding environment. They could then predict the various cell firing patterns under different circumstances depending on the variables changed. In this way, the authors evaluated the neuronal firing patterns of the STN, GP externa, GPi, and thalamus during simulation of three states: (1) normal conditions, in which GPi output to the thalamus is irregular with minimal effects on thalamic cells; (2) parkinsonian conditions, during which GPi cells, with output to the thalamus, fire in bursts at a tremor frequency, resulting in disruption of the processing capabilities of the thalamus; and (3) conditions of STN DBS in PD, causing subthalamopallidal projections that result in high-frequency tonic firing of the GPi, as opposed to the low-frequency bursting, which ultimately allows the thalamus to resume normal activity. From this model, the authors determined that STN DBS resulted in normalization of aberrant basal ganglia oscillations and thus abnormal basal ganglia output to the thalamus, ultimately restoring physiologic thalamic relay capabilities (Hahn and McIntyre, 2010).

Additional models have since been developed to further elucidate the role that STN DBS has on GPi bursting and subsequent thalamic processing. In 2010, Hahn and McIntyre (2010) looked at a model similar to that of Rubin and Terman, however, they attempted to parameterize a subthalamopallidal network model incorporating presumed cortical and striatal inputs thought to influence abnormal beta rhythms within the basal ganglia. They did this by training the model to fit *in vivo* microelectrode recordings from the basal ganglia of parkinsonian non-human primates (Hahn and McIntyre, 2010). As a result, the authors sought to more accurately predict the dynamic, multi-step cortico-striatal-thalamic network in a DBS model for PD. This complex analysis demonstrated that normalization of aberrant GPi bursting depends on the volume of STN tissue activated and may require a threshold reduction of bursting for therapeutic effects. It also reinforced the principle that extensive signaling pathways and networks, rather than isolated cell-to-cell interactions, play a large role in the etiology of disease states, as evidenced by the cortical and striatal inputs to the basal ganglia, which were reflected by the model. Therefore, using computational modeling systems, our understanding of the pathophysiology of diseases can be improved, which may in turn, allow us to more effectively treat diseases.

One further example of how computational modeling can be used to represent and predict multi-faceted systems within the brain is seen in a study by Humphries and Gurney (2012). They also utilized intricate models to assess the effects of STN DBS on the basal ganglia in PD (Humphries and Gurney, 2012). The authors hypothesized that STN DBS resulted in both increased and decreased firing rates within the basal ganglia output nuclei, contributing to the therapeutic effects of treatment. In their model, they replicated the diversification of responses from a primate STN DBS study, and showed that the mixed basal ganglia output responses underwent a step-wise change with therapeutic DBS frequencies (>100 Hz), which did not occur in optogenetic models of direct STN stimulation. They concluded that the efficacy of DBS was due to mixed effects of stimulation resulting in a combination of both stimulatory and inhibitory output from the basal ganglia in response to electrical STN stimulation unique to DBS at therapeutic thresholds. Once again, this highlights the complexity of processes concomitantly occurring as a result of DBS, leading to widespread network effects.

Volume of Tissue Activated

Another computational modeling technique that has played a critical role in our understanding of the effects of DBS is the concept of visualizing the extent of tissue that is influenced by DBS electrode stimulation, or the volume of tissue activated (**Figure 2**; Sweet et al., 2014b). In 2006, Miocinovic et al. (2006) developed a computational model in parkinsonian macaques of STN DBS. This model predicted the pattern of axonal activation during electrode stimulation

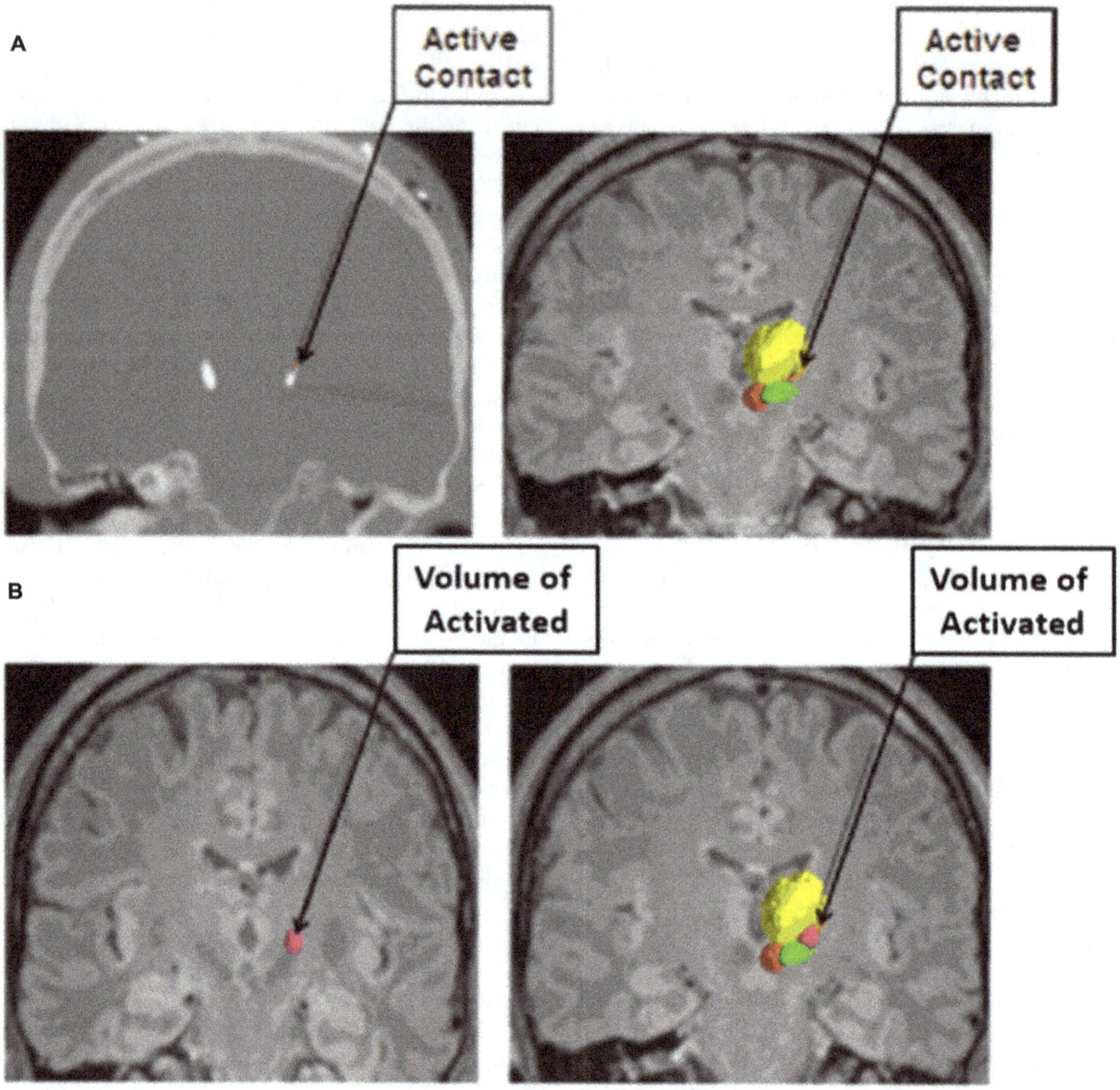

FIGURE 2 | Volume of Tissue Activated as determined from an anatomical model based on imaging data from subjects who have undergone deep brain stimulation (DBS) coupled with finite element modeling (FEM) to calculate the spread of electrical current through the tissue from the active electrode contact. (A) The active contact of each electrode was determined from postoperative programming sessions, and was defined as the cathodal electrode for either monopolar or bipolar stimulation. The active contact is shown on a postoperative computed tomography (CT) scan (left) and on image fusion on magnetic resonance imaging (MRI; right). **(B)** The volume of tissue activated was calculated from each patient's specific stimulation parameter settings by using a custom Python-based program from Python libraries. The volume of tissue activated is shown in dark pink alone (left) and in conjunction with the contored nuclei (right). The relevant nuclei were contored and include the thalami *(yellow)*, the red nuclei *(red)*, and the STN *(green)*; the active contact and the volume of tissue activated were also contored *(pink)*. Adapted from Sweet et al. (2014a).

of the STN, and demonstrated that while both STN and GPi fibers were activated, only activation of the STN neurons correlated with clinically therapeutic stimulation (Miocinovic et al., 2006).

The method by which such computational modeling systems determine the volume of tissue activated involves finite element modeling (FEM). FEM combines an anatomical model based on imaging data from subjects who have undergone DBS with an electrical model to calculate the electrical field from the DBS electrode. The FEM data can then be used to calculate the voltage spread of the electrical stimulation. This depends on the location of the electrode and the composition of the surrounding tissue, which is in turn evaluated by the electrode capacitance and impedance, as well as by the stimulation parameters used with programming of the electrode. Ultimately, the voltage distribution within the tissue is established from the FEM and the total amplitude of current is divided between the contacts of the electrode (Butson and McIntyre, 2005, 2008; Miocinovic et al., 2006). Axonal activation can then be predicted by again using an anatomical model to distribute axons in a grid around the DBS electrode and calculating the voltage spread produced by each active contact to find the threshold for generating an action potential within each surrounding axon. The volume of tissue activated is then predicted from the relationship between the electrical field and the evoked action potentials in the axon models (Butson and McIntyre, 2008).

Such modeling algorithms are not only able to accurately predict the volume of tissue activated, but can also determine its effect on clinical outcome. Maks et al. (2009) evaluated 10 patients with PD who underwent unilateral STN DBS using conventional preoperative imaging and intraoperative neurophysiology. The results were then superimposed to a brain atlas and fused with postoperative imaging of the electrodes and the volume of tissue activated calculated with a diffusion tensor stimulation model, followed by assessment of clinical outcomes. The authors found that the therapeutic benefits of stimulation were greatest with the active contacts near the dorsal border of the STN. Similarly, in 2011, Mikos et al. (2011) used computational modeling to analyze of the association between the volume of tissue activated and verbal fluency in PD patients who underwent STN DBS, finding a subtle decline in verbal fluency with stimulation of non-motor regions of the STN. Thus the volume of tissue activated can be assessed relative to the surrounding anatomy in the brain to better determine which structures are actively being stimulated in an effort to improve patient outcomes.

Limitations of Computational Modeling

It should be noted that there are limitations to computational modeling techniques. With respect to the modeling of network activity, numerous simplifications and assumptions are made and are therefore limitations of the model. For instance, the input and output connections to and from the basal ganglia likely ignore many fiber tracts in order to focus on the pathways under investigation. As a result, networks that are potentially involved in sensorimotor signals to the thalamus may also be neglected (Rubin and Terman, 2004). In addition, field effects and variations due to electrode positioning are also ignored, and each cell is treated as a single compartment, again simplifying the model substantially (Rubin and Terman, 2004; Hahn and McIntyre, 2010). Many of these models also look at an open-loop system, studying the effects of a unidirectional pathway or network. However, in actuality, there are likely closed-loop, feedback interactions that are not represented with such models (Hahn and McIntyre, 2010).

Similarly, calculations for the determination of the volume of tissue activated are also based on several assumptions and simplifications regarding the properties of the activated neurons. Preliminary studies to calculate the volume of tissue activated were initially based on the properties of rat STN neurons. Attempts were then made to approximate *in vivo* conditions of Parkinson macaques. In addition, activated neuronal populations were presumed to be uniform in their membrane dynamics, myelination, morphology, and projection pattern. Yet we know such homogeneity does not exist *in vivo*. As a result, the true thresholds for producing action potentials and thus the overall volume of tissue activated could vary somewhat compared to the predicted model. Finally, studies investigating the volume of tissue activated looked at the white matter tracts surrounding the STN that were felt to be the most likely contributing tracts to the therapeutic effects of STN DBS, while many other nearby tracts were ignored. Also ignored were the potential effects of antridromic stimulation of afferent fibers projecting to the STN and the effects of adjacent glial cells that could influence the extracellular environment and thus the effects of current spread and axonal activation (Miocinovic et al., 2006).

Additional Engineering Developments

Novel Stimulation Parameters

Many of the computational models predicting network activity with DBS have looked at the effects of high-frequency stimulation. In fact, as demonstrated by Humphries and Gurney (2012), the therapeutic effects of DBS are thought to occur with continuous stimulation at frequencies greater than 100 Hz. However, altering the parameters of the stimulation delivered could have significant results. Computational analyses using predictive models of stimulation have demonstrated that the volume of tissue activated is determined by both the stimulation parameters and the physical properties of the electrodes (Butson and Mcintyre, 2006). This has substantial implications regarding the importance of modulating stimulation settings to influence patient outcomes. Studies exploring innovative stimulation parameters such as high-frequency or patterned stimulation may have additional benefits compared to conventional stimulation. Moreover, such novel patterns of stimulation may be more effective in disrupting abnormal beta band oscillations within the cortico-basal ganglia network that are thought to be involved in the symptomatology of PD (Hurtado et al., 1999; Meijer et al., 2011,; Grant and Lowery, 2013; Kang and Lowery, 2013; McIntyre and Foutz, 2013).

Closed-Loop DBS and Current Steering

The delivery of stimulation can also be affected by the design of implanted DBS electrodes. New types of electrodes with recording capabilities have been studied such that changes in the environment surrounding the electrode can be assessed. Such changes include the recording of local field potentials, which could be used to correlate beta band oscillations with activity and posture in PD patients (Quinn et al., 2015) or even the characteristic chemical composition of the environment (Bennet et al., 2016). Recording electrodes such as these would then transmit the information to a pulse generator capable of analyzing the data, which would in turn deliver stimulation in response to the recorded information (Quinn et al., 2015; Bennet et al., 2016). This closed-loop responsive form of stimulation, may ultimately be used to further impact patient outcomes.

The volume of tissue activated can also be manipulated with changes in electrode design. For instance, as discussed by Butson and McIntyre (2008), shaping the volume of tissue activated by selectively activating specific fiber tracts via "current-steering" may better alleviate symptoms experienced by patients due to their disease. For example, in situations in which traditional STN DBS produces both therapeutic effects as well as concurrent side effects due to the undesired activation of adjacent fiber tracts like the internal capsule, current steering could be applied. This would enable directing the spread of current to avoid the activation of certain nearby structures, while activating the intended target. Currently utilized DBS electrodes have four cylindrical contacts, yet new electrode designs with more contacts of different shapes, capable of delivering stimulation in specific and variable configurations, are being developed (**Figure 3**; Van Dijk et al., 2015). These designs take advantage of the innumerable possible electrode orientations to maximize the efficacy of stimulation with surrounding anatomical structures (**Figure 3**; Beriault et al., 2012; Van Dijk et al., 2015). This notion of current-steering has given rise to multiple investigations (Contarino et al., 2014; Bour et al., 2015; Timmerman et al., 2015; Willsie and Dorval, 2015) and combining these engineering designs with computational models, such as those looking at the volume of tissue activated, could also prove to be useful in surgical planning and subsequent electrode programming. However, additional studies with long-term follow-up will be necessary to better determine the efficacy of such technologies.

Advanced Neuroimaging Technologies

Diffusion-Weighted Imaging and Tractography

The development of sophisticated imaging techniques has also enhanced our understanding of the complex circuitry of neural networks in the brain and the role of DBS in influencing such networks. As previously discussed, many of the effects of DBS are likely due to the involvement of white matter tracts comprising interconnected functional systems traveling between various intracranial structures. Neuroimaging modalities measuring metabolism and blood flow have demonstrated diffuse patterns of seemingly distant regions of the brain being simultaneously activated with DBS, thus supporting this notion of stimulation affecting widespread connectivity (Mayberg, 1997; Grafton et al., 2006; Laxton et al., 2010; Kahan et al., 2012; Figee et al., 2013). However, these studies do not directly show the actual white matter pathways thought to be involved.

Visualization of such fibers is now in part feasible with the use of diffusion-weighted imaging (DWI) MRI sequencing and tractography. DWI is a mode of MRI that illustrates the spontaneous diffusion of water within the brain. Since water diffuses easily along cell barriers rather than across them, one can assume that the diffusion of water throughout the brain represents the anatomical course of neuronal axons. Thus, by assessing water diffusivity in living tissue, the approximate location of axonal pathways can be estimated, and the likelihood of their connections to various structures can be established (Henderson, 2012; Klein, 2013; Auriat et al., 2015). From DWI, a diffusion tensor can be established within a given voxel on MRI. A diffusion tensor can take a perfectly spherical shape

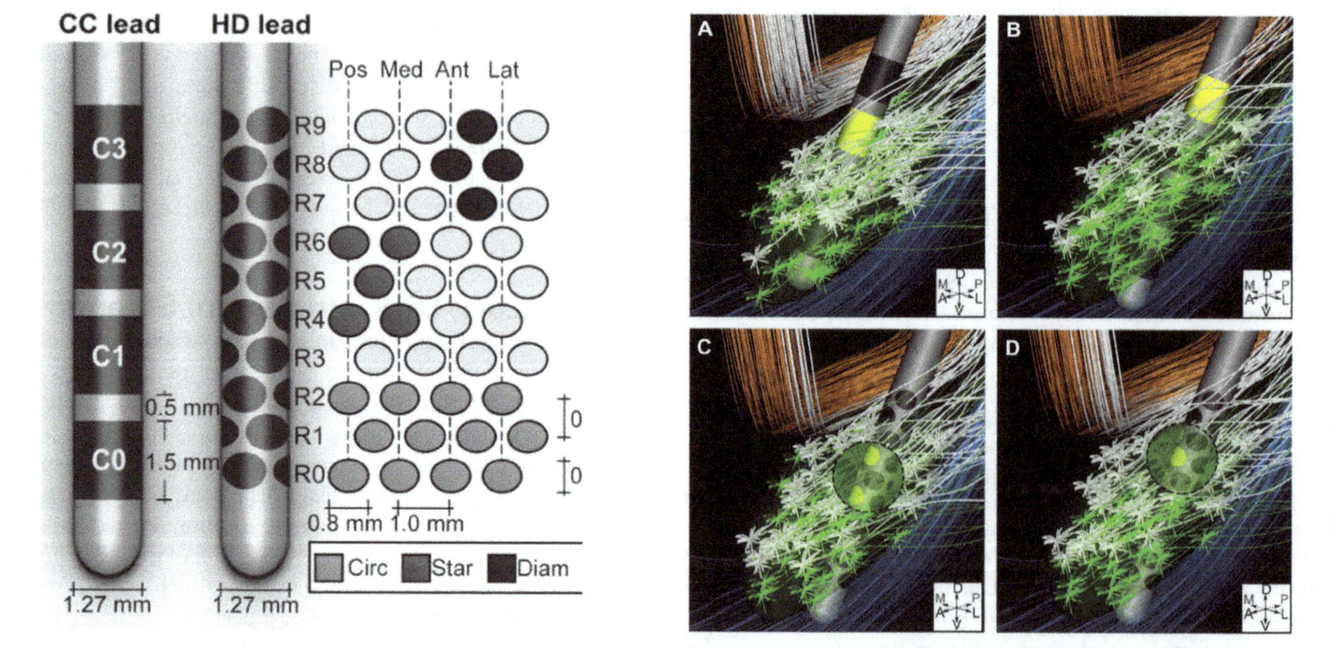

FIGURE 3 | Left: Conventional cylindrical four contact lead (CC) compared to high density lead design (HD). Right: An example of diffuse fiber activation with conventional DBS **(A,B)** vs. selective activation of fiber tracts with current steering **(C,D)**. Reprinted with permissions from Van Dijk et al. (2015).

when there is no water diffusion, such as the cerebrospinal fluid within a ventricle (**Figure 4**; Klein, 2013). However, the tensor can also become cylindrically-shaped when the water is diffusing in a given direction, such as along an axon as part of a group of white matter fibers (**Figure 4**; Klein, 2013). The more directions that are added to the DWI sequencing, the more specific the directionality of the diffusion tensor of a given voxel becomes. From the diffusion tensors, which are derived from DWI sequences, comes diffusion tensor imaging (DTI), which provides a voxel-to-voxel based estimation of the three-dimensional orientation of an axonal fiber (Auriat et al., 2015).

However, DTI has numerous limitations. Firstly, each diffusion tensor is only an estimation of the approximate directionality of water within a given voxel. As such, each tensor is only representative of a small portion of a single axonal fiber, and thus is not a representation of the entire axon or a group of axons comprising a fiber tract. Therefore, DTI may not even depict the actual anatomical course of a neuronal axon. As a result, any interpretation of the course of an axon or group of axons from DTI is relatively subjective (Auriat et al., 2015). Furthermore, DTI is limited by its technical acquisition, including poor resolution of images, poor signal-to-noise ratio, involuntary movements from subjects, and other related variables (Henderson, 2012).

A natural extension of DTI that attempts to correct for its limitations is fiber tractography. While DTI approximates the main nerve fiber direction within a given voxel, tractography attempts to assess all the voxels between two or more regions of interest in an effort to discern the entire course of axons comprising a white matter fiber tract (Klein, 2013). In order to achieve this, tractography uses the DWI data and a series of algorithms to produce a proposed fiber tract. By defining starting and ending seeds, or regions of interest, post-imaging analysis can be performed using various computer software platforms to determine the predominant fiber pathways coursing between the assigned seeds. However, it should be noted that tractography results are highly dependent upon the algorithms used, and larger white matter tracts are easier to visualize than smaller, unknown tracts (Coenen et al., 2012; Klein, 2013). In addition, sharply decussating tracts may be more difficult to identify than tracts without sudden or significant changes in direction (Coenen et al., 2012).

Thus tractography provides an anatomical three-dimensional model of white matter fiber tracts. There are two types of tractography, deterministic and probabilistic. Deterministic tractography is the more straightforward of the two and involves a streamline algorithm based on thresholds for collinearity of primary diffusion direction among adjacent voxels to establish a putative axonal pathway. These algorithms, such as FACT (fiber assignment by continuous tracking) create continuous tubular structures that are representative of white matter tracts between two or more regions of interest (**Figures 5**, **6**; Sweet et al., 2014b). However, this is an all-or-none calculation, and not all of the tracts identified using this technique will in fact exist, which again represents a substantial limitation. There is also, as noted above, particular ambiguity in areas with less anisotropy such as decussating fibers (Coenen et al., 2012; Klein, 2013). Thus, deterministic tractography works well for highly anisotropic tensors, but may be quite inaccurate for areas with less anisotropy. While any potential error in estimation may be evident for well-established white matter tracts, such as the corticospinal tract, the degree of inaccuracy is indeterminable for tracts that are not well established. Therefore, adding to

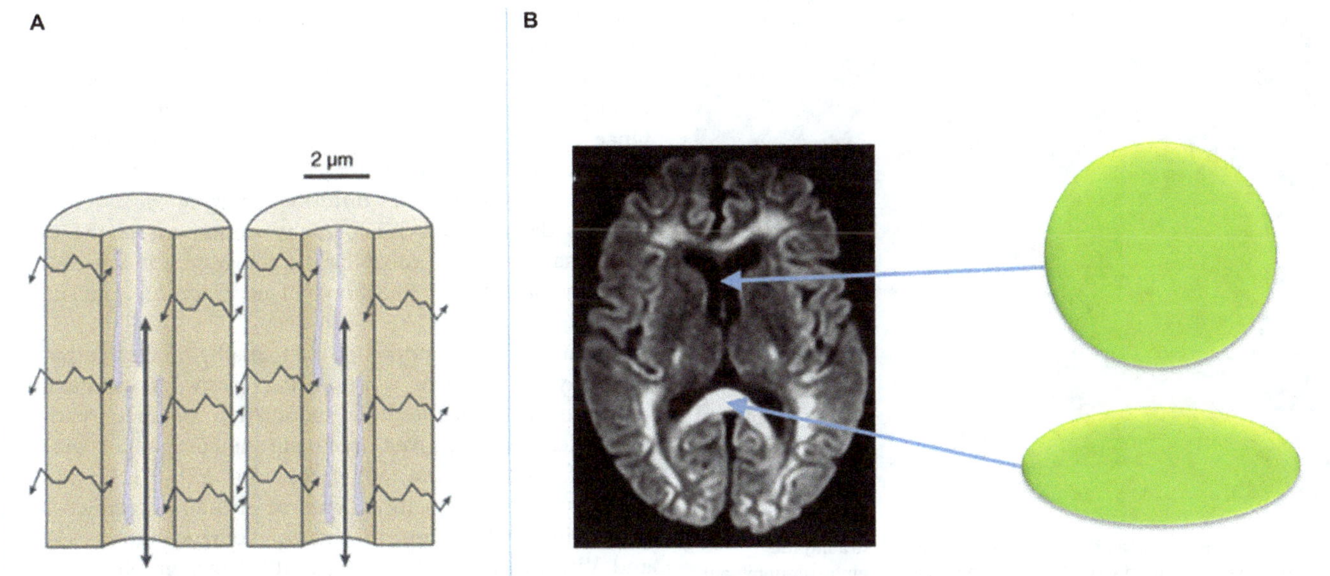

FIGURE 4 | Diffusion of water along cellular barriers in brain rather than across them (A), and examples of tensors with isotropic diffusion in CSF (represented by sphere) and anisotropic diffusion in callosal fibers (B). Adapted from Klein (2013).

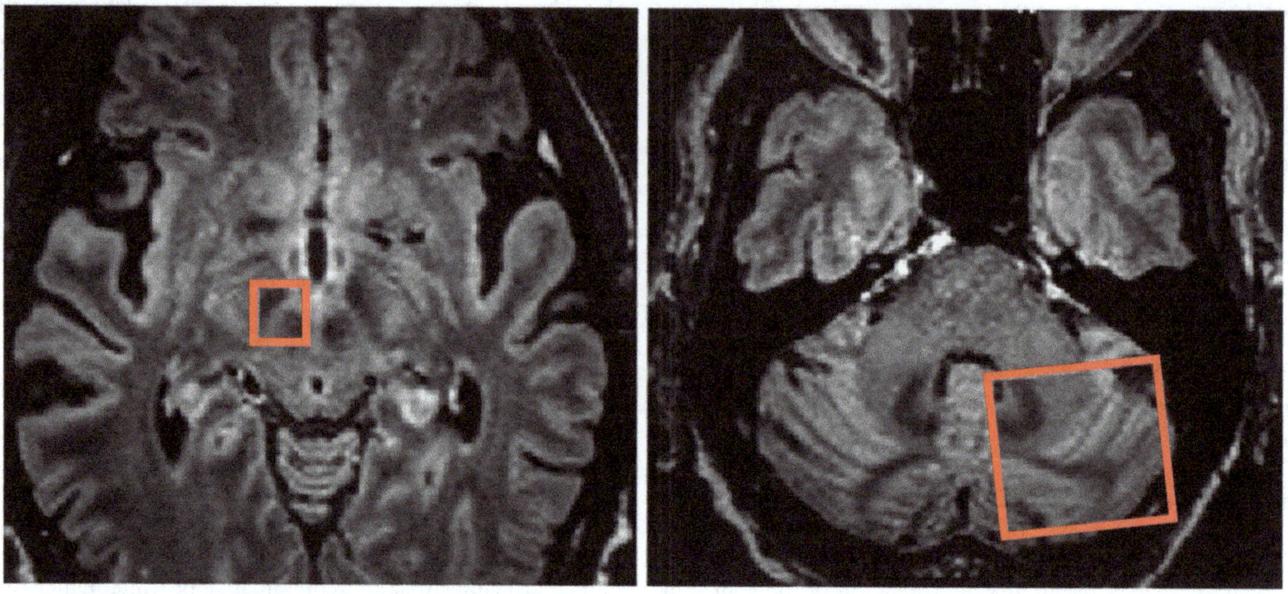

FIGURE 5 | Regions of interest (red boxes) shown on MRI in axial planes to include the right subthalamic nucleus (STN) and Red Nucleus and the contralateral cerebellar hemisphere for investigation of white matter tracts traversing between the two regions of interest. Adapted from Sweet et al. (2014a).

the above limitations of deterministic tractograpy, is the major disadvantage that the error or confidence in the estimation of a tracts is unknown (Coenen et al., 2014).

In contrast, probabilistic tractography attempts to overcome the limitations of deterministic tractography by explicitly characterizing the confidence with which connections may be established through the diffusion data itself (Coenen et al., 2012). Thus, probabilistic tractography uses advanced mathematical algorithms to produce an output of connection probability values to determine the statistical probability of a fiber tract running through a given set of voxels or between two anatomic structures based on the diffusion model (Coenen et al., 2012; Klein, 2013). This often requires the use of computer software programs such as FSL, which calculate and produce a color scale to indicate the probability of a given streamline connecting a start point to other voxels within the brain (Coenen et al., 2014). The same predictability could only be done with deterministic tractography by performing the fiber tracking on multiple patients and combining the results to determine a probability (Coenen et al., 2014). Once again, the primary limitation of tractography is its intrinsic nature of estimating the course and location of a fiber tract from the diffusion imaging data. However, whereas deterministic tractography cannot assess the degree of estimation error, probabilistic tractography is able to more precisely predict the likelihood of accuracy of a given fiber tract.

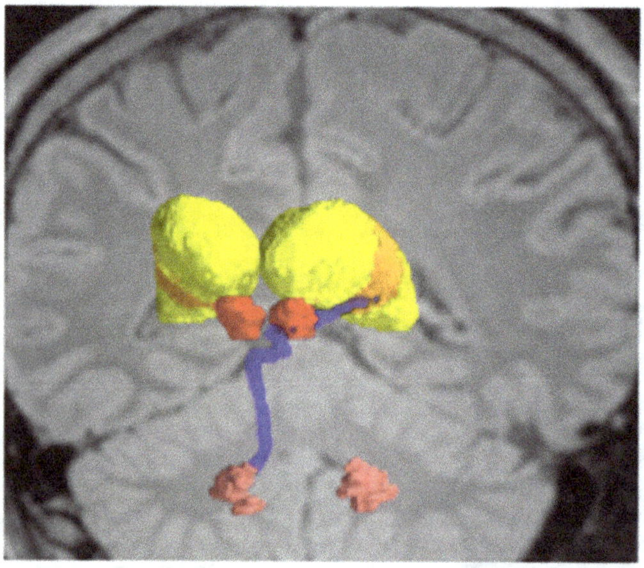

FIGURE 6 | Deterministic fiber tractography, demonstrating the dentatothalamaic tract (DTT; blue) in patients with tremor-predominant Parkinson's disease (PD). The relevant nuclei were contored and include the thalami *(yellow)*, the red nuclei *(red)*, and the dentate nuclei *(peach)*. Data from from Sweet et al. (2014a).

From a DBS standpoint, tractography makes it possible not only to visualize white matter pathways in the brain, but also to postulate how modulation of these pathways might lead to improved treatment outcomes. For example, both of the common DBS targets for PD (STN and GPi) are gray matter structures, and stimulation of either target results in notable improvement in motor symptoms (Walter and Vitek, 2004; Follett et al., 2010). Tractography has made it possible to view the axonal pathways surrounding each structure that may also be activated, such as subthalamopallidal and pallidothalamic pathways, as well as other connections to regions of the cortex, thalamus, and brainstem (Vanegas-Arroyave et al., 2016) and this activation may be responsible to some degree for the therapeutic effects of DBS. Similarly, studies assessing white matter tracts associated with the VIM thalamus, such as the dentantothalamic tract, indicate changes in tremor patients compared to controls that may account for some of the efficacy of DBS of this target (Klein et al., 2011). By identifying specific white matter pathways like the dentothalamic tract, which is thought to play a role in the pathogenesis of tremor, it is possible to determine whether there is any benefit to tract-specific targeting using DBS (Kwon et al., 2011; Klein et al., 2012; Coenen et al., 2014; Sweet et al., 2014b; Schlaier et al., 2015). In the same way, a better understanding of the involvement of white matter tracts in the pathophysiology of disease using tractography techniques can help direct future therapies. Using tractography to examine fiber networks in the brain of patients with psychiatric or cognitive disorders may allow identification of new targets in the brain for the treatment of various disorders. For example, Gutman et al. (2009) used DTI and probabilistic tractography to investigate two DBS white matter targets for the treatment of depression, the subcallosal cingulum bundle and the anterior limb of the internal capsule, and concluded that these targets are involved in distinct neural networks that overlap, explaining the benefit of DBS of each target in patients with depression. Likewise, Fernandes et al. (2015) used advanced tractography combined with whole-brain anatomical parcellation to establish connectivity "fingerprints" of successful and unsuccessful DBS targets for chronic pain, a technique which offers promise for discovery of new neuromodulation targets for other neuropsychological disorders. Boccard et al. (2016) used probabilistic tractography to demonstrate that connectivity with medial forebrain bundle and precuneus were associated with good and bad outcome, respectively, among patients treated with DBS of the anterior cingulate for chronic pain. The targeting of temporal fiber pathways for disorders of memory and cognition is also actively under investigation (Hamani et al., 2007; Laxton et al., 2010; Suthana et al., 2012; Miller et al., 2015). Incorporating tractography imaging techniques to better visualize neural pathways may prove to be invaluable in such targeting endeavors.

Resting-State Functional Connectivity MRI and Connectonomics

It is also worth discussing additional imaging technologies that have been developed to further assess connectivity, such as resting-state functional-connectivity MRI (rs-fcMRI). This technique allows for the visualization of neural networks within the brain by assessing fluctuations in blood oxygenation (Fox et al., 2014). Spontaneous alterations in the BOLD has been correlated with known functional networks within the brain, and may demonstrate continuous activity between various intracranial regions, thus representing connectivity (Faria et al., 2012). Such networks have been shown to be active in the absence of sensorimotor or cognitive tasks in fMRI studies, and deactivate during such goal-directed tasks (Ongur et al., 2010). As a result, these pathways have been termed the default-mode network (DMN) and are implicated in ongoing, default functions of the brain (Ongur et al., 2010). Thus, rs-fcMRI allows us to assess the DMN in patients as a surrogate for connectivity. Moreover, rs-fcMRI also enables visualization of brain structures more easily than tractography, which is derived from DWI MRI sequences rather than structural MRI sequencing. This also allows for structural connectivity-based parcellation to be incorporated into the imaging analysis. The parcellated functional connectivity approach is a natural extension of rs-fcMRI due to the spatial dimensionality visible in rs-fcMRI. This entails identifying brain structures and clustering voxels around such structures (Faria et al., 2012). This results in a more clearly depicted relationship between functional connectivity and structural anatomy. Such analysis can be taken a step further to include multi-modal analysis, combining DWI-based connectivity with rs-fcMRI connectivity using a parcel-to-parcel approach (Faria et al., 2012).

Data from rs-fcMRI pertaining to the DMN can be used to help draw conclusions regarding the wiring diagram of the brain, or the connectome. By modeling the DMN derived from BOLD signals on rs-fcMRI, lesions or disruptions of connections can be replicated to determine the resultant impact such changes would produce on the DMN (Hart et al., 2016). Thus by weakening specific projection fibers, as one might see in injuries induced by traumatic brain injury, one can predict the resultant effects this wound have on the connectome as a whole (Hart et al., 2016). Similarly, by strengthening certain connections, we can speculate as to the impact that DBS might have on the connectome or DMN.

Limitations of Connectivity Analyses

However, like any novel modality, limitations in both tractography and rs-fcMRI do exist. With respect to tractography, as previously discussed, the visualization of fiber tracts is based on numerous assumptions regarding the diffusion properties of water within the brain. Firstly, the premise of tractography relies on the presumption that the spontaneous flow of water in the brain only occurs along the course of an axon. Moreover, the tensors are themselves estimations of the mean vector of water diffusivity within a given voxel. Lastly, the mathematical algorithms that generate proposed fiber tracts are at best educated estimations of the presence of a given tract.

In addition, limitations of rs-fcMRI should also be noted. While there is a demonstrable correlation between rs-fcMRI and white matter connections, rs-fcMRI is still a surrogate for connectivity based on a suspected DMN. In addition, the exact causal relationship between two or more regions with increased BOLD can only be postulated, and polysynaptic interactions may play a larger role then suspected. This could thus be a misrepresentation of a particular connection or relationship in the brain, which could be misleading if used for target guidance in DBS (Fox et al., 2014).

Integration of Novel Technologies and Future Applications in Target Selection

Ultimately, the integration of computational modeling techniques and novel imaging technologies can perhaps be used to validate hypotheses regarding mechanisms of disease states and implicated networks, and thus aid in the discovery of new surgical targets. For example, in a study by Sweet et al. (2014b), patients with advanced PD who underwent STN DBS were assessed using deterministic tractography from preoperative imaging to identify fiber pathways extending between the cerebellum and the basal ganglia believed to be associated with the pathophysiology of the tremor component of PD. The findings from the tractography were then combined with postoperative computational modeling to determine the volume of tissue activated based on the therapeutic electrode contacts. The study showed that in patients with tremor-predominant PD, the volume of tissue activated tended to involve the dentatothalamic tract (**Figure 7**; Sweet et al., 2014b), supporting the idea that this tract contributes to tremor in PD. The findings also suggest that specific targeting of the dentatothalamic tract may better alleviate symptoms in tremor-predominant patients, and may thus represent a form of patient-specific DBS targeting.

Other studies have similarly integrated computational modeling, tractography, and patient outcomes. Specifically, the dentatothalamic tract has been assessed in PD and ET patients by several groups, using both deterministic and probabilistic tractography (Klein et al., 2012; Coenen et al., 2014; Sweet et al., 2014b; Schlaier et al., 2015), and combined with computational models to further validate this concept of patients-specific targeting to treat tremor symptomatology. Outcome data from patient-specific targeting techniques can also be combined with computational models to construct a probabilistic stimulation atlas that incorporates advanced computational modeling with clinical outcomes to determine the ideal target based on a patient's particular symptoms (Butson et al., 2011). Though further studies are needed, tractography and predictive modeling modalities may be able to be used to rather directly target specific pathways in a patient-specific manner .

Finally, the combination of computational models of electric field patterns with tractography could help us to better predict which specific white matter tracts are being activated for the treatment of psychiatric, cognitive, and neurologically-mediated disorders. Lujan et al. (2013), combined probabilistic tractography and electrical field modeling to help predict connectivity in patients with depression. The authors looked at white matter tracts within the subcallosal cingulum bundle who underwent DBS to look at which electrodes would be the most useful in treatment of the depression based on the pattern of current delivery and activation of the associated fibers using computational modeling. Similarly, Coenen et al. (2012) demonstrated the involvement of the medial forebrain bundle in depression using tractography, and utilized computational modeling to show how a new DBS target stimulating the medial forebrain bundle would potentially activate more white matter tracts associated with the pathophysiology of the disease than currently investigated targets. As more disease entities are studied for potential treatment using DBS, such as other psychiatric disorders, memory and cognitive dysfunction, and epilepsy (Fisher et al., 2010; Sankar et al., 2014; Miller et al., 2015), the

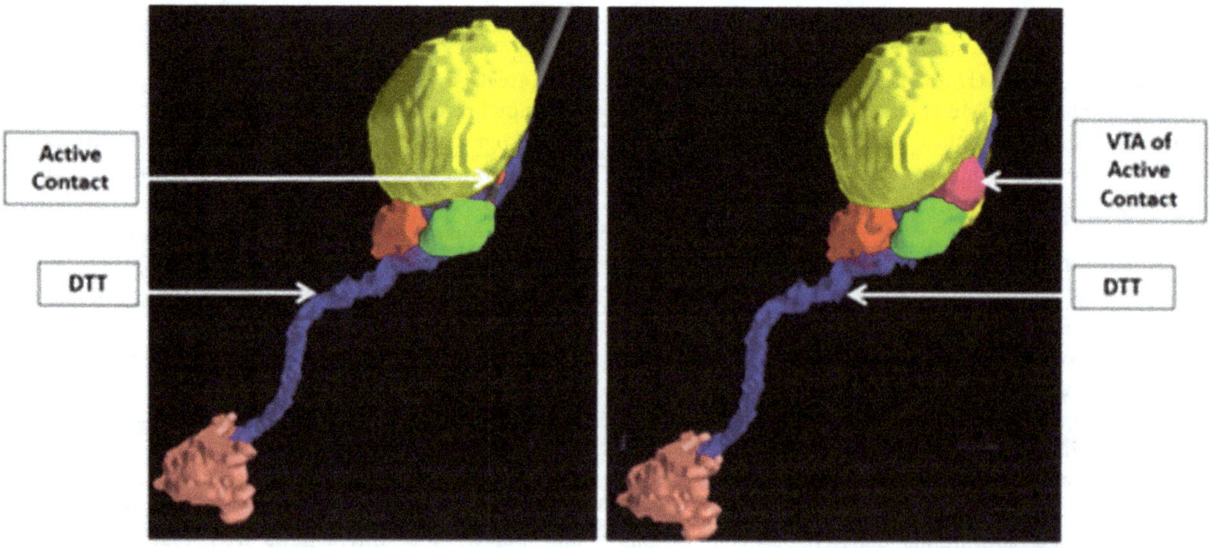

FIGURE 7 | Integration of computer modeling techniques and tractography to demonstrate that the volume of tissue activated of the active STN electrode contact includes the DTT in patients with tremor-predominant PD. The relevant nuclei were contored and include the globus pallidus and putamen *(blue)*, the thalami *(yellow)*, the red nuclei *(red)*, the STN *(green)*, and the dentate nuclei *(peach)*. Data from Sweet et al. (2014a).

applications for these techniques will undoubtedly grow as well.

CONCLUSION

Improvements in surgical targeting, computational modeling, engineering, and neuroimaging techniques have greatly enhanced our understanding of the pathophysiology of various diseases, allowing for the effective treatment of such conditions using DBS. In the future, it is likely that these novel technologies will have further applications in DBS surgery, including patient-specific targeting and the discovery of new targets for the treatment of neurological, psychiatric, and even cognitive disorders.

AUTHOR CONTRIBUTIONS

JPM, JAS, JP, and FG wrote and edited the article.

ACKNOWLEDGMENTS

This project was supported by the National Institutes of Health (NIH/NCATS CTSA KL2TR000440). The authors thank Cameron McIntyre, PhD for his contribution to the review.

REFERENCES

Aboshch, A., Yacoub, E., Ugurbil, K., and Harel, N. (2010). An assessment of current brain targets for deep brain stimulation surgery with susceptibility-weighted imaging at 7 tesla. *Neurosurgery* 67, 1745–1756; discussion 1756. doi: 10.1227/NEU.0b013e3181f74105

Acar, F., Miller, J. P., Berk, M. C., Anderson, G., and Burchiel, K. J. (2007). Safety of anterior commissure-posterior commissure-based target calculation of the subthalamic nucleus in functional stereotactic procedures. *Stereotact. Funct. Neurosurg.* 85, 287–291. doi: 10.1159/000107361

Auriat, A. M., Borich, M. R., Snow, N. J., Wadden, K. P., and Boyd, L. A. (2015). Comparing a diffusion tensor and non-tensor approach to white matter fiber tractography in chronic stroke. *Neuroimage Clin.* 7, 771–778. doi: 10.1016/j.nicl.2015.03.007

Balachandran, R., Mitchell, J. E., Dawant, B. M., and Fitzpatrick, J. M. (2009). Accuracy evaluation of microTargeting Platforms for deep-brain stimulation using virtual targets. *IEEE Trans. Biomed. Eng.* 56, 37–44. doi: 10.1109/TBME.2008.2002110

Bennet, K. E., Tomshine, J. R., Min, H. K., Manciu, F. S., Marsh, M. P., Paek, S. B., et al. (2016). A diamond-based electrode for detection of neurochemicals in the human brain. *Front. Hum. Neurosci.* 10:102. doi: 10.3389/fnhum.2016.00102

Beriault, S., Xiao, Y., Bailey, L., Collins, D. L., Sadikot, A. F., and Pike, G. B. (2012). Towards computer-assisted deep brain stimulation targeting with multiple active contacts. *Med. Image Comput. Comput. Assist. Interv.* 15, 487–494. doi: 10.1007/978-3-642-33415-3_60

Bewernick, B. H., Kayser, S., Sturm, V., and Schlaepfer, T. E. (2012). Long-term effects of nucleus accumbens deep brain stimulation in treatment-resistant depression: evidence for sustained efficacy. *Neuropsychopharmacology* 37, 1975–1985. doi: 10.1038/npp.2012.44

Bjarkam, C. R., Cancian, G., Glud, A. N., Ettrup, K. S., Jørgensen, R. L., and Sørensen, J. C. (2009). MRI-guided stereotaxic targeting in pigs based on a stereotaxic localizer box fitted with an isocentric frame and use of SurgiPlan computer-planning software. *J. Neurosci. Methods* 183, 119–126. doi: 10.1016/j.jneumeth.2009.06.019

Blomstedt, P., Hariz, G. M., Hariz, M. I., and Koskinen, L. O. (2007). Thalamic deep brain stimulation in the treatment of essential tremor: a long-term follow-up. *Br. J. Neurosurg.* 21, 504–509. doi: 10.1080/02688690701552278

Boccard, S. G., Fernandes, H. M., Jbabdi, S., Van Hartevelt, T. J., Kringelbach, M. L., Quaghebeur, G., et al. (2016). Tractography study of deep brain stimulation of the anterior cingulate cortex in chronic pain: key to improve the targeting. *World Neurosurg.* 86, 361.e3–370.e3. doi: 10.1016/j.wneu.2015.08.065

Bour, L. J., Lourens, M. A., Verhagen, R., de Bie, R. M., van den Munckhof, P., Schuurman, P. R., et al. (2015). *Brain Stimul.* 8, 730–741. doi: 10.1016/j.brs.2015.02.002

Burchiel, K., Anderson, V. C., Favre, J., and Hammerstad, J. P. (1999). Comparison of pallidal and subthalamic nucleus deep brain stimulation for advanced Parkinson's disease: results of a randomized, blinded pilot study. *Neurosurgery* 45, 1375–1382; discussion 1382–1384. doi: 10.1097/00006123-199912000-00024

Butson, C. R., Cooper, S. E., Henderson, J. M., Wolgamuth, B., and McIntyre, C. C. (2011). Probabilistic analysis of activation volumes generated during deep brain stimulation. *Neuroimage* 54, 2096–2104. doi: 10.1016/j.neuroimage.2010.10.059

Butson, C. R., and McIntyre, C. C. (2005). Tissue and electrode capacitance reduce neural activation volumes during deep brain stimulation. *Clin. Neurophysiol.* 116, 2490–2500. doi: 10.1016/j.clinph.2005.06.023

Butson, C. R., and Mcintyre, C. C. (2006). Role of electrode design on the volume of tissue activated during deep brain stimulation. *J. Neural. Eng.* 3, 1–8. doi: 10.1088/1741-2560/3/1/001

Butson, C. R., and McIntyre, C. C. (2008). Current Steering to control the volume of tissue activated during deep brain stimulation. *Brain Stimul.* 1, 7–15. doi: 10.1016/j.brs.2007.08.004

Castro, F. J., Pollo, C., Meuli, R., Maeder, P., Cuisenaire, O., Cuadra, M. B., et al. (2006). A cross validation study of deep brain stimulation targeting: from experts to atlas-based, segmentation-based and automatic registration algorithms. *IEEE Trans. Med. Imaging* 25, 1440–1450. doi: 10.1109/tmi.2006.882129

Chen, S. Y., Tsai, S. T., Hung, H. Y., Lin, S. H., Pan, Y. H., and Lin, S. Z. (2011). Targeting the subthalamic nucleus for deep brain stimulation–a comparative study between magnetic resonance images alone and fusion with computed tomographic images. *World Neurosurg.* 75, 132–137; discussion 122–134, 129–131. doi: 10.1016/j.wneu.2010.09.009

Cho, Z. H., Min, H. K., Oh, S. H., Han, J. Y., Park, C. W., and Lee, K. H. (2010). Direct visualization of deep brainstimulation targets in Parkinson disease with the use of 7-tesla magnetic resonance imaging. *J. Neurosurg.* 113, 639–647. doi: 10.3171/2010.3.JNS091385

Coenen, V. A., Allert, N., Paus, S., Kronenburger, M., Urbach, H., and Mädler, B. (2014). Modulation of the cerebello-thalamo-cortical network in thalamic deep brain stimulation for tremor: a diffusion tensor imaging study. *Neurosurgery* 75, 657–669; discussion 669–670. doi: 10.1227/NEU.0000000000000540

Coenen, V. A., Mädler, B., Schiffbauer, H., Urbach, H., and Allert, N. (2011a). Individual fiber anatomy of the subthalamic region revealed with diffusion tensor imaging: a concept to identify the deep brain stimulation target for tremor suppression. *Neurosurgery* 68, 1069–1075; discussion 1075–1066. doi: 10.1227/NEU.0b013e31820a1a20

Coenen, V. A., Schlaepfer, T. E., Maedler, B., and Panksepp, J. (2011b). Cross-species affective functions of the medial forebrain bundle-implications for the treatment of affective pain and depression in humans. *Neurosci. Biobehav. Rev.* 35, 1971–1981. doi: 10.1016/j.neubiorev.2010.12.009

Coenen, V. A., Schlaepfer, T. E., Allert, N., and Madler, B. (2012). Diffusion tensor imaging and neuromodulation: DTI as key technology for deep brain stimulation. *Int. Rev. Neurobiol.* 107, 207–234. doi: 10.1016/B978-0-12-404706-8.00011-5

Contarino, M. F., Bour, L. J., Verhagen, R., Lourens, M. A., de Bie, R. M., van den Munckhof, P., et al. (2014). Directional steering: a novel approach to deep brain stimulation. *Neurology* 83, 1163–1169. doi: 10.1212/WNL.0000000000000823

Deuschl, G., Schade-Brittinger, C., Krack, P., Volkmann, J., Schäfer, H., Bötzel, K., et al. (2006). A randomized trial of deep-brain stimulation for Parkinson's disease. *N. Engl. J. Med.* 355, 896–908. doi: 10.1056/NEJMoa060281

D'haese, P. F., Cetinkaya, E., Konrad, P. E., Kao, C., and Dawant, B. M. (2005). Computer-aided placement of deep brain stimulators: from planning to intraoperative guidance. *IEEE Trans. Med. Imaging* 24, 1469–1478. doi: 10.1109/tmi.2005.856752

Dougherty, D. D., Rezai, A. R., Carpenter, L. L., Howland, R. H., Bhati, M. T., O'Reardon, J. P., et al. (2015). A randomized sham-controlled trial of deep brain stimulation of the ventral capsule/ventral striatum for chronic treatment-resistant depression. *Biol. Psychiatry* 78, 240–248. doi: 10.1016/j.biopsych.2014.11.023

Duay, V., Bresson, X., Castro, J. S., Pollo, C., Cuadra, M. B., and Thiran, J. P. (2008). An active contour-based atlas registration model applied to automatic subthalamic nucleus targeting on MRI: method and validation. *Med. Image Comput. Comput. Assist. Interv.* 11, 980–988. doi: 10.1007/978-3-540-85990-1_118

Faria, A. V., Joel, S. E., Zhang, Y., Oishi, K., van Zjil, P. C., Miller, M. I., et al. (2012). Atlas-based analysis of resting-state functional connectivity: evaluation for reproducibility and multi-modal anatomy-function correlation studies. *Neuroimage* 61, 613–621. doi: 10.1016/j.neuroimage.2012.03.078

Fernandes, H. M., Van Hartevelt, T. J., Boccard, S. G. J., Owen, S. L. F., Cabral, J., Deco, G., et al. (2015). Novel fingerprinting method characterizes the necessary and sufficient structural connectivity from deep brain stimulation electrodes for a successful outcome. *New J. Phys.* 17:015001. doi: 10.1088/1367-2630/17/1/015001

Figee, M., Wielaard, I., Mazaheri, A., and Denys, D. (2013). Neurosurgical targets for compulsivity: what can we learn from acquired lesions? *Neurosci. Biobehav. Rev.* 37, 328–339. doi: 10.1016/j.neubiorev.2013.01.005

Fisher, R., Salanova, V., Witt, T., Worth, R., Henry, T., Gross, R., et al. (2010). Electrical stimulation of the anterior nucleus of thalamus for treatment of refractory epilepsy. *Epilepsia* 51, 899–908. doi: 10.1111/j.1528-1167.2010.02536.x

Follett, K. A., Weaver, F. M., Stern, M., Hur, K., Harris, C. L., Luo, P., et al. (2010). Pallidal versus subthalamic deep-brain stimulation for Parkinson's disease. *N. Engl. J. Med.* 362, 2077–2091. doi: 10.1056/NEJMoa0907083

Fox, M. D., Buckner, R. L., Liu, H., Chakravarty, M. M., Lozano, A. M., and Pascual-Leone, A. (2014). Resting-state networks link invasive and noninvasive brain stimulation across diverse psychiatric and neurological diseases. *Proc. Natl. Acad. Sci. U S A* 111, E4367–E4375. doi: 10.1073/pnas.1405003111

Fukaya, C., Sumi, K., Otaka, T., Obuchi, T., Kano, T., Kobayashi, K., et al. (2010). Nexframe frameless stereotaxy with multitract microrecording: accuracy evaluated by frame-based stereotactic X-ray. *Stereotact. Funct. Neurosurg.* 88, 163–168. doi: 10.1159/000313868

Galvan, A., Devergnas, A., and Wichmann, T. (2015). Alterations in neuronal activity in basal ganglia-thalamocortical circuits in the parkinsonian state. *Front. Neuroanat.* 9:5. doi: 10.3389/fnana.2015.00005

Grafton, S. T., Turner, R. S., Desmurget, M., Bakay, R., Delong, M., Vitek, J., et al. (2006). Normalizing motor-related brain activity: subthalamic nucleus stimulation in Parkinson disease. *Neurology* 66, 1192–1199. doi: 10.1212/01.wnl.0000214237.58321.c3

Grant, P. F., and Lowery, M. M. (2013). Simulation of cortico-basal ganglia oscillations and their suppression by closed loop deep brain stimulation. *IEEE Trans. Neural Syst. Rehabil. Eng.* 21, 584–594. doi: 10.1109/TNSRE.2012.2202403

Greenberg, B. D., Malone, D. A., Friehs, G. M., Rezai, A. R., Kubu, C. S., Malloy, P. F., et al. (2006). Three-year outcomes in deep brain stimulation for highly resistant obsessive-compulsive disorder. *Neuropsychopharmacology* 31, 2384–2393. doi: 10.1038/sj.npp.1301165

Guo, T., Parrent, A. G., and Peters, T. M. (2007). Surgical targeting accuracy analysis of six methods for subthalamic nucleus deep brain stimulation. *Comput. Aided Surg.* 12, 325–334. doi: 10.1080/10929080701730987

Gutman, D. A., Holtzheimer, P. E., Behrens, T. E. J., Johansen-Berg, H., and Mayberg, H. S. (2009). A tractography analysis of two deep brain stimulation white matter targets for depression. *Biol. Psychiatry* 65, 276–282. doi: 10.1016/j.biopsych.2008.09.021

Hahn, P. J., and McIntyre, C. C. (2010). Modeling shifts in the rate and pattern of subthalamopallidal network activity during deep brain stimulation. *J. Comput. Neurosci.* 28, 425–441. doi: 10.1007/s10827-010-0225-8

Hamani, C., McAndrews, M. P., Cohn, M., Oh, M., Zumsteg, D., Sharpiro, C. M., et al. (2007). Memory enhancement induced by hypothalamic/fornix deep brain stimulation. *Ann. Neurol.* 63, 119–123. doi: 10.1002/ana.21295

Hamani, C., Pilitsis, J., Rughani, A. I., Rosenow, J. M., Patil, P. G., Slavin, K. S., et al. (2014). Deep brain stimulation for obsessive-compulsive disorder: systematic review and evidence-based guideline sponsored by the American Society for Stereotactic and Functional Neurosurgery (ASSFN) and the Congress of Neurological Surgeons (CNS) and Endorsed by the CNS and American Association of Neurological Surgeons (AANS). *Neurosurgery* 75, 327–333. doi: 10.1227/NEU.0000000000000499

Hamel, W., Fietzek, U., Morsnowski, A., Schrader, B., Herzog, J., Weinert, D., et al. (2003). Deep brain stimulation of the subthalamic nucleus in Parkinson's disease: evaluation of active electrode contacts. *J. Neurol. Neurosurg. Psychiatry* 74, 1036–1046. doi: 10.1136/jnnp.74.8.1036

Hart, M. G., Ypma, R. J. F., Romero-Garcia, R., Price, S. J., and Suckling, J. (2016). Graph theory analysis of complex brain networks: new concepts in brain mapping applied to neurosurgery. *J. Neurosurg.* 124, 1665–1678. doi: 10.3171/2015.4.JNS142683

Hashimoto, T., Elder, C. M., Okun, M. S., Patrick, S. K., and Vitek, J. L. (2003). Stimulation of the subthalamic nucleus changes the firing pattern of pallidal neurons. *J. Neurosci.* 23, 1916–1923.

Henderson, J. M. (2012). "Connectomicsurgery": diffusion tensorimaging (DTI) tractography as a targeting modality for surgical modulation of neural networks. *Front. Integr. Neurosci.* 6:15. doi: 10.3389/fnint.2012.00015

Holtzheimer, P. E., Kelley, M. E., Gross, R. E., Filkowski, M. M., Garlow, S. J., Barrocas, A., et al. (2012). Subcallosal cingulate deep brain stimulation for treatment-resistant unipolar and bipolar depression. *Arch. Gen. Psychiatry* 69, 150–158. doi: 10.1001/archgenpsychiatry.2011.1456

Huff, W., Lenartz, D., Schormann, M., Lee, S. H., Kuhn, J., Koulousakis, A., et al. (2010). Unilateral deep brain stimulation of the nucleus accumbens in patients with treatment-resistant obsessive-compulsive disorder: outcomes after one year. *Clin. Neurol. Neurosurg.* 112, 137–143. doi: 10.1016/j.clineuro.2009.11.006

Humphries, M. D., and Gurney, K. (2012). Network effects of subthalamic deep brain stimulation drive a unique mixture of responses in basal ganglia output. *Eur. J. Neurosci.* 36, 2240–2251. doi: 10.1111/j.1460-9568.2012.08085.x

Hurtado, J. M., Gray, C. M., Tamas, L. B., and Sigvardt, K. A. (1999). Dynamics of tremor-related oscillations in the human globus pallidus: a single case study. *Proc. Natl. Acad. Sci. U S A* 96, 1674–1679. doi: 10.1073/pnas.96.4.1674

Joel, D., and Weiner, I. (1997). The connections of the primate subthalamic nucleus: indirect pathways and the open-interconnected scheme of basal ganglia-thalamocortical circuitry. *Brain Res. Brain Res. Rev.* 23, 62–78. doi: 10.1016/s0165-0173(96)00018-5

Johnson, M. D., Miocinovic, S., McIntyre, C. C., and Vitek, J. L. (2008). Mechanisms and targets of deep brain stimulation in movement disorders. *Neurotherapeutics* 5, 294–308. doi: 10.1016/j.nurt.2008.01.010

Kahan, J., Mancini, L., Urner, M., Friston, K., Hariz, M., Holl, E., et al. (2012). Therapeutic subthalamic nucleus deep brain stimulation reverses cortico-thalamic coupling during voluntary movements in Parkinson's disease. *Plos One* 7:e50270. doi: 10.1371/journal.pone.0050270

Kang, G., and Lowery, M. M. (2013). Interaction of oscillations and their suppression via deep brain stimulation, in a model of the cortico-basal ganglia network. *IEEE Trans. Neural Syst. Rehabil. Eng.* 21, 244–253. doi: 10.1109/TNSRE.2013.2241791

Kennedy, S. H., Giacobbe, P., Rizvi, S. J., Placenza, F. M., Nishikawa, Y., Mayberg, H. S., et al. (2011). Deep brain stimulation for treatment-resistant depression: follow-up after 3 to 6 years. *Am. J. Psychiatry* 168, 502–510. doi: 10.1176/appi.ajp.2010.10081187

Kern, D. S., and Kumar, R. (2007). Deep brain stimulation. *Neurologist* 13, 237–252. doi: 10.1097/NRL.0b013e3181492c48

Klein, J. C. (2013). "Diffusion imaging in tremor," in *Mechanisms and Emerging Therapies in Tremor Disorders*, eds G. Grimaldi and M. Manto (Springer New York, NY: Springer Science+Business Media New York), 391–401.

Klein, J. C., Barbe, M. T., Seifried, C., Baudrexel, S., Runge, M., Maarouf, M., et al. (2012). The tremor network targeted by successful VIM deep brain stimulation in humans. *Neurology* 78, 787–795. doi: 10.1212/WNL.0b013e318249f702

Klein, J. C., Lorenz, B., Kang, J. S., Baudrexel, S., Seifried, C., van de Loo, S., et al. (2011). Diffusion tensor imaging of white matter involvement in essential tremor. *Hum. Brain Mapp.* 32, 896–904. doi: 10.1002/hbm.21077

Kocabicak, E., Temel, Y., Höllig, A., Falkenburger, B., and Tan, S. K. H. (2015). Current perspectives on deep brain stimulation for severe neurological and psychiatric disorders. *Neuropsychiatr. Dis. Treat.* 11, 1051–1066. doi: 10.2147/NDT.s46583

Krack, P., Batir, A., Van Blercom, N., Chabardes, S., Fraix, V., Ardouin, C., et al. (2003). Five-year follow-up of bilateral stimulation of the subthalamic nucleus in advanced Parkinson's disease. *N. Engl. J. Med.* 349, 1925–1934. doi: 10.1056/nejmoa035275

Kringelbach, M. L., Jenkinson, N., Owen, S. L. F., and Aziz, T. Z. (2007). Translational principles of deep brain stimulation. *Nat. Rev. Neurosci.* 8, 623–635. doi: 10.1038/nrn2196

Kupsch, A., Benecke, R., Müller, J., Trottenberg, T., Schneider, G. H., Poewe, W., et al. (2006). Pallidal deep-brain stimulation in primary generalized or segmental dystonia. *N. Eng. J. Med.* 355, 1978–1990.

Kwon, H. G., Hong, J. H., Hong, C. P., Lee, D. H., Ahn, S. H., and Jang, S. H. (2011). Dentatorubrothalamic tract in human brain: diffusion tensor tractography study. *Neuroradiology* 53, 787–791. doi: 10.1007/s00234-011-0878-7

Lambert, C., Zrinzo, L., Nagy, Z., Lutti, A., Hariz, M., Foltynie, T., et al. (2012). Confirmation of functional zones within the human subthalamic nucleus: patterns of connectivity and sub-parcellation using diffusion weighted imaging. *Neuroimage* 60, 83–94. doi: 10.1016/j.neuroimage.2011.11.082

Laxton, A. W., Tang-Wai, D. F., McAndrews, M. P., Zumsteg, D., Wennberg, R., Keren, R., et al. (2010). A phase I trial of deep brain stimulation of memory circuits in Alzheimer's disease. *Ann. Neurol.* 68, 521–534. doi: 10.1002/ana.22089

Leksell, L. (1949). Stereotaxic apparatus for intra-cerebral surgery. *Acta Chir. Scand.* 99, 229–233.

Limousin, P., Krack, P., Pollak, P., Benazzouz, A., Ardouin, C., Hoffmann, D., et al. (1998). Electrical stimulation of the subthalamic nucleus in advanced Parkinson's disease. *N. Engl. J. Med.* 339, 1105–1111. doi: 10.1056/NEJM199810153391603

Lozano, A. M., Dostrovsky, J., Chen, R., and Ashby, P. (2002). Deep brain stimulation for Parkinson's disease: disrupting the disruption. *Lancet Neurol.* 1, 225–231. doi: 10.1016/s1474-4422(02)00101-1

Lozano, A. M., Mayberg, H. S., Giacobbe, P., Hamani, C., Craddock, R. C., and Kennedy, S. H. (2008). Subcallosal cingulate gyrus deep brain stimulation for treatment-resistant depression. *Biol. Psychiatry* 64, 461–467. doi: 10.1016/j.biopsych.2008.05.034

Lujan, J. L., Chaturvedi, A., Choi, K. S., Holtzheimer, P. E., Gross, R. E., Mayberg, H. S., et al. (2013). Tractography-activation models applied to subcallosal cingulate deep brain stimulation. *Brain Stimul.* 6, 737–739. doi: 10.1016/j.brs.2013.03.008

Maks, C. B., Butson, C. R., Walter, B. L., Vitek, J. L., and McIntyre, C. C. (2009). Deep brain stimulation activation volumes and their association with neurophysiological mapping and therapeutic outcomes. *J. Neurol. Neurosurg. Psychiatry* 80, 659–666. doi: 10.1136/jnnp.2007.126219

Mallet, L., Polosan, M., Jaafari, N., Baup, N., Welter, M. L., Fontaine, D., et al. (2008). Subthalamic nucleus stimulation in severe obsessive-compulsive disorder. *N. Engl. J. Med.* 359, 2121–2134. doi: 10.1056/NEJMoa0708514

Malone, D. A. Jr., Dougherty, D. D., Rezai, A. R., Carpenter, L. L., Friehs, G. M., Eskandar, E. N., et al. (2009). Deep brain stimulation of the ventral capsule/ventral striatum for treatment-resistant depression. *Biol. Psychiatry* 65, 267–275. doi: 10.1016/j.biopsych.2008.08.029

Mayberg, H. S. (1997). Limbic-cortical dysregulation: a proposed model of depression. *J. Neuropsychiatry Clin. Neurosci.* 9, 471–481. doi: 10.1176/jnp.9.3.471

Mayberg, H. S., Lozano, A. M., Voon, V., McNeely, H. E., Seminowicz, D., Hamani, C., et al. (2005). Deep brain stimulation for treatment-resistant depression. *Neuron* 45, 651–660. doi: 10.1016/j.neuron.2005.02.014

McIntyre, C. C., and Foutz, T. J. (2013). Computational modeling of deep brain stimulation. *Handb. Clin. Neurol.* 116, 55–61. doi: 10.1016/B978-0-444-53497-2.00005-X

McIntyre, C. C., Mori, S., Sherman, D. L., Thakor, N. V., and Viteck, J. L. (2004). Electric field stimulating influence generated by deep brain stimulation of the subthalamic nucleus. *Clin. Neurophysiol.* 115, 589–595. doi: 10.1016/j.clinph.2003.10.033

Meijer, H. G., Krupa, M., Cagnan, H., Lourens, M. A., Heida, T., Martens, H. C., et al. (2011). From Parkinsonian thalamic activity to restoring thalamic relay using deep brain stimulation: new insights from computational modeling. *J. Neural. Eng.* 8:066005. doi: 10.1088/1741-2560/8/6/066005

Mikos, A., Bowers, D., Noecker, A. M., Mcintyre, C. C., Won, M., Chaturvedi, A., et al. (2011). Patient-specific analysis of the relationship between the volume of tissue activated during DBS and verbal fluency. *Neuroimage* 54, S238–S246. doi: 10.1016/j.neuroimage.2010.03.068

Miller, J. P., Sweet, J. A., Bailey, C. M., Munyon, C. N., Luders, H. O., and Fastenau, P. S. (2015). Visual-spatial memory may be enhanced with theta burst deep brain stimulation of the fornix: a preliminary investigation with four cases. *Brain* 138, 1833–1842. doi: 10.1093/brain/awv095

Miocinovic, S., Parent, M., Butson, C. R., Hahn, P. J., Russo, G. S., Vitek, J. L., et al. (2006). Computational analysis of subthalamic nucleus and lenticular fasciculus activation during therapeutic deep brain stimulation. *J. Neurophysiol.* 96, 1569–1580. doi: 10.1152/jn.00305.2006

Nuttin, B., Cosyns, P., Demeulemeester, H., Gybels, J., and Meyerson, B. (1999). Electrical stimulation in anterior limbs of internal capsules in patients with obsessive-compulsive disorder. *Lancet* 354:1526. doi: 10.1016/s0140-6736(99)02376-4

Nuttin, B. J., Gabriels, L. A., Cosyns, P. R., Meyerson, B. A., Andreewitch, S., Sunaert, S. G., et al. (2003). Long-term electrical capsular stimulation in patients with obsessive-compulsive disorder. *Neurosurgery* 52, 1263–1272. doi: 10.1227/01.neu.0000064565.49299.9a

Ongur, D., Lundy, M., Greenhouse, I., Shinn, A. K., Menon, V., Cohen, B. M., et al. (2010). Default mode network abnormalities in bipolar disorder and schizophrenia. *Psychiatry Res.* 183, 59–68. doi: 10.1016/j.pscychresns.2010.04.008

Panov, F., Gologorsky, Y., Connors, G., Tagliati, M., Miravite, J., and Alterman, R. L. (2013). Deep brain stimulation in DYT1 dystonia: a 10-year experience. *Neurosurgery* 73, 86–93. doi: 10.1227/01.neu.0000429841.84083.c8

Quinn, E. J., Blumenfeld, Z., Velisar, A., Koop, M. M., Shreve, L. A., Trager, M. H., et al. (2015). Beta oscillations in freely moving Parkinson's subjects are attenuated during deep brain stimulation. *Mov. Disord.* 30, 1750–1758. doi: 10.1002/mds.26376

Rezai, A. R., Kopell, B. H., Gross, R. E., Vitek, J. L., Sharan, A. D., Limousin, P., et al. (2006). Deep brain stimulation for Parkinson's disease: surgical issues. *Mov. Disord.* 21, S197–S218. doi: 10.1002/mds.20956

Robinson, R. A., Taghva, A., Liu, C. Y., and Apuzzo, M. L. (2013). Surgery of the mind, mood and consciousnes: an idea in evolution. *World Neurosurg.* 80, S2–S26. doi: 10.1016/j.wneu.2013.08.002

Rubin, J. E., and Terman, D. (2004). High frequency stimulation of the subthalamic nucleus eliminates pathological thalamic rhythmicity in a computaional model. *J. Comput. Neurosci.* 16, 211–235. doi: 10.1023/b:jcns.0000025686.47117.67

Sankar, T., Lipsman, N., and Lozano, A. M. (2014). Deep brain stimulation for disorders of memory and cognition. *Neurotherapeutics* 11, 527–534. doi: 10.1007/s13311-014-0275-0

Schiefer, T. K., Matsumoto, J. Y., and Lee, K. H. (2011). Moving forward: advances in the treatment of movement disorders with deep brain stimulation. *Front. Integr. Neurosci.* 5:69. doi: 10.3389/fnint.2011.00069

Schlaier, J., Anthofer, J., Steib, K., Fellner, C., Rothenfusser, E., Brawanski, A., et al. (2015). Deep brain stimulation for essential tremor: targeting the dentato-rubro-thalamic tract? *Neuromodulation* 18, 105–112. doi: 10.1111/ner.12238

Schuurman, P. R., Bosch, D. A., Bossuyt, P. M., Bonsel, G. J., van Someren, E. J., de Bie, R. M., et al. (2000). A comparison of continuous thalamic stimulation and thalamotomy for suppression of severe tremor. *N. Engl. J. Med.* 342, 461–468. doi: 10.1056/nejm200002173420703

Sturm, V., Lenartz, D., Koulousakis, A., Treuer, H., Herholz, K., Klein, J. C., et al. (2003). The nucleus accumbens: a target for deep brain stimulation in obsessive-compulsive- and anxiety-disorders. *J. Chem. Neuroanat.* 26, 293–299. doi: 10.1016/j.jchemneu.2003.09.003

Suthana, N., Haneef, Z., Stern, J., Mukamel, R., Behnke, E., Knowlton, B., et al. (2012). Memory enhancement and deep-brain stimulation of the entorhinal area. *N. Engl. J. Med.* 366, 502–510. doi: 10.1056/NEJMoa1107212

Sweet, J. A., Walter, B. L., Gunalan, K., Chaturvedi, A., Mcintyre, C. C., and Miller, J. P. (2014a). Fiber tractography of the axonal pathways linking the basal ganglia and cerebellum in Parkinson disease: implications for targeting in deep brain stimulation. *J. Neurosurg.* 120, 988–996. doi: 10.3171/2013.12.jns131537

Sweet, J. A., Walter, B. L., Munyon, C., and Miller, J. P. (2014b). Multi-tract orthogonal microelectrode localization of the subthalamic nucleus: description of a novel technique. *Neurosurgery* 2, 240–245. doi: 10.1227/neu.0000000000000295

Tewari, A., Jog, R., and Jog, M. S. (2016). The striatum and subthalamic nucleus as independent and collaborative structures in motor control. *Front. Syst. Neurosci.* 10:17. doi: 10.3389/fnsys.2016.00017

Timmerman, L., Jain, R., Chen, L., Maarouf, M., Barbe, M. T., Allert, N., et al. (2015). Multiple-source current steering in subthalamic nucleus deep brain stimulation for Parkinson's disease (the VANTAGE study): a non-randomised, prospective, multicentre, open-label study. *Lancet Neurol.* 14, 693–701. doi: 10.1016/S1474-4422(15)00087-3

Van Dijk, K. J., Verhagen, R., Chaturvedi, A., McIntyre, C. C., Bour, L. J., Heida, C., et al. (2015). A novel lead design enables selective deep brain stimulation of neural populations in the subthalamic region. *J. Neural. Eng.* 12:046003. doi: 10.1088/1741-2560/12/4/046003

Van Hartevelt, T. J., Cabral, J., Moller, A., FitzGerald, J. J., Green, A. L., Aziz, T. Z., et al. (2015). Evidence from a rare case study for Hebbian-like changes in structural connectivity induced by long-term deep brain stimulation. *Front. Behav. Neurosci.* 9:167. doi: 10.3389/fnbeh.2015.00167

Vanegas-Arroyave, N., Lauro, P. M., Huang, L., Hallett, M., Horovitz, S. G., Zaghloul, K. A., et al. (2016). Tractography patterns of subthalamic nucleus deep brain stimulation. *Brain.* 139, 1200–1210. doi: 10.1093/brain/aww020

Vidailhet, M., Vercueil, L., Houeto, J. L., Krystkowiak, P., Benabid, A. L., Cornu, P., et al. (2005). Bilateral deep-brain stimulation of the globus pallidus in primary generalized dystonia. *N. Engl. J. Med.* 352, 459–467. doi: 10.1056/nejmoa042187

Vidailhet, M., Vercueil, L., Houeto, J. L., Krystkowiak, P., Lagrange, C., Yelnik, J., et al. (2007). Bilateral, pallidal, deep-brain stimulation in primary generalised dystonia: a prospective 3 years follow-up study. *Lancet Neurol.* 6, 223–229. doi: 10.1016/s1474-4422(07)70035-2

Volkmann, J., Allert, N., Voges, J., Weiss, P. H., Freund, H. J., and Sturm, V. (2001). Safety and efficacy of pallidal or subthalamic nucleus stimulation in advanced PD. *Neurology* 56, 548–551. doi: 10.1212/wnl.56.4.548

Volkmann, J., Wolters, A., Kupsch, A., Müller, J., Kühn, A. A., Schneider, G. H., et al. (2012). Pallidal deep brain stimulation in patients with primary generalised or segmental dystonia: 5-year follow-up of a randomised trial. *Lancet Neurol.* 11, 1029–1038. doi: 10.1016/S1474-4422(12)70257-0

Walter, B. L., and Vitek, J. L. (2004). Surgical treatment for Parkinson's disease. *Lancet Neurol.* 3, 719–728. doi: 10.1016/S1474-4422(04)00934-2

Williams, A., Gill, S., Varma, T., Jenkinson, C., Quinn, N., Mitchell, R., et al. (2010). Deep brain stimulation plus best medical therapy versus best medical therapy alone for advanced Parkinson's disease (PD SURG trial): a randomised, open-label trial. *Lancet Neurol.* 9, 581–591. doi: 10.1016/s1474-4422(10)70093-4

Willsie, A. C., and Dorval, A. D. (2015). Computational field shaping for deep brain stimulation with thousands of contacts in a novel electrode geometry. *Neuromodulation* 18, 542–550; discussion 550–551. doi: 10.1111/ner.12330

16

In vivo Exploration of the Connectivity between the Subthalamic Nucleus and the Globus Pallidus in the Human Brain using Multi-Fiber Tractography

Sonia Pujol[1]*, Ryan Cabeen[2], Sophie B. Sébille[3], Jérôme Yelnik[3], Chantal François[3], Sara Fernandez Vidal[3,4], Carine Karachi[3,5], Yulong Zhao[6], G. Rees Cosgrove[7], Pierre Jannin[6], Ron Kikinis[1] and Eric Bardinet[3,4]

[1] Surgical Planning Laboratory, Department of Radiology, Brigham and Women's Hospital, Harvard Medical School, Boston, MA, USA, [2] Department of Computer Science, Brown University, Providence, RI, USA, [3] Institut du Cerveau et de la Moëlle Epinière, INSERM U 1127, CNRS UMR 7225, Sorbonne Universités, University of Paris 06, UMR S 1127, Paris, France, [4] Centre de Neuro-Imagerie de Recherche, Institut du Cerveau et de la Moëlle Epinière, Paris, France, [5] Department of Neurosurgery, Pitié-Salpêtrière Hospital, Paris, France, [6] LTSI, Inserm UMR 1099 – Université de Rennes, Rennes, France, [7] Department of Neurosurgery, Brigham and Women's Hospital, Harvard Medical School, Boston, MA, USA

***Correspondence:**
Sonia Pujol
spujol@bwh.harvard.edu

The basal ganglia is part of a complex system of neuronal circuits that play a key role in the integration and execution of motor, cognitive and emotional function in the human brain. Parkinson's disease is a progressive neurological disorder of the motor circuit characterized by tremor, rigidity, and slowness of movement. Deep brain stimulation (DBS) of the subthalamic nucleus and the globus pallidus pars interna provides an efficient treatment to reduce symptoms and levodopa-induced side effects in Parkinson's disease patients. While the underlying mechanism of action of DBS is still unknown, the potential modulation of white matter tracts connecting the surgical targets has become an active area of research. With the introduction of advanced diffusion MRI acquisition sequences and sophisticated post-processing techniques, the architecture of the human brain white matter can be explored *in vivo*. The goal of this study is to investigate the white matter connectivity between the subthalamic nucleus and the globus pallidus. Two multi-fiber tractography methods were used to reconstruct pallido-subthalamic, subthalamo-pallidal and pyramidal fibers in five healthy subjects datasets of the Human Connectome Project. The anatomical accuracy of the tracts was assessed by four judges with expertise in neuroanatomy, functional neurosurgery, and diffusion MRI. The variability among subjects was evaluated based on the fractional anisotropy and mean diffusivity of the tracts. Both multi-fiber approaches enabled the detection of complex fiber architecture in the basal ganglia. The qualitative evaluation by experts showed that the identified tracts were in agreement with the expected anatomy. Tract-derived measurements demonstrated relatively low variability among subjects. False-negative tracts demonstrated the current limitations of both methods for clinical decision-making. Multi-fiber tractography methods combined with state-of-the-art diffusion MRI data have the potential to help identify white matter tracts connecting DBS targets in functional neurosurgery intervention.

Keywords: diffusion MRI, subthalamic nucleus, globus pallidus, multi-fiber tractography, deep brain stimulation, human neuroanatomy

INTRODUCTION

Deep brain stimulation (DBS) is an efficient neurosurgical treatment to alleviate motor symptoms, levodopa-induced motor fluctuations, and dyskinesia in Parkinson's disease patients (Benabid et al., 1987; Krack and Hariz, 2013). The subthalamic nucleus (STN) and globus pallidus pars interna (GPi) have been established as effective targets (Wagle Shukla and Okun, 2014; Fasano and Lozano, 2015). Both nuclei are components of a large segregated cortical-subcortical network and DBS is likely to activate white matter fiber tracts connecting the targeted regions (Ashby et al., 1999; Gradinaru et al., 2009). As Parkinson's disease is increasingly being viewed as a circuit disorder (DeLong and Wichmann, 2007; Lanciego et al., 2012), recent studies have investigated the changes in neural activity induced by DBS in the diseased circuits (McIntyre and Hahn, 2010). The white matter pathways that connect the STN and the globus pallidus (GP) include two sets of fibers: inhibitory pallido-subthalamic fibers that project from the globus pallidus pars externa (GPe) to the STN and excitatory subthalamo-pallidal fibers that project from the STN to the GPi and the GPe (Parent, 1995; Hamani et al., 2004). Tract tracing studies using invasive markers have been used in animal experiments to map the circuitry of these fibers (Shrink et al., 1996). In non-human primates, the pallido-subthalamic pathway presents with a complex topographical organization, with the pallidal input from the GPe extending over the entire rostrolateral two-thirds of the STN (Parent and Hzrati, 1995). Subthalamic neurons projecting to the GPe are predominantly located in the dorsolateral two-thirds of the STN whereas neurons projecting to the GPi are confined to the ventromedial third of the nucleus (Parent and Hzrati, 1995; Alkemade et al., 2015). Experimental studies in monkeys have demonstrated the subdivision of the basal ganglia into three functional motor, limbic and associative territories arising from the cerebral cortex (Haber et al., 1993; François et al., 1994; Karachi et al., 2005; Haynes and Haber, 2013). However, such studies cannot be reproduced in living humans. Magnetic resonance imaging (MRI) enables non-invasive exploration of the basal ganglia, and plays a critical role in the planning and execution of DBS (Dormont et al., 2010; De Celis Alonso et al., 2015). In the past decades, the introduction of diffusion MRI (dMRI) and subsequent development of tractography techniques have opened up the possibility to map the architecture of the brain white matter *in vivo* (Le Bihan et al., 1986; Basser et al., 1994; Pierpaoli and Basser, 1996; Mori et al., 1999). The analysis and interpretation of dMRI data using tractography tools have the potential to bring clinically relevant information for the planning and execution of DBS intervention (Henderson, 2012; Torres et al., 2014; Calabrese, 2016). In recent years, exploratory studies on the use of diffusion tensor imaging based on the single tensor model of diffusion for investigating white matter fibers connecting DBS targets have demonstrated promising findings (Barkhoudarian et al., 2010; Lemaire et al., 2011; Coenen et al., 2014; Rozanski et al., 2014; Sweet et al., 2014; Avecillas-Chasin et al., 2016; Vanegas-Arroyave et al., 2016). However, the tensor model can only identify a single fiber population within a voxel (Alexander et al., 2007). High angular resolution diffusion imaging (HARDI) acquisition sequences combined with sophisticated diffusion modeling approaches have been introduced to enable detection of multiple fiber orientations in complex neuroanatomical regions (Alexander, 2005). Such advanced techniques have been used for mapping white matter connections in the basal ganglia using dMRI data acquired on 7.0 Tesla scanners on healthy subjects and post-mortem specimens (Lenglet et al., 2012; Plantinga et al., 2014). While 7.0 Tesla scanners provide greater contrast than 3.0 Tesla scanners, such high-field MR scanners are not yet part of clinical routine. Through the Human Connectome Project (HCP) funded by the U.S. National Institutes of Health, cutting-edge neuroimaging data acquired on healthy young adults have been made publicly available to the scientific community. The HCP dMRI datatests include HARDI multi-shell data acquired on 3.0 Tesla scanners with customized coils and advanced dMRI acquisition sequences (David et al., 2013). Recent studies on HCP dMRI data have demonstrated the possibility to reconstruct the anatomical connectivity of complex pathways such as the orbitofrontothalamic fibers of passage using multi-fiber diffusion models (Makris et al., 2015). In this paper, we propose to investigate the connectivity between the subthalamic nucleus and the globus pallidus using two multi-fiber tractography approaches on five HCP subjects.

MATERIALS AND METHODS

Anatomical Objective

Our study focused on the white matter anatomical connectivity between the STN and the GP. Fibers interconnecting these two regions consist of subthalamo-pallidal projections from the STN to the GPi and the GPe, and pallido-subthalamic projections from the GPe to the STN (Hamani et al., 2004). As these fibers cross the

Abbreviations: DBS, deep brain stimulation; dMRI, diffusion MRI; GP, globus pallidus; GPe, globus pallidus pars externa; GPi, globus pallidus pars interna; HCP, Human Connectome Project; MC, multi-compartment; MSMT-CSD, multi-shell multi-tissue constrained spherical deconvolution; PD, Parkinson's disease; ROI, region of interest; STN, subthalamic nucleus.

internal capsule in their trajectory, we included the tractography reconstruction of the pyramidal pathway.

MRI Data Acquisition

We used the structural and dMRI datasets from five healthy subjects of the Human Connectome Project (**Table 1**). The data were acquired by the Washington University, University of Minnesota, and Oxford University (WU-Minn) HCP Consortium (Van Essen et al., 2013). All HCP subjects were scanned on the Connectome Skyra, which is a customized Siemens 3.0 Tesla Skyra scanner using a 32-channel head coil and a customized gradient set. The structural scans included T1-weighted and T2-weighted data that were acquired with the following parameters: T1-weighted: TE = 2.14 ms, TR = 2,400 ms, voxel size = 0.7 mm; T2-weighted: TE = 565 ms, TR = 3,200 ms, voxel size = 0.7 mm. The diffusion-weighted scans were acquired using a single-shot 2D spin-echo multiband Echo Planar Imaging (EPI) sequence. Each dMRI dataset consisted of 270 diffusion weighted images distributed equally over 3 shells defined with b-values of 1,000 s/mm^2, 2,000 s/mm^2, and 3,000 s/mm^2, and nominal voxel size of 1.25 mm isotropic (Sotiropoulos et al., 2013; Uğurbil et al., 2013). All five HCP diffusion-weighted imaging datasets used in this study had been pre-processed for intensity normalization, eddy-current, patient-motion and EPI distortion correction and co-registered to the anatomical scans (Glasser et al., 2013; Andersson and Sotiropoulos, 2015a,b).

TABLE 1 | HCP subjects.

Subject	HCP Id	Age range	Sex
1	100307	26–30	Female
2	100408	31–35	Male
3	101915	31–35	Female
4	103414	22–25	Female
5	106016	31–35	Female

The table presents the characteristics of the five healthy subjects of the Human Connectome Project that were used in the study.

MRI Data Post-processing

The tractography pipeline for the reconstruction of the targeted fascicles consisted of three steps: first, the segmentation of anatomical regions of interest, second the estimation of models based on the diffusion signal at each voxel, and third, the reconstruction and selection of the tracts.

Segmentation of Regions of Interest

We defined two sets of anatomical regions-of-interest (ROIs) on the T1-weighted images for tractography purpose. A first set of ROIs for the reconstruction of the subthalamo-pallidal and pallido-subthalamic fibers was defined in the STN, GPe, and GPi. A second set of ROIs for the pyramidal tract was defined in the primary motor cortex, internal capsule and cerebral peduncles. Both sets of ROIs were generated within the 3D Slicer open-source platform for medical research (Fedorov et al., 2012). In the first set of ROIs, as the contours of the STN, GPe, and GPi were not directly visible in the T1-weighted images, we used an automated atlas-based segmentation approach implemented in the pyDBS software (D'Albis et al., 2015) (**Figure 1**). The method uses the Yeb Atlas, a unique 3D histological and deformable atlas of the basal ganglia that comprises 3D meshes of 80 structures identified on histological stainings from a post-mortem specimen (Yelnik et al., 2007). For each subject, 3D meshes of the STN, GPe, and GPi were generated from the T1-weighted images by deforming the Yeb Atlas using a global-to-local registration approach (Bardinet et al., 2009). The meshes were then voxelized in 3D Slicer to create ROIs with 0.3 mm voxel size for the tractography algorithms. In addition, the contours of the GPe and GPi were manually edited to integrate the anatomical information contained in the dMRI data. The meshes of the edited structures were then re-generated from the edited labelmaps using the Marching Cubes algorithm (Lorensen and Cline, 1987). In the second set of ROIs, the primary motor cortex was annotated by positioning fiducials in the pre-central gyrus of a volume-rendered image of the T1-weighted scan. The cerebral peduncles and posterior limb of the internal capsule were manually segmented in axial cross-sections of the directionally encoded color map derived from the diffusion-weighted images in 3D Slicer.

Multi-Fiber Models

We used two different multi-fiber approaches to estimate the orientation of white matter fibers from the diffusion-weighted signal arising at each voxel: a multi-compartment (MC) model and a multi-shell multi-tissue constrained spherical deconvolution (MSMT-CSD) method.

The MC approach uses the ball-and-stick model to represent the diffusion-weighted signal as arising from a sum of multiple anisotropic components, a single isotropic diffusion compartment and volume fractions thereof (Behrens et al., 2007). We fitted the ball-and-stick model to the dMRI data using a using a Bayesian estimation procedure implemented in FSL XFibres (Jenkinson et al., 2012). Parameter settings included the continuous exponential approach for multi-shell data and a maximum of three fiber compartments per voxel. **Figure 2A** shows an example of 3D visualization of the principal directions of diffusion at each voxel identified using the MC method.

The MSMT-CSD method uses a continuous distribution of fiber orientations at each voxel. In this approach, the diffusion-weighted signal arising from different fibers population is represented as an integral over the distribution of fiber orientations, and therefore can be expressed as the spherical convolution of the fiber Orientation Distribution Function (fODF) and the diffusion-weighted signal profile from a single fiber orientation (Tournier et al., 2004). We estimated the fODF at each voxel with a maximum of eight spherical harmonics using the MSMT-CSD algorithm implemented in the Mrtrix software (Jeurissen et al., 2014). **Figure 2B** shows an example of 3D visualization of the principal directions of diffusion at each voxel identified using the MSMT-CSD approach.

Fiber Tracking Algorithms

For the MC approach, deterministic tractography was performed using a fiber tracking method similar to the eXTended multi-fiber streamline tractography approach (Qazi et al., 2009), which

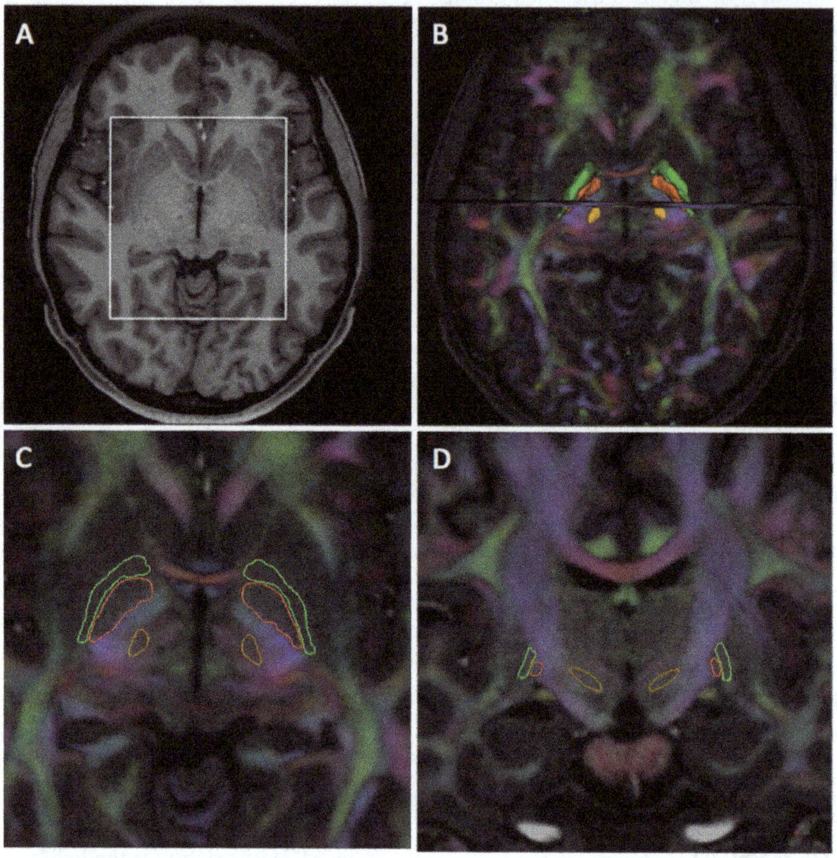

FIGURE 1 | Segmentation of the STN, GPi, and GPe in HCP subject 100307. (A) Axial T1-weighted image. **(B)** 3D superior view of surface models of the STN (light orange), GPi (dark orange), GPe (green) with axial and coronal T1-weighted images overlaid on directionally encoded color (DEC) map. **(C)** Axial T1-weighted image overlaid on DEC map with outlined contours of the STN, GPi, and GPe. **(D)** Coronal T1-weighted image overlaid on DEC map with outlined contours of the STN, GPi, and GPe. The view presented in **(C)** corresponds to the ROI (white square) defined in **(A)**. The view presented in **(D)** corresponds to the coronal image displayed in **(B)**.

consisted of a custom implementation used in combination with a model-based estimation framework for interpolation (Cabeen et al., 2013). The fiber tracking algorithm used a step size of 0.5 mm and 25 seeds per voxel, which were placed in a one-voxel neighborhood surrounding each ROI. The ball-and-stick diffusion models were interpolated using a data-adaptative kernel regression framework (Cabeen et al., 2013, 2016). The framework used clustering-based optimization and two parameters: spatial bandwidth, which controls the smoothness of the interpolation, and model selection, which controls the number of estimated compartments. In this study, we used a spatial bandwidth of 1.0 mm and model selection parameter $\lambda = 0.9999$, corresponding to up to three fiber compartments. Tracking was terminated upon reaching a target ROI, when the angle changed more than 55°, or when a compartment's volume fraction dropped below 0.05.

For the MSMT-CSD approach, whole brain probabilistic anatomically constrained tractography (Smith et al., 2012) was performed with the following parameters: 10 millions tracts, step length, 0.625 mm; curvature threshold, 45°; minimum tract length, 10 mm; maximum tract length, 250 mm; and fiber orientation distribution amplitude cut-off, 0.1. The spherical-deconvolution informed filtering of tractograms (SIFT) was applied to reduce the number of streamlines to five millions to provide a biologically meaningful estimate of structural connection density by removing false positive tracts (Smith et al., 2013). The tracts of interest in the resulting whole-brain tractogram were isolated using MrTrix.

In the rest of the paper, we designate the MC deterministic tractography approach as MC-det and the MSMT-CSD probabilistic approach as CSD-prob.

Tract Selection Strategy

The following section describes the tract selection strategy chosen for the MC-det and CSD-prob methods. In the MC-det approach, tractography seeds for the STN-GPi pathway were placed in one voxel shells surrounding both STN and GPi ROIs, and tracks were terminated with reaching either ROI. For the STN-GPe pathway, tractography seeds were placed in one voxel shells surrounding both STN and GPe ROIs, tracks were allowed to pass through the GPi and were terminated with reaching either the STN or the GPe ROI. For the pyramidal tract, tractography was

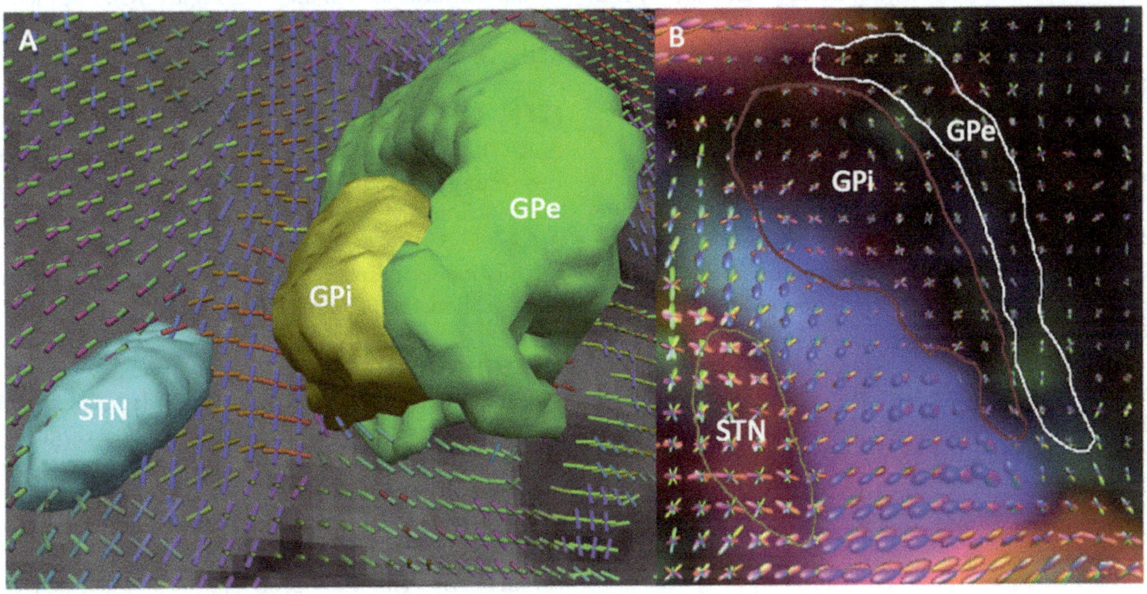

FIGURE 2 | 3D visualization of the principal directions of diffusion computed by the MC and MSMT-CSD diffusion models in HCP subject 100307. **(A)** MC model. The figure shows a 3D coronal view of the ball-and-stick glyphs representing the two principal directions of diffusion at each voxel. The glyphs are overlaid on a coronal T1-weighted image with 3D models of the STN (cyan), GPi (yellow), and GPe (green). **(B)** MSMT-CSD model. The figure shows a 3D superior view of the spherical harmonics glyphs representing the principal directions of diffusion. The glyphs are overlaid on a DEC map with contours of the STN (yellow), GPi (dark brown), and GPe (white).

seeded in three ROIs: white matter neighboring the precentral gyrus, the posterior limb of the internal capsule, and cerebral peduncle. Pyramidal fibers were retained only if they intersected all three ROIs and did not intersect either the GPi or GPe ROIs. The reconstructed tracts were visualized as streamlines with 3D Slicer.

In the CSD-prob approach, after whole brain tractography reconstruction, fibers passing through the STN, GPi, and GPe were selected for STN-GPi pathway, and fibers passing through the STN and GPe were selected for the STN-GPe pathway. Fibers passing through the motor cortex, the posterior limb of the internal capsule and the cerebral peduncles were selected for the pyramidal tract. Tract density maps (TDMs) were then calculated for all reconstructed pathways (Calamante et al., 2010), and the tracts were visualized as volume-rendered TDM images using the GPU-based volume rendering functionality of 3D Slicer.

Evaluation of the Tractography Reconstructions

Evaluation by Anatomical Experts

The qualitative evaluation of the anatomical accuracy of the tracts was performed by four experts in human neuroanatomy that include two neuroanatomists, a neurosurgeon and a neuroradiologist. For each subject, subthalamo-pallidal, pallido-subthalamic, and pyramidal tracts reconstructed using the MC-det and the CSD-prob methods were loaded into the 3D Slicer platform, along with the 3D models of the subthalamic nucleus and globus pallidus. The tracts and 3D models were overlaid on T1-weighted images, T2-weighted images and directionally encoded color maps. The experts reviewed the reconstructed white matter tracts using the interactive 3D visualization functionalities of the software. Each reviewer could adjust the transparency of the tracts and models, select which tract to view and which to hide, zoom in and out, and rotate the tracts to best demonstrate anatomical relationships between the different structures. The evaluation of the tracts was performed using four criteria: the topographical localization of each tract; the starting and ending regions of the fascicles; the specific shape of the fascicles, e.g., fanning shape of the pyramidal pathway from the cortex to the internal capsule; the relationships between the different bundles, e.g., comb organization of the subthalamic fasciculus and pyramidal tract. These criteria were used to evaluate the anatomical accuracy of the tracts based on the similarity between the tractography reconstructions and known neuroanatomy. The experts assigned a score ranging from 5 (excellent) to 1 (poor) averaged on the criteria used for the review of each fascicle.

Tract-Derived Measurements

In order to assess the variability among subjects, we calculated the fractional anisotropy (FA) and mean diffusivity (MD) of the envelope of the tracts reconstructed by both methods. For the MC-det method, the envelopes of the tracts were generated by converting the streamlines into voxelwise binary labelmaps, with label = 1 when a tract had been detected and label = 0 when no tract was detected. For the CSD-prob method, the TDM volumes were thresholded to remove voxels with probability values lower than 0.05 and the resulting maps were converted into binary labelmaps. For each subject, we calculated the FA and MD volumes from the dMRI data using the 3D Slicer software, and we computed the mean and standard deviation of the FA and MD values inside the envelopes of the MCM-det and CSD-prob tracts.

Statistical Analysis

We performed a statistical analysis of the scores given by the judges and the tract-derived measurements. For each tract, we calculated the mean and standard deviation of the average scores given by the four judges for the MC-det and CSD-prob methods to estimate the variability in the anatomical accuracy of the reconstructed tracts across subjects. In order to assess the level of agreement among the four judges, we computed the intraclass correlation coefficient (ICC) of the scores for each tractography method. In addition, we characterized the distribution of FA and MD values for each tract using box plots to evaluate the variability of tract-derived metrics among subjects.

RESULTS

The subthalamo-pallidal, pallido-subthalamic, and pyramidal tract were successfully identified on all five subjects using the MC-det and CSD-prob methods. **Figures 3**, **4**, and **5** show individual tractography reconstructions of the three pathways in a single subject. **Figure 5** shows the crossings of the pyramidal tract with subthalamo-pallidal and pallido-subthalamic tracts. **Figure 6** shows combined MC-det and CSD-prob tractography reconstruction of the subthalamo-pallidal and pallido-subthalamic tracts in three subjects, and illustrates the agreement between methods. Overall, the neuroanatomists rated the reconstructed tracts as consistent with the expected anatomy. **Table 2** presents the results of the qualitative evaluation of the tracts. The average and standard deviation of the scores for the STN-GPe, STN-GPi, and PT were 3.3 ± 0.2, 3.7 ± 0.3, and 3.5 ± 0.2, respectively. In addition, the calculation of the ICC showed a good agreement among judges for both tractography methods: the ICC for the MCM-Det method was 0.70 with 95% confidence interval of (0.39–0.97) and the ICC for the CSD-det methods was 0.79 with 95% confidence interval of (0.51–0.98). **Figure 7** shows the box plots of the tract-derived measurements computed for each tract and each method. Results show a relatively low variability of FA and MD values among subjects, and similar distributions of FA and MD values between methods.

STN-GPE Connections

In both the MC-det and CSD-prob methods, the majority of fibers interconnecting the STN and the GPe crossed the anterior two-thirds of the posterior limb of the internal capsule. This finding is in agreement with the presence of the descending pyramidal tract in the remaining third of the posterior limb. Most fibers reconstructed using the MC-det method emerged from the mediodorsal part of the GPe, while the central and ventral parts presented less fibers (**Figure 3A**). Fibers reconstructed using the CSD-prob connected the STN to both the mediodorsal and medioventral aspects of the GPe (**Figure 3C**). The method did not identify fibers on the upper most part of the mediodorsal aspect of the GPe.

STN-GPi Connections

Both the MC-det and CSD-prob methods identified tracts connecting the STN to the GPi. Most of the tracts arose from the ventromedial aspect of the STN (**Figures 3B,D**). The MC-det method detected a smaller number of tracts arising from the mediodorsal aspect of the STN (**Figure 3B**) compared to the CSD-prob method (**Figure 3D**).

Pyramidal Tracts

The pyramidal pathway was correctly depicted by the MC-det method (**Figure 4A**) and CSD-prob method (**Figure 4B**) at the level of the posterior limb of the internal capsule and cerebral peduncles. Lateral projections of the pyramidal pathway arising from the hand, face, lips and tongue area were identified by both the MC-det (**Figure 4A**) and the CSD-prob approach (**Figure 4B**). The CSD-prob approach identified a relatively smaller number of projections to most lateral lips and tongue area, and included false positive tracts belonging to the corpus callosum (**Figure 4B**). The streamline visualization of MC-det reconstructed tracts enabled three-dimensional depiction of the crossings of subthalamo-pallidal and pallido-subthalamic fibers with the descending pyramidal tract at the level of the internal capsule (**Figure 5**). Fibers crossings showed the comb fascicles organization (**Figures 5B,C**) (Nauta and Mehler, 1966).

DISCUSSION

This paper presents an exploratory study on the white matter connectivity between the subthalamic nucleus and the globus pallidus on healthy subjects data from the Human Connectome Project. We have shown that using multi-fiber modeling approaches and high-resolution multi-shell dMRI data at 3.0 Tesla, it is possible to detect complex fiber architecture in the basal ganglia. We chose to analyze the data using two different multi-fiber methods in order to confirm that our findings were not a method-related artifact. The results show that both approaches enabled the reconstruction of subthalamo-pallidal and pallido-subthalamic fibers. The review by four neuroanatomy experts demonstrated that overall the reconstructed tracts where in agreement with known anatomy. The main advantage of the MC-det and CSD-prob methods arises from the use of advanced multi-fiber models which enable the identification of complex anatomical configurations in voxels where multiple fiber population cross, such as at the intersection of the descending pyramidal tract with the pallido-subthalamic and subthalamo-pallidal fibers. However, both approaches also present some disadvantages. The MCM-det approach relies on the ball-and-stick model that is limited in the detection of fanning tracts. The volume rendered images of the TDMs generated by the CSD-prob methods can be difficult to interpret. In addition, both deterministic and probabilistic tractography methods propagate streamlines

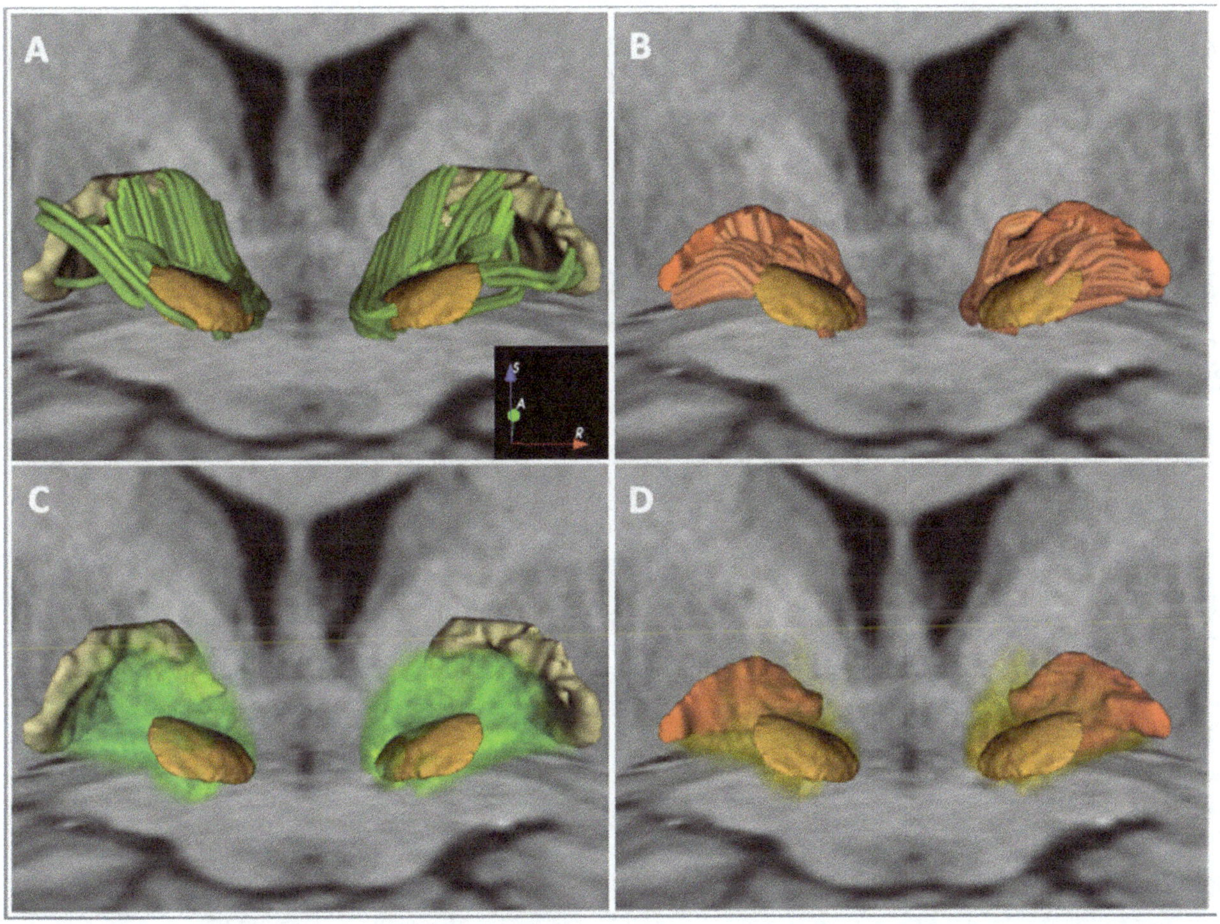

FIGURE 3 | White matter connectivity between the STN and the GP in HCP subject 100307. The figure shows an anterior 3D view of MC-det tracts represented as streamlines (top row) and CSD-prob tracts represented as volume-rendered tract density maps (bottom row). The tracts are superimposed on an axial T1-weighted image at the level of the cerebral peduncles and a coronal T1-weighted image at the level of the anterior commissure, along with 3D surface models of the STN (light orange), GPi (dark orange), and GPe (light yellow). **(A)** and **(C)** show tracts interconnecting the STN and the GPe. **(B)** and **(D)** show tracts interconnecting the STN and the GPi.

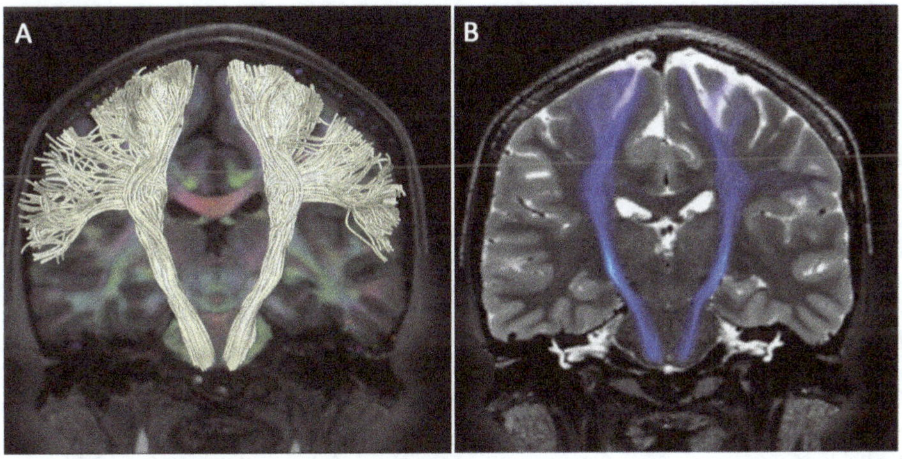

FIGURE 4 | Pyramidal pathway in HCP subject 100307. The figure shows the tractography reconstruction of pyramidal white matter fibers arising from the pre-central gyrus. **(A)** Pyramidal pathway (white) reconstructed using the MC-det approach. The tracts are displayed on a DEC map overlaid on a coronal T1-weighted image. **(B)** Pyramidal pathway (blue) reconstructed using the CSD-prob approach. The tracts are displayed on a coronal T2-weighted image.

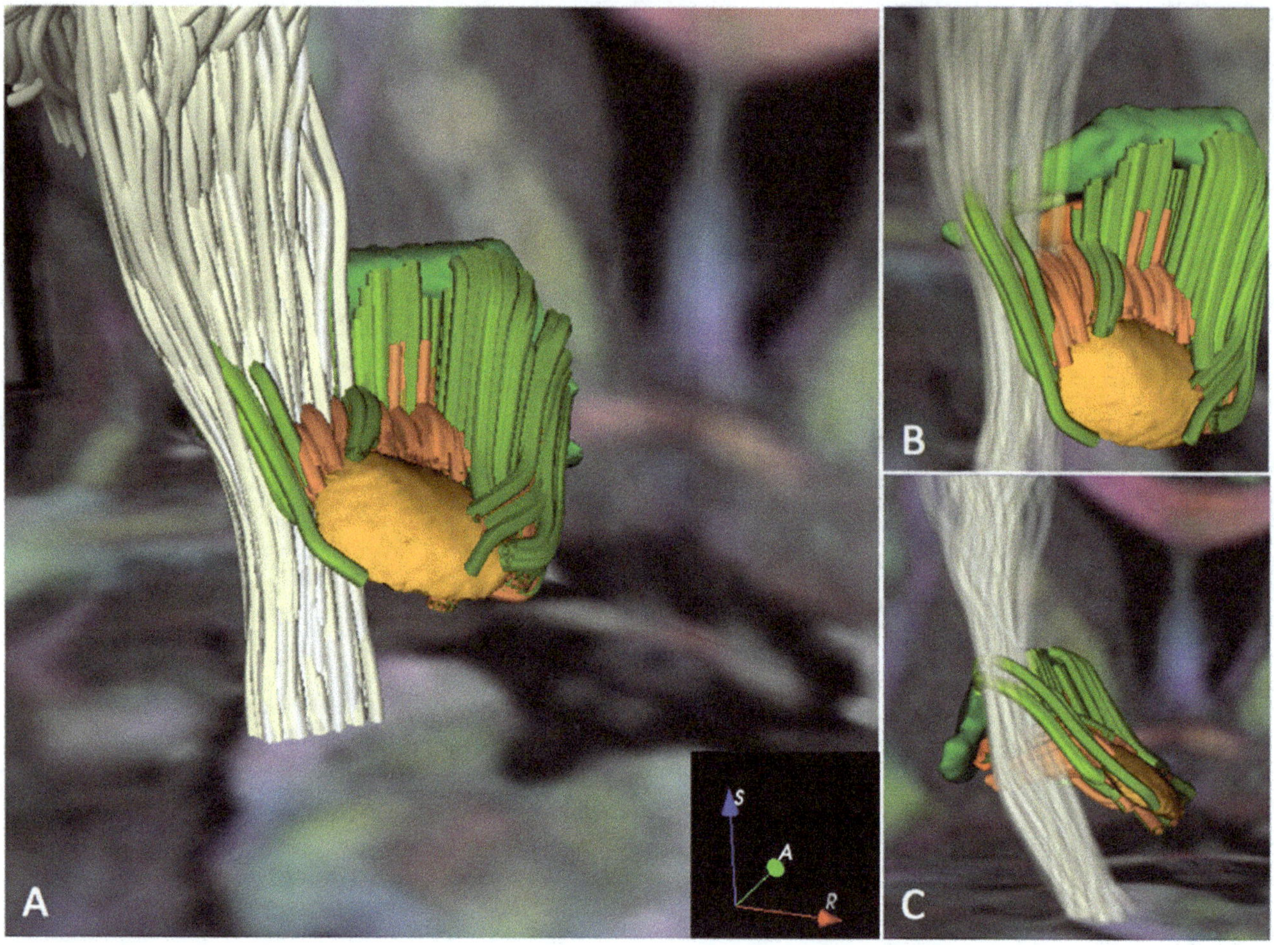

FIGURE 5 | Crossings of the pyramidal pathway with subthalamo-pallidal and pallido-subthalamic fibers (MC-det approach) in HCP subject 100307. The figure shows 3D postero-superior views of the intersection of the pyramidal pathway (white streamlines) with fibers interconnecting the STN and the GPi (dark orange streamlines) and fibers interconnecting the STN and the GPe (dark green streamlines). An axial T1-weighted image at the level of the cerebral peduncles and a coronal T1-weighted image at the level of the anterior commissure with 3D surface models of the STN (light orange), GPi (dark orange), and GPe (green) are displayed for anatomical reference. A DEC map is overlaid on the T1-weighted images. The opacity and number of pyramidal fibers displayed in **(A)** have been reduced in **(B)** and **(C)** to enable the visualization of the crossings of the motor pathway with fibers interconnecting the STN with the GPi and GPe.

by considering only directional information at the voxel level and ambiguities can occur in complex anatomical regions.

While we used two advanced multi-fiber models and high-quality data, the tractography results still present some limitations. First, the majority of pallido-subthalamic and subthalamo-pallidal fibers identified by the MC-det approach were located on the ventral aspect of the STN. **(Figures 3A,B)**, and the streamlines seem to stop just before entering the nucleus (**Figure 5**). A potential explanation of the absence of tracts on the dorsal aspect of the STN can be given by the presence of the H2 field of Forel where the lenticular fasciculus and the ansa lenticular merge to form a dense bundle of fibers (Dejerine, 1901). The lenticular fasciculus projects from the GPi, crosses the internal capsule, reaches the H2 and H fields of Forel, and courses superiorly and anteriorly through H1 field of Forel to enter the thalamus. The ansa lenticularis projects infero-medially from the GPi, crosses the internal capsule, travels towards the STN and turns superiorly to pass through H and H1 before entering the thalamus. As the focus of our study was to investigate the connectivity between the STN and the GP, we did not include the tractography reconstruction of these two pathways. However, the anatomical complexity of the ansa lenticularis and the lenticular fasciculus and their close proximity to the pallido-subthalamic and subthalamo-pallidal fibers might have affected the anatomical accuracy of the tractography results and introduced false-negative tracts. The apparent distance between the extremities of the streamlines and the nuclei visible in **Figure 5** is likely due to the generation of the tractography ROIs. The ROIs were voxelized from the 3D meshes of the nuclei, which had been generated from a high-resolution histological atlas with 0.16 mm × 0.16 mm × 0.41 mm voxel size. During the voxelization process, we used as a reference the T1-weigthed HCP scan resampled to 0.3 mm. The difference

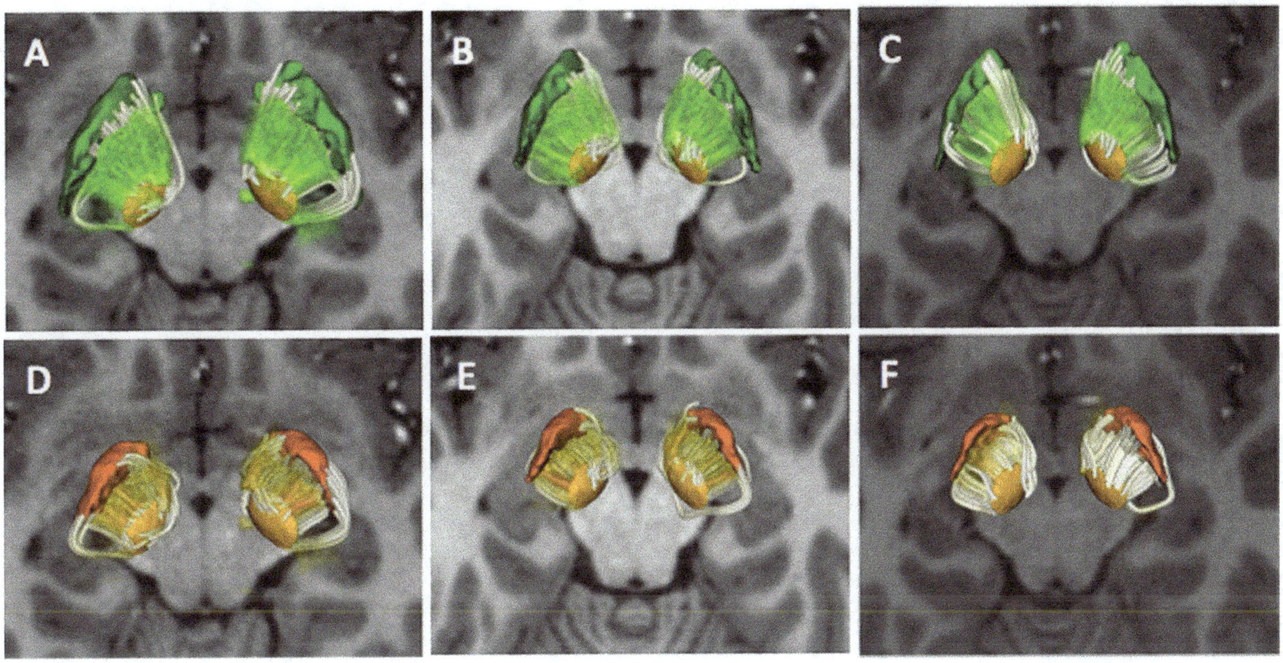

FIGURE 6 | Combined deterministic and probabilistic tractography reconstructions. The figure shows a superior 3D view of the deterministic and probabilistic tracts interconnecting the STN and the GPe (top row) and STN and GPi (bottom row) in three subjects (**A–D**: HCP 100408; **B–E**: HCP:101915; **C–F**: HCP 103414). The MC-det tracts are represented as streamlines (white) and the CSD-prob tracts are represented as volume-rendered imaged (green, orange). The tracts are superimposed on an axial T1-weighted image at the level of the cerebral peduncles with 3D surface models of the STN (light orange), GPi (dark orange), and GPe (green).

in voxel size between the original mesh and the voxelized ROI likely introduced a few tenth of millimeters difference that may explain the visual gap between the extremities of the tracts and the nuclei.

Second, we observed a discrepancy between the two methods in the tractography reconstruction of fibers interconnecting the STN and the GPe. Tracts generated using the MC-det approach were mostly located on the upper dorsal part of the GPe while tracts generated using the CSD-prob approach were located in the ventrolateral and mediolateral part of the GPe. The MC-det approach used a ball-and-stick model for the detection of crossings fibers. However, the model presents limitations for the detection of fanning fibers, which may be encountered within the globus pallidus (Sotiropoulos et al., 2012). In addition, the relatively smaller number of fibers detected by both methods may be due to the presence of the striato-pallido-nigral pathway crossing the pallidum. Striato-pallido-nigral fibers arise from the striatum, travel through the GPe and the GPi and cross the internal capsule to reach the substantia nigra (Percheron et al., 1984). Pallido-subthalamic and subthalamo-pallidal fibers within the GPe and GPi are likely to be less dense that striato-pallido-nigral fibers, which might explain the smaller number of fibers detected (Percheron et al., 1984). In addition, the CSD-prob approach included in the descending pyramidal pathway false positive tracts belonging to the corpus callosum. This limitation is likely due to the high number of kissing fibers along the trajectory of the pyramidal tract, and its close location to the corpus callosum.

Finally, despite the high-resolution of the HCP dMRI data, the difference in scale between the microscopic size of myelinated axons and the macroscopic 1.25 mm voxel size of the diffusion-weighted images remains significant. As a consequence, each voxel is likely to contain multiple axons belonging to several different pathways. Further studies are needed to investigate the complex spatial relationship between the pallido-subthalamic and subthalamo-pallidal fibers with the ansa lenticularis, lenticular fasciculus and striato-pallido-nigral pathway. Future work will include the tractography reconstruction of these complex pathways as well as their crossings with the internal capsule, and will explore the use of a higher number of compartments in the MC-det method and a larger number of harmonics of the CSD-prob methods (Tournier et al., 2012).

While the continuous refinement of mathematical models of diffusion and fiber tracking techniques enables the non-invasive exploration of the connectivity of the human white matter, dMRI tractography remains a research tool. Studies have demonstrated that dMRI tractography presents limitations for neurosurgical decision-making in the resection of brain gliomas (Pujol et al., 2015). The false-negative findings of our exploratory work demonstrate that tractography cannot currently replace electrophysiology mapping or intra-operative MR imaging in functional neurosurgery. However, as the technology continues

TABLE 2 | Summary of the qualitative evaluation of the reconstructed tracts.

Tract	Subject 1	Subject 2	Subject 3	Subject 4	Subject 5	Average (*SD*)
STN-GPe	3.6	3.3	3.5	3.1	3	3.3 (0.2)
STN-GPi	4.1	3.5	3.5	3.6	3.9	3.7 (0.3)
PT	3.8	3.2	3.5	3.5	3.4	3.5 (0.2)

The table presents the average review score of the tracts interconnecting the STN and the GPe (STN-GPe), tracts interconnecting the STN and the GPi (STN-GPi), and the pyramidal tract (PT) for each subject. The scores were given using a scale of 1–5 (1 – poor, 2 – fair, 3 – good, 4 – very good, and 5 – excellent).

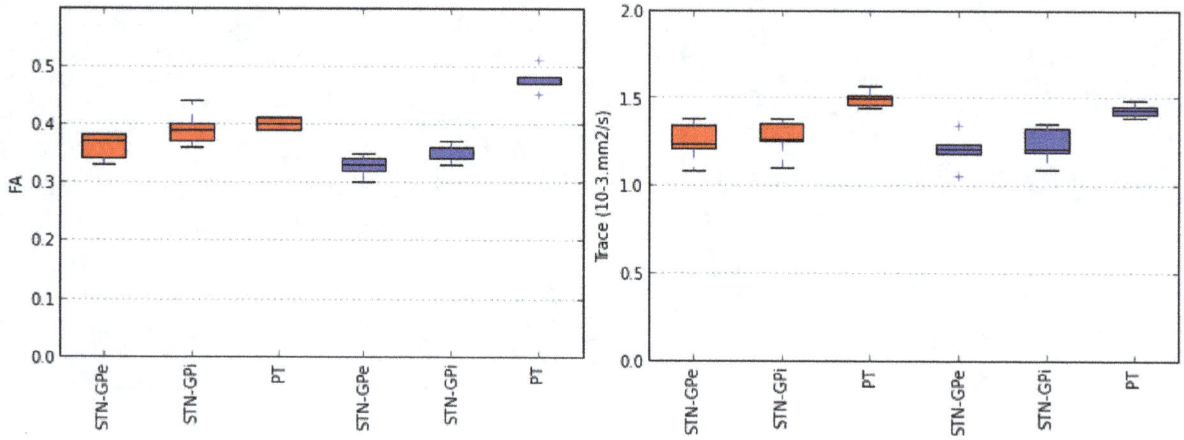

FIGURE 7 | Variability in tract-derived measurements. The figure presents box plots of fractional anisotropy (FA) and mean diffusivity (MD) of tracts interconnecting the STN and the GPe (STN-GPe), tracts interconnecting the STN and the GPi (STN-GPi) and pyramidal tract (PT). The lines in each box correspond to the median, interquartile range, minimum and maximum values of the tract-derived measurements. Tracts identified by the MCM-det method are represented in red. Tracts identified by the CSD-prob methods are represented in blue.

to progress, dMRI tractography has the potential to become part of the apparatus of brain mapping tools to help understand the clinical effects of DBS interventions. The HCP datasets used in this study have been acquired with optimized multiband pulse sequences on a customized Siemens 3T Connectome scanner and pre-processed for noise removal and artifacts minimization. The HCP dMRI scans represent the state-of-the-art dMRI data currently available in brain research, and are expected to represent the clinical dMRI scans that will be available in neurosurgery departments in the upcoming years. Our preliminary study aimed at exploring the tractography reconstructions that could become available to assist with pre-surgical planning of DBS intervention in neurosurgery clinics in the near future.

CONCLUSION

We have presented a pilot study on the connectivity between the subthalamic nucleus and the globus pallidus using two multi-fiber tractography approaches on dMRI data acquired on five healthy subjects of the Human Connectome Project. Our analysis revealed that multi-fiber tractography enables three-dimensional visualization of complex neuroanatomical fibers in the basal ganglia. However, false-negative tracts have demonstrated the current limitations of the techniques. As progresses are continuously being made in the development of advanced mathematical models of diffusion and fiber tracking algorithms, dMRI tractography has the potential to become a useful component of the brain mapping apparatus available to clinicians for functional neurosurgery intervention.

AUTHOR CONTRIBUTIONS

Substantial contributions to the conception or design of the work: SP, EB, JY, CF, PJ, and RK. Substantial contributions to the data analysis: SP, RC, SBS, SFV, YZ, EB, and RK. Substantial contributions to the interpretation of data with anatomical expertise: SP, JY, CF, GRC, and RK. Substantial contributions to drafting the work: SP, RC, SBS, RK, and EB. Substantial contributions to revising the work: SP, RC, SBS, JY, CF, SFV, CK, YZ, GRC, PJ, RK, and EB. Agreement to be accountable for all aspects of the work in ensuring that questions related to the accuracy or integrity of any part of the work are appropriately investigated and resolved: all authors SP, RC, SBS, JY, CF, SFV, CK, YZ, GRC, PJ, RK, and EB.

FUNDING

This work was partially funded by the Neuroimage Analysis Center (NIH P41EB015902), the National Center for Image-Guided Therapy (NIH P41EB015898), the Institut des

Neurosciences Translationnelles (ANR-10-IAIHU-06), and the Infrastructure d'Avenir en Biologie Santé (ANR-11-INBS-0006). SBS was supported by the Bettencourt Schueller Foundation and the Investments for the Future program of the French National Agency for Research (ANR-10-EQPX-15). Data were provided by the Human Connectome Project, WU-Minn Consortium (Principal Investigators: David Van Essen and Kamil Ugurbil (U54MH091657) funded by the 16 NIH Institutes and Centers that support the NIH Blueprint for Neuroscience Research; and by the McDonnell Center for Systems Neuroscience at Washington University.

REFERENCES

Alexander, A. L., Lee, J. E., Lazar, M., and Field, A. S. (2007). Diffusion tensor imaging of the brain. *Neurotherapeutics* 4, 316–329. doi: 10.1016/j.nurt.2007.05.011

Alexander, D. C. (2005). Multiple-fiber reconstruction algorithms for diffusion MRI. *Ann. N. Y. Acad. Sci.* 1046, 113–133. doi: 10.1196/annals.1340.018

Alkemade, A., Schnitzker, A., and Forstmann, B. U. (2015). Topographic organization of the human and non-human primate subthlamic nucleus. *Brain Struct. Funct.* 220, 3075–3086. doi: 10.1007/s00429-015-1047-2

Andersson, J. L., and Sotiropoulos, S. N. (2015a). Non-parametric representation and prediction of single- and multi-shell diffusion-weighted MRI data using Gaussian processes. *Neuroimage* 15, 166–176. doi: 10.1016/j.neuroimage.2015.07.067

Andersson, J. L., and Sotiropoulos, S. N. (2015b). An integrated approach to correction for off-resonance effects and subject movement in diffusion MR imaging. *Neuroimage* 125, 1063–1078. doi: 10.1016/j.neuroimage.2015.10.019

Ashby, P., Kim, Y. J., Kumar, R., Lang, A. E., and Lozano, A. M. (1999). Neurophysiological effects of stimulation throughelectrodes in the human subthalamic nucleus. *Brain* 122(Pt 10), 1919–1931. doi: 10.1093/brain/122.10.1919

Avecillas-Chasin, J. M., Rascón-Ramírez, F., and Barcia, J. A. (2016). Tractographical model of the cortico-basal ganglia and corticothalamic connections: improving our understanding of deep brain stimulation. *Clin. Anat.* 29, 481–492. doi: 10.1002/ca.22689

Bardinet, E., Bhattacharjee, M., Dormont, D., Pidoux, B., Malandain, G., and Schüpbach, M. (2009). A three-dimensional histological atlas of the human basal ganglia. II. Atlas deformation strategy and evaluation in deep brain stimulation for Parkinson disease. *J. Neurosurg.* 110, 208–219. doi: 10.3171/2008.3.17469

Barkhoudarian, G., Klochkov, T., Sedrak, M., Frew, A., Gorgulho, A., Behnke, E., et al. (2010). A role of diffusion tensor imaging in movement disorder surgery. *Acta Neurochir.* 152, 2089–2095. doi: 10.1007/s00701-010-0742-2

Basser, P. J., Mattiello, J., and Le Bihan, D. (1994). Estimation of the effective self-diffusion tensor from the NMR spin echo. *J. Magn. Reson.* 103, 247–254. doi: 10.1006/jmrb.1994.1037

Behrens, T. E., Berg, H. J., Jbabdi, S., Rushworth, M. F., and Woolrich, M. W. (2007). Probabilistic diffusion tractography with multiple fibre orientations: what can we gain? *Neuroimage* 34, 144–155. doi: 10.1016/j.neuroimage.2006.09.018

Benabid, A. L., Pollak, P., Louveau, A., Henry, S., and de Rougemont, J. (1987). Combined (thalamotomy and stimulation) stereotactic surgery of the VIM thalamic nucleus for bilateral Parkinson disease. *Appl. Neurophysiol.* 50, 344–346.

Cabeen, R. P., Bastin, M. E., and Laidlaw, D. H. (2013). Estimating constrained multi-fiber diffusion MR volumes by orientation clustering. *Med. Image Comput. Comput. Assist. Interv.* 16(Pt 1), 82–89.

Cabeen, R. P., Bastin, M. E., and Laidlaw, D. H. (2016). Kernel regression estimation of fiber orientation mixtures in diffusion MRI. *Neuroimage* 127, 158–172. doi: 10.1016/j.neuroimage.2015.11.061

Calabrese, E. (2016). Diffusion Tractography in brain stimulation surgery: a review. *Front. Neuroanat.* 10:45. doi: 10.3389/fnana.2016.00045

Calamante, F., Tournier, J.-D., Jackson, G. D., and Connelly, A. (2010). Track-density imaging (TDI): super-resolution white matter imaging using whole-brain track-density mapping. *Neuroimage* 53, 1233–1243. doi: 10.1016/j.neuroimage.2010.07.024

Coenen, V. A., Allert, N., Paus, S., Kronenbürger, M., Urbach, H., and Mädler, B. (2014). Modulation of the cerebello-thalamo-cortical network in thalamic deep brain stimulation for tremor: a diffusion tensor imaging study. *Neurosurgery* 75, 657–69; discussion 669–670. doi: 10.1227/NEU.0000000000000540

D'Albis, T., Haegelen, C., Essert, C., Fernández-Vidal, S., Lalys, F., and Jannin, P. (2015). PyDBS: an automated image processing workflow for deep brain stimulation surgery. *Int. J. Comput. Assist. Radiol. Surg.* 10, 117–128. doi: 10.1007/s11548-014-1007-y

De Celis Alonso, B., Hidalgo-Tobón, S. S., Menéndez-González, M., Salas-Pacheco, J., and Arias-Carrión, O. (2015). Magnetic resonance techniques applied to the diagnosis and treatment of Parkinson's disease. *Front. Neurol.* 6:146. doi: 10.3389/fneur.2015.00146

Dejerine, J. (1901). *Anatomie des Centres Nerveux.* Paris: Rueff et Cie.

DeLong, M., and Wichmann, T. (2007). Circuits and circuits disorders of the basal ganglia. *Arch. Neurol.* 64, 20–24. doi: 10.1001/archneur.64.1.20

Dormont, D., Seidenwurm, D., Galanaud, D., Cornu, P., Yelnik, Y., and Bardinet, E. (2010). Neuroimaging and deep brain stimulation. *AJNR Am. J. Neuroradiol.* 31, 15–23. doi: 10.3174/ajnr.A1644

Fasano, A., and Lozano, A. M. (2015). Deep brain stimulation for movement disorders: 2015 and beyond. *Curr. Opin. Neurol.* 28, 423–436. doi: 10.1097/WCO.0000000000000226

Fedorov, A., Beichel, R., Kalpathy-Cramer, J., Finet, J., Fillion-Robin, J. C., and Pujol, S. (2012). 3D Slicer as an image computing platform for the Quantitative Imaging Network. *Magn. Reson. Imaging* 30, 1323–1341. doi: 10.1016/j.mri.2012.05.001

François, C., Yelnik, J., Percheron, G., and Tandé, D. (1994). Calbindin D-28k as a marker for the associative cortical territory of the striatum in macaque. *Brain Res.* 633, 331–336. doi: 10.1016/0006-8993(94)91557-1

Glasser, M. F., Sotiropoulos, S. N., Wilson, J. A., Coalson, T. S., Fischl, B., and Andersson, J. L. (2013). The minimal preprocessing pipelines for the Human Connectome Project. *Neuroimage* 80, 105–124. doi: 10.1016/j.neuroimage.2013.04.127

Gradinaru, V., Mogri, M., Thompson, K., Henderson, J., and Deisseroth, K. (2009). Optical deconstruction of parkinsonian neural circuitry. *Science* 324, 354–359. doi: 10.1126/science.1167093

Haber, S. N., Lynd-Balta, E., and Mitchell, S. J. (1993). The organization of the de- scending ventral pallidal projections in the monkey. *J. Comp. Neurol.* 329, 111–128. doi: 10.1002/cne.903290108

Hamani, C., Saint-Cyr, J. A., Fraser, J., Kaplitt, M., and Lozano, A. M. (2004). The subthalamic nucleus in the context of movement disorders. *Brain* 127(Pt 1), 4–20. doi: 10.1093/brain/awh029

Haynes, W. I., and Haber, S. N. (2013). The organization of prefrontal-subthalamic inputs in primates provides an anatomical substrate for both functional specificity and integration: implications for Basal Ganglia models and deep brain stimulation. *J. Neurosci.* 33, 4804–4814. doi: 10.1523/JNEUROSCI.4674-12.2013

Henderson, J. M. (2012). "Connectomic surgery": diffusion tensor imaging (DTI) tractography as a targeting modality for surgical modulation of neural networks. *Front. Integr. Neurosci.* 6:15. doi: 10.3389/fnint.2012.00015

Jenkinson, M., Beckmann, C. F., Behrens, T. E., Woolrich, M. W., and Smith, S. M. (2012). Fsl. *Neuroimage* 62, 782–790. doi: 10.1016/j.neuroimage.2011.09.015

Jeurissen, B., Tournier, J.-D., Dhollander, T., Connelly, A., and Sijbers, J. (2014). Multi-tissue constrained spherical deconvolution for improved analysis of multi-shell diffusion MRI data. *Neuroimage* 103, 411–426. doi: 10.1016/j.neuroimage.2014.07.061

Karachi, C., Yelnik, J., Tande, D., Tremblay, L., Hirsch, E. C., and François, C. (2005). The pallidosubthalamic projection: an anatomical substrate for nonmotor functions of the subthalamic nucleus in primates. *Mov. Disord.* 20, 172–180. doi: 10.1002/mds.20302

Krack, P., and Hariz, M. I. (2013). Deep brain stimulation in Parkinson's disease: reconciliation of evidence-based medicine with clinical practice. *Lancet Neurol.* 12, 25–26. doi: 10.1016/S1474-4422(12)70270-3

Lanciego, J. L., Luquin, N., and Obeso, J. A. (2012). Functional neuroanatomy of the basal ganglia. *Cold Spring Harb. Perspect. Med.* 2:a009621. doi: 10.1101/cshperspect.a009621

Le Bihan, D., Breton, E., Lallemand, D., Grenier, P., Cabanis, E., and Laval-Jeantet, M. (1986). MR imaging of intravoxel incoherent motions: application to diffusion and perfusion in neurologic disorders. *Radiology* 161, 401–407. doi: 10.1148/radiology.161.2.3763909

Lemaire, J. J., Cosnard, G., Sakka, L., Nuti, C., Gradkowski, W., Mori, S., et al. (2011). White matter anatomyof the human deep brain revisited with high resolution DTI fibre tracking. *Neurochirurgie* 57, 52–67. doi: 10.1016/j.neuchi.2011.04.001

Lenglet, C., Abosch, A., Yacoub, E., De Martino, F., Sapiro, G., and Harel, N. (2012). Comprehensive in vivo mapping of the human basal ganglia and thalamic connectome in individuals using 7T MRI. *PLoS ONE* 7:e29153. doi: 10.1371/journal.pone.0029153

Lorensen, W. E., and Cline, H. E. (1987). "Marching cubes: a high resolution 3D surface construction algorithm," in *Proceedings of the 14th Annual Conference on Computer Graphics and Interactive Techniques, SIGGRAPH'87*, Anaheim, CA, 163–169. doi: 10.1145/37401.37422

Makris, N., Rathi, Y., Mouradian, P., Bonmassar, G., Papadimitriou, G., and Ing, W. I. (2015). Variability and anatomical specificity of the orbitofrontothalamic fibers of passage in the ventral capsule/ventral striatum (VC/VS): precision care for patient-specific tractography-guided targeting of deep brain stimulation (DBS) in obsessive compulsive disorder (OCD). *Brain Imaging Behav.* doi: 10.1007/s11682-015-9462-9 [Epub ahead of print].

McIntyre, C. C., and Hahn, P. J. (2010). Network perspectives on the mechanisms of deep brain stimulation. *Neurobiol. Dis.* 38, 329–337. doi: 10.1016/j.nbd.2009.09.022

Mori, S., Crain, B. J., Chacko, V. P., and van Zijl P. C. (1999). Three-dimensional tracking of axonal projections in the brain by magnetic resonance imaging. *Ann. Neurol.* 45, 265–269.

Nauta, W. J., and Mehler, W. R. (1966). Projections of the lentiform nucleus in the monkey. *Brain Res.* 1, 3–4. doi: 10.1016/0006-8993(66)90103-X

Parent, A. (1995). *Human Neuroanatomy*, 9th Edn. Baltimore, MD: Williamns& Wilkinsl, 795–863.

Parent, A., and Hzrati, L. N. (1995). Functional anatomy of the basal ganglia. II. The place of subthlamic nucleus, and external pallidum in the basal ganglia circuitry. *Brain Res. Rev.* 20, 128–154. doi: 10.1016/0165-0173(94)00008-D

Percheron, G., Yelnik, J., and François, C. (1984). A Golgi analysis of the primate globus pallidus. III. Spatial organization of the striato-pallidal complex. *J. Comp. Neurol.* 227, 214–227. doi: 10.1002/cne.902270207

Pierpaoli, C., and Basser, P. J. (1996). Toward a quantitative assessment of diffusion anisotropy. *Magn. Reson. Med.* 36, 893–906. doi: 10.1002/mrm.1910360612

Plantinga, B. R., Temel, Y., Roebroeck, A., Uludağ, K., Ivanov, D., Kuijf, M. L., et al. (2014). Ultra-high field magnetic resonance imaging of the basal ganglia and related structures. *Front. Hum. Neurosci.* 8:876. doi: 10.3389/fnhum.2014.00876

Pujol, S., Wells, W., Pierpaoli, C., Brun, C., Gee, J., and Cheng, G. (2015). The DTI challenge: toward standardized evaluation of diffusion tensor imaging tractography for neurosurgery. *J. Neuroimaging* 25, 875–882. doi: 10.1111/jon.12283

Qazi, A. A., Radmanesh, A., O'Donnell, L., Kindlmann, G., Peled, S., and Whalen, S. (2009). Resolving crossings in the corticospinal tract by two-tensor streamline tractography: method and clinical assessment using fMRI. *Neuroimage* 47, T98–T106. doi: 10.1016/j.neuroimage.2008.06.034

Rozanski, V. E., Vollmar, C., Cunha, J. P., Tafula, S. M. N., Ahmadi, S. A., and Patzig, M. (2014). Connectivity patterns of pallidal DBS electrodes in focal dystonia: a diffusion tensor tractography study. *Neuroimage* 84, 435–442. doi: 10.1016/j.neuroimage.2013.09.009

Shrink, E., Bevan, M. D., Bolam, J. P., and Smith, Y. (1996). The subthalamic nucleus and the external pallidum: two tightly interconnected structures that control the output of the basal ganglia in the monkey. *Neuroscience* 73, 335–357. doi: 10.1016/0306-4522(96)00022-X

Smith, R. E., Tournier, J.-D., Calamante, F., and Connelly, A. (2012). Anatomically-constrained tractography: improved diffusion MRI streamlines tractography through effective use of anatomical information. *Neuroimage* 62, 1924–1938. doi: 10.1016/j.neuroimage.2012.06.005

Smith, R. E., Tournier, J.-D., Calamante, F., and Connelly, A. (2013). SIFT: Spherical-deconvolution informed filtering of tractograms. *Neuroimage* 67, 298–312. doi: 10.1016/j.neuroimage.2012.11.049

Sotiropoulos, S. N., Behrens, T. E., and Jbabdi, S. (2012). Ball and rackets: inferring fibre fanning from diffusion-weighted MRI. *Neuroimage* 60, 1412–1425. doi: 10.1016/j.neuroimage.2012.01.056

Sotiropoulos, S. N., Jbabdi, S., Xu, J., Andersson, J. L., Moeller, S., Auerbach, E. J., et al. (2013). Advances in diffusion MRI acquisition and processing in the Human Connectome Project. *Neuroimage* 80, 125–143. doi: 10.1016/j.neuroimage.2013.05.057

Sweet, J. A., Walter, B. L., Gunalan, K., Chaturvedi, A., McIntyre, C. C., and Miller, J. P. (2014). Fiber tractography of the axonal pathways linking the basal ganglia and cerebellum in Parkinson disease: implications for targeting in deep brain stimulation. *J. Neurosurg.* 120, 988–996. doi: 10.3171/2013.12.JNS131537

Torres, C. V., Manzanares, R., and Sola, R. G. (2014). Integrating diffusion tensor imaging-based tractography into deep brain stimulation surgery: a review of the literature. *Stereotact. Funct. Neurosurg.* 92, 282–290. doi: 10.1159/000362937

Tournier, J. D., Calamante, F., and Connelly, A. (2012). MRtrix: diffusion tractography in crossing fiber regions. *Int. J. Imaging Syst. Technol.* 22, 53–66. doi: 10.1002/ima.22005

Tournier, J. D., Calamante, F., Gadian, D. G., and Connelly, A. (2004). Direct estimation of the fiber orientation density function from diffusion-weighted MRI data using spherical deconvolution. *Neuroimage* 23, 1176–1185. doi: 10.1016/j.neuroimage.2004.07.037

Uğurbil, K., Xu, J., Auerbach, E. J., Moeller, S., Vu, A. T., Duarte-Carvajalino, J. M., et al. (2013). Pushing spatial and temporal resolution for functional and diffusion MRI in the Human Connectome Project. *Neuroimage* 80, 80–104. doi: 10.1016/j.neuroimage.2013.05.012

Van Essen, D. C., Smith, S. M., Barch, D. M., Behrens, T. E., Yacoub, E., Ugurbil, K., et al. (2013). The WU-Minn human connectome project: an overview. *Neuroimage* 80, 62–79. doi: 10.1016/j.neuroimage.2013.05.041

Vanegas-Arroyave, N., Lauro, P. M., Huang, L., Hallett, M., Horovitz, S. G., Zaghloul, K. A., et al. (2016). Tractography patterns of subthalamic nucleus deep brain stimulation. *Brain* 139(Pt 4), 1200–1210. doi: 10.1093/brain/aww020

Wagle Shukla, A., and Okun, M. S. (2014). Surgical treatment of Parkinson's disease: patients, targets, devices, and approaches. *Neurotherapeutics* 11, 47–59. doi: 10.1007/s13311-013-0235-0

Yelnik, J., Bardinet, E., Dormont, D., Malandain, G., Ourselin, S., and Tandé, D. (2007). A three-dimensional, histological and deformable atlas of the human basal ganglia. I. Atlas construction based on immunohistochemical and MRI data. *Neuroimage* 34, 618–638. doi: 10.1016/j.neuroimage.2006.09.026

17

Weight Change after Subthalamic Nucleus Deep Brain Stimulation in Patients with Isolated Dystonia

Weibin He[1], Hongxia Li[2], Yijie Lai[3], Yunhao Wu[3], Yiwen Wu[2], Adolfo Ramirez-Zamora[4], Wei Yi[1] and Chencheng Zhang[3]**

[1] Department of Neurosurgery, Renmin Hospital, Wuhan University, Wuhan, China, [2] Department of Neurology, Ruijin Hospital, Shanghai Jiao Tong University School of Medicine, Shanghai, China, [3] Department of Functional Neurosurgery, Ruijin Hospital, Shanghai Jiao Tong University School of Medicine, Shanghai, China, [4] Fixel Center for Neurological Diseases, University of Florida, Gainesville, FL, United States

***Correspondence:**
Wei Yi
weiyi.renmin@whu.edu.cn
Chencheng Zhang
i@cczhang.org

Purpose: Deep brain stimulation of the subthalamic nucleus (STN-DBS) is an effective treatment method for advanced Parkinson's disease (PD) and isolated dystonia and provides marked improvement of major motor symptoms. In addition, non-motor effects have been reported including weight gain (WG) in patients with PD after STN-DBS. However, it is still unclear whether patients with isolated dystonia also experience WG.

Methods: Data from 47 patients with isolated dystonia who underwent bilateral STN-DBS surgery between October 2012 and June 2019 were retrospectively collected. The severity of dystonia was assessed via the Burke–Fahn–Marsden Dystonia Rating Scale (BFMDRS). Changes in the body mass index (BMI) and BFMDRS score were analyzed using paired Student's *t*-tests. Regression analysis was performed to identify factors that affected the BMI after surgery.

Results: Postoperative WG was observed in 78.7% of patients. The percentage of overweight and obese patients increased from 25.5% (before STN-DBS) to 48.9% (at the last follow-up). The mean BMI and mean percentage change in BMI increased by 1.32 ± 1.83 kg/m^2 ($P < 0.001$) and 6.28 ± 8.34%, respectively. BMI increased more in female than in male patients. At the last follow-up, BFMDRS movement and disability scores improved by 69.76 ± 33.23% and 65.66 ± 31.41%, respectively (both $P < 0.001$). The final regression model analysis revealed that sex and preoperative BMI alone were independently associated with BMI change ($P < 0.05$).

Conclusions: STN-DBS is associated with postoperative WG with patients with isolated dystonia. WG is more prominent in female patients and is associated with preoperative weight but not with the efficacy of STN-DBS on motor symptoms.

Keywords: isolated dystonia, subthalamic nucleus, deep brain stimulation, Burke-Fahn-Marsden dystonia rating scale, weight gain

INTRODUCTION

In recent decades, deep brain stimulation (DBS) has been applied to treat many disorders, such as advanced stages of Parkinson's disease (PD), intractable essential tremor, complicated segmental and generalized dystonia, and neuropsychiatric diseases (1, 2). DBS may improve patients' quality of life and result in desired therapeutic effects such as reduced tremor, dyskinesia, and stiffness in patients with PD (3, 4). However, DBS can also cause adverse events (5) and side effects (e.g., cognitive and emotional changes) (6–8) in some patients.

Interestingly, many researchers have reported that weight gain (WG) is common in patients with PD after DBS of the subthalamic nucleus (STN-DBS) (9). This is concerning because WG may lead to additional health complications such as obesity and diabetes (6). Some potential mechanisms underlying WG in patients with PD after STN-DBS treatment have been suggested, including the improvement of resting tremor and dyskinesias, reduction in energy expenditure (EE), changes in eating behavior and food intake, perturbations of homeostatic control, changes in hormone and neurotransmitter systems, and improvement in motor function; however, the exact mechanism underlying WG remains unknown (9).

Dystonia is characterized by sustained and involuntary muscular contractions, which result from dysfunction of the cortico-striato-thalamo-cortical circuitry. Dystonia can be classified according to the involved body distribution: focal, segmental, multifocal, generalized, and hemidystonia, or according to the etiology: inherited (proven genetic origin), acquired (known specific cause), and idiopathic (unknown cause) (10). Dystonia is the third most common movement disorder after PD and essential tremor (11). It is highly disabling and can seriously affect patients' quality of life. Recent studies have demonstrated that DBS of either the STN or globus pallidus internus (GPi) is an efficient treatment option for dystonia (12–16). A dual-target, crossover sham-controlled study has directly compared the clinical effects of GPi and STN stimulations in patients with dystonia, which indicated that the STN was a more effective target for dystonia than the GPi (17). STN-DBS is believed to improve the repetitive motions, abnormal posture, and quality of life of refractory patients with isolated dystonia (12, 13, 15, 18–21). The motor outcomes of STN-DBS in the treatment of dystonia have been extensively studied (12–16, 18–21). However, little is known about the effects of STN-DBS on non-motor (e.g., weight changes) symptoms in dystonia.

A thorough review of the available literature revealed that only one study has investigated WG in patients with isolated dystonia after STN-DBS, which only included nine patients (22). Given that there are significant differences in the pathophysiology and clinical manifestations of dystonia and PD (23), we investigated WG in patients with isolated dystonia who underwent STN-DBS at our center. Our center was one of the early explorers to the use of STN as a DBS target to treat isolated dystonia, which allowed us to study weight changes of a larger sample of patients with isolated dystonia after STN-DBS (24). Information on adverse events can help to better define the populations that will most benefit from STN-DBS. Thus, careful attention must be devoted to the investigation of WG after STN-DBS for the treatment of dystonia. To the best of our knowledge, this is the first study to explore the association between weight change and symptomatic improvement after STN-DBS in patients with dystonia.

MATERIALS AND METHODS

Participants

Patients with isolated dystonia [with normal brain magnetic resonance imaging (MRI) scans] (10) who were treated with bilateral STN-DBS between August 2012 and May 2019 were included in the present study. Patients were diagnosed with isolated dystonia by movement disorder specialists and admitted to the Department of Functional Neurosurgery, Ruijin Hospital, Shanghai Jiao Tong University School of Medicine, Shanghai. All patients, in the absence of secondary causes, presented with marked symptoms, despite optimal pharmacologic treatment. Except for dystonia, all patients presented without other neurological deficiencies. The exclusion criteria were as follows: diabetes and thyroid disease, nutritional intervention received in addition to routine care, unexplained weight change, severe metabolic disease (chronic gastroenteritis, liver dysfunction, malignant tumors, other consumptive diseases, and others), severe dysphagia, history of operations (esophagectomy, bowel resection, gastrectomy, and others), active mental illness (depression, schizophrenia, and others), other brain surgery, and postoperative complications (cerebral hemorrhage, infection, and others). Patients' age ranged from 18 to 75 years. To gain insight into the etiology (idiopathic or inherited) of patients with isolated dystonia, we performed whole-exome sequencing. Thirteen patients underwent genetic testing, whereas 34 declined genetic testing. This study was approved by the ethics committee of Ruijin Hospital. Written informed consent from all patients was obtained for participation in this study.

Data Collection

We used a structured questionnaire (32 questions) about their family and personal history, focusing on metabolic syndrome, diabetes, access to nutrition counseling, and body mass index (BMI) data. Patients with recent (<1 month) Burke–Fahn–Marsden Dystonia Rating Scale (BFMDRS) data received questionnaires via email or express delivery. The remaining patients received clinical routine outpatient follow-ups with this particular additional questionnaire. We retrospectively collected the following pre- and post-DBS data from Ruijin Hospital database of surgical patients: BFMDRS scores, weight, height, age at surgery, disease duration, and sex. Videos of BFMDRS scores were recorded by an evaluator who did not know the patient's neurostimulation status at baseline and the last follow-up postoperatively. Data from the evaluations were obtained by other evaluators (HXL and WBH) who were blinded tothe patients' names and stimulation status, using standardized scoring criteria. According to the Chinese standard "WS/T 428-2013: Criteria of weight for adults," we classified patients into the four following groups: low weight (BMI < 18.5 kg/m^2), normal weight ($18.5 \leq$ BMI < 24.0 kg/m^2), overweight ($24.0 \leq$ BMI $<$ 28.0 kg/m^2), and obese (BMI ≥ 28.0 kg/m^2).

Surgical Procedure

Patients underwent standard bilateral stereotactic STN-DBS implantation procedures. MRI (1.5 T SIGNA or 3 T

HDx; General Electric Company, Boston, MA, USA) and macrostimulation were used for STN targeting. Quadripolar DBS electrodes (serial number, 3387; Medtronic, Minneapolis, MN, USA or serial number, 3389; Medtronic, Minneapolis, MN, USA or L301; PINS, Beijing, China or L302; PINS, Beijing, China) were implanted under local anesthesia for precise monitoring of motor function and adverse effects using macrostimulation. An implantable pulse generator (Kinetra 7428; Medtronic or 37612; Medtronic or G101A; PINS or G102R; PINS) was implanted subclavicularly under general anesthesia. Electrode placement was validated using postoperative MRI or CT.

Statistical Analyses

IBM SPSS Statistics for Windows version 22.0 (IBM Corp., Armonk, NY, USA) was used for data analysis. We analyzed changes in BMI, BFMDRS movement scale (BFMDRS-MS), and BFMDRS disability scale (BFMDRS-DS) using a paired Student's *t*-test or independent samples *t*-test. A one-way analysis of variance (ANOVA) was used to analyze the influence of body fat distribution on the percentage change in BMI. Multivariate linear regression was performed to evaluate the association between clinical/demographic characteristics and percentage change in BMI following surgery. The latter was regarded as dependent variables. Independent variables included sex (binary variable, where male = 0, and female = 1), age at surgery (years), preoperative BMI, time interval after surgery (months), preoperative BFMDRS-MS, and percentage change in BFMDRS-MS following surgery. All continuous data are presented as the means ± standard deviations and ranges. We report two-tailed *P*-values along with 95% confidence intervals. We selected a significance threshold of $P = 0.05$ and adjusted the significance levels for multivariate linear regression using the Benjamini–Hochberg procedure to account for multiple testing.

RESULTS

Patient Characteristics

In total, 54 patients with isolated dystonia underwent bilateral STN-DBS surgery within the study period. Seven patients were excluded due to a lack of follow-up, and 47 (87%) were included in the final analysis. The results of the 13 patients who underwent genetic testing were as follows: 10 patients with idiopathic isolated dystonia, 2 patients with TOR1A (DYT1)-positive isolated dystonia, and 1 patient with THAP1 (DYT6)-positive isolated dystonia. Thirty-four patients who refused genetic testing were diagnosed with unknown (inherited or idiopathic) isolated dystonia. The body distribution of 47 patients was as follows: generalized ($N = 14$), multifocal ($N = 17$), segmental ($N = 5$), and focal ($N = 11$). These 47 patients (23 women and 24 men) were 50.62 ± 15.02 years old at the time of the operation (range, 21 to 73 years), and the average follow-up time after surgery was 39.89 ± 26.25 months (range, 4 to 83 months). The average time from diagnosis to surgery was 11.98 ± 7.68 years. The preoperative medications were as follows: 40 patients were treated with botulinum toxin, 8 with clonazepam, 17 with trihexyphenidyl, 12 with tiapride, 8 with haloperidol, 18 with baclofen, and 2 with levodopa and benserazide hydrochloride. Patient demographics and clinical data are summarized in **Table 1**.

TABLE 1 | Demographics and dystonia- and DBS-related information.

Demographics characteristics	Isolated dystonia
No.	47
Distribution, generalized/multifocal/segmental/focal	14/17/5/11
Axis: neck and trunk/limbs: lower, upper/face: eyes and mouth/speech and swallowing	25/29/23/11
Sex, M/F	24/23
Age at surgery (years)	
Mean ± SD	50.62 ± 15.02
Range	21-73
History of disease (years)	
Mean ± SD	11.98 ± 7.68
Range	0.57-31.66
Follow-up time (years)	
Mean ± SD	3.32 ± 2.21
Range	0.36-6.96

DBS, deep brain stimulation; SD, standard deviation.

TABLE 2 | Effect of STN stimulation on BMI at baseline and at the last follow-up in 47 patients.

BMI groups	Score (kg/m², mean ± SD)		*P*
	Before surgery	After surgery	
All patients ($n = 47$)	22.64 ± 3.09	23.95 ± 2.94	<0.001
Female patients ($n = 23$)	21.93 ± 2.18	23.95 ± 2.46	<0.001
Male patients ($n = 24$)	23.32 ± 3.68	23.97 ± 3.41	0.03

STN, subthalamic nucleus; BMI, body mass index; SD, standard deviation.

Changes in Body Weight

Changes in BMI are summarized in **Table 2** and **Figure 1**. Compared with the baseline, 78.7% of the 47 patients exhibited postoperative WG at the final follow-up. The percentage of overweight or obese patients increased from 25.5 to 48.9%. The mean BMI of all patients increased by 1.32 ± 1.83 kg/m^2 (22.64 ± 3.09 kg/m^2 before surgery vs. 23.95 ± 2.94 kg/m^2 after surgery; $P < 0.001$, $n = 47$), and the mean increase in BMI increase was 6.28 ± 8.34%. The mean BMI of female patients increased significantly more than that of male patients (2.02 ± 2 and 0.65 ± 1.38 kg/m^2 for female and male, respectively; $P = 0.009$).

Similarly, the mean percentage change in BMI increased significantly more in female than in male patients (9.54 ± 9.32% and 3.15 ± 5.93%, respectively; $P = 0.007$). There was no significant difference in clinical characteristics between male and female patients (see **Table 3**). Patients were divided into three groups according to the age: <40 ($N = 13$), 40–60 ($N = 19$), and over 60 years ($N = 15$). One-way ANOVA showed no difference in percentage change in BMI among the three groups [$F_{2,45} = 0.909$, $P = 0.410$]. Considering the different follow-up times, patients were divided into four groups according to the follow-up

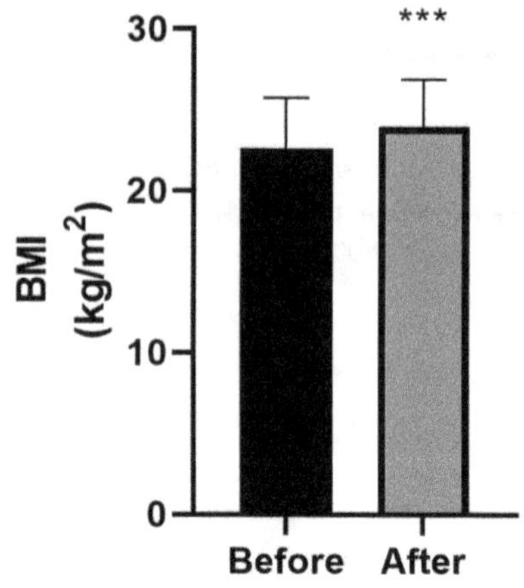

FIGURE 1 | Body mass index (BMI) at baseline and final follow-up ($n = 47$). Bars represent the mean + standard deviation score. The asterisk indicates that the comparison with the preoperative score was statistically significant (***$P < 0.001$).

TABLE 3 | Clinical characteristics of male and female subjects.

Parameters	Female	Male	P
Preoperative BMI (kg/m^2)	21.93 ± 2.18	23.32 ± 3.68	0.121
Postoperative BMI (kg/m^2)	23.95 ± 2.46	23.97 ± 3.41	0.975
Age at surgery (years)	51.09 ± 15.63	50.17 ± 14.73	0.836
Follow-up time (years)	3.00 ± 2.35	3.63 ± 2.07	0.333
Disease duration (years)	11.63 ± 8.06	12.32 ± 7.45	0.764
Preoperative BFMDRS-MS	27.80 ± 18.66	31.13 ± 23.79	0.598
Postoperative BFMDRS-MS	8.91 ± 9.16	8.02 ± 10.68	0.760
Preoperative BFMDRS-DS	9.39 ± 6.40	11.13 ± 6.17	0.349
Postoperative BFMDRS-DS	3.13 ± 3.32	2.79 ± 2.60	0.698

BMI, body mass index; BFMDRS, Burke–Fahn–Marsden Dystonia Rating Scale; BFMDRS-MS, BFMDRS movement score; BFMDRS-DS, Burke–Fahn–Marsden Dystonia Rating Scale disability score.

time: <1 ($N = 13$), 1–3 ($N = 8$), 3–5 ($N = 11$), and more than 5 years ($N = 16$). One-way ANOVA showed no difference in the percentage change in BMI [$F_{3,44} = 0.850$, $P = 0.474$], BFMDRS-MS [$F_{3,44} = 0.558$, $P = 0.646$], and BFMDRS-DS [$F_{3,44} = 0.296$, $P = 0.828$] among the three groups.

Changes in the Burke–Fahn–Marsden Dystonia Rating Scale

The changes in the BFMDRS scores are shown in **Table 4** and **Figure 2**. Compared with those at baseline, the BFMDRS-MS and BFMDRS-DS were lower at the final follow-up. The BFMDRS-MS was reduced by 69.76 ± 33.23% (a score of 29.5 ± 21.27 before surgery vs. 8.46 ± 9.87 after surgery; $P < 0.001$, $n = 47$); for BFMDRS-DS, this was 65.66 ± 31.41% (a score of 10.28 ± 6.28 before surgery vs. 2.96 ± 2.95 after surgery; $P < 0.001$, $n = 47$).

Factors Associated With Body Mass Index Gain

In the univariate linear regression analysis, age at surgery, follow-up period, baseline BFMDRS-MS, and percentage change in BFMDRS-MS were not associated with percentage change in BMI ($P > 0.05$; see **Table 5**); thus, we only added sex and preoperative BMI to the multivariate linear regression model. These were both independently associated with an increase in BMI ($P < 0.05$; see **Table 6**).

TABLE 4 | Effects of STN stimulation on BFMDRS disability scores at baseline and last follow-up in patients with isolated dystonia.

Scale	Score (mean ± SD)		P
	Before surgery ($n = 47$)	After surgery ($n = 47$)	
BFMDRS-MS	29.5 ± 21.27	8.46 ± 9.87	<0.001
BFMDRS-DS	10.28 ± 6.28	2.96 ± 2.95	<0.001

SD, standard deviation; BFMDRS, Burke–Fahn–Marsden Dystonia Rating Scale; BFMDRS-MS, BFMDRS movement score; BFMDRS-DS, BFMDRS disability score.

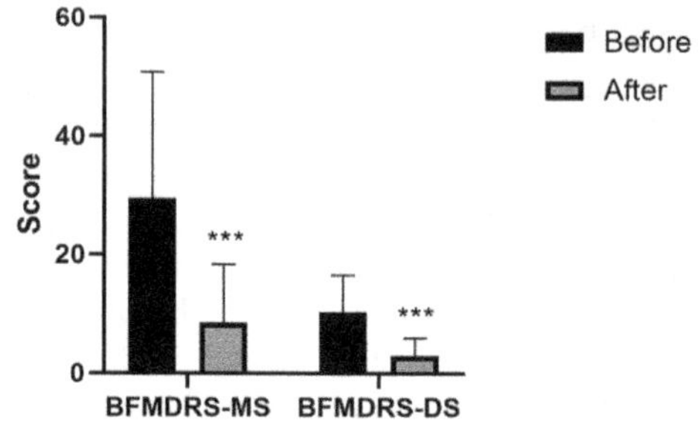

FIGURE 2 | Burke–Fahn–Marsden Dystonia Rating Scale (BFMDRS) movement scores and disability scores at baseline and final follow-up ($n = 47$). Bars represent the mean + standard deviation score. Asterisks indicate where the comparisons between final follow-up score and preoperative score were statistically significant (***$P < 0.001$). BFMDRS-MS, BFMDRS movement score; BFMDRS-DS, BFMDRS disability score.

According to the distribution of dystonia, the 47 patients with dystonia were divided into four groups, as follows: focal ($n = 11$), segmental ($n = 5$), multifocal ($n = 17$), and generalized (with or without eyelid involvement) ($n = 14$). The one-way ANOVA indicated no difference in the percentage change of BMI before and after operation [$F_{3,43} = 0.465$, $P = 0.708$] or BFMDRS-MS [$F_{3,43} = 0.484$, $P = 0.695$]. Patients were divided into two groups according to their dyskinesias, as follows: group 1, with limb involvement ($n = 30$); and group 2, without limb involvement ($n = 17$). The results of the independent samples t-test revealed no difference in the percentage change in BMI ($P = 0.346$) or BFMDRS-MS ($P = 0.477$) between the two groups.

Five patients in whom only the eyelids were affected were regarded as one group, and the other patients (with or without eyelid involvement) ($n = 42$) were regarded as another group. The results of an independent samples t-test revealed no difference in the percentage change in BMI ($P = 0.862$) or BFMDRS-MS ($P = 0.499$) between the two groups.

DISCUSSION

In this study, we confirmed that patients with isolated dystonia typically exhibit WG after STN-DBS. Overall, 78.7% of the patients exhibited postoperative WG at the final follow-up. The

TABLE 5 | Clinical and demographic predictors of changes in BMI after surgery.

Parameters	Coefficient	Standard error	Beta	*t*	*P*
Sex (female)	6.389	2.259	0.387	2.817	0.007*
Age at surgery (years)	−0.072	0.082	−0.129	−0.871	0.388
Pre-surgical BMI	−1.104	0.367	−0.409	−3.009	0.004*
Disease duration (years)	0.167	0.160	0.154	1.042	0.303
Time interval after surgery (years)	0.756	0.551	0.200	1.372	0.177
Pre-surgical BFMDRS-MS	0.015	0.058	0.039	0.261	0.795
Percent change in BFMDRS-MS scores (%)	−0.014	0.037	−0.058	−0.386	0.701

*BMI, body mass index; BFMDRS-MS, Burke–Fahn–Marsden Dystonia Rating Scale movement score. *$P < 0.05$.*

proportion of patients that were overweight or obese increased from 25.5% before surgery to 48.9% in the final follow-up period.

There was a significant correlation between WG and sex, whereby the mean BMI of female patients increased significantly more than that of male patients after surgery. Considering that the average age of female patients at surgery was 51 years, this association may be associated with changes in menopausal hormones (25). This correlation has been previously identified for patients with PD who underwent STN-DBS (26). There is evidence showing that female patients with PD gain disproportionate amounts of fat mass after STN-DBS, while WG in men was driven by both fat-free mass and fat mass (27, 28). In this study, the percentage of overweight or obese female patients increased by 34.8% (8.7% before surgery vs. 43.5% after surgery), while that of men increased by 12% (42% before vs. 54% after surgery). In this context, it is also important to assess the changes in body composition after STN-DBS.

We found that the average percentage reduction in BFMDRS-MS was 69.76 ± 33.23%. However, the baseline BFMDRS-MS and percentage change in BFMDRS-MS were not associated with WG. There are three possible explanations for this result. First, BFMDRS-MS evaluates not only the limbs and trunk but also the eyes, the mouth, speech, swallowing, and the neck; thus, the affected body part may not be associated with resting EE (REE). There were only three patients with low weight before the operation, which may also indicate that the slight movement disorder before the operation had little effect on the patients' REE. Second, patients were able to perform larger movements and were more mobile after the operation than before the operation, which should theoretically increase EE. This may offset the reduced EE caused by improved motor symptoms. Of course, since we did not evaluate the free-living EE in a calorimetric chamber, the decrease in total daily EE due to the reduction in dyskinesias is uncertain. Third, we regrouped the patients three times (according to the distribution of the dystonia, dyskinesias, and involvement of the eyelids) and analyzed the subgroups separately. There were no differences in the percentage change of postoperative BMI and BFMDRS-MS between subgroups. Initially, we assumed that there would be no difference in postoperative physical activity in patients with involvement of only the eyelids before and after surgery and that there would be no difference in REE or free-living EE before and after surgery in this subgroup. However, the BMI of these patients differed before and after surgery. Therefore, the observed WG

TABLE 6 | Clinical and demographic predictors of changes in BMI after surgery.

	Coefficient	Standard error	Beta	*t*	*P*
Sex	5.115	2.200	0.310	2.325	0.025*
Pre-surgical BMI	−0.913	0.360	−0.339	−2.540	0.015*

*BMI, body mass index. *$P < 0.05$.*

may result from changes in the central regulation of energy metabolism caused by STN-DBS. Concerning WG after STN-DBS in patients with PD, various studies have discovered no correlation between WG and changes in the Unified Parkinson Disease Rating Scale III score (28, 29). For future studies, it will be important to measure REE and free-living EE. Moreover, the reduction in EE may be due to the reduction in sustained or intermittent muscle contractions; however, changes in the central regulation of energy metabolism caused by direct STN-DBS may also be involved.

Indeed, previous studies have illustrated that a change in body weight is the direct result of STN-DBS on the regulation of the dietary and metabolic nucleus (in the lateral region of the thalamus and the marginal portion of the STN) (30–34). STN-DBS may have a regional effect on the hypothalamic–pituitary–adrenal homeostatic control of EE by diffusion of the electrical pulse to the hypothalamus (35, 36). Results of the direct effects of STN-DBS on hypothalamic catabolic/anabolic regulators including blood cortisol (36), ghrelin, neuropeptide Y, and leptin peptides (37–39) remain inconsistent and require further study. Therefore, the improvement of motor symptoms in dystonia is insufficient to explain WG after STN-DBS.

The balance between energy intake and EE determines weight change. However, there are no data on the difference in pre- and postoperative energy intake for STD-DBS in patients with isolated dystonia. Notably, a number of researchers have observed that WG after STN-DBS in patients with PD could result from increased sensitivity to food reward cues (40) and changes in eating behavior, including higher food intake, increased appetite, binge eating, or cravings (41–45). However, there have also been reports of no significant changes in the quality or quantity of daily food intake after surgery (41, 46). These inconsistencies could be explained by inaccuracies in food intake measurements. Patients with PD display a large amount of interindividual variation of non-motor symptoms including autonomic dysfunction, olfactory hypoxia, mood disturbances, sleep disorders, and gastrointestinal dysfunction. However, the association of non-motor symptoms with body weight and daily food intake in patients with PD has not been confirmed, and findings have often been contradictory (47, 48). Patients with dystonia also show non-motor symptoms including pain, cognitive, and sleep disturbances (8); therefore, the association between non-motor symptoms and weight change in patients with dystonia deserves further study.

The limitations of the current study include its retrospective study design and the absence of a control group. As this was a retrospective study, relevant preoperative data (hormonal and dietary diaries represent) are not available. We did not prospectively collect the patients' movement scores and BMI information during multiple follow-ups. Despite the follow-up time in our study, ranging from 4 to 83 months, previous studies have revealed that patients with isolated dystonia can achieve near-maximum improvement in motor scores and remain relatively stable for 3 months after STN-DBS (13). Despite a wide age range and different follow-up times, the one-way ANOVA showed no difference in the percentage change in BMI, BFMDRS-MS, and BFMDRS-DS in different subgroups. Nevertheless, the conclusions that can be drawn from this study are limited by the heterogeneity of isolated dystonia, age range of patients, and follow-up time. In the future, a larger sample size is required to study weight change after STN-DBS in patients with isolated dystonia, as well as to explore the mechanisms underlying WG after treatment. Also, due to the heterogeneity of isolated dystonia and the relatively small number of dystonia patients, we do not have data on the GPI-DBS matching STN-DBS group. Therefore, we did not use the GPI-DBS treatment group as the control group. Interestingly, the WG in patients with PD after STN-DBS was more significant than that in patients with PD after GPI-DBS (22).

Large-scale systematic studies are required to determine the reasons for postoperative weight change. Future studies should also focus on changes in non-motor symptoms, food intake, and EE (resting/free-living) after STN-DBS in patients with isolated dystonia. In addition, those patients in whom sustained or intermittent muscle contractions has little to no effect on the range of physical activity (such as those with dystonia involving only the eyelids) warrant further study. Such patients may be better disease models for studying weight change after STN-DBS. Their postoperative REE and free-living EE should be similar before and after STN-DBS, which should help elucidate reasons (such as changes in energy metabolism caused by direct stimulation), other than the improvement of motor symptoms, that lead to postprocedural weight change.

CONCLUSIONS

To our knowledge, this is the first report to investigate changes in body weight after STN-DBS in patients with isolated dystonia. We found that STN-DBS is an effective treatment to relieve symptoms of isolated dystonia, but that it may cause postoperative WG, especially in female patients. Such WG was correlated with preoperative weight, but not to DBS treatment efficacy of, for example, motor symptoms. Clinical teams must be more careful in choosing STN as a therapeutic target for DBS in patients with dystonia who are overweight or obese, especially women. Although this is the first case investigating change in body weight after STN-DBS in patients with isolated dystonia, more studies and long-term follow-ups are needed to determine the mechanisms underlying WG after STN-DBS operation.

ETHICS STATEMENT

The studies involving human participants were reviewed and approved by the ethical committee of Ruijin Hospital. The patients/participants provided their written informed consent to participate in this study.

AUTHOR CONTRIBUTIONS

WH: research project execution, statistical analysis design and execution, and manuscript writing of the first draft. HL: research project execution, and statistical analysis execution. YL and YuW: statistical analysis design and execution. YiW: research project conception and organization, statistical analysis design, review, critique, and manuscript review and critique. AR-Z: research project conception and organization, statistical analysis design, review, critique, and manuscript review and critique. WY and CZ: research project conception and organization, statistical analysis design, review, critique, and manuscript review and critique. All authors contributed to the article and approved the submitted version.

ACKNOWLEDGMENTS

We thank all of the participants who took part in our study.

REFERENCES

1. Okun MS. Deep-brain stimulation for parkinson's disease. *N Engl J Med.* (2012) 367:1529–38. doi: 10.1056/NEJMct1208070
2. Koeglsperger T, Palleis C, Hell F, Mehrkens JH, Bötzel K. Deep brain stimulation programming for movement disorders: current concepts and evidence-Based strategies. *Front Neurol.* (2019) 10:410. doi: 10.3389/fneur.2019.00410
3. Zhou H, Wang L, Zhang C, Qiu X, Hu W, van der Stelt O, et al. Acute effects of subthalamic deep brain stimulation on motor outcomes in parkinson's disease; 13 year follow up. *Front Neurol.* (2019) 10:689. doi: 10.3389/fneur.2019.00689
4. Ramirez-Zamora A, Ostrem JL. Globus pallidus interna or subthalamic nucleus deep brain stimulation for parkinson disease: a review.

JAMA Neurol. (2018) 75:367–72. doi: 10.1001/jamaneurol.2017.4321

5. Zhang J, Wang T, Zhang CC, Zeljic K, Zhan S, Sun BM, et al. The safety issues and hardware-related complications of deep brain stimulation therapy: a single-center retrospective analysis of 478 patients with parkinson's disease. *Clin Interv Aging.* (2017) 12:923–8. doi: 10.2147/CIA.S130882
6. Guimarães J, Matos E, Rosas MJ, Vieira-Coelho A, Borges N, Correia F, et al. Modulation of nutritional state in parkinsonian patients with bilateral subthalamic nucleus stimulation. *J. Neurol.* (2009) 256:2072–8. doi: 10.1007/s00415-009-5252-x
7. Fasano A, Daniele A, Albanese A. Treatment of motor and non-motor features of parkinson's disease with deep brain stimulation. *Lancet Neurol.* (2012) 11:429–42. doi: 10.1016/S1474-4422(12)70049-2
8. Eggink H, Szlufik S, Coenen MA, van Egmond ME, Moro E, Tijssen MAJ. Non-motor effects of deep brain stimulation in dystonia: a systematic review. *Parkinsonism Relat Disord.* (2018) 55:26–44. doi: 10.1016/j.parkreldis.2018.06.024
9. Steinhardt J, Münte TF, Schmid SM, Wilms B, Brüggemann N. A systematic review of body mass gain after deep brain stimulation of the subthalamic nucleus in patients with parkinson's disease. *Obes Rev.* (2020) 21:e12955. doi: 10.1111/obr.12955
10. Albanese A, Bhatia K, Bressman SB, Delong MR, Fahn S, Fung VSC, et al. Phenomenology and classification of dystonia: a consensus update. *Mov Disord.* (2013) 28:863–73. doi: 10.1002/mds.25475
11. Defazio G. The epidemiology of primary dystonia: current evidence and perspectives. *Eur J Neurol.* (2010) 17 Suppl. 1:9–14. doi: 10.1111/j.1468-1331.2010.03053.x
12. Liu Y, Zhu G, Jiang Y, Wang X, Chen Y, Meng F, et al. Comparison of short-Term stimulation of the globus pallidus interna and subthalamic nucleus for treatment of primary dystonia. *World Neurosurg.* (2019) 123:e211–e7. doi: 10.1016/j.wneu.2018.11.137
13. Lin S, Wu Y, Li H, Zhang C, Wang T, Pan Y, et al. Deep brain stimulation of the globus pallidus internus versus the subthalamic nucleus in isolated dystonia. *J Neurosurg.* (2019) 2019:1–12. doi: 10.3171/2018.12.JNS181927
14. Balint B, Mencacci NE, Valente EM, Pisani A, Rothwell J, Jankovic J, et al. Dystonia. *Nat Rev.* (2018) 4:25. doi: 10.1038/s41572-018-0039-y
15. Deng ZD, Li DY, Zhang CC, Pan YX, Zhang J, Jin H, et al. Long-term follow-up of bilateral subthalamic deep brain stimulation for refractory tardive dystonia. *Parkinsonism Relat. Disord.* (2017) 41:58–65. doi: 10.1016/j.parkreldis.2017.05.010
16. Ostrem JL, Racine CA, Glass GA, Grace JK, Volz MM, Heath SL, et al. Subthalamic nucleus deep brain stimulation in primary cervical dystonia. *Neurology.* (2011) 76:870–8. doi: 10.1212/WNL.0b013e31820f2e4f
17. Schjerling L, Hjermind LE, Jespersen B, Madsen FF, Brennum J, Jensen SR, et al. A randomized double-blind crossover trial comparing subthalamic and pallidal deep brain stimulation for dystonia. *J Neurosurg.* (2013) 119:1537–45. doi: 10.3171/2013.8.JNS13844
18. Cao C, Pan Y, Li D, Zhan S, Zhang J, Sun B. Subthalamus deep brain stimulation for primary dystonia patients: a long-term follow-up study. *Mov Disord.* (2013) 28:1877–82. doi: 10.1002/mds.25586
19. Ostrem JL, San Luciano M, Dodenhoff KA, Ziman N, Markun LC, Racine CA, et al. Subthalamic nucleus deep brain stimulation in isolated dystonia: a 3-year follow-up study. *Neurology.* (2017) 88:25–35. doi: 10.1212/WNL.0000000000003451
20. Zhan S, Sun F, Pan Y, Liu W, Huang P, Cao C, et al. Bilateral deep brain stimulation of the subthalamic nucleus in primary meige syndrome. *J Neurosurg.* (2018) 128:897–902. doi: 10.3171/2016.12.JNS16383
21. Xu W, Li H, Zhang C, Sun B, Wu Y, Li D. Subthalamic nucleus stimulation in pediatric isolated dystonia: a 10-Year follow-up. *Can J Neurol Sci.* (2020) 47:328–35. doi: 10.1017/cjn.2020.32
22. Mills KA, Scherzer R, Starr PA, Ostrem JL. Weight change after globus pallidus internus or subthalamic nucleus deep brain stimulation in parkinson's disease and dystonia. *Stereotact Funct Neurosurg.* (2012) 90:386–93. doi: 10.1159/000340071
23. Shetty AS, Bhatia KP, Lang AE. Dystonia and parkinson's disease: what is the relationship? *Neurobiol Dis.* (2019) 132:104462. doi: 10.1016/j.nbd.2019.05.001
24. Sun B, Chen S, Zhan S, Le W, Krahl SE. Subthalamic nucleus stimulation for primary dystonia and tardive dystonia. *Acta Neurochir Suppl.* (2007) 97:207–14. doi: 10.1007/978-3-211-33081-4_23
25. Zhu D, Chung HF, Pandeya N, Dobson AJ, Kuh D, Crawford SL, et al. Body mass index and age at natural menopause: an international pooled analysis of 11 prospective studies. *Eur. J. Epidemiol.* (2018) 33:699–710. doi: 10.1007/s10654-018-0367-y
26. Foubert-Samier A, Maurice S, Hivert S, Guelh D, Rigalleau V, Burbaud P, et al. A long-term follow-up of weight changes in subthalamic nucleus stimulated parkinson's disease patients. *Rev Neurol.* (2012) 168:173–6. doi: 10.1016/j.neurol.2011.04.006
27. Macia F, Perlemoine C, Coman I, Guehl D, Burbaud P, Cuny E, et al. Parkinson's disease patients with bilateral subthalamic deep brain stimulation gain weight. *Mov Disord.* (2004) 19:206–12. doi: 10.1002/mds.10630
28. Montaurier C, Morio B, Bannier S, Derost P, Arnaud P, Brandolini-Bunlon M, et al. Mechanisms of body weight gain in patients with parkinson's disease after subthalamic stimulation. *Brain.* (2007) 130:1808–18. doi: 10.1093/brain/awm113
29. Locke MC, Wu SS, Foote KD, Sassi M, Jacobson CE, Rodriguez RL, et al. Weight changes in subthalamic nucleus vs globus pallidus internus deep brain stimulation: results from the cOMPARE parkinson disease deep brain stimulation cohort. *Neurosurgery.* (2011) 68:1233–7; discussion 7–8. doi: 10.1227/NEU.0b013e31820b52c5
30. Berthoud HR. Multiple neural systems controlling food intake and body weight. *Neurosci Biobehav Rev.* (2002) 26:393–428. doi: 10.1016/S0149-7634(02)00014-3
31. Haegelen C, Rouaud T, Darnault P, Morandi X. The subthalamic nucleus is a key-structure of limbic basal ganglia functions. *Med Hypotheses.* (2009) 72:421–6. doi: 10.1016/j.mehy.2008.07.065
32. Lardeux S, Pernaud R, Paleressompoulle D, Baunez C. Beyond the reward pathway: coding reward magnitude and error in the rat subthalamic nucleus. *J Neurophysiol.* (2009) 102:2526–37. doi: 10.1152/jn.91009.2008
33. Rouaud T, Lardeux S, Panayotis N, Paleressompoulle D, Cador M, Baunez C. Reducing the desire for cocaine with subthalamic nucleus deep brain stimulation. *Proc Natl Acad Sci USA.* (2010) 107:1196–200. doi: 10.1073/pnas.0908189107
34. Wise RA. Forebrain substrates of reward and motivation. *J Comp Neurol.* (2005) 493:115–21. doi: 10.1002/cne.20689
35. Lipp A, Tank J, Trottenberg T, Kupsch A, Arnold G, Jordan J. Sympathetic activation due to deep brain stimulation in the region of the sTN. *Neurology.* (2005) 65:774–5. doi: 10.1212/01.wnl.0000174436.36399.ca
36. RuŽička E, Nováková L, Jech R, Urgošík D, RuŽička F, Haluzík M. Decrease in blood cortisol corresponds to weight gain following deep brain stimulation of the subthalamic nucleus in parkinson's disease. *Stereot Funct Neurosurg.* (2012) 90:410–1. doi: 10.1159/000341707
37. Escamilla-Sevilla F, Pérez-Navarro MJ, Muñoz-Pasadas M, Sáez-Zea C, Jouma-Katati M, Piédrola-Maroto G, et al. Change of the melanocortin system caused by bilateral subthalamic nucleus stimulation in parkinson's disease. *Acta Neurol Scand.* (2011) 124:275–81. doi: 10.1111/j.1600-0404.2010.01469.x
38. Markaki E, Ellul J, Kefalopoulou Z, Trachani E, Theodoropoulou A, Kyriazopoulou V, et al. The role of ghrelin, neuropeptide y and leptin peptides in weight gain after deep brain stimulation for parkinson's disease. *Stereotact Funct Neurosurg.* (2012) 90:104–12. doi: 10.1159/000335045
39. Novakova L, Haluzik M, Jech R, Urgosik D, Ruzicka F, Ruzicka E. Hormonal regulators of food intake and weight gain in parkinson's disease after subthalamic nucleus stimulation. *Neuro Endocrinol Lett.* (2011) 32:437–41.
40. Aiello M, Eleopra R, Foroni F, Rinaldo S, Rumiati RI. Weight gain after sTN-DBS: the role of reward sensitivity and impulsivity. *Cortex.* (2017) 92:150–61. doi: 10.1016/j.cortex.2017.04.005
41. Barichella M, Marczewska AM, Mariani C, Landi A, Vairo A, Pezzoli G. Body weight gain rate in patients with parkinson's disease and deep brain stimulation. *Mov Disord.* (2003) 18:1337–40. doi: 10.1002/mds.10543
42. Castrioto A, Lhommée E, Moro E, Krack P. Mood and behavioural effects of subthalamic stimulation in parkinson's disease. *Lancet.* (2014) 13:287–305. doi: 10.1016/S1474-4422(13)70294-1

43. Sauleau P, Le Jeune F, Drapier S, Houvenaghel JF, Dondaine T, Haegelen C, et al. Weight gain following subthalamic nucleus deep brain stimulation: a pET study. *Mov Disord.* (2014) 29:1781–7. doi: 10.1002/mds.26063
44. Serranová T, Jech R, Dušek P, Sieger T, RuŽička F, Urgošík D, et al. Subthalamic nucleus stimulation affects incentive salience attribution in parkinson's disease. *Mov Disord.* (2011) 26:2260–6. doi: 10.1002/mds.23880
45. Serranová T, Sieger T, Dušek P, RuŽička F, Urgošík D, RuŽička E, et al. Sex, food and threat: startling changes after subthalamic stimulation in parkinson's disease. *Brain Stimul.* (2013) 6:740–5. doi: 10.1016/j.brs.2013.03.009
46. Tuite PJ, Maxwell RE, Ikramuddin S, Kotz CM, Kotzd CM, Billington CJ, et al. Weight and body mass index in parkinson's disease patients after deep brain stimulation surgery. *Parkinson Rel Disord.* (2005) 11:247–52. doi: 10.1016/j.parkreldis.2005.01.006
47. Aiello M, Eleopra R, Rumiati RI. Body weight and food intake in parkinson's disease. A review of the association to non-motor symptoms. *Appetite.* (2015) 84:204–11. doi: 10.1016/j.appet.2014.10.011
48. Fabbri M, Guedes LC, Coelho M, Simão D, Abreu D, Rosa MM, et al. Subthalamic deep brain stimulation effects on odor identification in parkinson's disease. *Eur J Neurol.* (2015) 22:207–10. doi: 10.1111/ene.12396

18

Evolution of Globus Pallidus Targeting for Parkinson's and Dystonia Deep Brain Stimulation: A 15-Year Experience

Vanessa M. Holanda [1], Robert Stephen Eisinger [2], Leonardo Almeida [2], Takashi Tsuboi [3], Huimin Wang [2], Michael S. Okun [2], Wissam Deeb [4], Addie Patterson [2], Aparna Wagle Shukla [2], Janine Lobo Lopes [2] and Kelly Douglas Foote [2]*

[1] Department of Neurosurgery, Center of Neurology and Neurosurgery Associates (NeuroCENNA), Beneficencia Portuguesa of São Paulo Hospital, São Paulo, Brazil, [2] Department of Neurology, Norman Fixel Institute for Neurological Diseases, University of Florida Health, Gainesville, FL, United States, [3] Department of Neurology, Nagoya University, Nagoya, Japan, [4] Department of Neurology, University of Massachusetts Medical School, Worcester, MA, United States

***Correspondence:**
Janine Lobo Lopes
janinelobolopes@ufl.edu

Objective: The aim of this study is to evaluate the evolution of GPi DBS targeting.

Methods: This retrospective, single-center study included patients implanted with GPi DBS leads for dystonia or PD during the years 2004 to 2018 at the University of Florida Fixel Institute for Neurological Diseases. Each patient underwent a high-resolution targeting study on the day prior to the surgery, which was fused with a high resolution CT scan that was acquired on the day of the procedure. Intraoperative target location was selected using a digitized 3D Schaltenbrand-Bailey atlas. All patients underwent a high-resolution head CT scan without contrast approximately one month after lead implantation and accurate measurement of neuroanatomical lead position was acquired after fusion of pre-operative and post-operative image studies.

Results: We analyzed 253 PD patients with 352 leads and 80 dystonia patients with 141 leads. During 15 years of follow-up, lead locations in the PD group migrated more laterally ($\beta = 0.09$, $p < 0.0001$), posteriorly [slope (β) = 0.04, $p < 0.05$], and dorsally ($\beta = 0.07$, $p < 0.001$), whereas leads in the dystonia group did not significantly change position aside from a trend in the dorsal direction ($\beta = 0.06$, $p = 0.053$).

Conclusion: The evolving target likely results from multiple factors including improvements in targeting techniques and clinical feedback intraoperatively and post-operatively. Our demonstrates the potential importance of a systematic post-operative DBS lead measurement protocol to ensure quality control and to inform and optimize DBS programming.

Keywords: deep brain stimulation, globus pallidus, targeting, dystonia, Parkinson's disease

INTRODUCTION

Deep brain stimulation (DBS) is a surgical therapy that uses a neurostimulator and one or multiple brain leads to modulate specific neural circuits (1). Modulation of the globus pallidus internus (GPi) is a well-established and highly effective therapeutic option for appropriately selected patients with Parkinson's disease (PD) and for patients with severe dystonia that is refractory to optimized medical therapy (2, 3). GPI DBS has the potential to improve both hypokinetic and hyperkinetic disorders (4). Although the antiparkinsonian effects of GPi DBS are well recognized, there remains debate about the underlying therapeutic mechanism (5) and the ideal position for lead implantation within the target. The posterolateral, somatosensory region of the GPi has been one of the most consistently utilized areas and has shown robust benefits across studies (3, 6, 7).

Despite established efficacy and safety, the clinical response to DBS may at times be variable among patients and dependent on a variety of factors including patient selection, appropriate target selection, and adequate surgical planning. Okun et al. (2005) evaluated causes of DBS failures in patients referred to tertiary movement disorders centers (8). Nearly half of the patients had sub optimally placed DBS electrodes, and 17% had leads that were not programmable. Half of the cohort required lead revision (8). Although several factors may influence lead placement, appropriate surgical planning is critical to the process.

In both PD and dystonia, accurate DBS targeting is a primary determinant of outcomes (9) and the evolution of improved direct targeting techniques over the last two decades has provided more effective stimulation with fewer side effects. The aim of this study is to evaluate the evolution of GPi DBS targeting over time through analysis of a large, single-center cohort.

METHODS

This is an IRB-approved, retrospective, single-center study including patients implanted with GPi DBS leads for dystonia or PD during the years 2004–2018 at the University of Florida Fixel Institute for Neurological Diseases. Informed consent was obtained. We confirm that we have read the Journal's position on issues involved in ethical publication and affirm that this work is consistent with those guidelines.

The standard-of-care surgical approach has been previously described by our group (10). On the day prior to the surgery, each patient underwent a high-resolution 3 Tesla MRI direct targeting study. The image study included a Gadolinium enhanced MPRAGE sequence and a Fast Gray Matter Acquisition T1 Inversion Recovery sequence (FGATIR), which was introduced in 2009. On the day of the procedure, a high resolution CT scan was acquired after the Cosman-Roberts-Wells (CRW) frame was attached to the patient's head. Both the MRI and the CT images were fused and intraoperative target location was selected using a digitized Schaltenbrand-Bailey atlas (11). The atlas was manually fitted to each patient's pre-operative imaging using three-dimensional (3D) scaling, shifting, and rotating. All patients underwent a high-resolution head CT scan without contrast approximately 1 month after implantation. This image study was fused to the pre-operative targeting MRI, which allowed accurate measurement of neuroanatomical lead position. Planned and measured lead positions were reverse normalized based on individual atlas-fits in order to place all leads within the Schaltenbrand-Bailey atlas coordinate space for comparison across patients. We analyzed the PD and dystonia cohorts separately. For analysis, we dropped the sign of the lateral position to combine data from the left and right hemispheres. Absolute error in all three dimensions and 3D Euclidean error was computed.

Data were filtered to remove outliers defined by a z-score greater than or less than three standard deviations away from the mean with respect to the final planned positions or measured positions in the lateral, A-P, and axial dimensions. Correlation analysis was used to identify associations between time (years) and variables of interest including lead positions and errors in final positions. The significance level was set at an alpha of 0.05. The statistical software R was used for all analyses.

RESULTS

Patient Characteristics

A total of 253 PD patients with 352 leads and 80 dystonia patients with 141 leads were included after outlier analysis led to exclusion of 10 patients. Within the PD group, 152 patients had unilateral implants and 101 patients had bilateral implants. Within the dystonia group, 13 patients had unilateral implants and 67 patients had bilateral implants. Ages at the time of surgery were 63.61 +/− 9.12 (M +/− SD) years in the PD group and 44.40 +/− 21.94 years in the dystonia group.

Evolution of the Lead Positioning and Error

During 15 years of follow-up, lead locations in the PD group migrated more laterally (β = 0.09, p < 0.0001; **Figure 1A**), posteriorly [slope (β) = 0.04, p < 0.05; **Figure 1B**], and dorsally (β = 0.07, p < 0.001; **Figure 1C**), whereas leads in the dystonia group did not significantly change position aside from a trend in the dorsal direction (β = 0.06, p = 0.053; **Figures 1D–F**). Similar lateral (β = 0.11, p < 0.0001) and posterior (β = 0.09, p < 0.0001) shifts in the PD group were also found in the intraoperative planned coordinates whereas the axial shift (β = 0.02, p = 0.34) was not. However, the intraoperative planned coordinates for the lateral position in the dystonia group showed a small but significant shift more laterally with time (β = 0.05, p < 0.05).

Absolute error significantly decreased over time in the PD group for the lateral (β = −0.04, p < 0.01; **Figure 2A**), A-P (β = −0.04, p < 0.001; **Figure 2B**), and axial (β = −0.05, p < 0.001; **Figure 2C**) directions leading to a reduction in overall 3D Euclidean error of about 0.08 mm per year (p < 0.0001; **Figure 2D**). In the dystonia group, error did not significantly reduce over time (**Figures 2E–H**). The average lead position from 2004–2006 to 2016–2018 for Parkinson's disease and dystonia in axial, coronal, and sagittal planes was shown in **Supplementary Figure 1**.

DISCUSSION

To our knowledge this is the first study evaluating long-term accuracy and evolution of GPi DBS targeting, though there are many studies evaluating the effectiveness of GPi DBS (12, 13). There is a paucity of data regarding errors in lead location measurement or of errors in surgical placement. It is well known in stereotactic surgery that the further away a target is from the midline, the higher the predicted error may be (14),

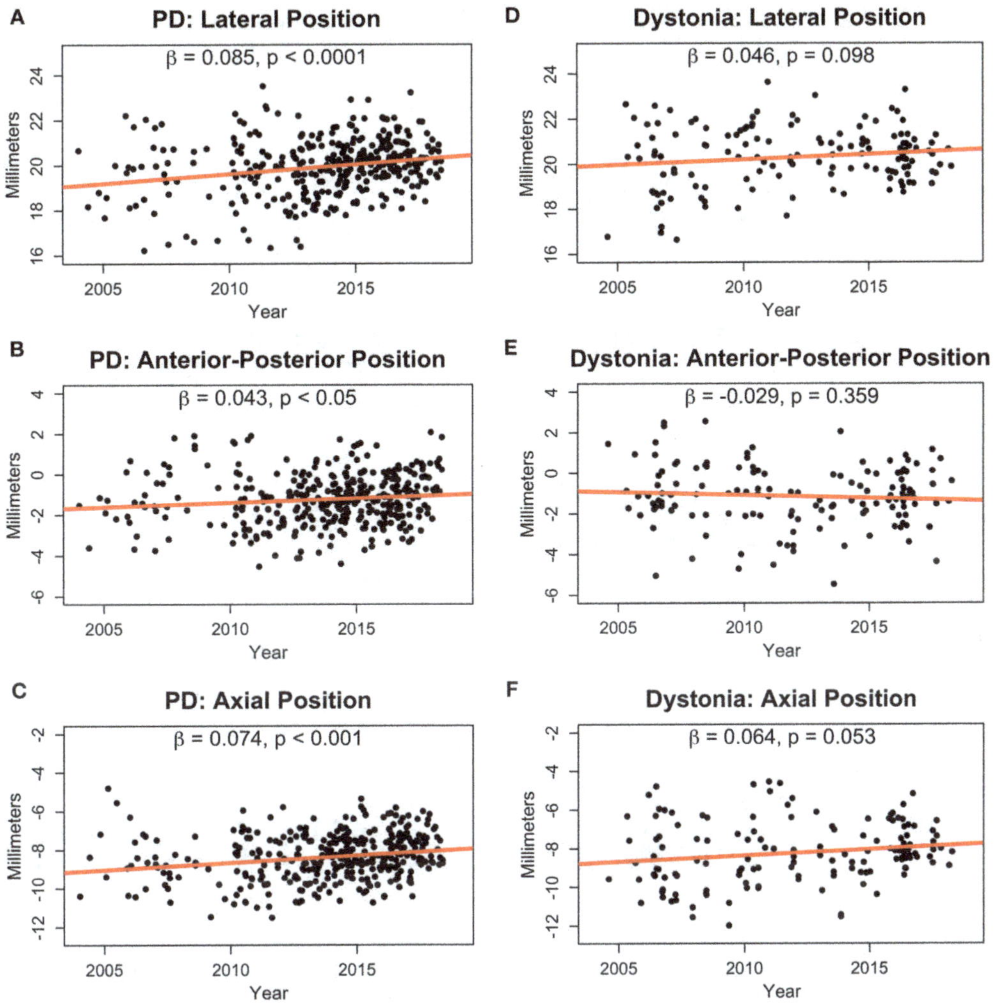

FIGURE 1 | Normalized lead positions in millimeters for PD **(A–C)** and dystonia **(D–F)** patients in the lateral **(A,D)**, anterior-posterior **(B,E)**, and axial **(C,F)** dimensions shown from 2004 to 2018. Slopes (β) and p-values are shown for linear fits in all plots.

especially if the targeting procedure is based only on indirect targeting relative to the mid-commissural point. Improvement of DBS targeting software and high resolution brain imaging [e.g., FGATIR, quantitative susceptibility mapping] has improved our ability to clearly identify and directly target neuroanatomical structures (15–17). The FGATIR sequence was introduced in 2009 and its combination of high resolution (1 x 1 x 1 mm voxel), 1 mm slice thickness and high contrast, enabled better visualization of the GPi borders, leading to a more precise location of the target (15). These improvements have likely contributed to the diminishing rate of GPi-DBS targeting errors during the more recent years of this cohort.

Evolution of the final lead placement may also be a result of technique refinement, including reasons beyond the advent of high-resolution MRI. For instance, clinical feedback from outpatient programming sessions may play a role as lateral placement decreases the likelihood of inadvertent internal capsule stimulation and widens the therapeutic window for DBS programming, an aspect particularly important in dystonia patients, who often require larger volumes of tissue activation to control their symptoms chronically (18). These patients are also more prone to stimulation-induced side effects. In addition, dystonia patients may require DBS earlier and require it for a longer time given the younger mean age at implantation. Dystonia patients commonly require higher settings and higher charge densities over time for chronic symptom control (19–22). This is the largest study to examine the evolution of GPi targeting over a period of 15 years, and it reinforces the potential importance of an interdisciplinary team and the clinical feedback directed from neurologists to neurosurgeons. We highlight that during these 15 years, there was consistency in our team in terms of senior neurosurgeon and senior neurology programmer. Clinical feedback relating lead locations to outcomes is particularly important for refining lead placements to maximize benefits while minimizing adverse effects of DBS (23). Surgical teams that do not receive such clinical feedback regarding their patients' post-operative lead locations relative to their clinical outcomes fail to exploit an important tool for DBS quality improvement and will likely have less optimal surgical outcomes.

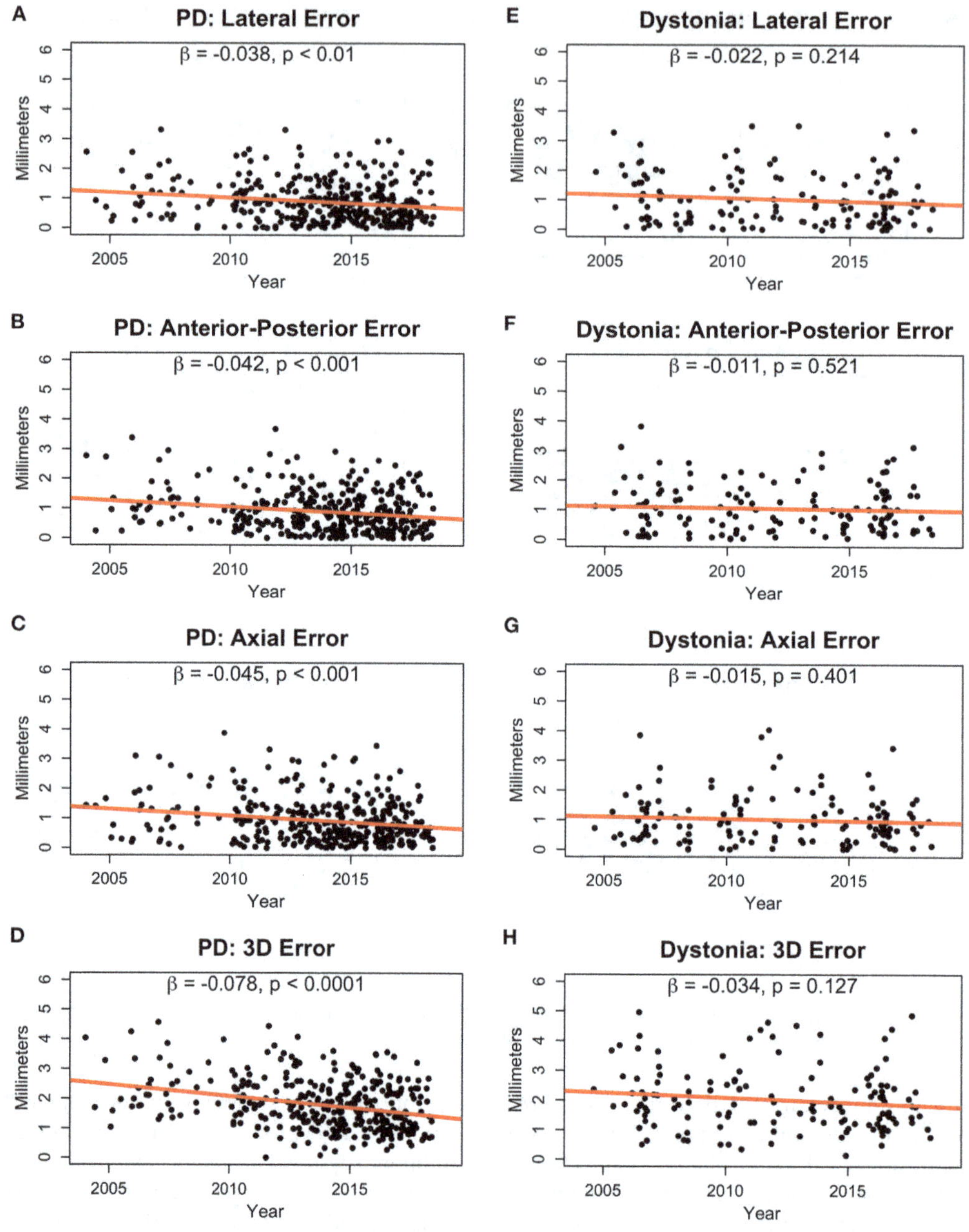

FIGURE 2 | Absolute error in lead positions in millimeters for PD **(A–C)** and dystonia **(E–G)** patients in the lateral **(A,E)**, anterior-posterior **(B,F)**, and axial **(C,G)** dimensions shown from 2004 to 2018. 3D Euclidean distance in the PD **(D)** and dystonia groups **(H)** are also shown. Slopes (β) and p-values are provided for linear fits in all plots.

There are some hypotheses for why the GPi targets moved through the years: (1) For the lateral move, it was mainly related to the neurological team feedback requiring more "room" to work. Over the years, due to the progression of the dystonia and Parkinson's disease, the DBS programming may require amplitude and pulse width increase to control the motor symptoms. (2) For the dorsal move, it could be related to the surgeon's cautious with deep vessels, which are commonly seen inferiorly to the GPi.

There are particular limitations of this analysis that should be mentioned. This is a single center study. As previously described by our group, microelectrode recording (MER) is part of our surgical approach. Thus, adjustments of the coordinates based on MER and intra operative stimulation can play an important role in the final location of the lead. The retrospective nature of the study can introduce bias related to record keeping, though this bias is partially offset by the large number of patients included. The different size of the heads between the patients can be a limitation; however, the planned and measured lead positions were reverse normalized to individual atlas-fits to place all leads within the Schaltenbrand-Bailey atlas coordinate space to enable more meaningful comparison across patients.

In summary, this is the first single tertiary center study to show the longitudinal evolution of targeting in GPi DBS. The evolving target likely results from multiple factors including improvements in targeting techniques and clinical feedback intraoperatively and post-operatively. Our results also demonstrate the potential importance of a systematic post-operative DBS lead measurement protocol to ensure quality control and to inform and optimize DBS programming. More precise targeting of the GPi with patient-specific modeling can potentially predict effectiveness by representing the volume of tissue activated. This strategy can aid in predicting optimal stimulation parameters, more efficiently maximizing therapeutic benefit and reducing adverse effects. Future studies incorporating a larger, multi-center dataset might be useful to corroborate the findings of this analysis and help to establish useful guidelines for improving electrode placement and global outcomes in movement disorders patients.

ETHICS STATEMENT

The studies involving human participants were reviewed and approved by UF Institutional Review Board. The patients/participants provided their written informed consent to participate in this study.

AUTHOR CONTRIBUTIONS

VH: conception, organization and execution of research project, review and critique of statistical analysis, and writing the first draft of the manuscript. RE and TT: conception, organization and execution of research project, design, execution, review and critique of statistical analysis, and writing the first draft of the manuscript. LA: conception, organization and execution of research project, review and critique of statistical analysis, and review and critique of manuscript. HW: execution of research project, design, execution, review and critique of statistical analysis, and writing the first draft of the manuscript. MO and KF: conception of research project, review and critique of statistical analysis, and review and critique of manuscript. WD and AP: organization and execution of research project, review and critique of statistical analysis, and review and critique of manuscript. AW: review and critique of statistical analysis, and review and critique of manuscript. JL: review of manuscript. All authors contributed to the article and approved the submitted version.

ACKNOWLEDGMENTS

All former Movement Disorders fellows at UF who assisted in precise measurements of each patient after DBS surgery. We would like to acknowledge the UF INFORM database and the Parkinson's Foundation Center of Excellence and support from Tyler's Hope for a Dystonia Cure.

REFERENCES

1. Williams NR, Okun MS. Deep brain stimulation (DBS) at the interface of neurology and psychiatry. *J Clin Invest.* (2013) 123:4546–56. doi: 10.1172/JCI68341
2. Odekerken VJ, van Laar T, Staal MJ, Mosch A, Hoffmann CFE, Nijssen PCG, et al. Subthalamic nucleus versus globus pallidus bilateral deep brain stimulation for advanced Parkinson's disease (NSTAPS study): a randomised controlled trial. *The Lancet Neurology.* (2013) 12:37–44. doi: 10.1016/S1474-4422(12)70264-8
3. Barow E, Neumann WJ, Brucke C, Huebl J, Horn A, Brown P, et al. Deep brain stimulation suppresses pallidal low frequency activity in patients with phasic dystonic movements. *Brain: J Neurol.* (2014) 137:3012–24. doi: 10.1093/brain/awu258
4. Udupa K, Chen R. The mechanisms of action of deep brain stimulation and ideas for the future development. *Progress in Neurobiology.* (2015) 133:27–49. doi: 10.1016/j.pneurobio.2015.08.001
5. Lozano AM, Lipsman N. Probing and regulating dysfunctional circuits using deep brain stimulation. *Neuron.* (2013) 77:406–24. doi: 10.1016/j.neuron.2013.01.020
6. Vayssiere N, van der Gaag N, Cif L, Hemm S, Verdier R, Frerebeau P, et al. Deep brain stimulation for dystonia confirming a somatotopic organization in the globus pallidus internus. *J Neurosurg.* (2004) 101:181–8. doi: 10.3171/jns.2004.101.2.0181
7. Vidailhet M, Yelnik J, Lagrange C, Fraix V, Grabli D, Thobois S, et al. Bilateral pallidal deep brain stimulation for the treatment of patients with dystonia-choreoathetosis cerebral palsy: a prospective pilot study. *Lancet Neurol.* (2009) 8:709–17. doi: 10.1016/S1474-4422(09)70151-6
8. Okun MS, Tagliati M, Pourfar M, Fernandez HH, Rodriguez RL, Alterman RL, et al. Management of referred deep brain stimulation failures: a retrospective analysis from 2 movement disorders centers. *Arch Neurol.* (2005) 62:1250–5. doi: 10.1001/archneur.62.8.noc40425
9. Okun MS, Fernandez HH, Wu SS, Darrow LK, Bowers D, Bova F, et al. Cognition and mood in Parkinson's disease in subthalamic nucleus versus globus pallidus interna deep brain stimulation: the COMPARE trial. *Ann Neurol.* (2009) 65:586–95. doi: 10.1002/ana.21596
10. Morishita T, Hilliard JD, Okun MS, Neal D, Nestor KA, Peace D, et al. Postoperative lead migration in deep brain stimulation surgery: Incidence, risk factors, and clinical impact. *PLoS ONE.* (2017) 12. doi: 10.1371/journal.pone.0183711
11. Morishita T, Foote KD, Burdick AP, Katayama Y, Yamamoto T, Frucht SJ, et al. Identification and management of deep brain stimulation intra- and postoperative urgencies and emergencies. *Parkinsonism Relat Disord.* (2010) 16:153–62. doi: 10.1016/j.parkreldis.2009.10.003
12. Sudhyadhom A, Okun MS, Foote KD, Rahman M, Bova FJ, A. Three-dimensional deformable brain atlas for DBS targeting. I methodology for atlas creation and artifact reduction open. *Neuroimag J.* (2012) 6:92–8.
13. Ide S, Kakeda S, Yoneda T, Moriya J, Watanabe K, Ogasawara A, et al. Internal structures of the globus pallidus in patients with parkinson's disease: evaluation with phase difference-enhanced imaging. *Magn Reson Med Sci.* (2016) 16:304–10. doi: 10.2463/mrms.mp.2015-0091
14. Walsh RA, Sidiropoulos C, Lozano AM, Hodaie M, Poon YY, Fallis M, et al. Bilateral pallidal stimulation in cervical dystonia: blinded evidence of benefit beyond 5 years. *Brain: J Neurol.* (2013) 136:761–9. doi: 10.1093/brain/awt009
15. Volkmann J, Mueller J, Deuschl G, Kühn AA, Krauss JK, Poewe W, et al. Pallidal neurostimulation in patients with medication-refractory cervical

dystonia: a randomised, sham-controlled trial. *Lancet Neurol.* (2014) 13:875–84. doi: 10.1016/S1474-4422(14)70143-7

16. Starr PA, Martin AJ, Ostrem JL, Talke P, Levesque N, Larson PS. Subthalamic nucleus deep brain stimulator placement using high-field interventional magnetic resonance imaging and a skull-mounted aiming device: technique and application accuracy. *J Neurosurg.* (2010) 112:479–90. doi: 10.3171/2009.6.JNS081161
17. Sudhyadhom A, Haq IU, Foote KD, Okun MS, Bova FJ. A high resolution and high contrast MRI for differentiation of subcortical structures for DBS targeting: the Fast Gray Matter Acquisition T1 Inversion Recovery (FGATIR). *Neuroimage.* (2009) 47:T44–52. doi: 10.1016/j.neuroimage.2009.04.018
18. Liu T, Eskreis-Winkler S, Schweitzer AD, Chen W, Kaplitt MG, Tsiouris AJ, et al. Improved subthalamic nucleus depiction with quantitative susceptibility mapping. *Radiology.* (2013) 269:216–23. doi: 10.1148/radiol.13121991
19. Gross RE, McDougal ME. Technological advances in the surgical treatment of movement disorders. *Curr Neurol Neurosci Rep.* (2013) 13:371. doi: 10.1007/s11910-013-0371-2
20. Vidailhet M, Vercueil L, Houeto JL, Krystkowiak P, Benabid AL, Cornu P, et al. Bilateral deep-brain stimulation of the globus pallidus in primary generalized dystonia. *N Engl J Med.* (2005) 352:459–67. doi: 10.1056/NEJMoa042187
21. Rawal PV, Almeida L, Smelser LB, Huang H, Guthrie BL, Walker HC. Shorter pulse generator longevity and more frequent stimulator adjustments with pallidal DBS for dystonia versus other movement disorders. *Brain Stimul.* (2014) 7:345–9. doi: 10.1016/j.brs.2014.01.008
22. Almeida L, Martinez-Ramirez D, Ahmed B, Deeb W, Jesus SD, Skinner J, et al. A pilot trial of square biphasic pulse deep brain stimulation for dystonia: The BIP dystonia study. *J Mov Disord.* (2017) 32:615–8. doi: 10.1002/mds.26906
23. Yianni J, Nandi D, Shad A, Bain P, Gregory R, Aziz T. Increased risk of lead fracture and migration in dystonia compared with other movement disorders following deep brain stimulation. *J Clin Neurosci.* (2004) 11:243–5. doi: 10.1016/j.jocn.2003.10.003

19

The Efficacy of Intraoperative Passive Language Mapping for Glioma Surgery

Kohei Kanaya [1,2], Takumi Mitsuhashi [3], Takafumi Kiuchi [2] and Sumio Kobayashi [2]*

[1] Department of Neurosurgery, Shinshu University School of Medicine, Matsumoto, Japan, [2] Department of Neurosurgery, Iida Municipal Hospital, Nagano, Japan, [3] Department of Neurosurgery, Juntendo University, Tokyo, Japan

***Correspondence:**
Kohei Kanaya
kanaya@shinshu-u.ac.jp

Background: Recently, electrocorticographic (ECoG) studies have emphasized the importance of gamma band-based functional mapping in the presurgical localization of the eloquent cortex. Passive functional mapping using ECoG signals provides a reliable method for identifying receptive language areas without many of the risks and limitations associated with electrical cortical stimulation. We report a surgical case of left temporal malignant glioma with intraoperative passive language mapping.

Case Description: A 78-year-old woman was diagnosed with left temporal glioma with inspection of her language difficulty. MRI showed a left temporal tumor measuring 74.6 × 50.0 × 51.5 mm in size. Real-time CortiQ-based mapping using high-gamma activity by word-listening and story-listening tasks was performed. Significant listening task-evoked high gamma activities were detected in 5 channels in the superior temporal gyrus and one channel in the middle temporal gyrus. The tumor was grossly removed except for the region corresponding to listening task-evoked high gamma activities. Postoperatively, the patient's symptoms of language comprehension difficulty improved, and no new neurological deficits were observed.

Conclusion: Intraoperative passive language mapping was successfully performed, and the patient's language function was well-preserved. Intraoperative passive language mapping, which is applicable in a short time and under general anesthesia, can be an important tool for detecting language areas.

Keywords: cortiq, awake craniotomy, intraoperative passive language mapping, real-time, high-gamma activity, glioma

INTRODUCTION

Electrical cortical stimulation (ECS) mapping remains the gold standard for presurgical localization of brain function (1). Awake craniotomy is the only established method to intraoperatively verify the preservation of language function (2); however, precise functional mapping is still difficult in patients with language deficits (3). ECS has shortcomings, as it is time-consuming and may evoke after-discharges or seizures (4).

Recently, electrocorticographic (ECoG) studies have emphasized the importance of gamma band-based functional mapping in the presurgical localization of the eloquent cortex (5). Passive ECoG-based mapping is set to become one of the most important novel tools in presurgical functional mapping (4).

We report an elderly patient with left temporal glioma evaluated with intraoperative passive language mapping. Tumor removal was successfully performed, preserving her language function.

CASE DESCRIPTION

Initial Presentation

A previously healthy 78-year-old woman noticed a worsening of language difficulty and visited our hospital. CT showed a calcified lesion on the left temporal lobe (**Figure 1A**), and MRI revealed an intra-axial tumor showing high T2 signal and heterogeneous enhancement and a cystic component located medially (**Figures 1B,C**). The tumor was located in the inferior temporal and middle temporal regions and the fusiform gyrus and 74.6 × 50.0 × 51.5 mm (AP × LR × HT) in size. Preoperative fMRI could not show the Wernicke area clearly because of the large tumor and perifocal edema. Preoperatively, she had fluent aphasia, naming disorder, and difficulty in language comprehension.

Awake craniotomy was abandoned as a possibility considering her aphasia and age. Tumor removal with passive language mapping under general anesthesia was planned to remove as much of the tumor as possible to preserve her language function.

Intraoperative Passive Language Mapping and Surgery

We used a 20-channel ECoG grid with a 3-mm electrode diameter and a 10-mm interelectrode distance (Unique Medical), together with 4-channel strip electrodes. The exposed brain surface and grid were captured by a digital camera before resection (**Figures 2A,B**). Real-time CortiQ-based mapping (g.tec medication engineering GmbH, Austria) using high-gamma activity by word-listening (e.g., moon, book, flog, cake, etc.,) and Japanese story-listening tasks was performed. The listening tasks were delivered without sound for 20 s (rest phase) and then delivered sounds for 20 s (active phase). The active phase was composed of meaning and meaningless sounds. The rest and active phases were repeated alternately six times. The sampling rate was 1,200 Hz with a g.HIamp (g.tec medical engineering GmbH, Austria). The analysis was performed by MATLAB 2015a at 60–90 and 110–140 Hz, and over 25% task/rest band power was defined as significant. Anesthesia was maintained with propofol, muscle relaxant, and fentanyl. A bispectral index (BIS) monitor was used to assess the depth of anesthesia and it was maintained with a high BIS level (70–90) during passive language mapping. Significant listening task-evoked high gamma activities were detected (**Figure 2C**). We analyzed 5 channels in the superior temporal gyrus and one channel in the middle temporal gyrus that were most meaningful for the auditory and Wernicke areas (**Figure 3A**). The tumor was totally removed except for the region corresponding to the listening task-evoked high gamma activities in the middle temporal gyrus and was suspected to be a lower-grade glioma (**Figure 3B**).

Postoperative Course

The patient's postoperative course was uneventful, and her symptoms of language comprehension difficulty improved, although, her naming disorder was unchanged. Postoperative MRI showed gross total resection of the enhancing component (**Figure 4**). A diagnosis of anaplastic oligodendroglioma (WHO grade 3) was made, and postoperative irradiation and chemotherapy (temozolomide) were performed. She was followed for 1 year without any new neurological deficits or radiological signs of recurrence.

DISCUSSION

ECS has been the gold standard for functional mapping for decades (4). It is widely accepted that the application of conventional ECS methods produces specific and reliable outcomes at defined sites and that neurosurgical resective strategies guided by this method can eliminate or minimize sensorimotor and linguistic postoperative deficits (6, 7). Awake craniotomy is usually performed in patients aged 15–65 years, although, awake craniotomy is not only specified by age (8). Recently, there have been some reports that awake craniotomy can be successfully performed for elderly and younger patients (9–11); however, the procedure can be difficult to apply for patients with severe aphasia, intellectual disability, or psychiatric disorders, and elderly and younger patients who cannot tolerate awake craniotomy (12, 13). Furthermore, ECS has noteworthy limitations that include substantial time requirements (14, 15) and an increased risk for induced pathological brain activity, such as after-discharges or seizures (16, 17).

Gamma oscillation may be induced by synchronized activity of γ-aminobutyric acidergic (GABAergic) interneurons in the population network playing an important role in controlling the timing of action potential generation in pyramidal cells (18–21). Several researches have revealed that gamma-band power is positively correlated with neuronal firing rates (22–24).

Tamura et al. reported that the dynamics of oscillatory neuronal activity on ECoG have been proposed as potential neurophysiological indicators. Among these oscillatory changes, augmentation of high gamma activity from ∼60 to 140 Hz was assumed to reflect localized cortical processing. Therefore, high gamma activity may be a strong candidate for an index of local cortical activation, and passive language mapping has possibilities of detecting physiological mechanisms related to language in the human brain (3).

Swift et al. reported that the qualitative comparison between cortical sites identified by ECoG and ECS shows a high concordance. However, the authors emphasized that it is important to evaluate language function by not only ECoG mapping but also other modalities, such as ECS, although, passive functional mapping using ECoG signals provides a fast, robust, and reliable method for identifying receptive language areas without many of the risks and limitations associated with ECS (4).

Wang et al. reported that electrode sites showing task-related high-gamma augmentation were spatially concordant with, but more extensive than, the language areas suggested by

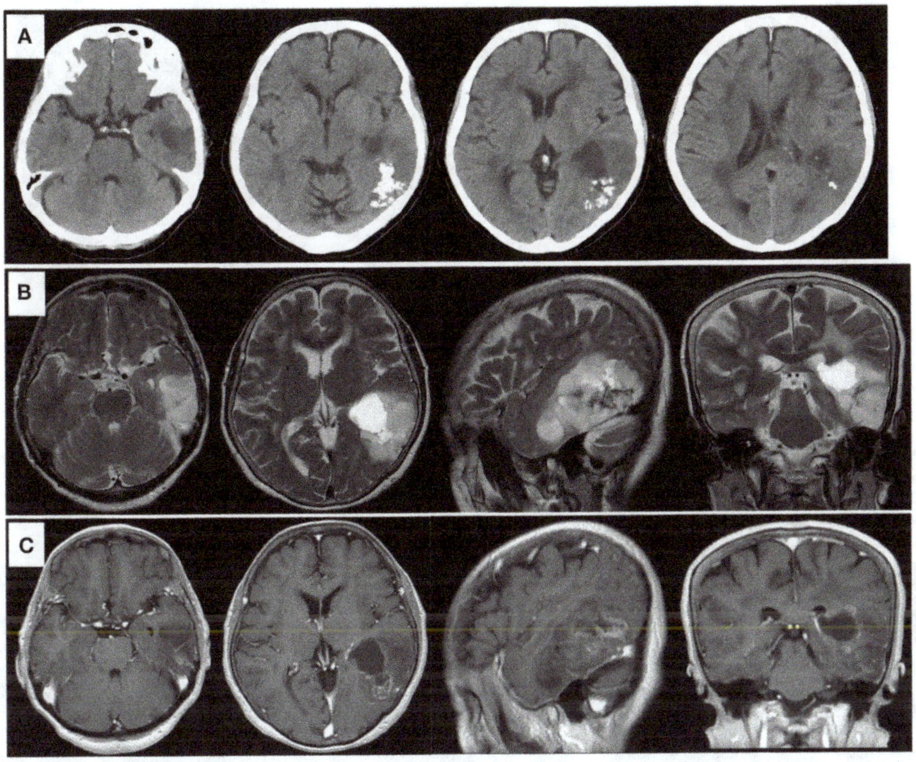

FIGURE 1 | Preoperative computed tomography showing calcified and cystic lesions in the left temporal lobe **(A)**. MR images showing high intensity in the left temporal lobe on T2-weighted image **(B)** and heterogeneous enhanced lesion on gadolinium-enhanced T1- weighted image **(C)**.

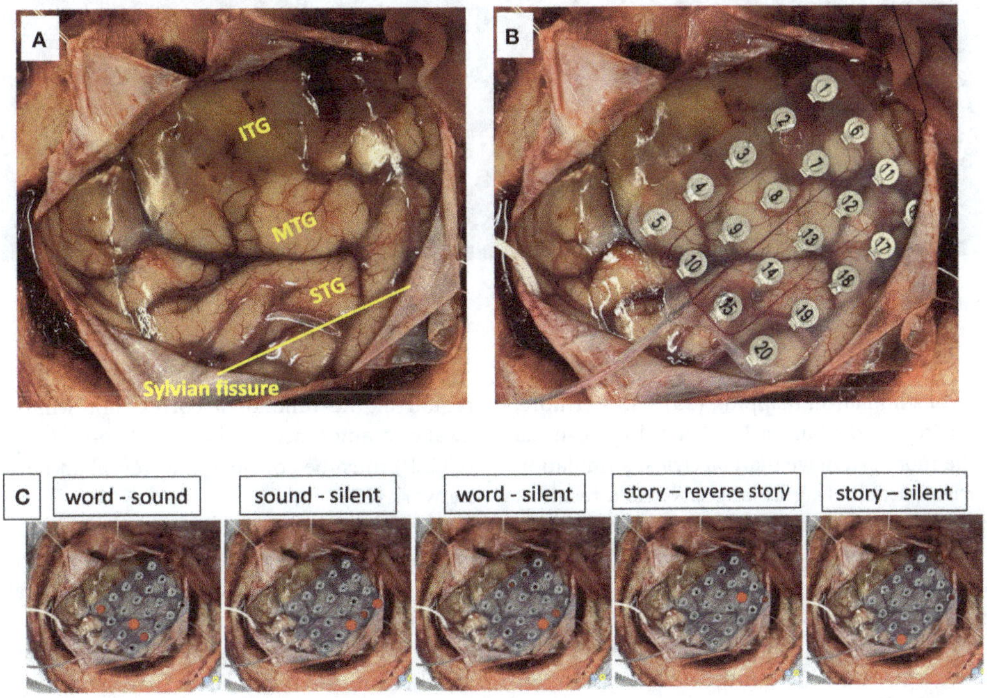

FIGURE 2 | The exposed brain surface **(A)** and a 20-channel ECoG grid placement **(B)** before resection. Red bubble meaning significant listening task-evoked high gamma activities in each task during passive language mapping **(C)**. STG, superior temporal gyrus; MTG, middle temporal gyrus; ITG, inferior temporal gyrus.

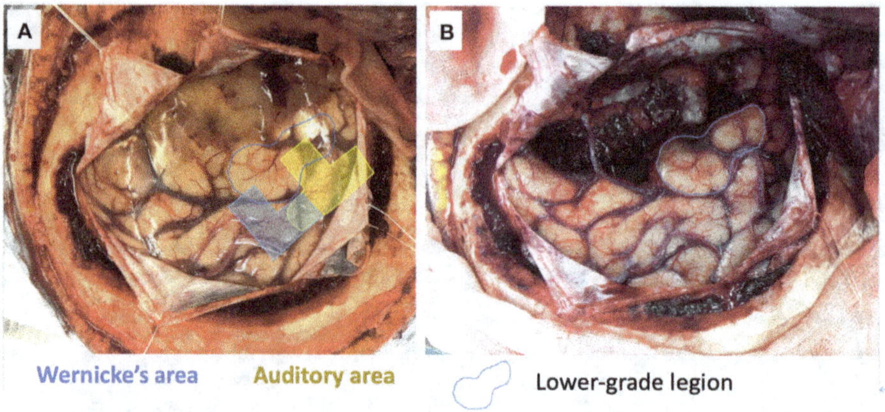

FIGURE 3 | 5 channels in the superior temporal gyrus and one channel in the middle temporal gyrus meaning the auditory (yellow) and Wernicke (blue) areas **(A)**. The gross tumor removal except for the lower-grade lesion in the middle temporal gyrus (blue circle) **(B)**.

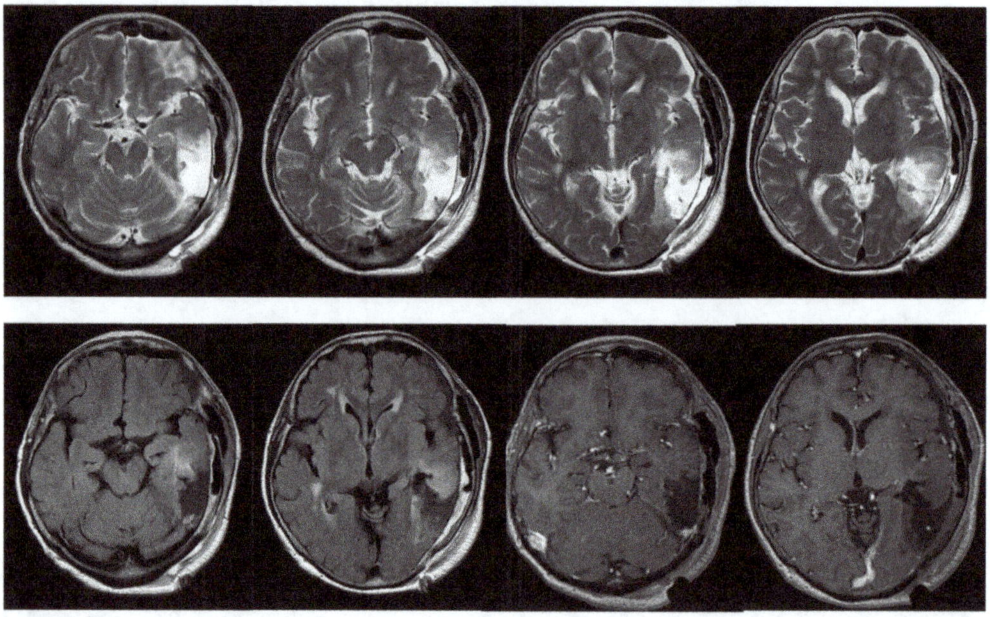

FIGURE 4 | Postoperative MRI showing gross total removal of the tumor.

gold standard electrical stimulation mapping (25). Furthermore, Asano and Gotman reported that task-related high-gamma augmentation may be more extensive than electrical stimulation in localizing the cortex participating in language. As a result of this increased sensitivity, task-related high-gamma augmentation could involve a more extensive area than the region that, if removed, would result in clinically noteworthy language deficits (26). Therefore, we speculated that the possibility of postoperative language functional preservation can be higher when ECoG-positive regions are left intact. The reason for the improvement of the language comprehension could be the preservation and the decompression of the auditory and Wernicke areas. However, ECoG can be identified only in the region of the functional cortex, not white matter. Therefore, awake craniotomy and/or cortico-cortical evoked potential (CCEP) must be considered to reveal and preserve the language network (27).

It is noteworthy that passive language mapping was successfully performed under general anesthesia, and language function preservation was achieved postoperatively in the present case. Pre and postoperative language functions were evaluated using the Standard Language Test of Aphasia (SLTA) which is widely administered in Japan (28). The SLTA is a comprehensive Japanese language test battery including 26 subtests for language comprehension, speaking, reading comprehension, writing, and calculation abilities.

The influence of general anesthesia should be considered when passive functional mapping under general anesthesia is done. Suzuki et al. (29) reported that the amplitudes of corticocortical evoked potential were increased in accordance with BIS level, and there were statistically significant differences between the awake (>80 BIS level) and anesthesia (<65 BIS level) states. However, to our best knowledge, there were no articles about a correlation between passive functional mapping and the depth of general anesthesia. We speculated that functional language mapping can be affected by the depth of anesthesia, therefore, anesthesia was maintained with a high BIS level in the present case. Further, studies about the influences of anesthesia on passive functional mapping are necessary to evaluate the intraoperative passive functional mapping accurately.

A limitation of this case report is that we do not know how the sensitivity and specificity of ECoG compared with ECS were in this case because ECS was not performed. We presume that passive language mapping will be widely applicable for the detection of brain function with the least stress for patients. We believe that real-time passive language mapping can be one of the most powerful tools to detect the region of the receptive-language function in brain surgery, especially for those who are not able to tolerate awake craniotomy.

CONCLUSION

We performed real-time CortiQ-based passive language mapping under general anesthesia for an elderly patient with left temporal glioma. The patient's language function was well-preserved postoperatively. Further, studies are necessary to investigate the efficacy of intraoperative passive language mapping.

ETHICS STATEMENT

Ethical review and approval was not required for the study on human participants in accordance with the local legislation and institutional requirements. Written informed consent to participate in this study was provided by the participants' legal guardian/next of kin. Written informed consent was obtained from the individual for the publication of any potentially identifiable images or data included in this article.

AUTHOR CONTRIBUTIONS

KK, TM, TK, and SK contributed conception and design of the study. KK wrote the first draft of the manuscript. TM, TK, and SK critically revised the final manuscript draft. All authors contributed to manuscript revision, read and approved the submitted version.

REFERENCES

1. Arya R, Roth C, Leach JL, Middeler D, Wilson JA, Vannest J, et al. Neuropsychological outcomes after resection of cortical sites with visual naming associated electrocorticographic high-gamma modulation. *Epilepsy Res.* (2019) 151:17–23. doi: 10.1016/j.eplepsyres.2019.01.011
2. Kanno A, Mikuni N. Evaluation of language function under awake craniotomy. *Neurol Med Chir.* (2015) 55:367–73. doi: 10.2176/nmc.ra.2014-0395
3. Tamura Y, Ogawa H, Kapeller C, Prueckl R, Takeuchi F, Anei R, et al. Passive language mapping combining real-time oscillation analysis with cortico-cortical evoked potentials for awake craniotomy. *J Neurosurg.* (2016) 125:1580–8. doi: 10.3171/2015.4.JNS15193
4. Swift JR, Coon WG, Guger C, Brunner P, Bunch M, Lynch T, et al. Passive functional mapping of receptive language areas using electrocorticographic signals. *Clin Neurophysiol.* (2018) 129:2517–24. doi: 10.1016/j.clinph.2018.09.007
5. Kapeller C, Korostenskaja M, Prueckl R, Chen PC, Lee KH, Westerveld M, et al. CortiQ-based real-time functional mapping for epilepsy surgery. *J Clin Neurophysiol.* (2015) 32:e12–22. doi: 10.1097/WNP.0000000000000131
6. Haglund MM, Berger MS, Shamseldin M, Lettich E, Ojemann GA. Cortical localization of temporal lobe language sites in patients with gliomas. *Neurosurgery.* (1994) 34:567–76. doi: 10.1227/00006123-199404000-00001
7. Sanai N, Mirzadeh Z, Berger MS. Functional outcome after language mapping for glioma resection. *N Engl J Med.* (2008) 358:18–27. doi: 10.1056/NEJMoa067819
8. Kayama T. Guidelines committee of the Japan awake surgery conference. the guidelines for awake craniotomy guidelines committee of the Japan awake surgery conference. *Neurol Med Chir.* (2012) 52:119–41. doi: 10.2176/nmc.52.119
9. Grossman R, Nossek E, Sitt R, Hayat D, Shahar T, Barzilai O, et al. Outcome of elderly patients undergoing awake-craniotomy for tumor resection. *Ann Surg Oncol.* (2013) 20:1722–8. doi: 10.1245/s10434-012-2748-x
10. Lohkamp LN, Mottolese C, Szathmari A, Huguet L, Beuriat PA, Christofori I, et al. Awake brain surgery in children-review of the literature and state-of-the-art. *Childs Nerv Syst.* (2019) 35:2071–7. doi: 10.1007/s00381-019-04279-w
11. Lohkamp LN, Beuriat PA, Desmurget M, Cristofori I, Szathmari A, Huguet L, et al. Awake brain surgery in children-a single-center experience. *Childs Nerv Syst.* (2020) 36:967–74. doi: 10.1007/s00381-020-04522-9
12. Chitoku S, Otsubo H, Harada Y, Jay V, Rutka JT, Weiss SK, et al. Extraoperative cortical stimulation of motor function in children. *Pediatr Neurol.* (2001) 24:344–50. doi: 10.1016/S0887-8994(01)00264-8
13. Korostenskaja M, Chen PC, Salinas CM, Westerveld M, Brunner P, Schalk G, et al. Real-time functional mapping: potential tool for improving language outcome in pediatric epilepsy surgery. *J Neurosurg Pediatr.* (2014) 14:287–95. doi: 10.3171/2014.6.PEDS13477
14. Hamberger MJ. Cortical language mapping in epilepsy: a critical review. *Neuropsychol Rev.* (2007) 17:477–89. doi: 10.1007/s11065-007-9046-6
15. Ritaccio AL, Brunner P, Schalk G. Electrical stimulation mapping of the brain: basic principles and emerging alternatives. *J Clin Neurophysiol.* (2018) 35:86–97. doi: 10.1097/WNP.0000000000000440
16. Qian T, Zhou W, Ling Z, Gao S, Liu H, Hong B. Fast presurgical functional mapping using task-related intracranial high gamma activity. *J Neurosurg.* (2013) 119:26–36. doi: 10.3171/2013.2.JNS12843
17. Corley JA, Nazari P, Rossi VJ, Kim NC, Fogg LF, Hoeppner TJ, et al. Cortical stimulation parameters for functional mapping. *Seizure.* (2017) 45:36–41. doi: 10.1016/j.seizure.2016.11.015
18. Cobb SR, Buhl EH, Halasy K, Paulsen O, Somogyi P. Synchronization of neuronal activity in hippocampus by individual GABAergic interneurons. *Nature.* (1995) 378:75–8. doi: 10.1038/378075a0
19. Fries P, Nikolić D, Singer W. The gamma cycle. *Trends Neurosci.* (2007) 30:309–16. doi: 10.1016/j.tins.2007.05.005
20. Hasenstaub A, Shu Y, Haider B, Kraushaar U, Duque A, McCormick DA. Inhibitory postsynaptic potentials carry synchronized

frequency information in active cortical networks. *Neuron.* (2005) 47:423–35. doi: 10.1016/j.neuron.2005.06.016

21. Traub RD, Cunningham MO, Gloveli T, LeBeau FE, Bibbig A, Buhl EH, et al. GABA-enhanced collective behavior in neuronal axons underlies persistent gamma-frequency oscillations. *Proc Natl Acad Sci U S A.* (2003) 100:11047–52. doi: 10.1073/pnas.1934854100
22. Manning JR, Jacobs J, Fried I, Kahana MJ. Broadband shifts in local field potential power spectra are correlated with singleneuron spiking in humans. *J Neurosci.* (2009) 29:13613–20. doi: 10.1523/JNEUROSCI.2041-09.2009
23. Nir Y, Fisch L, Mukamel R, Gelbard-Sagiv H, Arieli A, Fried I, et al. Coupling between neuronal firing rate, gamma LFP, and BOLD fMRI is related to interneuronal correlations. *Curr Biol.* (2007) 17:1275–85. doi: 10.1016/j.cub.2007.06.066
24. Ray S, Crone NE, Niebur E, Franaszczuk PJ, Hsiao SS. Neural correlates of high-gamma oscillations (60–200 Hz) in macaque local field potentials and their potential implications in electrocorticography. *J Neurosci.* (2008) 28:11526–36. doi: 10.1523/JNEUROSCI.2848-08.2008
25. Wang Y, Fifer MS, Flinker A, Korzeniewska A, Cervenka MC, Anderson WS, et al. Spatial-temporal functional mapping of language at the bedside with electrocorticography. *Neurology.* (2016) 86:1181–9. doi: 10.1212/WNL.0000000000002525
26. Asano E, Gotman J. Is electrocorticography-based language mapping ready to replace stimulation? *Neurology.* (2016) 86:1174–6. doi: 10.1212/WNL.0000000000002533
27. Saito T, Tamura M, Muragaki Y, Maruyama T, Kubota Y, Fukuchi S, et al. Intraoperative cortico-cortical evoked potentials for the evaluation of language function during brain tumor resection: initial experience with 13 cases. *J Neurosurg.* (2014) 121:827–38. doi: 10.3171/2014.4.JNS131195
28. Brain Function Test Committee. *Japan Society for Higher Brain Dysfunction. The Standard Language Test of Aphasia.* Tokyo: Sinkoh Igaku Shuppansha (2003).
29. Suzuki Y, Enatsu R, Kanno A, Yokoyama R, Suzuki H, Tachibana S, et al. The influence of anesthesia on corticocortical evoked potential monitoring network between frontal and temporoparietal cortices. *World Neurosurg.* (2019) 123:e685–92. doi: 10.1016/j.wneu.2018.11.253

20

Fixed-Life or Rechargeable Battery for Deep Brain Stimulation: Preference and Satisfaction in Chinese Patients with Parkinson's Disease

Xian Qiu [1,2†], Tingting Peng [1,2†], Zhengyu Lin [1], Kaiwen Zhu [1], Yuhan Wang [1], Bomin Sun [1], Keyoumars Ashkan [3], Chencheng Zhang [1] and Dianyou Li [1*]*

[1] Department of Nursing, Ruijin Hospital, Shanghai Jiao Tong University School of Medicine, Shanghai, China, [2] Department of Neurosurgery, Ruijin Hospital, Shanghai Jiao Tong University School of Medicine, Shanghai, China, [3] Department of Neurosurgery, King's College Hospital, London, United Kingdom

***Correspondence:**
Chencheng Zhang
i@cczhang.org
Dianyou Li
ldy11483@rjh.com.cn

† These authors have contributed equally to this work

Introduction: DBS is a widely used therapy for PD. There is now a choice between fixed-life implantable pulse generators (IPGs) and rechargeable IPGs, each having advantages and disadvantages. This study aimed to evaluate the preference and satisfaction of Chinese patients with Parkinson's disease (PD) who were treated with deep brain stimulation (DBS).

Materials and Methods: Two hundred and twenty PD patients were treated with DBS and completed a self-reported questionnaire to assess their long-term satisfaction and experience with the type of battery they had chosen and the key factors affecting these choices. The survey was performed online and double-checked for completeness and accuracy.

Results: The median value of the postoperative duration was 18 months. The most popular way for patients to learn about DBS surgery was through media (79/220, 35.9%) including the Internet and television programs. In total, 87.3% of the DBS used rechargeable IPGs (r-IPG). The choice between rechargeable and non-rechargeable IPGs was significantly associated with affordability ($\chi^2_{(1)} = 19.13, p < 0.001$). Interestingly, the feature of remote programming significantly affected patients' choices between domestic and imported brands ($\chi^2_{(1)} = 16.81, p < 0.001$). 87.7% of the patients were satisfied with the stimulating effects as well as the implanted device itself. 40.6% of the patients with r-IPGs felt confident handling devices within 1 week after discharge. More than half of the patients checked their batteries every week. The mean interval for battery recharge was 4.3 days. 57.8% of the patients spent around 1 h recharging, and 71.4% of them recharged the battery independently.

Conclusions: Most patients were satisfied with their choice of IPGs. The patients' economic status and the remote programming function of the device were the two most critical factors in their decision. The skill of recharging the IPG was easy to master for most patients.

Keywords: deep brain stimulation, movement disorders, patient satisfaction, Parkinsion's disease, rechargeable implantable pulse generator

INTRODUCTION

Deep brain stimulation (DBS) is a well-established neurosurgical treatment for advanced Parkinson's disease (PD), which achieves its therapeutic effects by the delivery of continuous electrical current to the target structure, circuitry, or network implicated in disease pathophysiology. The electric power comes from an implantable pulse generator (IPG), which was initially designed to be non-rechargeable. Depending on the patient's diagnosis and DBS parameter settings, the fixed-life batteries need to be replaced 3–5 years after implantation. Battery depletion is the most common reason for additional surgery in DBS patients (1, 2). Although IPG replacement is a minor surgical procedure compared to primary brain surgery, multiple IPG replacements over the course of the patient's treatment and illness can pose an increased health risk, such as an elevated post-implantation infection risk and wound healing problems (3).

The rechargeable-IPG was developed in 2008 and outperformed the IPG with fixed-life batteries in various ways (4). First, patients with DBS need fewer IPG replacement surgeries due to battery depletion, thereby reducing surgical-related health risks. Second, rechargeable batteries are less subject to induce unexpected clinical changes, such as a worsening of PD symptoms, whereas the current of fixed-life batteries gets irregular as they are gradually exhausted. Third, rechargeable batteries are smaller in size. The frequency and duration of the IPG battery recharging procedure depend on the power of the DBS needed to manage the PD symptoms of a patient. However, patients are required to check the battery status and need to regularly recharge the battery using a handheld device. The recharging procedure, though not difficult to perform by healthy persons, can be challenging for patients with PD as most of them are elderly with various levels of motor and cognitive deficits (5).

Other technological advances during the past decade have also been incorporated into present-day DBS systems to provide clinicians with more flexible and personalized treatment options. As a result, neurologists and neurosurgeons are facing the challenge of selecting the most appropriate DBS system and treatment for a given patient. They need to make a clinical decision based on many factors, such as lead geometry, the specific DBS target, the amount of current needed for the patient, and the nature of the programming platform of different device brands (6). Other relevant factors include the patients' overall health status, medical history, level of social support available, socioeconomic status, the health care insurance plan, and their psychomotor ability both to deal with the IPG battery recharging procedure and to use modern interactive devices.

The preference of the patients and concerns about how the DBS treatment may impact their daily activities have received little attention in previous studies (5). Most studies have focused on DBS safety and efficacy, but the patient's perspective on the DBS treatment delivered and the reasons for choosing or accepting a specific DBS system remain an important but under-recognized topic. For example, only a few studies performed in Europe have demonstrated that patients with PD preferred rechargeable IPG batteries over fixed-life batteries (7–9). This situation is problematic because patient preference and satisfaction are important for treatment acceptance, treatment compliance, and the further development of next generation of DBS systems. This study aimed to shed more light on patients' perspectives, including their IPG preference and the reasons that drive their choice (e.g., patient affordability, DBS, and IPG device features) of either rechargeable or fixed-life IPG batteries. We also explored preferences for the use of either an imported brand or domestic rechargeable IPG. To address these questions, we examined patient satisfaction and IPG choices in a large cohort of Chinese patients with PD treated with DBS.

MATERIALS AND METHODS

Participants

A total of 768 patients diagnosed with idiopathic PD who underwent DBS surgery at our hospital were contacted and invited to participate in this study. At the time of their DBS surgery, the patients had been offered a choice of receiving an IPG that was either non-rechargeable (nr-IPG) or rechargeable (r-IPG). They were also given a choice of receiving either an imported (Medtronic) or domestic (PINS and SceneRay) brand IPG. Each IPG option had been fully explained and discussed with patients. In China, the costs of surgery were primarily covered by the patient's health insurance, but the costs of DBS hardware were only partly covered. In general, r-IPGs were substantially more expensive than nr-IPGs and international IPG devices were slightly more expensive than domestic made devices. An illustration of the international and domestic brands of IPG devices used in this study can be found in **Supplementary Figure 1**. The study was approved by the Ethical Committee of Ruijin Hospital. Written informed consent was completed by all participants.

Survey Questionnaire

An internet-based survey questionnaire (powered by www.wjx.cn) was developed to evaluate the patients' perceptions, expectations, and experiences with the DBS treatment and the IPG device they chose (r-IPGs vs. nr-IPGs and international vs. domestic brands). The questionnaire focused on the patients' satisfaction with the DBS treatment and the IPG of choice as well as four aspects of possible concern (patient affordability, prospect of further required surgeries to replace the battery, requirement for recharging the battery, and battery size) and the sources of information (e.g., clinical advice, electronic media) the patients considered in making decisions. Several extra questions were included in the questionnaire for patients with r-IPGs to collect their experiences with the battery recharging procedure, including how often they checked the battery capacity and the frequency, duration, and ease of recharging, as well as the occurrences that they forgot or were unable to recharge. The patients indicated their answers using a forced-choice dichotomous format or a 4- or 5-point Likert scale. The questionnaire was distributed via the online chat platform WeChat. Participants completed the questionnaire after having received at least 8 months of DBS treatment. In most cases, it took no more than 30 min to complete the questionnaire.

Data Processing and Statistical Analysis

The survey question answers were first organized into dichotomous variables (e.g., sex, satisfaction rate), categorical nominal variables (e.g., sources of information used by patients to make their choice), categorical ordinal variables (e.g., patient affordability, frequency, and duration of recharging procedure, frequency of battery capacity checks), and continuous variables (e.g., age). We then computed descriptive statistics consisting of frequencies and percentages, measures of central tendency (median or mean), and measures of variation [interquartile range (IQR) or standard deviation].

Initially, two separate one-sample binomial tests of proportions were performed to ascertain that the patients' choice-preference decisions for r-IPGs or nr-IPGs, as well as for an international or domestic device, which were not made at random but differed significantly from chance (50%).

Fisher's exact test was performed to assess the significance of the association between patient satisfaction rate (satisfied vs. unsatisfied) and the type of IPG (r-IPG vs. nr-IPG). The patient's affordability or budget consisted of 4 ordinal categories (<100,000 RMB, 100,000–200,000 RMB, 200,000–300,000 RMB, and >300,000 RMB). The Fisher-Freeman-Halton Test was used to assess the relationship between patient's affordability and the choice of r-IPG vs. nr-IPG.

Fisher's exact test to assess the relationship between affordability and the choice of r-IPG vs. nr-IPG. We used Pearson's or Yates' continuity corrected Chi-squared test to evaluate the influencing factors for patients' choices of international vs. domestic manufacturers in the r-IPG group, and to compare the satisfaction rate between patients with r-IPG and nr-IPG. A p-value < 0.05 was considered significant. Data were analyzed with SPSS (version 23.0; Amonk, NY: IBM). Continuous variables were expressed as Mean ± SD or median value with interquartile range (IQR). Categorical variables were presented as frequencies (%).

RESULTS

Patient Sample Characteristics

Two hundred and twenty patients with PD (135 men, 85 women; age: 62.8 ± 9.8 years) out of 768 patients contacted responded to the survey, yielding a response rate of 28.6%. The median duration of postoperative DBS treatment was 18 (IQR: 8–36) months (**Table 1**).

Patient Preference

In the patient sample (n = 220), 192 (87%) patients used r-IPGs (**Table 1**). The remaining 28 (13%) patients chose to use nr-IPGs for their DBS treatment. In addition, 142 (65%) patients chose a device from an imported manufacturer (Medtronic), whereas 78 (36%) patients preferred a device from a domestic manufacturer (PINS or SceneRay). Two one-sample binomial tests of proportions (expressed in percentages) confirmed that the patients' choice-preference decisions (i.e., 87% favoring r-IPGs and 65% international devices) were significantly different from that could be expected by chance (50%) (z = 8.8 and 11.0, both $p < 0.001$).

TABLE 1 | Patient sample characteristics (N = 220).

Characteristics	Total	r-IPG	nr-IPG
Gender			
Men (n, %)	135 (61%)	114 (59%)	21 (75%)
Women (n, %)	85 (39%)	78 (41%)	7 (25%)
Age, year (mean ± SD)	62.8 ± 9.8	62.5 ± 9.8	64.4 ± 10.0
Follow-up, month (median, IQR)	18 (8–36)	19 (9–38)	15.5 (5.25–26.5)
Origin of DBS system manufacturer			
International (Medtronic)	142	136	6
Domestic (PINS or SceneRay)	78	56	22

Patient's Sources of DBS Information

The two most common reasons for patients' preference-choice and making a decision prior to surgery were digital media (web sites, television) (36% of all patients) and primary care physicians who referred the patients to our DBS center (36%). A substantial portion of patients (26%) reported having gained information about DBS by word of mouth from other patients with PD treated with DBS in our center.

Factors Affecting Patient's Choice for r-IPG or nr-IPG

We evaluated four factors (patient affordability, prospect of further required surgeries to replace the battery, requirement for recharging the battery, and battery size), which the patients might have considered when choosing a specific IPG. The affordability consisted of four ordinal categories (<100 thousand RMB, 100–200 thousand RMB, 200–300 thousand RMB, and >300 thousand RMB) (**Figure 1**). A 4 × 2 Chi-squared test to assess the association between patients' affordability and patients' choice could not be performed because one cell was empty in the contingency table analyzed (i.e., there were no patients with the highest budget available who had chosen for an nr-IPS) (**Figure 1A**).

Nevertheless, a two-sample binomial test of proportions showed that patients with the two highest personal budgets were over-represented among the patients who had chosen an r-IPG (72% of the 192 patients) and under-represented among the patients who opted for an nr-IPG (32% of the 28 patients) ($z = 4.2, p < 0.0001$) (**Figure 1B**). Alternatively, patients with the two lowest budgets were under-represented among the patients who opted for an r-IPG (28%) and over-represented among the patients who chose to use an nr-IPG (68%) (z = 4.2, p < 0.0001). These results indicate that a significant association existed between patient affordability and choice to use either an r-IPG or an nr-IPG device.

In response to the survey questions about the factors that were of concern for patients' in making their choice, the personal financial costs involved were perceived as a "concern" or "serious concern" by 82% (23/28) of the patients who chose an nr-IPG, whereas the corresponding percentage was 61% (117/192) for the patients who preferred to use an r-IPG. A two-sample

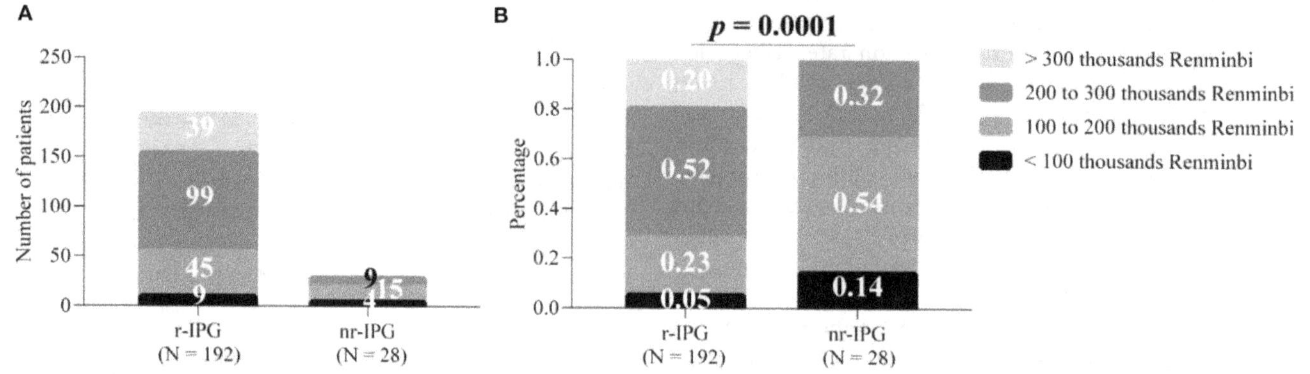

FIGURE 1 | Patient budgets for deep brain stimulation and implanted pulse generators (IPGs). The budgets are divided into four levels. Data are presented as either absolute numbers **(A)** or percentages **(B)**. A *p*-value < 0.05 is considered statistically significant. r-IPG, rechargeable IPG; nr-IPG, non-rechargeable IPG.

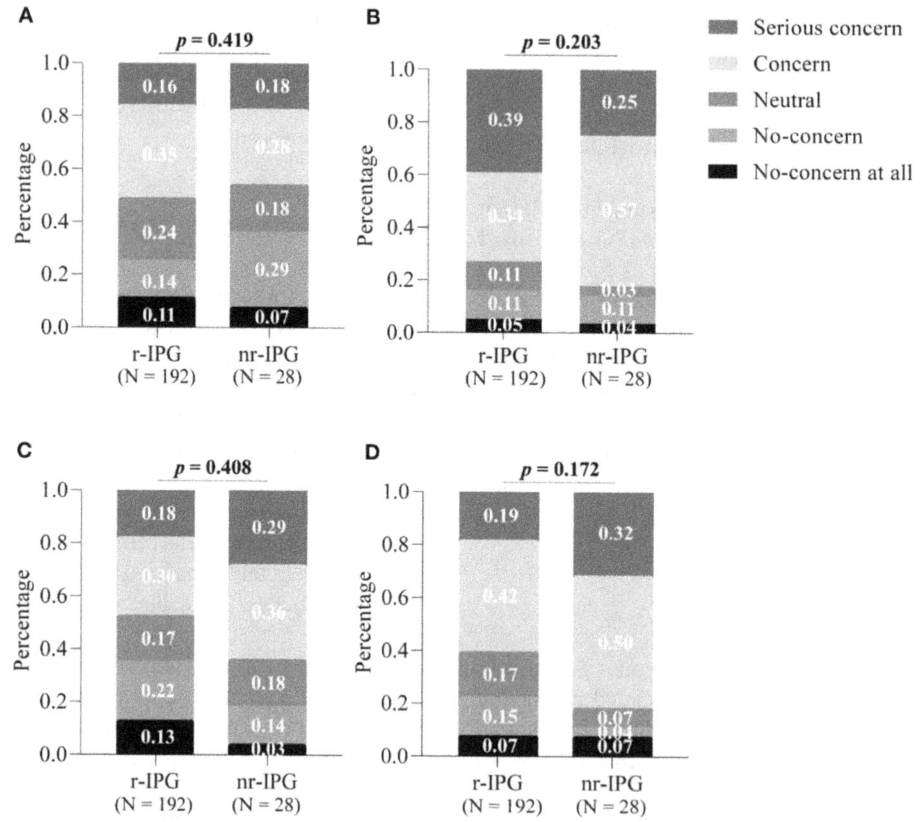

FIGURE 2 | Factors influencing patient's choice between a rechargeable (r-IPG) and non-rechargeable (nr-IPG) implanted pulse generator. **(A)** Battery size; **(B)** the need for further surgery to replace the battery; **(C)** the need for recharging the battery; and **(D)** economic issues. Patients' attitudes toward these factors were divided into five levels in the questionnaire: "No concern at all", "No concern", "Neutral", "Concern", and "Serious concern". Data are presented as percentages. A *p*-value < 0.05 is considered statistically significant.

binomial test showed that these two sample proportions differed significantly from each other ($z = 2.2, p = 0.031$) (**Figure 2D**).

The proportions of patients who indicated "concern" or "serious concern" at the prospect of further surgeries to replace the battery (**Figure 2A**), the need for recharging the battery (**Figure 2B**), and the size of the battery (**Figure 2C**) was substantial (ranging from 50% of all patients concerned about the prospect of battery recharging to 74% concerning about the need for further surgeries), but the proportions did not differ significantly between the patients with either an r-IPG or an nr-IPG ($z = 1$, $p = 0.310$; $z = 1.6$, $p = 0.114$; $z = 0.6$, $p = 0.553$, respectively).

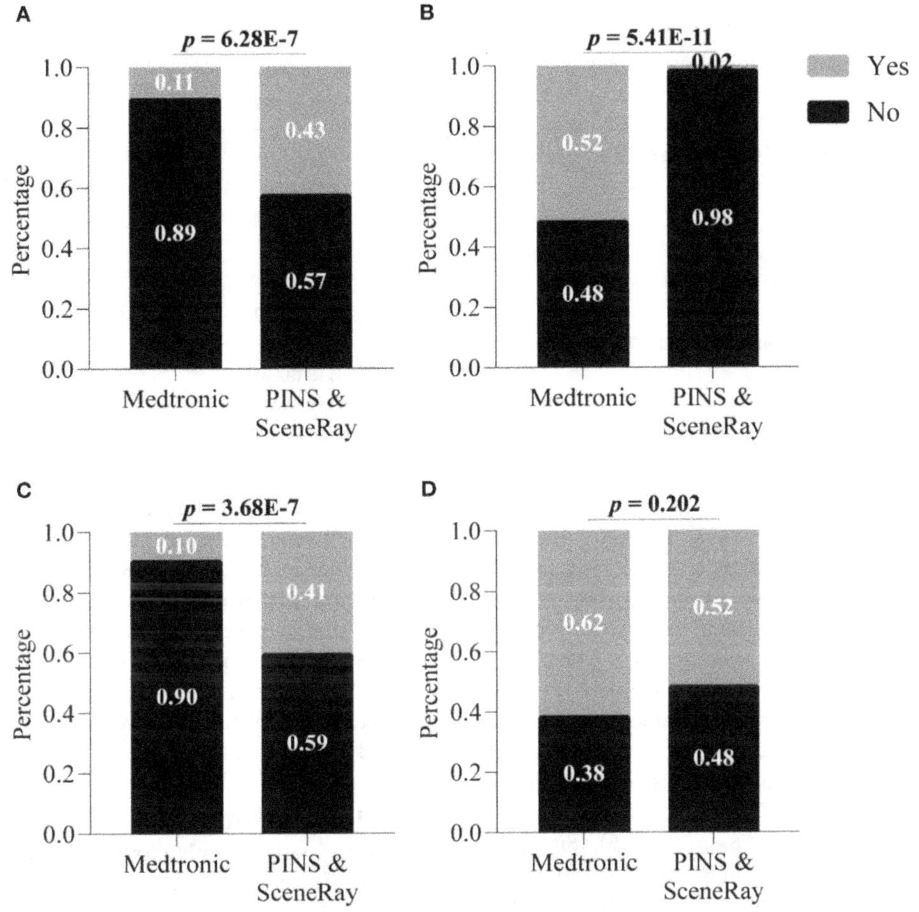

FIGURE 3 | Factors influencing patient's choice between imported and domestic rechargeable implanted pulse generator (r-IPG). **(A)** Budget issue; **(B)** international reputation; **(C)** remote programming feature; and **(D)** convenience of postoperative management. Data are presented as percentages. A p-value < 0.05 is considered statistically significant.

Factors Affecting Patient's Choice for Imported or Domestic r-IPG

We examined four factors (patient affordability, the international reputation of DBS manufacturer, DBS remote programming product feature, medical advice) that the patients might have considered when choosing between an imported r-IPG or domestic r-IPG. Among the 192 patients who preferred the use of an r-IPG, 136 (71%) patients chose a device from the international manufacturer (Medtronic) and 56 (29%) chose a device from one of the domestic manufacturers (PINS or SceneRay). A one-sample binomial test indicated that the patient's choice (i.e., 71% of patients favored an imported r-IPG) was not made at random (50%) ($z = 5.8$, $p < 0.001$).

Figure 3 illustrates the patients' answers ("yes" or "no") about whether they considered the above-mentioned four factors in making their decision to use an imported or domestic r-IPG. A two-sample binomial test showed that the proportion of affirmative ("yes") answers to the question of whether the patients considered their budget was significantly lower among patients who preferred an imported r-IPG (11% of the 136 patients) than those who chose a domestic r-IPG (43% of the 56 patients) ($z = 5.0$, $p < 0.0001$) (**Figure 3A**). The proportion of affirmative answers regarding the attention to remote DBS programming product features was significantly lower among the patients who preferred an imported r-IPG than those who opted for a domestic one (10 vs. 41%, $z = 5.0$, $p < 0.0001$) (**Figure 3C**).

In contrast, the proportion of affirmative answers concerning the international reputation of the DBS manufacturer was significantly higher among the patients who chose an imported r-IPG than those who preferred a domestic r-IPG (52 vs. 2%, $z = 6.5$, $p < 0.0001$) (**Figure 3B**). Finally, the proportion of affirmative answers to the question as to whether medical advice had played a role in the patients' choice was relatively higher in patients who chose an imported brand but did not differ significantly from those choosing a domestic r-IPG (62 vs. 52%, $z = 1.3$, $p = 0.2002$) (**Figure 3D**).

TABLE 2 | Patient satisfaction as a function of the type of IPG ($N = 220$).

Questions	Group	
	r-IPG ($n = 192$)	nr-IPG ($n = 28$)
1. Are you still satisfied with the choice of your device?		
Yes	169 (88.0%)	24 (85.7%)
No	23 (12.0%)	4 (14.3%)
1.1. If not, please specify.		
The stimulating effects did not meet your expectation.	18 (9.4%)	4 (14.3%)
Others	5 (2.6%)	0
2. Would you choose the same type of your device today?		
Yes	178 (92.7%)	26 (92.9%)
No	14 (7.3%)	2 (7.1%)

Patient Satisfaction

Overall, the majority of patients (88%, 193/220) reported being satisfied with the DBS treatment and the type of IPG device chosen. A minor portion of patients (10%, 22/220) was not satisfied and reported that their expectations of the stimulating effects of DBS treatment were not met. The patient satisfaction rate was 88% among patients with an r-IPG and 86% among patients with an nr-IPG (**Table 2**). Statistical analysis on the frequency data demonstrated that there was no significant association between patient satisfaction (satisfied vs. unsatisfied) and the type of IPG chosen (r-IPG vs. nr-IPG) (Fisher exact test value = 0.76, $p > 0.05$). Similarly, within the r-IPG patient group, no significant association was observed between patient satisfaction and the manufacturer (imported vs. domestic) of the IPG device (Fisher exact test value = 0.72, $p > 0.05$). Finally, 93% (178/192) of the patients with r-IPGs and 93% (26/28) of the patients with nr-IPGs indicated that they would choose the same type of device again (**Table 2**). A group of PD patients at late-stage (13 out of 14 = 92.8%) with a median duration of postoperative DBS treatment being 22 (IQR: 3–36) months were satisfied with their choice of r-IPG.

Patient Experience With Battery Recharging Procedure

The patients' experiences with the battery recharging procedure are summarized in **Table 3**. The majority of the r-IPG patients (71%, 137/192) were able to perform the battery recharge procedure by themselves. The remaining patients (29%, 55/192), however, were unable to conduct the procedure independently and needed assistance from another person, usually, their spouse, to check and recharge the battery. Furthermore, most patients or their partners (93%) felt confident managing the r-IPG device (**Table 3**). Almost half of the patients (41%) felt confident managing the r-IPG device within 1 week after being discharged from the hospital. Yet, it took more than 4 weeks for another large portion of the patients (34%) to become proficient in using the device. More than half of the patients (64%) checked the battery every week, and most patients (92%) preferred to recharge when the battery level was still over 50%. The mean interval between subsequent battery recharging procedures was 4.3 days. For most patients (58%), it took about 1 h to complete the recharging procedure. Notably, about 8% of the patients reported that they were unable to recharge the battery on at least one occasion, and more than half of them failed to resolve the technical problem involved. Furthermore, 19% of the patients reported that they forgot to recharge the battery at least once (**Table 3**).

Mobility in Patients Living With an r-IPG

Most of the patients with an r-IPG (73%) had not traveled since receiving it, and 89% did not return to work postoperatively (**Table 4**). Among those patients who did travel and went on vacation at least once after surgery (27%), the majority (78%) were able to recharge during the vacation. In daily life, most patients (93%) preferred to sit or lie down while recharging the battery (**Table 4**).

DISCUSSION

To the best of our knowledge, this study included the largest cohort of patients with PD ($N = 220$) to report satisfaction with DBS treatment and the choice of IPG. In this study, most patients (87%) preferred the use of r-IPGs over nr-IPGs for their DBS treatment. Most patients (65%) also preferred an IPG device from an imported brand (Medtronic) over a domestic IPG (PINS or SceneRay). The patients' choice (i.e., 87% chose r-IPGs and 65% chose the imported brand) was significantly different from what would be expected by chance (50%), indicating that the patients had made active, deliberate binary choices among the different options given to them.

The patients accessed information about the DBS treatment for PD prior to their referral to specialized DBS medical care in three primary ways (electronic media, medical advice, word-of-mouth from other patients). The patients' budget for DBS treatment turned out to be the major factor that affected their choice to use either an r-IPG or nr-IPG device. Patients with a relatively low budget tended to choose a cheaper, nr-IPG

TABLE 3 | Patients' experiences with battery recharging procedure ($N = 192$).

Questions	Number (%)
1. Do you feel confident using your r-IPG?	
No	14 (7.3%)
Yes	178 (92.7%)
1.1. If yes, how long did it take to feel confident?	
Within 1 week	78 (40.7%)
1–2 weeks	27 (14.1%)
2–4 weeks	8 (4.2%)
More than 4 weeks	65 (34.0%)
2. How frequently do you check the battery capacity of your r-IPG?	
Everyday	35 (18.2%)
Every week	123 (64.1%)
Every 2 weeks	6 (3.1%)
Every 4 weeks	17 (8.9%)
Every year	11 (5.7%)
3. Have you ever forgotten to recharge your r-IPG?	
No	156 (81.3%)
Yes	36 (18.7%)
4. How frequently do you recharge your r-IPG?	
Everyday	49 (25.5%)
2–4 days	28 (14.6%)
5–7 days	115 (59.9%)
5. How frequently do you recharge your recharger?	
Everyday	15 (7.8%)
Every week	104 (54.2%)
Every 2 weeks	31 (16.1%)
Every 4 weeks	37 (19.3%)
Not fixed	5 (2.6%)
6. At what level of battery capacity do you usually recharge your r-IPG?	
75–100%	101 (52.6%)
75–50%	76 (39.6%)
<50%	15 (7.8%)
Warning sign	0
7. How long does recharging usually take?	
<15 min	9 (4.7%)
15–30 min	37 (19.3%)
30–45 min	35 (18.2%)
45–60 min	40 (20.8%)
More than 60 min	71 (37.0%)
8. Do you check and recharge your r-IPG yourself?	
No	55 (28.6%)
Yes	137 (71.4%)
9. Have you ever been unable to recharge your battery?	
No	176 (91.7%)
Yes	16 (8.3%)
9.1. if yes, could you solve the problem on your own?	
No	11 (68.9%)
Yes	5 (31.2%)

TABLE 4 | Mobility in patients living with a rechargeable IPG ($N = 192$).

Questions	Number (%)
1. Have you ever traveled since your DBS surgery?	
No	141 (73.4%)
Yes	51 (26.6%)
1.1. If yes, have you ever recharged during the vacation?	
No	11 (21.6%)
Yes	40 (78.4%)
2. Do you continue to work after DBS surgery?	
No	170 (88.5%)
Yes	22 (11.5%)
2.1. If yes, have you ever recharged during work?	
No	21 (95%)
Yes	1 (5%)
3. Are you ambulatory during recharging?	
No	178 (92.7%)
Yes	14 (7.3%)

device. Patient's affordability, international reputation of the manufacturer, and the remote programming product feature also affected the choice of the manufacturer of the IPG device (imported or domestic). The patients' choices were not affected by the medical advice given by their primary care physicians. These results highlighted the role of the patient's economic status as a major non-clinical factor in choosing how the treatment was conducted (10).

The majority of patients (88%) reported being satisfied with the DBS treatment effects and the type of IPG device used. This result aligned with a 3 month follow-up study in patients with movement disorders ($N = 21$) treated with DBS using r-IPGs (9). This follow-up study reported an overall patient satisfaction rate of 83%. In a retrospective study, similar favorable patient experiences were observed in a group of patients with movement disorders ($N = 35$) whose DBS surgeries (using r-IPGs) had been completed for 21 months on average (5). In keeping with the latter study, most patients with an r-IPG in the present study were also able to learn the recharging procedure easily and rapidly. Additionally, no negative correlation was found between age and a patient's ability to handle the recharging procedure (5), although ~30% of patients with an r-IPG did require help from caregivers in our study. Interestingly, several patients only checked their batteries every year, meaning that they recharged the IPG frequently but did not check the IPG status as frequently. In most cases, power depletion did not cause irreversible consequences. Although it was not reported in these participants, there was one patient who got aspiration pneumonia during the power-off period.

Inability to recharge the IPG could be annoying and might induce serious adverse consequences. In our study, most problems were caused by malfunctioning power banks that needed to be replaced. One patient reported that the device was shut down unexpectedly, and the program controller was used to restart the IPG. Another case involved an elderly patient, whose new caregiver at the nursing home failed to recharge the IPG because of unfamiliarity.

Research about patient satisfaction by Timmermann et al. described a small prospective patient satisfaction cohort ($N = 21$)

during a 3 month follow-up (9). Jakobs et al. reported another small retrospective group ($N = 35$) with a more extensive follow-up (mean value of 21.2 months) (5). Their work together indicates that there was no significant association between the satisfaction rate and the number of training sessions. These two studies included a small number of patients with PD, dystonia, and essential tremor together into the analysis. Similarly, Jakobs et al. also pointed out that the majority of patients who claimed a lack of confidence after the training program had only participated in only one single session. They, therefore, proposed at least two training sessions for patients (5). In our study, 178 (92.7%) patients felt confident of using their IPG, and such a high rate of satisfaction was probably because our patients and their caregivers were encouraged to participate in two training sessions: one before discharge and one at 1 week after discharge. Patient satisfaction was reported by 31 patients in which 12 received r-IPGs as their initial implants (11). Interestingly, these patients were more satisfied with their IPGs compared with patients who previously had an nr-IPG implanted. In our study, 26 patients had IPG replacement surgery, and 18 out of 26 patients switched from an nr-IPG to an r-IPG and were satisfied with the results. The remote programming function, decreased chances of IPG replacement were the driving force for these 18 patients to change IPG type. The reasons for the eight patients who did not undergo the switch of IPG type were primarily economic concerns and inabilities in DBS self-management. This study did not explore the satisfaction rates among different products but the therapy efficacy was found to be the dominating factor contributing to patients' general satisfaction.

Our results demonstrate that patient affordability had a significant impact on the choice of IPG type in Chinese PD patients. It was estimated that more than 223,000 EUR could be saved over nearly 8 years in 1,499 patients if they were all implanted with r-IPG instead of nr-IPG (12). However, reimbursement policies differ across countries and cities. DBS therapy remains a substantial financial burden for many families as DBS electrodes and IPG are only partly reimbursed by insurance in China. The impact of insurance policies as well as other factors such as the individual life expectancy should be elucidated in future cost-effective investigations.

Previous studies raised the challenging question of how device-aided treatment could be managed in late-stage PD patients (13, 14). In our study, 92.8% of late-stage PD patients were satisfied with the choice of r-IPG. In the meantime, only one patient complained about the tediousness of recharging the battery. The IPG replacement may require an in-hospital admission of a few days and a surgical intervention under total/local anesthesia depending on the patient's compliance. Using the r-IPG could avoid IPG-replacement for these late-stage PD patients, and this was the main reason why r-IPD was preferred by the PD caregivers in our study. Most late-stage PD patients in the study lived at home with their family members, such as a spouse, children, and the r-IPG management was taken care of by their family.

We recognize some limitations in this study. First, as a cross-sectional study, we were not able to identify how the patient's satisfaction developed over time as the disease progressed. Second, the high costs of the DBS treatment could be a financial burden for many families in China which might result in a selection bias. In addition, socioeconomic factors are largely different across regions. Thus, the result of our study may only be generalizable in well-developed regions in China. The education level of the PD patients could also be explored in the future. Finally, in this study, we only analyzed the patients' attitude toward different types of IPG and the recharging process but not an extended assessment for other aspects such as the LEDD. Given the necessity of clinical improvement and the importance of patient satisfaction, we believe that further long-term follow-up studies are needed.

CONCLUSION

In conclusion, we found that most patients were satisfied with their choice of IPG. The financial status of patients and the remote programming product feature were the two most critical factors in their decision. The skill required to use a rechargeable IPG was also easily mastered by most patients.

ETHICS STATEMENT

The studies involving human participants were reviewed and approved by Ruijin Ethical Committee. The patients/participants provided their written informed consent to participate in this study.

AUTHOR CONTRIBUTIONS

KA, CZ, and DL: study conception and design. XQ, TP, ZL, and YW: data collection. ZL and YW: data analysis. XQ, ZL, and CZ: draft writing. All authors critical comments.

ACKNOWLEDGMENTS

We thank Ms. Kaile Zhang, Dr. Luciano Furlanetti, and Mrs. Xinmeng Xu for support in this study.

REFERENCES

1. Kumar N, Murgai A, Jog M. Neurological worsening after implantable pulse generator replacement. *Can J Neurol Sci.* (2019) 46:1–6. doi: 10.1017/cjn.2019.51
2. Niemann M, Schneider G, Kühn A, Vajkoczy P, Faust K. Clinical efficacy of bilateral deep brain stimulation does not change after implantable pulse generator replacement but the impedances do: a prospective study. *Neuromodulation.* (2020) 23:530–6. doi: 10.1111/ner.13022
3. Thrane J, Sunde N, Bergholt B, Rosendal F. Increasing infection rate in multiple implanted pulse generator changes in movement disorder patients treated with deep brain stimulation. *Stereotact Funct Neurosurg.* (2014) 92:360–4. doi: 10.1159/000365576
4. Hitti F, Vaughan K, Ramayya A, McShane B, Baltuch G. Reduced long-term cost and increased patient satisfaction with rechargeable implantable pulse generators for deep brain stimulation. *J Neurosurg.* (2018) 131:799–806. doi: 10.3171/2018.4.JNS172995
5. Jakobs M, Kloß M, Unterberg A, Kiening K. Rechargeable internal pulse generators as initial neurostimulators for deep brain stimulation in patients with movement disorders. *Neuromodulation.* (2018) 21:604–10. doi: 10.1111/ner.12748
6. Okun M. Tips for choosing a deep brain stimulation device. *JAMA Neurol.* (2019) 76:749–50. doi: 10.1001/jamaneurol.2019.0849
7. Furlanetti L, Raslan A, Khaleeq T, Hasegawa H, Ashkan K. Fixed-life or rechargeable battery for deep brain stimulation: a prospective long-term study of patient's preferences. *Stereotact Funct Neurosurg.* (2019) 98:1–5. doi: 10.1159/000505700
8. Khaleeq T, Hasegawa H, Samuel M, Ashkan K. Fixed life or rechargeable battery for deep brain stimulation: which do patients prefer? *Neuromodulation.* (2019) 22:1–4. doi: 10.1111/ner.12810
9. Timmermann L, Schüpbach M, Hertel F, Wolf E, Eleopra R, Franzini A, et al. A new rechargeable device for deep brain stimulation: a prospective patient satisfaction survey. *Eur Neurol.* (2013) 69:193–9. doi: 10.1159/000342236
10. Zafar S, Peppercorn J. Patient financial assistance programs: a path to affordability or a barrier to accessible cancer care? *J Clin Oncol.* (2017) 35:2113–6. doi: 10.1200/JCO.2016.71.7280
11. Waln O, Jimenez-Shahed J. Rechargeable deep brain stimulation implantable pulse generators in movement disorders: patient satisfaction and conversion parameters. *Neuromodulation.* (2014) 17:425–30; discussion 430. doi: 10.1111/ner.12115
12. Rizzi M, Messina G, Penner F, D'Ammando A, Muratorio F, Franzini A. Internal pulse generators in deep brain stimulation: rechargeable or not? *World Neurosurg.* (2015) 84:1020–9. doi: 10.1016/j.wneu.2015.05.028
13. Limousin P, Foltynie T. Long-term outcomes of deep brain stimulation in Parkinson disease. *Nat Rev Neurol.* (2019) 15:9. doi: 10.1038/s41582-019-0145-9
14. Fabbri M, Zibetti M, Rizzone MG, Giannini G, Borellini L, Stefani A, et al. Should we consider deep brain stimulation discontinuation in late-stage Parkinson's disease? *Mov Disord.* (2020) 35:9. doi: 10.1002/mds.28091

Permissions

All chapters in this book were first published by Frontiers; hereby published with permission under the Creative Commons Attribution License or equivalent. Every chapter published in this book has been scrutinized by our experts. Their significance has been extensively debated. The topics covered herein carry significant findings which will fuel the growth of the discipline. They may even be implemented as practical applications or may be referred to as a beginning point for another development.

The contributors of this book come from diverse backgrounds, making this book a truly international effort. This book will bring forth new frontiers with its revolutionizing research information and detailed analysis of the nascent developments around the world.

We would like to thank all the contributing authors for lending their expertise to make the book truly unique. They have played a crucial role in the development of this book. Without their invaluable contributions this book wouldn't have been possible. They have made vital efforts to compile up to date information on the varied aspects of this subject to make this book a valuable addition to the collection of many professionals and students.

This book was conceptualized with the vision of imparting up-to-date information and advanced data in this field. To ensure the same, a matchless editorial board was set up. Every individual on the board went through rigorous rounds of assessment to prove their worth. After which they invested a large part of their time researching and compiling the most relevant data for our readers.

The editorial board has been involved in producing this book since its inception. They have spent rigorous hours researching and exploring the diverse topics which have resulted in the successful publishing of this book. They have passed on their knowledge of decades through this book. To expedite this challenging task, the publisher supported the team at every step. A small team of assistant editors was also appointed to further simplify the editing procedure and attain best results for the readers.

Apart from the editorial board, the designing team has also invested a significant amount of their time in understanding the subject and creating the most relevant covers. They scrutinized every image to scout for the most suitable representation of the subject and create an appropriate cover for the book.

The publishing team has been an ardent support to the editorial, designing and production team. Their endless efforts to recruit the best for this project, has resulted in the accomplishment of this book. They are a veteran in the field of academics and their pool of knowledge is as vast as their experience in printing. Their expertise and guidance has proved useful at every step. Their uncompromising quality standards have made this book an exceptional effort. Their encouragement from time to time has been an inspiration for everyone.

The publisher and the editorial board hope that this book will prove to be a valuable piece of knowledge for researchers, students, practitioners and scholars across the globe.

List of Contributors

Elizabeth W. Pang and O. C. Snead III
Division of Neurology, Hospital for Sick Children, Toronto, ON, Canada
Neurosciences and Mental Health, SickKids Research Institute, Toronto, ON, Canada
Department of Paediatrics, Faculty of Medicine, University of Toronto, Toronto, ON, Canada

Yupeng Wu, Yong Wang, Yibao Wang and Shaowu Ou
Department of Neurosurgery, The First Affiliated Hospital of China Medical University, Shenyang, China

Dandan Sun
Department of Cardiovascular Ultrasound, The First Affiliated Hospital of China Medical University, Shenyang, China

Ardian Hana, Hans Boecher-Schwarz and Frank Hertel
National Service of Neurosurgery, Centre Hospitalier de Luxembourg, Luxembourg City, Luxembourg

Anisa Hana
Internal Medicine, Erasmus University of Rotterdam, Rotterdam, Netherlands

Georges Dooms
Service of Neuroradiology, Centre Hospitalier de Luxembourg, Luxembourg City, Luxembourg

András Jakab
Center for Magnetic Resonance Imaging Research, University Children's Hospital, Zürich, Switzerland
Computational Imaging Research Lab, Department of Biomedical Imaging and Image-Guided Therapy, Medical University of Vienna, Vienna, Austria

Beat Werner, Ernst Martin and Ruth O'Gorman Tuura
Center for Magnetic Resonance Imaging Research, University Children's Hospital, Zürich, Switzerland

Marco Piccirelli
Department of Neuroradiology, University Hospital Zürich, Zürich, Switzerland

Kázmér Kovács
Department of Biomedical Imaging and Laboratory Science, University of Debrecen, Debrecen, Hungary

John S. Thornton and Tarek Yousry
University College London Institute of Neurology, London, UK

Gabor Szekely
Computer Vision Laboratory, ETH Zürich, Zürich, Switzerland

Peter S.-P. Hung
Institute of Medical Science, Faculty of Medicine, University of Toronto, Toronto, ON, Canada

David J. Hayes
Krembil Research Institute, University Health Network, Toronto, ON, Canada

Mojgan Hodaie
Institute of Medical Science, Faculty of Medicine, University of Toronto, Toronto, ON, Canada
Krembil Research Institute, University Health Network, Toronto, ON, Canada
Division of Neurosurgery, Toronto Western Hospital and University of Toronto, Toronto, ON, Canada
Joint Department of Medical Imaging, University Health Network, Toronto, ON, Canada

Dave J. Hayes
Psychology Department and Neuroscience Program, Union College, Schenectady, NY, United States
Division of Brain, Imaging and Behaviour Systems Neuroscience and Division of Neurosurgery, Department of Surgery, Toronto Western Hospital, Krembil Research Institute, University Health Network, University of Toronto, Toronto, ON, Canada

David Q. Chen, Jidan Zhong, Brendan Behan and Matthew Walker
Division of Brain, Imaging and Behaviour Systems Neuroscience and Division of Neurosurgery, Department of Surgery, Toronto Western Hospital, Krembil Research Institute, University Health Network, University of Toronto, Toronto, ON, Canada

Ariel Lin
Psychology Department and Neuroscience Program, Union College, Schenectady, NY, United States

Danielle D. DeSouza
Department of Neurology and Neurological Sciences, Stanford University, Stanford, CA, USA

Karen D. Davis
Division of Brain, Imaging and Behavior-Systems Neuroscience, Krembil Research Institute, University Health Network, Toronto, ON, Canada
Institute of Medical Science, University of Toronto, Toronto, ON, Canada
Division of Neurosurgery, Toronto Western Hospital and Department of Surgery, University of Toronto, Toronto, ON, Canada

Zang-Hee Cho, Sang-Han Choi, Sung-Yeon Park, Chan-Woong Park and Young-Bo Kim
Neuroscience Research Institute, Gachon University of Medicine and Science, Incheon, South Korea

Je-Geun Chi
Neuroscience Research Institute, Gachon University of Medicine and Science, Incheon, South Korea
Department of Pathology, Seoul National University College of Medicine, Seoul, South Korea

Se-Hong Oh
Neuroscience Research Institute, Gachon University of Medicine and Science, Incheon, South Korea
Department of Radiology, School of Medicine, University of Pennsylvania, Philadelphia, PA, USA

Sun Ha Paek
Departments of Neurosurgery, Seoul National University College of Medicine, Seoul, South Korea

Fernando Calamante
The Florey Institute of Neuroscience and Mental Health, Melbourne, VIC, Australia
Department of Medicine, Austin Health and Northern Health, University of Melbourne, Melbourne, VIC, Australia

Limor Avivi-Arber and Massieh Moayedi
University of Toronto Centre for the Study of Pain, University of Toronto, Toronto, ON, Canada
Faculty of Dentistry, University of Toronto, Toronto, ON, Canada

Ze'ev Seltzer
University of Toronto Centre for the Study of Pain, University of Toronto, Toronto, ON, Canada
Faculty of Dentistry, University of Toronto, Toronto, ON, Canada
Department of Physiology, Faculty of Medicine, University of Toronto, Toronto, ON, Canada
Department of Anesthesiology, University Health Network, Toronto, ON, Canada
Central Institute of Mental Health, University of Heidelberg, Mannheim, Germany

Miriam Friedel
Mouse Imaging Centre, Hospital for Sick Children, Toronto, ON, Canada

Jason P. Lerch
Mouse Imaging Centre, Hospital for Sick Children, Toronto, ON, Canada
Medical Biophysics, Faculty of Medicine, University of Toronto, Toronto, ON, Canada

Karen D. Davis
University of Toronto Centre for the Study of Pain, University of Toronto, Toronto, ON, Canada
Department of Surgery, University of Toronto, Toronto, ON, Canada
Institute of Medical Science, University of Toronto, Toronto, ON, Canada
Division of Brain, Imaging and Behaviour - Systems Neuroscience, Krembil Research Institute, Toronto Western Hospital, University Health Network, Toronto, ON, Canada

Barry J. Sessle
University of Toronto Centre for the Study of Pain, University of Toronto, Toronto, ON, Canada
Faculty of Dentistry, University of Toronto, Toronto, ON, Canada
Department of Physiology, Faculty of Medicine, University of Toronto, Toronto, ON, Canada

Dylan J. H. A. Henssen
Department of Anatomy, Donders Institute for Brain Cognition and Behavior, Radboud University Medical Center, Nijmegen, Netherlands
Department of Neurosurgery, Radboud University Medical Center, Nijmegen, Netherlands

Erkan Kurt and Ronald H. M. A. Bartels
Department of Neurosurgery, Radboud University Medical Center, Nijmegen, Netherlands

Tamas Kozicz and Anne-Marie van Cappellen van Walsum
Department of Anatomy, Donders Institute for Brain Cognition and Behavior, Radboud University Medical Center, Nijmegen, Netherlands

Robert van Dongen
Department of Anaesthesiology, Pain and Palliative Care, Radboud University Medical Center, Nijmegen, Netherlands

Adam Waspe, Thomas Looi and Karolina Piorkowska
Centre for Image Guided Innovation and Therapeutic Intervention, The Hospital for Sick Children, Toronto, ON, Canada

James M. Drake
Centre for Image Guided Innovation and Therapeutic Intervention, The Hospital for Sick Children, Toronto, ON, Canada
Division of Neurosurgery, The Hospital for Sick Children, Toronto, ON, Canada

Timothy G. Dyster, Charles B. Mikell and Sameer A. Sheth
Functional and Cognitive Neurophysiology Laboratory, Department of Neurological Surgery, Columbia University Medical Center, New York Presbyterian Hospital, New York, NY, USA

Evan Calabrese
Center for In Vivo Microscopy, Department of Radiology, Duke University Medical Center, Durham, NC, USA

Jennifer A. Sweet, Jonathan Pace, Fady Girgis and Jonathan P. Miller
Department of Neurosurgery, University Hospitals Case Medical Center, Case Western Reserve University, Cleveland, OH, USA

Sonia Pujol and Ron Kikinis
Surgical Planning Laboratory, Department of Radiology, Brigham and Women's Hospital, Harvard Medical School, Boston, MA, USA

Ryan Cabeen
Department of Computer Science, Brown University, Providence, RI, USA

Sophie B. Sébille, Jérôme Yelnik and Chantal François
Institut du Cerveau et de la Moëlle Epinière, INSERM U 1127, CNRS UMR 7225, Sorbonne Universités, University of Paris 06, UMR S 1127, Paris, France

Sara Fernandez Vidal and Eric Bardinet
Institut du Cerveau et de la Moëlle Epinière, INSERM U 1127, CNRS UMR 7225, Sorbonne Universités, University of Paris 06, UMR S 1127, Paris, France
Centre de Neuro-Imagerie de Recherche, Institut du Cerveau et de la Moëlle Epinière, Paris, France

Carine Karachi
Institut du Cerveau et de la Moëlle Epinière, INSERM U 1127, CNRS UMR 7225, Sorbonne Universités, University of Paris 06, UMR S 1127, Paris, France
Department of Neurosurgery, Pitié-Salpêtrière Hospital, Paris, France

Yulong Zhao and Pierre Jannin
LTSI, Inserm UMR 1099 - Université de Rennes, Rennes, France

G. Rees Cosgrove
Department of Neurosurgery, Brigham and Women's Hospital, Harvard Medical School, Boston, MA, USA

Weibin He and Wei Yi
Department of Neurosurgery, Renmin Hospital, Wuhan University, Wuhan, China

Hongxia Li and Yiwen Wu
Department of Neurology, Ruijin Hospital, Shanghai Jiao Tong University School of Medicine, Shanghai, China

Yijie Lai and Yunhao Wu
Department of Functional Neurosurgery, Ruijin Hospital, Shanghai Jiao Tong University School of Medicine, Shanghai, China

Adolfo Ramirez-Zamora
Fixel Center for Neurological Diseases, University of Florida, Gainesville, FL, United States

Vanessa M. Holanda
Department of Neurosurgery, Center of Neurology and Neurosurgery Associates (NeuroCENNA), Beneficencia Portuguesa of São Paulo Hospital, São Paulo, Brazil

Robert Stephen Eisinger, Leonardo Almeida, Huimin Wang, Michael S. Okun, Addie Patterson, Aparna Wagle Shukla, Janine Lobo Lopes and Kelly Douglas Foote
Department of Neurology, Norman Fixel Institute for Neurological Diseases, University of Florida Health, Gainesville, FL, United States

Takashi Tsuboi
Department of Neurology, Nagoya University, Nagoya, Japan

Wissam Deeb
Department of Neurology, University of Massachusetts Medical School, Worcester, MA, United States

Kohei Kanaya
Department of Neurosurgery, Shinshu University School of Medicine, Matsumoto, Japan
Department of Neurosurgery, Iida Municipal Hospital, Nagano, Japan

Takumi Mitsuhashi
Department of Neurosurgery, Juntendo University, Tokyo, Japan

Takafumi Kiuchi and Sumio Kobayashi
Department of Neurosurgery, Iida Municipal Hospital, Nagano, Japan

Xian Qiu and Tingting Peng
Department of Nursing, Ruijin Hospital, Shanghai Jiao Tong University School of Medicine, Shanghai, China
Department of Neurosurgery, Ruijin Hospital, Shanghai Jiao Tong University School of Medicine, Shanghai, China

Zhengyu Lin, Kaiwen Zhu, Yuhan Wang, Bomin Sun, Chencheng Zhang and Dianyou Li
Department of Nursing, Ruijin Hospital, Shanghai Jiao Tong University School of Medicine, Shanghai, China

Keyoumars Ashkan
Department of Neurosurgery, King's College Hospital, London, United Kingdom

Index

www.ingramcontent.com/pod-product-compliance
Lightning Source LLC
LaVergne TN
LVHW060519210926
848485LV00005B/1109